AF761896

Figures available in three downloadable sizes (resolutions)

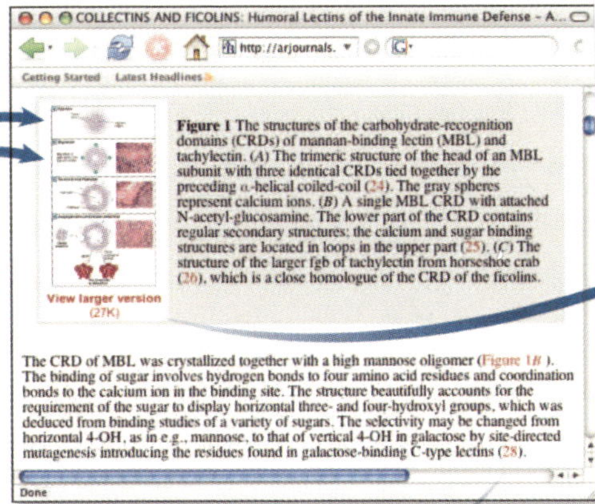

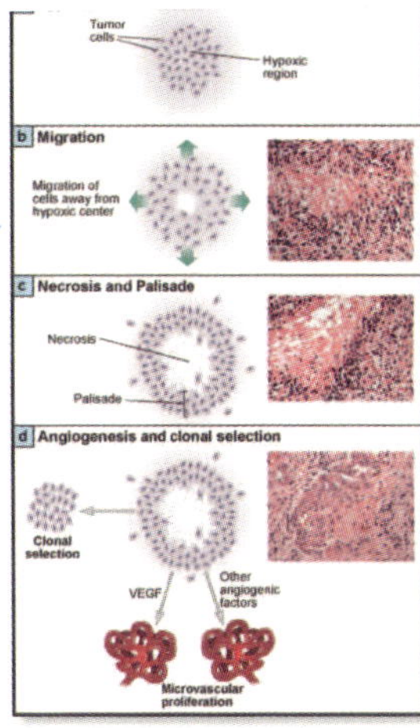

Citations in text link to references in bibliography

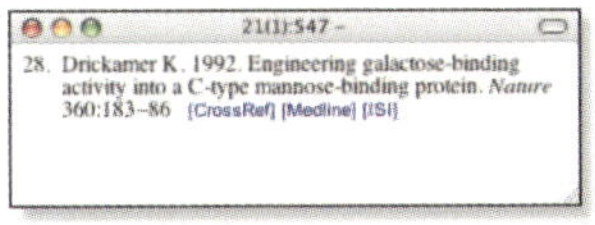

References in Annual Reviews chapter bibliography link out to sources of cited articles online

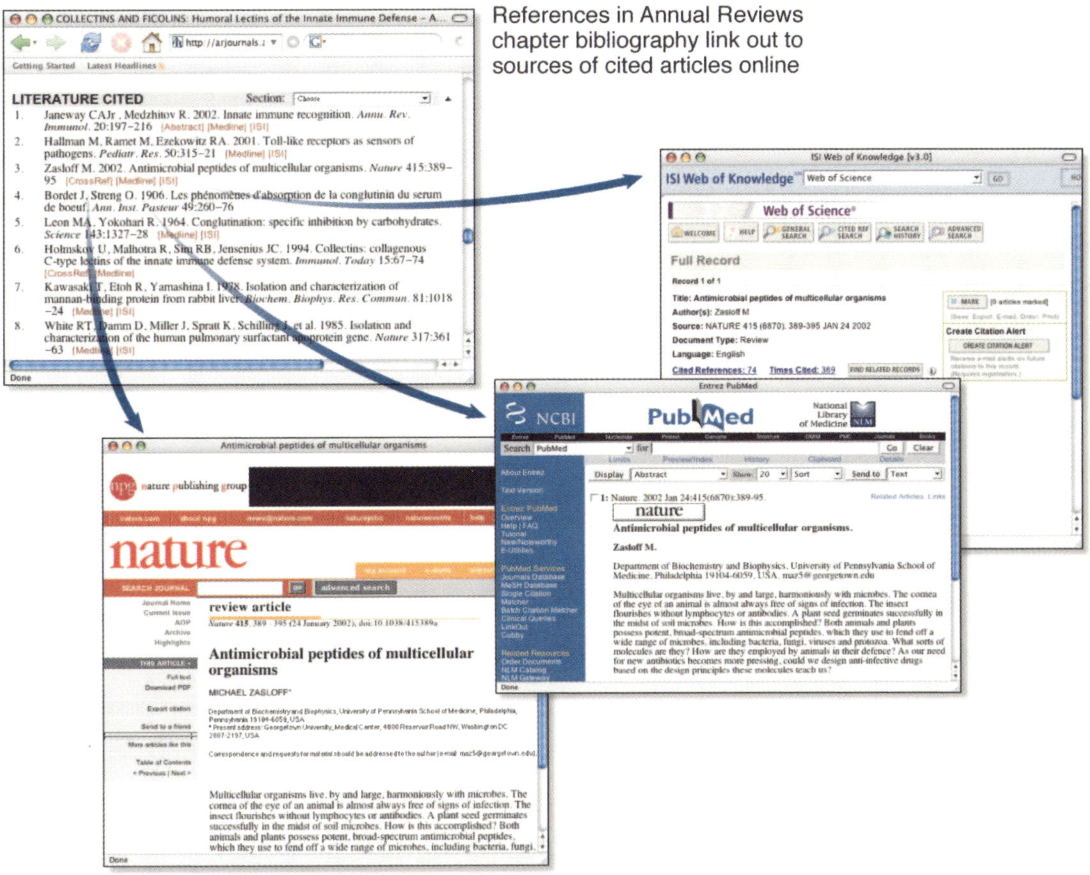

Annual Review of Pathology: Mechanisms of Disease

Production Editor: Joyce Tang
Bibliographic Quality Control: Mary A. Glass
Electronic Content Coordinator: Suzanne K. Moses
Subject Indexer: Cheri Walsh

Annual Review of Pathology: Mechanisms of Disease

Volume 1, 2006

Abul K. Abbas, *Co-Editor*
University of California, San Francisco

James R. Downing, *Co-Editor*
St. Jude Children's Research Hospital

Vinay Kumar, *Co-Editor*
University of Chicago

www.annualreviews.org • science@annualreviews.org • 650-493-4400

Annual Reviews
4139 El Camino Way • P.O. Box 10139 • Palo Alto, California 94303-0139

Annual Reviews
Palo Alto, California, USA

International Standard Serial Number: 1553-4006
International Standard Book Number: 0-8243-4301-8

TYPESET BY TECHBOOKS, FAIRFAX, VA
PRINTED AND BOUND BY QUEBECOR WORLD, KINGSPORT, TN

Preface

We, the Editorial Committee for the *Annual Review of Pathology*, introduce this new series with a strong sense of anticipation and excitement.

Although pathology (*pathos*, disease; *logos*, study of) is an old biomedical discipline, we think that there has never been a more rewarding and exciting time for students of pathology. Powerful new molecular, imaging, and biocomputational approaches; the availability of increasingly versatile and effective techniques to genetically modify cell lines and animals; and advances in the approaches for designing and analyzing the results of clinical trials have combined to create striking new opportunities for the direct study of human diseases, as well as for the development of increasingly sophisticated animal models of human disorders. Combined with the remarkable progress in our understanding of the biology of cells, tissues, and organisms that has occurred over the past 50 years, this set of new tools and approaches is enabling investigators from diverse scientific and medical disciplines to build on a strong foundation of basic science to tackle the challenges of human disease.

For these reasons we think that an Annual Reviews series devoted to mechanisms of disease is particularly timely. Our fundamental goal is to solicit articles that attempt to elucidate the biological underpinnings of disorders affecting diverse organ systems, while calling attention to key remaining "unsolved" aspects of such diseases. The focus then is clearly on biology and mechanisms, as it is our belief that we will understand disease manifestations, and stand a better chance of developing new and improved therapies, only if we better comprehend the underlying pathophysiology. Indeed, this series will succeed only if we are able to offer its readers robust bridges between fundamental biology and clinical medicine. Of course, the most useful bridges permit traffic in both directions. Accordingly, perhaps the most tangible reflection of success will be if basic scientists as well as clinicians find new and valuable insights in the articles in this series.

The Editors

Annual Review of Pathology: Mechanisms of Disease

Volume 1, 2006

Contents

INDEX

Related Articles

From the ***Annual Review of Biochemistry,*** Volume 74 (2005)

The Biochemistry of Parkinson's Disease
Mark R. Cookson

Applications of DNA Microarrays in Biology
Roland B. Stoughton

NOD-LRR Proteins: Role in Host-Microbial Interactions and Inflammatory Disease
Naohiro Inohara, Mathias Chamaillard, Christine McDonald, and Gabriel Nuñez

Regulation of Protein Function by Glycosaminoglycans–as Exemplified by Chemokines
T.M. Handel, Z. Johnson, S.E. Crown, E.K. Lau, M. Sweeney, and A.E. Proudfoot

Structure and Physiologic Function of the Low-Density Lipoprotein Receptor
Hyesung Jeon and Stephen C. Blacklow

Copper-Zinc Superoxide Dismutase and Amyotrophic Lateral Sclerosis
Joan Selverstone Valentine, Peter A. Doucette, and Soshanna Zittin Potter

From the ***Annual Review of Cell and Developmental Biology,*** Volume 21 (2005)

The Lymphatic Vasculature: Recent Progress and Paradigms
Guillermo Oliver and Kari Alitalo

Phagocytosis: At the Crossroads of Innate and Adaptive Immunity
Isabelle Jutras and Michel Desjardins

Stem Cell Niche: Structure and Function
Linheng Li and Ting Xie

The Great Escape: When Cancer Cells Hijack the Genes for Chemotaxis and Motility
John Condeelis, Robert Singer, and Jeffrey E. Segall

From the ***Annual Review of Genetics,*** Volume 39 (2005)

Drosophila as a Model for Human Neurodegenerative Disease
Julide Bilen and Nancy M. Bonini

A Mitochondrial Paradigm of Metabolic and Degenerative Diseases, Aging, and Cancer: A Dawn for Evolutionary Medicine
Douglas C. Wallace

From the ***Annual Review of Immunology,*** Volume 23 (2005)

How Neutrophils Kill Microbes
Anthony W. Segal

Role of C5A in Inflammatory Responses
Ren-Feng Guo and Peter A. Ward

Immunology of Multiple Sclerosis
Mireia Sospedra and Roland Martin

From the ***Annual Review of Medicine,*** Volume 56 (2005)

Myelodysplastic Syndrome
Wolf K. Hofmann and H. Phillip Koeffler

Post-Transplant Lymphoproliferative Disorders
Stephen Gottschalk, Cliona M. Rooney, and Helen E. Heslop

Endothelial Progenitor Cells
Aarif Y. Khakoo and Toren Finkel

New Concepts in Von Willebrand Disease
J. Evan Sadler

Endometriosis: New Genetic Approaches and Therapy
David H. Barlow and Stephen Kennedy

Severe Acute Respiratory Syndrome (SARS): A Year in Review
Danuta M. Skowronski, Caroline Astell, Robert C. Brunham, Donald E. Low, Martin Petric, Rachel L. Roper, Pierre J. Talbot, Theresa Tam, and Lorne Babiuk

DNA Repair Defects in Stem Cell Function and Aging
Youngji Park and Stanton L. Gerson

From the ***Annual Review of Physiology,*** Volume 67 (2005)

Molecular and Evolutionary Basis of the Cellular Stress Response
Dietmar Kültz

Lung Vascular Development: Implications for the Pathogenesis of Bronchopulmonary Dysplasia
Kurt R. Stenmark and Steven H. Abman

Surfactant Protein C Biosynthesis and Its Emerging Role in Conformational Lung Disease
Michael F. Beers and Surafel Mulugeta

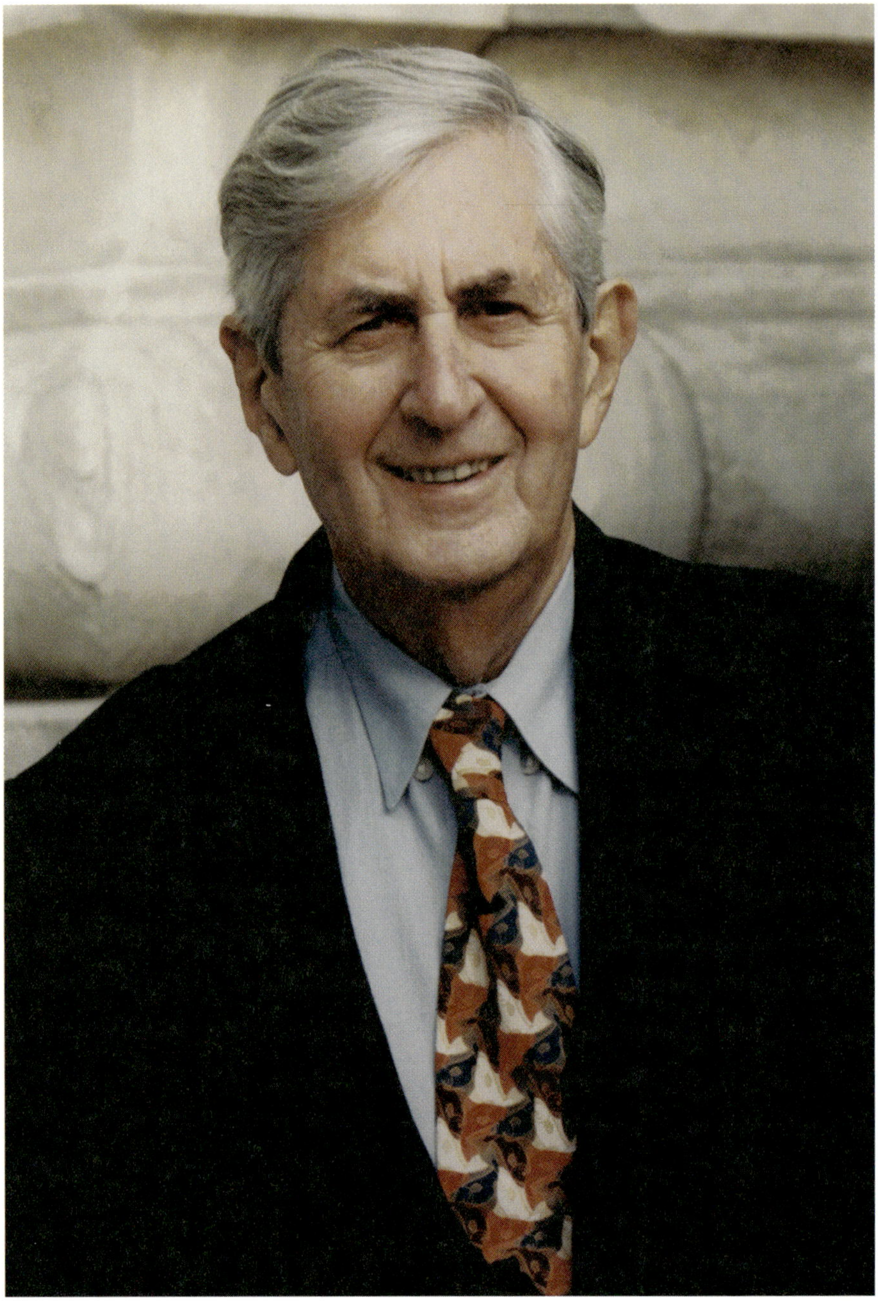

Morris J Karnovsky

A Pathologist's Odyssey

Morris J. Karnovsky

Department of Pathology, Harvard Medical School, Boston, Massachusetts 02115;
email: mkarnovsky@hms.harvard.edu

Annu. Rev. Pathol. Mech. Dis.
2006. 1:1–22

First published online as a Review in Advance on September 30, 2005

The *Annual Review of Pathology: Mechanisms of Disease* is online at pathmechdis.annualreviews.org

doi: 10.1146/annurev.pathol.1.110304.100140

1553-4006/06/0114-0001$20.00

I am honored to write the prefatory chapter for the inaugural volume of the Annual Review of Pathology: Mechanisms of Disease. *This publishing venture signals that pathology takes its rightful place alongside the other biomedical sciences.*

I thought it may be of interest to some to delineate how a circuitous path led me into a career in experimental pathology and to give some of the flavor of a past era in experimental approaches. Thus, my title.

EARLY DAYS

South Africa: An Education

I was born in Johannesburg, Republic of South Africa. My forebears immigrated to South Africa in the mid-to-late nineteenth century from Poland and Lithuania. I was educated at the King Edward VII High School. This was a public school run along the lines of the private (i.e., "public") schools of Britain. Despite its semifeudal atmosphere, it provided an excellent classical education, including four years of Latin—which I have unfortunately mostly forgotten, except for a few "tags," which I trot out on occasion to make an impression. There was, however, an excellent course in Modern Poetry, which provided a basis for much enjoyment in later years. The teacher was, not inappropriately, named Keats. Perhaps my greatest triumph at school was to score the winning, and only, try (goal) in a rugby match played against a rival school. (Years later, when I thought I might try out for the Harvard rugby team, my best friend promptly broke his leg at the first practice, and so, discretion being the better part of valor, and age telling, that was the end of athletic glory for both of us.)

Throughout school the teaching was in English, but we also had to learn Afrikaans, the other official language. (Regrettably, no black African language was required in those times.) I thoroughly enjoyed Afrikaans, in which I became quite fluent. It is a "modern" language with few irregular verbs and rules and with a rich literature descriptive of the landscapes, peoples, and flora and fauna of southern Africa.

During my high school years, I helped start an evening school for adult blacks. The headmaster, whom I had regarded as a conservative fellow, gave us students permission to use the school facilities even though, I am sure, this would not have met with approval from the governmental authorities if they had been aware of our venture. He was upset when one evening we had an influx of students and were short of space and so used his office as a classroom. I was called in to see him the next morning, but there was only an expression of mild displeasure and no retribution. On average we had approximately one hundred students who attended every session. In setting up this school, we consulted with Alan Paton, of *Cry the Beloved Country*, and my visit to see him left an indelible impression on me.

I entered the Medical School of the University of the Witwatersrand directly from high school, which is the British custom. I was interested in biology and not particularly interested in medicine, but as zoology or botany did not enthrall me, I chose to study medicine as a portal to the biological and biomedical sciences. After two years of medical school, an inspired program, created by the renowned anatomist and anthropologist Professor Raymond Dart, the head of the Anatomy Department and the discoverer of the first *Australopithecine* (the Taung child skull of *Australopithecus africanus*), enabled scientifically inclined students to drop out of medical school for a year or two and pursue a science degree.

Another influential member of the Department was Joseph Gillman, officially a histology lecturer, though he had wide-ranging interests in other fields. Gruff, irascible, and iconoclastic, Gillman inspired students constantly to question dogma and orthodoxy. I remember the shock when I was ushered into a large laboratory occupied by approximately eight students and was told that I was expected to produce a thesis in a year or two. We could pretty well do what we liked, courses were few, and the interests of the students were diverse. I decided to work in cytogenetics, and my thesis was on the chromosomes of a delightful little animal—the bush baby, or night ape (*Galago senegalensis moholi*). The work was done under the direction of my fellow students Sydney Brenner and Philip Tobias. Both were interested in the evolution of chromosome shape and number, and though only one year ahead of me, they knew more about cytogenetics than anyone on the faculty. Today, Brenner is a renowned molecular biologist and Nobel Laureate, and Tobias has an international reputation as a foremost anthropologist.

In those days the tissue-culture techniques for conducting cytogenetics had not been developed. To get useful spreads of chromosomes, one had to macerate the tissue in acetic acid and squash it between two glass slides—sometimes, in frustration, we would jump on the preparation, which was padded with books. The illustrations were made with a camera lucida. Some chromosome numbers published in that era were wrong because of the primitive techniques available. In addition to our laboratory studies, many of us spent enjoyable weekends camping in the countryside and hunting for fossils in caves and other rich sites under the direction of the eminent anthropologists Raymond Dart and Robert Broom and other paleoanthropologists on the faculty, as well as under the leadership of students such as Sydney Brenner and Phillip Tobias.

One of the highlights of the science program was the compulsory course History and Philosophy of Science taught by Brian Farrell, later of Oxford, who was a logical positivist. We became afficionados of L. Wittgenstein, B. Russell, J. Dewey, S.K. Langer, and A.N. Whitehead, and my readings by these authors, as well as by biologists J. Needham and C.H. Waddington, were important influences in my thinking about science, although I must admit that I was defeated by Wittgenstein's *Tractatus Logico-Philosophicus*.

As South Africa was rather remote from scientific centers, the students imposed a voluntary levy on themselves to import visiting luminaries from abroad. I remember particularly well the stimulating visit of C.H. Waddington, the eminent British embryologist, geneticist, and philosopher of science. One of our professors was a Marxist and a Lysenkoist, who also favored the eccentric (to my mind) therapeutic theories of the Russian physician A.D. Speransky; consequently, our philosophical discussions were at times quite rowdy yet good tempered.

Professor Dart had established on the roof of the medical school a colony of baboons, which was the first primate study center in Africa. I helped Joe Gillman take blood from these beasts—not an easy job. Our research and philosophical discussions in the laboratory beneath the colony were carried on with the symphonic accompaniment of the raucous calls of the baboons, of which Sydney Brenner gave a great imitation.

Interest in the history, philosophy, and nature of science has remained with me, and I find it curious that many of the students and faculty I encounter in the United States seem singularly disinterested in such matters. I would think that in these days when issues regarding science and society are at the forefront, some background thinking by scientists on the nature and limits of science would be useful.

After one or two years in the science program, most graduates resumed their medical studies, many now fired with the ambition of making their careers in basic science or academic medicine. The medical curriculum at that time was a classical one based on the Scottish model. The courses in the first year were botany, zoology, organic and inorganic chemistry, and physics. The classical organic chemistry laboratories (spot tests and so on) placed me in good stead in later years in developing cytochemical techniques. Dissecting dogfish, frogs, and rats in zoology and making meticulous drawings were quite enjoyable. Botany was not enthralling—a matter of plant identification and classification; there was no mention of evolution or adaptation. We had fun, however, in dumping huge specimens of various species that we had dug up in the veldt, and which took several students to move, at our professor's door; sometimes he was pleased, other times not. He was a patient man. The teaching of physics was dull; rolling balls up and down inclined planes on a sunny afternoon was tiresome. The second year consisted of gross anatomy, histology and embryology, physiology, and biochemistry (then known as physiological chemistry).

The year was greatly enlivened by the unforgettable laboratory teaching and inspiring lectures by Raymond Dart. During some of his lectures on evolution, the lecture hall would be filled with stuffed crocodiles, apes, large mammals, skulls, and skeletons so that there was scarcely room for the students as we stumbled over all this paraphernalia into our seats. The third year was devoted to bacteriology, surgical anatomy (a course taught by surgeons in which anatomy sprung alive and became relevant to clinical work), pathology, and pharmacology.

I did not find the Pathology Department at that time particularly inspiring, as it was very classical and descriptive in approach, although diagnostically sound. Nevertheless the subject matter interested me, and I began to read some papers and books on experimental pathology, although one of the professors tried to discourage me by saying that "work on animals was not relevant to the human." The text we used was so old-fashioned that the micrographs were round, as in nineteenth-century fashion. Remarkably, we attended autopsies or organ demonstrations almost every day during the school year, which was the duration of the course in Pathology, and there was an admirable museum available. The specimens were well preserved in natural color, and the relevant clinical history, microscopic slides, X rays, autopsy findings, etc. accompanied each specimen. One could cover a case or two a day and thus learn a good deal of pathology and medicine. If accompanied by a friend, each could take a turn in acting as an interlocutor. The museum was several stories tall and a spiral stairway was lined with shelves of specimens; thus one started at the top and spiraled one's way down through the realms of pathology as the days went by. In later years when I came to the United States, I learned that such museums were rather rare, were an expensive proposition to develop and maintain, and were regarded as somewhat out-of-date. I think, however, that they are useful teaching aids and regret their so-called obsolescence.

In pharmacology we had to learn how to write and read prescriptions written in Latin and how to dispense the medicines. Some of the graduates would likely practice in rural areas and would have to do their own dispensing, as no pharmacists would be available. I learned to grind powders and roll pills and dispense them in small round boxes. I made up and bottled all sorts of tinctures and elixirs, wrapping and sealing the bottles neatly in white paper. My father, who was a pharmacist, thought my skills in dispensing were acceptable but not "highly elegant."

A course in forensic pathology was intriguing but often a cause for queasiness. At the final exam each student was allotted a case to solve. I had a case of accidental poisoning. The remainder of the third year as well as the entire fourth, fifth, and sixth years were devoted to walking the wards—clerking in all aspects of clinical medicine and surgery as well as in the so-called subspecialties of obstetrics (I delivered more than one hundred babies), otolaryngology, dermatology, and so on. The best times were spent "hanging out" in what we called the casualty (also known as the emergency room in the United States) at night, on a voluntary basis, hoping to get a good case, which we could clerk and follow through the night and thereafter. As we got to know the staff, we were allowed to perform procedures, culminating, if one showed enough skill, in the performance of quite major surgeries, such as appendectomies (under supervision of course). Overall, the clinical training was excellent, and upon graduation we were equipped to handle most of what faced us as interns. However, the basic sciences were at times somewhat short-changed.

Although the faculty in general were not particularly activist in regard to the disparities and inequities existing between the South African whites and nonwhites, there were notable exceptions, such as Raymond Dart, Joseph Gillman, and his brother Teddy (Theodore). The student body was, by post-1950 South African standards, liberal and tolerant in outlook, with the exception of a hard core who opposed the relatively progressive attitude of the school allowing the presence of nonwhite students, who had been accepted since 1940, when Dart was Dean. However, the nonwhites could clerk patients only in the segregated nonwhite hospitals but not in the all-white hospitals. There were protests from some supporters of strict segregation against the presence of nonwhite students in the anatomy dissecting hall and at autopsy demonstrations, where, in both cases, cadavers of white women were on view. In the anatomy hall the protestors wanted the nonwhite students segregated to a separate room. Their request went nowhere. Professor Dart, the Department Chairman, offered instead to segregate the protestors. I cannot remember whether his offer was accepted. Unfortunately, nonwhite students were excluded by the Department of Pathology from the autopsy demonstrations when white female cadavers were visible. This led to protests from a considerable number of the student body.

The relatively liberal attitude of most students was conditioned to some extent by the presence of large numbers of ex-service men and women, many of whom had returned from World War II filled with idealism for a better South Africa. (South Africa had had a purely volunteer army because of a population that was divided in its support for the war against fascism. Many of those younger medical students who had not yet joined the armed services had been persuaded by officialdom that they would be of greater use if they first completed all or part of their medical training, particularly if they had close relatives already in the services; I was was one of them.)

Because of the influx of ex-service folk, our class was very large—220 students overall—but the administration and faculty dealt well with the logistical problems implicit in accommodating such a large group. An interesting consequence of the size of the class was that greater reliance was placed on the use of the nonwhite, segregated hospitals for clinical work, and so many of us were exposed to diseases, such as malnutrition, tuberculosis, syphilis, rickets, and pediatric gastroenteritis, that were rarely seen in the hospitals reserved for whites. Several of us realized that socioeconomic conditions, racism, and politics could determine the health and welfare of populations.

Thus we found inspiration in the teachings and practice of Sidney Kark, a graduate of our school, who propounded a multidisciplinary and multilevel approach to health care that comprised medical, social, economic, cultural, and political facets. He established a health care center at Pholela, in rural Zululand, which we attended during summer vacation. This center became a model for a national health system of primary care based on nonracial health centers, surprisingly supported by some far-seeing administrators in the government of Prime Minister Jan Smuts. (These concepts became the inspiration for Jack Geiger, a visiting medical student from the United States, later of Tufts University Medical School, to found the movement that led to the establishment of more than 800 health clinics in the United States.) Kark also started a course in social medicine, not under academic auspices, but at the request of, and partly organized by, some of my interested classmates. A cadre of students, including myself, were enthusiastic about this exciting, comprehensive approach to the delivery of health care, and some were desirous of making a career in the fields of social medicine and public health as conceived by Kark.

For my own part, I could not make up my mind between a career in academic medicine and this novel and intriguing alternative pathway. However, with the downfall of the Smuts government in 1948, and the advent of the Nationalists with their stringent concepts of Apartheid, the Karkian revolution in health care in South Africa virtually died, and many of my involved friends and colleagues emigrated for both political and professional reasons. Some carried the ideas of Kark abroad and promulgated them in diverse countries such as the United States, Israel, and the United Kingdom. As mentioned below,

I spent some time working in a clinic in an African township while I tried to decide my future career plans.

As the ironclad Apartheid rules came into effect, it became increasingly difficult for nonwhite students to be admitted to medical school. An onerous and drawn-out process had to be undertaken to gain permission for each student. The majority of the student body, as well as some of the faculty, participated in resistance meetings and demonstrations, and our student representative organizations were active in protest. These had some impact, both locally and globally, but were quite disruptive of the normal academic routine and atmosphere, yet they were obviously necessary.

I graduated M.B.B.Ch. [i.e., Bachelor of Medicine and Bachelor of Surgery (Ch., *Chirugia* in Latin, from the Greek *Cheirourgia*)] in 1950, and after internships in both medicine, at an all-white hospital, and surgery, at a nonwhite hospital, I felt the need to put my hands to work utilizing the theoretical and practical knowledge that I hoped I had learned. I worked for a while as a general practitioner in a clinic in an African township, and it was most satisfying practicing the many skills I had acquired in my training, including minor surgery, obstetrics (sometimes delivering babies in poorly-lit shanties), subspecialties such as dermatology, as well as general medicine. As a student I had spent a rotation at the clinic, so I knew the ropes. Eighty thousand Africans were packed into a few square miles, and poverty was rampant. It was somewhat dangerous for a white person to walk the streets, but wearing a white coat and carrying a stethoscope afforded protection. As in the hospital in which I had been a surgical intern, trauma was a major component of the cases we saw, especially on weekends, when there was intermittent chaos in the township owing to the drinking of potent and often illicit, or toxic, alcoholic brews. These concoctions, dispensed in bars known as shebeens, no doubt assuaged the loneliness and boredom of poor migrant workers, separated from their families left behind in rural areas, but led to the exacerbation of intertribal animosities with consequent ferocious fights, gang warfare, or random acts of violence. In addition to clubs and knives, a favorite weapon was a sharpened bicycle spoke inserted expertly into vital areas.

At that time we never saw cases of myocardial infarction, peptic ulcer, or appendicitis in the black population, although these were common in the white population. Blacks suffered from hypertension, diabetes, strokes, tuberculosis, venereal diseases, and malnutrition. Now, as I understand it, the emerging black middle class exhibits the diseases of Western "civilization." At the clinic I was under the tutelage of Mervyn Susser and Zena Stein, husband and wife, former prominent student leaders in opposition to Apartheid, and later luminaries in the fields of social medicine and public health and Chairpersons and Professors at Columbia University Medical School, respectively. They revolutionized clinical practice by introducing an appointment system—virtually unheard of until then for black Africans—and by keeping accurate vital records, which led to several significant publications in public health, particularly in regard to maternity care.

The clinic was supported financially in part by an annual "Rag," a carnival-like event in which the university students virtually took over the city for a day or two, with parades, floats, dances, and other rather wild activities. As students, Sydney Brenner and I were one year appointed as the official cameramen and made a movie that had several shots taken at weird angles, particularly by Syd—shades of *The Cabinet of Dr. Caligari*.

However, despite my enjoyment of clinical work, I gradually came to realize from my reading of the current literature that pathology and the nascent science of cell biology were what interested me. I saw pathology as a bridge between basic and clinical science. Furthermore, the political climate strengthened my belief that I should seek a career abroad.

London: Training in Pathology

I then went to London and became a trainee, first at the Central laboratories, Lewisham Hospital, which serviced a large area; then at the Department of Pathology at the Postgraduate Medical School, Hammersmith Hospital; and lastly at the Royal Cancer Hospital (now the Royal Marsden). I trained in morbid anatomy (histopathology) and all branches of laboratory medicine—hematology, bacteriology, and clinical chemistry. My Chief at the Royal Cancer Hospital was Rupert Willis, who had a marvelous biological and embryological approach to the evolution of tumors; his books are classics. Unfortunately, he became ill and Dr. Skelton took his place. Knowing of my interest in cytogenetics, he proposed that I study the recently discovered Barr body (sex chromatin). As is now well known, in the cells of the female one of the X chromosomes remains condensed during interphase and can be seen as a small clump of heterochromatin. This is not found in males. Our idea was to see if some of the diverse tissues found in teratomas from males showed such sexual dimorphism. To this end we obtained, from the London Hospital, which kept specimens for years, a series of teratomas found in the testes of horses gelded around the turn of the century. Unfortunately, the material was not sufficiently well preserved for our study. The famous cytogeneticist P.C. Koller had his laboratory close by, and as he was one of the heroes of my days in science in South Africa, it was a pleasure to visit with him.

I was impressed that the pathologists at the Royal Cancer Hospital made rounds on patients with the surgeons and that when a biopsy arrived for diagnosis we would go upstairs to the wards to examine the patient. In fact, some of the senior pathologists had patients directly under their care. It was also impressive that after surgery the surgeons would come to the pathology laboratories to go over the specimens with the pathologists, and some of the "old-timer" surgeons were pretty good gross pathologists. I was disappointed later when I came to the United States to find that the pathology laboratories were in the bowels of the basement and we rarely saw a patient.

One of my teachers at Hammersmith Hospital was A.G. Everson Pearse, who stimulated my interest in cytochemistry. He was a pioneer in the field and later the author of an authoritative textbook. The pathology staff quite frequently applied cytochemical methods in diagnostic work and research, which convinced me of the potential usefulness of this technology.

As it was rather difficult in those days to obtain a foothold in an academic department in the United Kingdom, particularly for someone from the "colonies," I decided, on the kindly advice of Lord Cohen of Birkenhead, President of the Royal College of Physicians and the premier physician in England, to try and obtain an academic position in the United States. During my interview with Lord Cohen I was offered a glass or two of sherry. I never before, nor since, have had the chance to imbibe at an interview. (As an aside, Lord Cohen's hobby was said to be crocheting doilies, which he was reputed to do while sitting in the House of Lords. When I visited him in his office in Liverpool, where he was Chairman of Medicine, I thought that he may have been crocheting, but his rooms were very dark and illuminated by a single light over his desk, so I was not sure.)

Boston: Nascent Research and Teaching

Shortly after my rather bizarre interview with Lord Cohen, I was surprised to see an advertisement in *The Lancet* for a residency in pathology at Massachusetts General Hospital—a most unusual occurrence. I applied forthwith, but I was rejected because another young pathologist [W.M. ("Whitey") Thurlbeck, I believe] from southern Africa had already been accepted to the program, and the Chief, Benjamin Castleman, did not think it was fair to have two residents from the same part of the world when positions for foreign candidates were scarce. However, Castleman kindly forwarded my application to Arthur T. Hertig, who was the Chairman of Pathology at Harvard Medical School. Hertig was looking for someone to replace Guido Majno to teach Medical Sciences 201ab, the seminal, historic, and comprehensive year-long course in all the basic sciences, including General Pathology, required of all the graduate (Ph.D.) students at Harvard Medical School and taught by junior faculty members assigned from each basic science department. The course, funded by the Commonwealth Fund, was an early and influential experiment in integrated teaching, which was later applied to the curricula for medical students. Hertig thought I would be suitable to replace Dr. Majno as I had a degree in Physiological Chemistry and knew some pathology and therefore could presumably hold my own with the basic scientists. He hired me sight unseen. As I also wanted to complete my residency training, I became, in 1955, an assistant resident pathologist at Beth Israel Hospital, afternoon and nights, and taught Medical Science 201ab in the mornings as a research fellow at the Central Pathology Department at the medical school. Carrying out these double duties was quite a task, especially as my scientific background was somewhat outdated—for instance, I had never seen a Warburg apparatus, which was then an example of big-time technology in biochemistry. To my amazement, no one had ever verified then or since that I hold any degrees whatsoever.

I learned a great deal trying to keep up with students and faculty. The course was the sole teaching responsibility of the young faculty representing each basic science, and we were expected to participate in all the activities, helping to teach each other's sections and laboratories. For instance, a biochemist helped me mount hands-on experiments, which the students conducted on chemical carcinogenesis in the liver or on aminonucleoside nephrosis, all studied with a multidisciplinary approach. For me, it was a formative experience and a lot of fun. I got to know the faculty, which led to good friendships and collaborations in the future. In learning the principles and concepts of general pathology, I was greatly indebted to my predecessor, friend, guide, and colleague, Guido Majno, who also introduced me to Lord Florey's great book, *Lectures in General Pathology* (1). I could not believe my good luck in having so fortuitously landed in such a hive of research and teaching.

Having completed my residency, I moved to the Central Pathology Department situated on the quadrangle at the medical school—a department responsible solely for teaching and research. Upon my arrival I found that a laboratory was not available, so I took refuge in a small room (10 feet by 20 feet) in the Department of Microbiology. My friendly neighbor was Dr. Albert Coons, who was then developing his now ubiquitous immunofluorescence techniques and who, in many discussions, reinforced my interest in cytochemistry, immunocytochemistry, and structure-function relationships.

My first laboratory was a rather modest affair. I had, as mentioned, little space and no equipment or grants. With no seed money (lavish or otherwise) in those days, I was obliged to scrounge equipment from my colleagues and hone my scavenging skills. For instance, I recovered from the garbage dump, which was located behind our building, an old, but rather elegant, brass and asbestos oven. I fixed and calibrated the primitive thermostat (a copper coil) and used the oven for 20 years.

My first few grant applications were rejected as I had a short publication track record and I lacked formal postdoctoral training. I guess I am essentially self-taught. Eventually, a pathology study section had some faith in me and I obtained modest funding. To supplement my income, I was also an Associate in Pathology at the then Peter Bent Brigham Hospital, under Gustave Dammin, signing out autopsies and walking a well-worn path between the Brigham and my laboratory on the quadrangle at the medical school.

Electron microscopy was then in its bloom as an exciting, new, and sexy technology for application in biology. Shortly after my arrival, Don W. Fawcett had been appointed as Chair of the Anatomy Department, so I asked him if I could become one of his trainees in electron microscopy. Unfortunately his roster was full, but he allowed me to become an unofficial trainee with free run of the department. Through the goodwill and friendship of the members of the department—Jean-Paul Revel, Susumo Ito, and Elizabeth Hay—I learned a great deal about electron microscopy. Later, Revel, Ito, and I became collaborators on several projects.

Fawcett assigned me to study the virally caused Lucké carcinoma, which occurs in the kidneys of the frog (*Rana pipiens*)—no doubt because I was a pathologist. As it was winter I had to palpate the kidneys of hundreds of dormant frogs, which were held in a cage under the ice in a lake. I only found three or so tumors, but they did not fix properly, nor embed well in methacrylate, which caused all sorts of distortions in the tissues—so-called explosions. I tried a variety of maneuvers such as polymerizing under UV light in the cold, at room temperature, on top of the manifold of Sus Ito's car, and on my furnace at home, all to no avail. I eventually ran out of tumor material. Such were the trials and tribulations of the early days in electron microscopy.

However, I was able to redeem part of the project some months later by using a different embedding medium that I imported from Switzerland (Vestopal-W, invented by E. Kellenberger, in whose laboratory I later worked). I showed that the proximal tubules of summer frogs, which were known to have secretory function, had high levels of enzymes supporting oxidative phosphorylation, which were markedly depleted in winter- and summer-starved frogs. There was no decrease in the latter two cases in the number of mitochondria, but marked disarray in organization of mitochondrial cristae (2, 3).

The proximal tubules of *Necturus maculosus*, like those of other species, reactively absorb many substances. Unlike other species however, the majority do not secrete spontaneously into their proximal tubular urine. Their proximal tubular cells had an anaerobic pattern similar to that of the winter- and summer-starved frogs, and their mitochondria in the proximal tubules, although numerous, had few cristae. In contrast, in both *Rana pipiens* and *Necturus maculosus*, oxidative enzymes and normal-appearing mitochondria were present in the distal tubules of both species. We concluded that secretion in the proximal tubule is accompanied by high oxidative phosphorylation, whereas reabsorptive processes are accompanied by glycolysis (4).

My early interest in cytochemistry as a tool for studying structure-function was heightened when, in an early paper, we were able to illuminate an ongoing discrepancy and dispute regarding the site of ammonia production in the kidney via the activity of glutaminase I, an enzyme for which we devised a novel cytochemical method. We found that there were species differences in the localization of the enzyme that could resolve discrepancies between biochemical data in one species and physiological data in another (5).

My first successful ultrastructural paper was one of the earliest studies of the fine structure of the osteoclast. It was rather foolhardy for beginners to attempt to cut bone, as diamond knives were not then available, so we used glass knives to cut thin sections of the relatively soft callus of healing experimental fractures (6).

Progress and promotion were slow. I was an instructor for four years. Arthur Hertig thought I would never get promoted unless I stopped my research and wrote and published instead. So in the final year of my four-year instructorship (a record tenure at that rank according to Hertig), I squeezed out some publications, which are mentioned above, and was on my way as an Assistant Professor—but I was on my way in more than one sense.

Geneva: Cholinesterases, Skiing, and Wine

In 1961 I had to leave the United States because my temporary visa had expired. Despite the best efforts of Harvard and several senators, I was required to spend two years abroad before re-entering the United States as an immigrant. Harvard kindly gave me a leave of absence, but without pay. Consequently, I spent two years in Geneva, Switzerland, at the Ecole de Medicine as a Collaborateur Scientifique. I worked in the Institutes of Histology and Embryology, Physiology, and Biophysics, under Professors Ch. Rouiller, J.M. Posternak and E. Kellenberger, respectively. My assigned project was to localize at the ultrastructural-level cholinesterase activity in heart muscle. Much biochemistry and physiology had been done in Posternak's department on these enzymes. I designed novel techniques utilizing specific substrates for localizing cholinesterases at the light (7) and ultrastructural levels (8) and found that they were present in the longitudinal elements of the sarcoplasmic reticulum and in the A-band, but not elsewhere. Previous work using a nonspecific substrate had localized cholinesterases to the M-band. We deemed this activity an organophosphate-resistant, nonspecific esterase (9). My light microscopic method for localizing cholinesterases (7) became popular with neurobiologists and is much cited, as is the ultrastructural method (8).

My new laboratory had a beautiful view of the Jura Mountains, and all the benchwork and the hood were handcrafted, but for some inexplicable reason there was no hot water, which had to be fetched in containers from down the corridor. This omission was later rectified. The electron microscopy was done in Kellenberger's laboratory. This was a fascinating place: As his laboratory was in the forefront of phage and bacterial structure and genetics, a succession of eminent scientists visited, including pioneers in molecular biology and genetics.

Kellenberger had built one of the earliest electron microscopes, and newcomers to the laboratory, like me, were assigned to use it. The resolution obtainable was that of a very bad light microscope or worse. After a day or two of struggling with this monster the joke played on the newcomer was revealed—nobody used the microscope because it was useless. Thus was the rite of passage passed.

Another embarrassment was when I was asked to give a demonstration to Roullier's group of my lead stain, which I had just developed (10). Nothing worked—it was a disconcerting disaster. I blamed the water in Geneva.

A peculiarity of Rouiller's laboratory was that after a paper was written it was locked away for a few months. Then it was reread and if Roullier and the author still liked it, it was sent off to a journal. In the meantime, if someone else had published on the same topic, then too bad! It did not seem to matter. I found this attitude quite admirable, but rather frustrating. While in Geneva I learned to ski (badly) and polished my skills as an oenophile. Roullier spoke limited English and my French was worse, so we began each day by reading Hemmingway's *The Old Man and the Sea* in our respective language to each another—a pleasant, if limited, way to learn. A compensation was that Roullier gave me tutelage in wines, in which he was expert. It was in Roullier's laboratory that I met Lelio Orci, who later succeeded him as chairperson.

Boston Regained

Despite the gratifying offer of a permanent position in Geneva, I decided to return to the hurly-burly of Harvard and American science, rejoining the Central Pathology Department in 1963. I gained tenure in 1965 and succeeded my predecessors Arthur T. Hertig and Benjamin Castleman as the Shattuck Professor of Pathological Anatomy in 1972. This is the oldest full-time professorship of pathology in the United States, founded in 1847 (funded then by the fees paid by the students) and endowed in 1853 by George Shattuck, Professor of Medicine.

Upon my return from Geneva, the direction of my research was partly determined in a serendipitous fashion. One of the most prestigious awards at Harvard Medical School are the annual Dunham Lectures, given to only foreign scientists, many of whom are, or become, Nobel Laureates. The week of the lectureships was, in the 1960s, celebrated in grand style and was considered one of the highlights of the year. It was traditional for a member of the junior faculty to "look after" the Dunham Lecturer, to act as chauffeur, general factotum, and to ensure that he or she made all appointments on time and did not get lost. I was assigned to be Lord Florey's shadow in 1965 when he was the Dunham Lecturer, and this turned out to be a most enjoyable and illuminating experience. Florey was the co-winner of the Nobel Prize in 1945, together with Fleming and Chain, for the discovery, purification, and therapeutic application of penicillin. We had many conversations about science. One of Lord Florey's main interests at that time, in fact the topic of one of his lectures, was the nature of the ultrastructural bases for the permeability of the microcirculation to macromolecules. In fact, so engrossing was the topic that, in driving my distinguished guest to the grand banquet held in his honor, I got so thoroughly lost we arrived somewhat late, much to the annoyance of the Chairman of the committee, a most distinguished biochemist and, I believe, ex-marine, who reprimanded me in military style—one of the low points of my career. Lord Florey was unfazed.

The tracers suitable for ultrastructural studies were, at that time, essentially limited to large molecules such as colloidal carbon and ferritin, the latter of which Florey had been using. He urged me to develop smaller tracers to study the passage of small molecules across the endothelium, which, as indicated below, I attempted to do.

RESEARCH OVERVIEW

I was a relatively late starter in a serious research career, but I believe the two threads running though most of my research (namely, the study of the structural components of cells and their functions and the analysis of how disease states change structure and function) were entwined early. Although to do this I frequently had to pioneer the invention and development of several technologies, I usually perceived these efforts as a necessary means of addressing problems and not as ends in themselves. My papers, I believe, reveal a meld of disciplines including cell biology, experimental pathology, biochemistry, and physiology, perhaps reflecting my lack of specialization in any one field. Such eclecticism is probably not possible in these days of hyperspecialization.

In summarizing some selective areas of research in which I have been engaged, I must admit that I have, not infrequently, merely indulged my curiosity, and sometimes my involvement in a topic has been accidental. On occasion, though, there has been a logical extension of a train of thought. I do not, for obvious reasons, provide a comprehensive review, but instead delineate a topic and provide a minimum of references that summarize our work. To those who have made important contributions to the area I deal with, I have referred to their papers on a highly selective basis; to those omitted, I apologize.

ULTRASTRUCTURAL TRACERS

Horseradish Peroxidase and the Diaminobenzidine Reaction

Werner Strauss (11) had used horseradish peroxidase (HRP) to study endocytic electron uptake at the light microscopic level, but benzidine, the electron donor in the peroxidase reaction used at that time to reveal the site of the enzyme, did not yield a sufficiently electron-opaque reaction product suitable for electron microscopy. HRP had the prospect of being a suitable tracer molecule: It is not highly charged, it is suitably small, and its peroxidatic activity could enhance sensitivity. I thought that a suitable substrate (electron donor) could be formulated, one that would yield an insoluble reaction product that would reduce osmium tetroxide and bind the reduced osmium. Modified benzidine, with additional amino groups, seemed to be a suitable candidate; 3,3′-diaminobenzidine (DAB) was the answer. Luckily, before I embarked on an organic synthesis, for which I was ill prepared, I found that DAB was commercially available as a reagent for detecting vanadium in milk. In the DAB-peroxidase reaction, HRP oxidizes DAB in the presence of H_2O_2 and converts it into an insoluble brown polymer; this polymer causes reduction of added osmium tetroxide, and the reduced osmium forms an insoluble electron-opaque precipitate at the site of the HRP. Thus, when HRP is injected into the bloodstream, the pathways that it takes to reach the tissues can be followed by fixing tissues at various times after injection and by performing the DAB reaction. Furthermore, HRP can be cross-linked to antibodies and other proteins for localization studies in vivo and in vitro.

It amuses me to think that the discovery of DAB and its usefulness in detecting peroxidatic activity may well be attributed to Sherlock Holmes (see *A Study in Scarlet*). In that story, Dr. Watson first meets Holmes when he visits the chemistry laboratory at St. Bartholomew's Hospital, London, and Holmes gleefully shows Watson his new reagent and method for detecting blood stains, no doubt because of the peroxidatic activity of the hemoglobin in red blood cells. Holmes' reaction yielded a brown precipitate, as does DAB: "[A] brownish dust was precipitated to the bottom of the glass jar." The forensic methods for detecting blood in the 1889s, the guaic, or the preferable benzidine reactions, yielded blue or blue-green colors, respectively.

In the first paper introducing this technique (12), we studied the passage of HRP through the glomerulus into the urine; as HRP is smaller than albumen, it readily crosses the glomerular basement membrane, passes through the epithelial slits, between the epithelial foot processes, and through the slit diaphragm, into the urinary space, where a considerable portion is absorbed by endocytotic uptake from the glomerular filtrate by the proximal tubular cells. This paper, which validated the methodology, is one of the most quoted in the biomedical literature, having been cited (according to The Institute for Scientific Information, Philadelphia) some 7000 times.

THE BLOOD-BRAIN BARRIER AND OTHERS

In another classic paper Thomas Reese and I (13) used the DAB-HRP method to establish for the first time that the cerebral endothelial cells form the structural basis for the so-called blood-brain barrier. The concept of a barrier between cerebral blood vessels and brain tissues had existed since the work of Paul Ehrlich in the late nineteenth century. He found that intravenously injected dyes failed to stain certain areas of the brain, whereas non-neural tissues were stained. It was not clear, however, until the high resolution obtainable with the electron microscope, as to whether the structural barrier was at the level of the endothelium, the basement membrane, astrocytes, or glial cells. We found that extensive tight junctions (zonulae occludentes) between the endothelial cells, and a paucity of endothelial vesicles, effectively prevented HRP from crossing the endothelium. This paper concentrated the attention of physiologists, morphologists, and pharmacologists on the cerebral endothelium as the site of the blood-brain barrier and also led to the construction of in vitro models utilizing endothelial cells in culture (14).

Eveline Schneeberger and I also defined the alveolar-capillary barrier (blood-air barrier) as residing at the tight junctions between the alveolar epithelial cells (15). Similarly, Elio Raviola and I defined a putative blood-thymus barrier, limited to the cortex, but not found in the medulla, but the mechanisms appeared complex and included impermeable cortical capillaries plus other factors (16).

VASCULAR PERMEABILITY

In contrast, in a paper published the same year, I found that HRP passed across the endothelium of the heart and skeletal muscle microcirculation apparently through incomplete junctions, or maculae (17), with a possible contribution from endothelial vesicles (18). We postulated that the incomplete junctions represented the small pores Pappenheimer (19; see also Reference 17) thought underlay the semipermeable properties of microcirculatory endothelia to macromolecules smaller than albumin. I think it is unreasonable to expect to find pores corresponding exactly in shape and size to those proposed by the physiologists. The theoretical pores are symmetrical, water-filled, equivalent pores, and it seems unlikely that a living endothelium would exhibit these exactly—it behaves as if it has such theoretical pores. Our paper (17) has been frequently quoted, but it must be admitted, however, that the relative roles of junctions (17) and/or Palade vesicles (18) in microcirculatory permeability are still a matter of some controversy.

GLOMERULAR PERMEABILITY AND THE SLIT DIAPHRAGM: THE "ZIPPER"

Following up on our initial studies on glomerular permeability to HRP (12), we utilized a variety of peroxidatic tracers of different sizes (HRP, myeloperoxidase, catalase), as well as endogenous plasma albumin and IgG (localized with specific antibodies labeled with HRP). Several of these studies were collaborations with Manjeri Venkatachalam and my dear friend, the late Ramzi Cotran. We concluded, in agreement with Caulfield and Farquar (20), that the glomerular basement membrane (GBM) was the major barrier to the passage of proteins into the urine. However, Graham Ryan and I emphasized that this concept pertained to conditions of normal blood flow (see below) (21, 22). Richard Rodewald and I studied in detail the fine structure of the slit diaphragm and found it consisted of a meshwork of struts and pores, somewhat resembling a zipper, by which name the structure has become known. The pores, we calculated, were of sufficient size, shape, and density to constitute a barrier to the passage of molecules the size of albumin or larger (23). In addition, we proposed that the slit pore also constituted a regulator of hydraulic flow (23).

In what has been referred to as a unique experiment (24), Graham Ryan and I restricted blood flow to the glomerulus and observed the distribution of plasma albumin tagged with HRP. Under normal-flow conditions, albumin was restricted by the GBM. Under low-flow conditions, albumin as well as larger molecules, such as IgG, passed into the urine (21, 22). When normal flow was restored, molecules were once again restricted by the GBM. We interpreted our results in terms of changes in molecular sieving, perhaps associated with concentration polarization and/or charge modulations in the GBM. However, Smithies (24) has lately adduced a novel hypothesis: that transport across the GBM is by diffusion and that in the above experiments the difference in concentration of albumin on the two sides of the GBM disappears because diffusion is no longer accompanied by the wash-out of Bowman's space that normally occurs as a result of flow of liquid.

In recent years, exciting new evidence for the role of the slit diaphragm in glomerular permeability is the remarkable discovery by Tryggvason and associates (25, 26) that a unique protein, nephrin, directly constitutes at least part of the structure of the slit diaphragm and, cogently, abnormal nephrin or its absence results in proteinuria and slit-pore defects (25, 26). This exciting work has opened a new chapter in the pathophysiology of glomerular filtration and nephrology.

It is gratifying to me that after many years of relative obscurity our earlier findings and hypotheses regarding the slit diaphragm now have considerable relevance. It is clear, however, that many issues remain unresolved. I am sure that in the near future the approaches of molecular physiology will unravel the mysteries of glomerular filtration.

FURTHER STUDIES ON THE RENAL GLOMERULUS

Over the years we maintained our ongoing interest in glomerular pathophysiology, including the development of methods for isolating and culturing glomerular cells—studies initated in my laboratory by Jeffrey Kreisberg and Richard Hoover. We showed that cells of apparent mesangial origin (27) were contractile, as had been postulated, but not proven, for many years. This function has been related to control of glomerular filtration via decrease in capillary surface area.

Jonathan Diamond and I developed a new model for studying focal and segmental glomerular sclerosis, in which an acute phase of proteinuria was followed by a latent phase, then a chronic phase, thus mimicking many aspects of human disease (28). In collaboration with Barry Brenner's group, we showed that the acute nephrotic phase is accompanied by severe morphologic injury and renal insufficiency. The nephrotic syndrome resolves, but it is accompanied by glomerular capillary hypertension, leading to recurrent proteinuria and glomerular sclerosis, which was alleviated by angiotensin 1–converting enzyme inhibitors (29). We postulated that glomerular hypertension led to glomerular sclerosis and renal failure after an episode of acute glomerular injury, in accordance with the bounteous experimental and clinical evidence produced by Brenner's group (see Reference 28).

GAP JUNCTIONS

Another electron-opaque tracer I introduced was the use of colloidal lanthanum. Using this tracer, Jean-Paul Revel and I succeeded in revealing the fine structure of electrotonic (so-called gap, close, or nexus) junctions (30). These junctions are the structural correlate of the electrophysiologically defined electrical synapses that occur in excitable tissues. We showed that these junctions, consisting of subunits in hexagonal arrays, also are formed by cells in nonexcitable tissues. We now know that they are basic to cell-cell communication. Viewed in light of more recent biochemical electron diffraction and crystallographic studies by others, our original model of this junction appears to have been quite perceptive. It is amusing that in our original paper we did not use the rather unsuitable, oxymoronic term gap junction (there is no real gap), although the introduction of that term has almost invariably been referenced to our original paper (30). We did, however, later use the term in an abstract and in seminars and at meetings, so we are partly to blame for following the fashion. Our original paper (30) is also a "citation classic."

REACTIVE OXYGEN SPECIES

When activated in phagocytosis polymorphonuclear leukocytes undergo a respiratory burst, generating reactive oxygen species such as H_2O_2, superoxide; some of which are bacteriocidal. In the 1970s, the exact sites where these reactive oxygen species are generated were, from biochemical data, somewhat controversial. The ultrastructural cytochemical approaches pursued by Richard Briggs, John Robinson, Manfred Karnovsky, and myself have been summarized (31). We designed two ultrastructural cytochemical methods for detecting H_2O_2 and found that it was generated at the site of contact with the bacterium at the surface membrane. As the bacterium is internalized by phagocytosis, the membrane of the phagosome (derived from the surface) is the site of H_2O_2 generation. Subsequently, we showed by a novel technique the similar generation sites of superoxide, a precursor of H_2O_2. We verified, at the ultrastructural level, the delivery of myeloperoxidase from cytoplasmic granules into the phagasome, which contains powerful mechanisms for bacteriocidal action. Marla Steinbeck, A.U. Khan, and I later demonstrated by devising a chemical trap method that leukocytes upon activation also generate singlet oxygen (32). The significance of this finding was not initally apparent as singlet oxygen is short lived. However, recently, Babior and associates (33) have shown that when antibodies are bound to the leukocyte cell surface, ozone (a potent and long-lived cidal agent) is generated from singlet oxygen.

IMMUNOGLOBULINS AND LYMPHOCYTE SURFACES

In the late 1960s Baruj Benacerraf, an eminent immunologist and Nobel Laureate, became chairman of our department and I found myself suddenly surrounded by immunologists, who tried valiantly, but with only partial success, to convert me to this intricate discipline. Luckily, Baruj allowed his faculty to pursue their own interests and did not bother them with administrative chores. I was fortunate to have fruitful collaborations with some of my immunologist colleagues, despite my recalcitrance in understanding their language. An extension of our interest in cell surface membranes, which arose from our work on activated leukocytes, included collaboration with our friend and colleague Emil Unanue on the distribution of immunoglobulins on lymphocyte surfaces and their behavior and fate after binding to cross-linking antibodies. Our studies are partly reviewed in Reference 34. By utilizing antibodies variously labeled with fluorescein, radioactive iodine, HRP, or hemocyanine in murine lymphocytes, we found that after anti-IgG antibody treatment, the IgG-antibody complexes form patches on the cell surface: This is a passive process due to movement of the receptors in the fluid membrane and their capture, cross-linking, and immobilization by the multivalent antibody. The patches are immobile and become anchored to the cytoskeleton through a transmembrane mechanism. Thereafter, the sweeping of the patches into a single large patch or cap situated at one pole of the cell requires metabolic energy and the participation of cytoskeletal and microtubular elements. Perturbation of the membrane by various agents that rendered it more or less fluid (e.g., the removal or addition of cholesterol, the insertion of free fatty acids) modified the process of capping. Basically, increasing fluidity inhibited capping.

Together with Abul Abbas (35) we mapped the inherent distribution of surface immunoglobulin on murine-B lymphocytes, thereby utilizing monovalent antibodies labeled with fluorescein. We then treated the cell surface with monovalent antibodies to fluorecein labeled with ferritin. The cell-surface distribution of the complexes was revealed by rapid freezing of pre-fixed cells and freeze-etching. We found that the surface Ig was in small clusters and interconnected networks and was compared with the expected random (Poisson) distribution. Surprisingly, we also found that the distribution was nonrandom to a high degree of statistical significance, suggesting organization in a specific manner. The functional significance of this microclustering was not elucidated. Perhaps it contributes to the efficiency of antibody binding. A parallel study on Ia-antigen distribution on murine-B cells showed a similar nonrandom distribution of microclusters of the antigen.

LIPID DOMAINS

Over the years, our laboratory has been interested in the mechanisms underlying various cell-surface phenomena that relate to physiological and pathological processes (discussed above). In collaboration with Richard Klausner, Alan Kleinfeld, and Eliezar Dawidowicz, we used free fatty acids (FFAs) as one class of probe to perturb structure and function at the cell surface. FFAs produced profound biological effects when incorporated into surface membranes. These effects included alteration of membrane-bound enzymatic activity, platelet aggregation, lymphocyte mitogenesis, surface receptor capping, and cell-substrate and cell-cell adhesion (see References 36, 37). These phenomena required explanation in terms of membrane structure. Thus, the interaction of FFAs with cell-surface membranes and lipid bilayers was studied by monitoring the emission polarization changes of the fluorescent probes 1,6-diphenyl-1,3,5,-hexatriene (DPH) and 8-anilino-1-naphthalene sulfonate (ANS) (38). The differential polarization effects of *cis*-unsaturated FFA versus *trans*-unsaturated and saturated FFA, when incorporated into plasma membranes as well as into mixed-phase vesicles, were similar. Using solution theory in mixed-phase vesicles, we understood the shift in the transition midpoint temperature to mean that *cis*-unsaturated FFA preferentially partitioned into fluid domains, whereas *trans*-unsaturated FFA and saturated FFA preferentially partitioned into solid-like domains.

The fluorescent lifetime of DPH in membranes and vesicles was measured using the phase-modulation technique. The results were analyzed in terms of site heterogeneity (38) and indicated that although DPH decay in single-phase vesicles was monoexponential, a considerable degree of heterogeneity was observed in mixed-phase vesicles and also in plasma membranes (with the exception of the erythrocyte membrane). These results, together with the FFA effects, were interpreted in terms of lipid domains (relatively fluid and gel-like) existing in membranes (38).

We theorized that the insertion of various FFA into specific domains caused perturbation of domain structure with consequent effects on the conformation, structure, and function of proteins embedded in those domains. In general, our working hypotheses were that *cis*-unsaturated FFA, or subtracted cholesterol, further fluidized gel-like domains and vice-versa for *trans*-unsaturated FFA, saturated FFA, and for added cholesterol. Many questions regarding the precise mechanisms involved remain unanswered. Nevertheless, the concept of membrane lipid domains originally put forward remains viable, perhaps in more modern terms, such as that of lipid rafts.

HEPARIN AND VASCULAR SMOOTH MUSCLE PROLIFERATION

In recent years, we became interested in the proliferation of vascular smooth muscle (VSMC) that occurs after vascular injury, particularly in arteries, for instance, following angioplasty, stent placement, or organ transplantation, and which is of considerable clinical import in these situations. Our studies are summarized in Reference 39. Many of these studies were performed by Elazer Edelman, Richard Hoover, and John Castellot. We initially surmised that an insult to the endothelium would lead to activation of the clotting cascade and the generation of thrombin, which is a mitogen. Thus inhibition of thrombin generation by administration of the antithrombin-III binding agent, heparin, should inhibit proliferation of VSMC. Somewhat to our surprise this turned out to be the case, initially in vivo after air drying or balloon injury of the aorta or carotid arteries [as shown by me and Alexander Clowes (40)]. (In proofing the paper we both failed to notice that our names were misspelled. This is embarrassing, as the paper has been cited often.) The inhibition of growth was also observed in vitro (see Reference 39). However, these were serendipitous findings, as removal of the antithrombin-III binding capacity of the heparin by a variety of means caused retention of the antiproliferative but lost the anticoagulative activities. This antiproliferative activity was novel for heparin, as other glygosaminoglygans were virtually inactive. Heparin is a structurally heterogeneous, highly charged (O- and N-sulfated and carboxylated) glycosaminoglycan consisting of varying repeating disaccharide units of alternating D-glucosamine and uronic acid sugars, including L-iduronic acid. The structural specificity of the latter lends special antiproliferative properties to the molecule.

The heparin antiproliferative activity was size dependent (hexamers were the minimum), and O-sulfation (but not N-sulfation) was required (whereas the anticoagulant activity required both). There are inhibitory effects early in the cell cycle and inhibition of expression of early response genes. The final block in the cell cycle was in early to late G1 and was fully reversible when the heparin or its derivatives were removed.

With John Castellot and Richard Hoover, we showed that the growth of glomerular mesangial cells, which resemble VSMC, was also inhibited by heparin (41). Furthermore, the chronic phase of our glomerular nephritis model referred to above (28), in which there is mesangial cell proliferation, was prevented by administration of a nonanticoagulant, antiproliferative heparin derivative, as well as by whole heparin (42), and proteinuria was markedly diminished.

We demonstrated that endothelial cells produce heparin-like molecules (heparan sulfates) that are antiproliferative for VSMC and render them unresponsive to growth factors (see Reference 39). Similarly, glomerular epithelial cells produce heparin-like molecules antiproliferative for mesangial cells (idem). We surmised (39) that in endothelial or glomerular epithelial cell injury, VSMC or mesangial cells, respectively, are released from nonresponsiveness to growth factors, as the heparin-like molecules are no longer secreted from the adjacent heparin-like molecule producers, the endothelial, or glomerular epithelial cells. Such modeling may also apply to smooth muscle proliferation occurring at other sites such as in the pulmonary vasculature and in bronchoproliferative diseases.

The mechanisms underlying the antiproliferative activity of heparin and similar molecules are complex and not clear. Heparin has anti-inflammatory effects; for instance, it blocks the adhesion of leukocytes to endothelia and their invasion into the artery or other tissues to provide a source of growth factors for VSMC proliferation. It does not appear to be effective by directly binding to growth factors nor by blocking binding to their cell receptors. Laurel Pukac of my laboratory found that serum and platelet-derived growth factor BB activate a heparin-sensitive pathway involving protein kinase C and raf-1 (43). Suppression of C-dependent mitogen-activated protein kinase activation appears to be a key element in the antimitogenic actions of heparin. In contrast, epidermal growth factor does not stimulate these kinases and acts through a heparin-insensitive pathway. However, no sole inhibitory mechanism has been unequivocally established, although several other signal transduction mechanisms have been suggested. For instance, in both VSMC and mesangial cells, heparin-sensitive, Ca^{2+}/calmodulin-dependent protein kinase has been demonstrated (44). Furthermore, the heparin-induced block in G1 to S phase, which we described above, is claimed to be caused by p27(kip1)-mediated inhibition of cyclin-dependent kinase 2 (44a).

CARDIAC TRANSPLANTATION AND GRAFT ARTERIOSCLEROSIS

VSMC proliferation is one of the characteristics of progressive graft arteriosclerosis, which is a leading cause of morbidity and mortality in organ transplants after the first postoperative year. David Adams and I developed the Lewis-to-F344 heterotopic rat cardiac transplant model to study these phenomena (45). These strains have minor histocompatibility differences, and the donor (Lewis) hearts, attached to the blood supply in the inguinal region, develop chronic rejection characterized by progressive graft arteriosclerosis and chronic inflammation in the myocardium. We showed that graft arteriosclerosis developed in well-defined stages: (*a*) early adherence of monocytes and T cells to the endothelial surface, proceeding to (*b*) subintimal infiltration of monocyte/macrophages and T-cells, and, finally, (*c*) a diffuse arterial concentric intimal thickening, predominately consisting of proliferating VSMC. This appeared to be an ideal model for studying the effects of a nonanticoagulant heparin on the development of the lesion and the inhibition of chronic rejection and graft arteriosclerosis. A large amount of nonanticoagulant heparin was required for administration over a period of months and this was prepared for us by the Institut Choay of Paris, France. Unfortunately, the large bottle of the white, fluffy powder that we received disappeared from our cold room overnight, obviously stolen by persons unknown, no doubt for nefarious purposes. We were thus unable to conduct this long-term experiment, so we investigated the roles of activated macrophages in the pathogenesis of graft arteriosclerosis.

In collaboration with Mary Russell, we showed that during development of lesions in rats on a normal diet, gene transcript levels in the donor hearts were significantly increased for the cytokine effectors associated with macrophage activation: interferon-γ, interleukin-6, monocyte chemoattractant protein-1 (MCP-1), macrophage colony stimulating factor, and the macrophage lectin Gal/GalNAc (46). These increased levels in gene transcripts were confined to the donor hearts and were not raised systemically in the tissues of the recipient rats, with the exception of interleukin-6. In several cases we confirmed cytochemically increased levels of the gene products in macrophages in the donor hearts.

We then inhibited the chronic inflammatory response in the donor hearts with a diet for the recipients deficient in essential fatty acids, which causes an increase in the ratio of Mead acid to arachidonate, which results in decreased prostaglandin and leukotriene synthesis and leukocyte functions. The diet deficient in essential fatty acids significantly decreased VSMC proliferation, graft arteriosclerosis, and the chronic inflammatory response (47). Gene transcript levels for MCP-1, interferon-γ, and CD4 were also significantly decreased compared with those levels in control hearts transplanted into hosts on a normal diet (48). We concluded that activated macrophage functions were major contributors to graft arteriosclerosis and VSMC proliferation.

TEACHING

I have always regarded teaching as an important component of my academic life. For almost 50 years I have taught general pathology to medical students, both as a lecturer and as a laboratory instructor. For 12 years I organized and ran the general pathology course. In the early days we had three mornings a week for a whole semester assigned to us and were able to perform experiments with the active participation of the students [e.g., aminonucleoside nephrosis, clearance of bacteria from the blood (with the collaboration of the microbiologists), anaphylactic shock, etc.]. We had lectures on the latest ongoing research in the laboratories of the faculty. Nowadays, unfortunately, owing to time constraints, the difficulties in obtaining permission for animal experiments, and the fashionable emphasis on clinical cases and "relevance," the general pathology course is but a shadow of its former self. I, and many of the students and faculty, do not find this situation intellectually satisfying.

I have noticed over the years a rather strange phenomenon: The more senior the faculty, the less teaching they do. Professors may give one or two lectures a year and this is regarded as fulfilling their responsibility for teaching. Chairpersons are not infrequently too busy having to be entrepreneurial, or having to deal with the exigencies imposed by managed care, to participate significantly in teaching. This is unfortunate: Students are being denied wisdom and experience. In the best of all worlds, professors should profess—that is, teach—their discipline.

As there was, and still is, a large nonmedical population, consisting of Ph.D. graduate students, post-doctoral fellows, and faculty at our institution, I felt there was a gap in their education and experience at medical school resulting from a lack of exposure to mechanisms of disease and the concepts of pathogenesis. As a consequence, together with my friend and colleague, the late Ramzi Cotran, and with generous financial support from the Josiah Macy, Jr., Foundation, we organized an experimental course in molecular pathology and mechanisms of disease to service these needs. This course, which ran annually for five years, proved to be immensely popular, and even senior faculty from a variety of disciplines, such as physics, engineering, and biochemistry, attended. Similar courses were thereafter instituted at other schools. Several students told me that being exposed to the content and philosophy of the course had profound impact on their research interests and, in several instances, had changed the direction of their careers into investigating disease processes—a most gratifying result.

Because I believe that general and experimental pathology meld with other disciplines, as they are eclectic in the application of techniques and approach, I was pleased to chair the first interdepartmental, interdisciplinary Ph.D. program at our school, namely that in cell and developmental biology, for a period of approximately 17 years. In fact, I regard myself as a sort of hybrid cell biologist and experimental pathologist. This experience in the program, besides broadening my own perspectives, enabled me to bring Ph.D. graduate students in a variety of disciplines into the orbit of disease mechanisms and pathogenesis.

CODA

One thing I have learned over the years is that sometimes it takes a long time for the significance of one's results and hypotheses to be fully recognized. This applies, for instance, to our work of several decades ago on the glomerular slit diaphragm (23), which now is recognized to be of considerable importance in glomerular filtration. The molecular nature of the structure, and its perturbation leading to proteinuria, is now being established (25, 26), reinforcing our original concepts that this structure plays a major role in filtration. Another instance is our concept of membrane lipid heterogeneity and lipid domains (38), which somehow never became popular when proposed in the 1970s, but which, in modern form, resonates, I like to think, in concepts such as that of lipid rafts and other membrane lipid heterogeneities. Patience is a virtue and sometimes a necessity. Occasionally, of course, we were plain wrong, as was later shown by us or others. An example is our initial reasoning as to the nature of the antiproliferative activity of heparin for VSMC. On the other hand, our papers on the blood-brain barrier (13), the gap junction (30), and the antiproliferative activity of heparin for VSMC (40) were fairly rapidly recognized for what they were worth, so one cannot complain.

I here provide an overview of the rather itinerant route by which I have evolved from the African veldt to the hallowed halls of Harvard. I have been extremely fortunate to have worked with talented collaborators and trainees, few of whom I have been able to mention, who have carried the load of work in many diverse areas of research. I am proud that more than two dozen have achieved prominent positions in academia and biomedical organizations. I am also grateful to have been amply supported by the National Institutes of Health. Overall, my rather hodge-podge career has been a lot of fun. However, I would add a cautionary note if any young pathologist should take my sort of career path as an exemplar. In this age of modern science—genomics, proteomics, and other "omics" of the future—I recommend a greater degree of specialization. Although I have enjoyed savoring many areas of pathobiology and cell biology, biomedical science today moves fast and is too complex for such an approach; one needs to concentrate more specifically in a discipline. However, to have as powerful an armamentarium as possible, I have always encouraged my students early in their careers to acquire expertise in the most basic of sciences—mathematics, physics, chemistry, molecular biology, biochemistry, genetics, and the like—before plunging into disease-related areas. This approach may, I hope, enable students both to adapt to new techniques and concepts and to turn attention to a variety of emerging problems as well as provide them with the flexibility to move into newer areas of research.

As indicated, I was much influenced by Florey and by his book on general pathology (1). As Frank Fenner wrote (49), Florey viewed pathology with the eye of an experimental physiologist and not purely as a morphologist, which was the fashion of the time. He also had a strong background in biochemistry. I hope I am not being overly sententious when I say that today the pathologist should have the piercing eye of a modern biologist. Furthermore, work beyond the relatively easy task of data collection is needed, e.g., understanding the implications of the data, insightful synthesis, and conceptualization.

Those in pathology, no matter how basic their research, should, I believe, always try to keep in mind the unique concept that pathology embodies above all other sciences—the Concept of Pathogenesis. With this concept in mind, I believe that pathologists can make a singular contribution in their study of disease states.

Lastly, I can say the following regarding my own Odyssey:

Heureux qui comme Ulysse, a fait un beau voyage.

Happy he who like Ulysses has made a glorious voyage.

Joachim du Bellay, 1559, *Les Regrets*

LITERATURE CITED

1. Florey H, ed. 1954. *Lectures in General Pathology.* Philadelphia/London: Saunders. 733 pp. 1st ed.
2. Karnovsky MJ, Himmelhoch SR. 1961. Seasonal and starvation-induced changes in the enzymatic pattern of the frog nephron. *Am. J. Physiol.* 201:781–85
3. Karnovsky MJ. 1963. The fine structure of mitochondria in the frog nephron correlated with cytochrome oxidase activity. *Exp. Mol. Pathol.* 2:347–66
4. Himmelhoch SR, Karnovsky MJ. 1961. Oxidative and hydrolytic enzymes in the nephron of *Necturus maculosus*. Histochemical, biochemical, and electron microscopical studies. *J. Biophys. Biochem. Cytol.* 9:893–908
5. Karnovsky MJ, Himmelhoch SR. 1961.The histochemical localization of glutaminase 1 activity in the kidney. *Am. J. Physiol.* 201:786–90
6. Gonzales F, Karnovsky MJ. 1961. Electron microscopical study of osteoclasts in healing fractures of rat bone. *J. Biophys. Biochem. Cytol.* 9:299–16
7. Karnovsky MJ, Roots L. 1964. A "direct-coloring" thiocholine method for cholinesterases. *J. Histochem. Cytochem.* 12:219–21
8. Karnovsky MJ. 1964.The localization of cholinesterase activity in rat cardiac muscle by electron microscopy. *J. Cell Biol.* 23:217–23
9. Karnovsky MJ, Hug K. 1963. The nature of the M band enzyme in rat ventricular muscle. *J. Cell Biol.* 19:255–60
10. Karnovsky MJ. 1961. Simple methods for staining with lead at high pH in electron microscopy. *J. Biophys. Biochem. Cytol.* 11:729–32
11. Strauss W. 1957. Segregation of an intravenously injected protein by "droplets" of the cells of rat kidney. *J. Biophys. Biochem. Cytol.* 3:1037–40
12. Graham RC Jr, Karnovsky MJ. 1966. The early stages of absorption of injected horseradish peroxidase in the proximal tubules of mouse kidney: Ultrastructural cytochemistry by a new method. *J. Histochem. Cytochem.* 14:291–302

13. Reese TS, Karnovsky MJ. 1967. Fine structural localization of a blood-brain barrier to exogenous peroxidase. *J. Cell Biol.* 34:207–17
14. Rutten MJ, Hoover RL, Karnovsky MJ. 1987. Electrical resistance and macromolecular permeability of brain endothelial monolayer culture. *Brain Res.* 425:301–10
15. Schneeberger-Keeley EE, Karnovsky MJ. 1968. The ultrastructural basis of alveolar-capillary permeability to peroxidase as a tracer. *J. Cell Biol.* 37:781–93
16. Raviola E, Karnovsky MJ. 1972. Evidence for a blood-thymus barrier using electron-opaque tracers. *J. Exp. Med.* 136:466–98
17. Karnovsky MJ. 1967. The ultrastructural basis of capillary permeability studied with peroxidase as a tracer. *J. Cell Biol.* 35:213–36
18. Palade GE, Bruns RR. 1968. Structural modifications of plasmalemmal vesicles. *J. Cell Biol.* 37:633–49
19. Landis EM, Pappenheimer JR. 1963. Exchange of substances through the capillary walls. In *Handbook of Physiology, Circulation*, ed. WF Hamilton, P Dow, 2:961–1034. Washington, DC: Am. Physiol. Soc.
20. Caulfield JP, Farquar MG. 1974. The permeability of glomerular capillaries to graded dextrans: Identification of the basement membrane as the primary filtration barrier. *J. Cell Biol.* 63:883–903
21. Ryan GB, Karnovsky MJ. 1976. Distribution of endogenous albumin in the rat glomerulus: Role of hemodynamic factors in glomerular barrier function. *Kidney Int.* 9:36–45
22. Ryan GB, Hein SJ, Karnovsky MJ. 1976. Glomerular permeability to proteins. Effects of hemodynamic factors on the distribution of endogenous immunoglobulin G and exogenous catalase in the rat glomerulus. *Lab. Invest.* 34:415–27
23. Rodewald R, Karnovsky MJ. 1974. Porous substructure of the glomerular slit diaphragm in the rat and the mouse. *J. Cell Biol.* 60:168–80
24. Smithies O. 2003. Why the kidney glomerulus does not clog: A gel permeation/diffusion hypothesis of renal function. *Proc. Natl. Acad. Sci. USA* 100:4108–13
25. Ruotsalainen V, Ljungberg P, Wartiovaara J, Lenkkeri U, Kestilä M, et al.1999. Nephrin is specifically located at the slit diaphragm of glomerular podocytes. *Proc. Natl. Acad. Sci. USA* 96:7962–67
26. Wartiovaara J, Överstedt L-G, Khoshnoodi J, Zhang J, Mäkelä E, et al. 2004. Nephrin strands contribute to a porous slit diaphragm scaffold as revealed by electron tomography. *J. Clin. Invest.* 114:1475–83
27. Ausiello DA, Kreisberg JI, Roy C, Karnovsky MJ. 1980. Contraction of cultured rat glomerular cells of apparent mesangial origin after stimulation with angiotensin 11 and arginine vasopressin. *J. Clin. Invest.* 65:754–60
28. Diamond JR, Karnovsky MJ. 1986. Focal and segmental glomerulosclerosis following a single intravenous dose of puromycin aminonucleoside. *Am. J. Pathol.* 122:481–87
29. Anderson S, Diamond JR, Karnovsky MJ, Brenner BM. 1988. Mechanisms underlying transition from acute glomerular injury to late glomerular sclerosis in a rat model of nephrotic syndrome. *J. Clin. Invest.* 82:1757–68
30. Revel JP, Karnovsky MJ. 1967. Hexagonal array of subunits in intecellular junctions of the mouse heart and liver. *J. Cell Biol.* 33:C7–12
31. Karnovsky MJ, Robinson JM, Briggs RT, Karnovsky ML. 1981. Oxidative cytochemistry in phagocytosis: the interface between structure and function. *Histochem. J.* 13:1–22
32. Steinbeck M, Khan AU, Karnovsky MJ. 1992. Intracellular singlet oxygen generation by phagocytosing neutrophils in response to particles coated with a chemical trap. *J. Biol. Chem.* 267:13425–33

33. Wentworth P, McDunn JE, Wentworth AD, Takeuchi C, Nieva J, et al. 2002. Evidence for anti-body catalyzed ozone formation in bacterial killing and inflammation. *Science* 298:2195–99
34. Unanue ER, Karnovsky MJ. 1973. Redistribution and fate of Ig complexes on surface of B lymphocytes: functional implications and mechanisms. *Transplant. Rev.* 14:184–210
35. Abbas AK, Ault KA, Karnovsky MJ, Unanue ER. 1975. Non-random distribution of surface immunoglobulin of murine B cells. *J. Immunol.* 114:1197–204
36. Karnovsky MJ, Kleinfeld AM, Hoover RL, Klausner RD. 1982. The concept of lipid domains in membranes. *J. Cell Biol.* 94:1–6
37. Karnovsky MJ, Kleinfeld AM, Hoover RL, Dawidowicz EA, MacItyre DE, et al. 1983. Lipid domains in membranes. *Ann. NY Acad. Sci.* 401:61–76
38. Klausner RD, Kleinfeld AM, Hoover RL, Karnovsky MJ. 1980. Lipid domains in membranes. Evidence from structural perturbations induced by free fatty acids and lifetime heterogeneity analysis. *J. Biol. Chem.* 255:1286–95
39. Karnovsky MJ, Edelman ER. 1994. Heparin/heparan sulphate regulation of vascular smooth muscle cell behaviour. In *Airways and Vascular Remodelling in Asthma and Cardiovascular Disease*, ed. C Page, J Black, pp. 45–70. London: Academic
40. Clowes AW, Karnovsky MJ. 1977. Suppression by heparin of smooth muscle cell proliferation in injured arteries. *Nature* 265:625–36
41. Castellot JJ, Hoover RL, Harper PA, Karnovsky MJ. 1985. Heparin and heparin-like species inhibit mesangial-cell proliferation. *Am. J. Pathol.* 120:427–35
42. Diamond JR, Karnovsky MJ. 1986. Nonanticoagulant protective effect of heparin in chronic aminonucleoside nephrosis. *Renal Physiol.* 3:366–74
43. Pukac LA, Carter JE, Morrison KS, Karnovsky MJ. 1997. Mechanisms of inhibition by heparin of PDGF stimulated MAP kinase activation in vascular smooth muscle cells. *J. Cell. Physiol.* 172:69–78
44. Xiao W, Liu Y, Templeton DM. 2005. Ca2+/Calmodulin-dependent protein kinase–II inhibition by heparin in mesangial cells. *Am. J. Physiol. Renal Physiol.* 288:F142–49
44a. Fasciano S, Patel RC, Handy I, Patel CV. 2005. Regulation of vascular smooth muscle proliferation by heparin: inhibition of cyclin-dependent kinase 2 activity by p27kip1. *J. Biol. Chem.* 280:15682–89
45. Adams DH, Tilney NL, Collins JJ Jr, Karnovsky MJ. 1992. Experimental graft arteriosclerosis. 1. The Lewis-to-F-344 model. *Transplantation* 53:1115–19
46. Russell ME, Wallace AF, Hancock WW, Sayegh MH, Adams DH, et al. 1995. Upregulation of cytokines associated with macrophage activation in the Lewis-to-F-344 chronic rejection model. *Transplantation* 59:572–78
47. Adams DH, Wyner LR, Steinbeck MJ, Karnovsky MJ. 1993. Inhibition of graft arteriosclerosis by modulation of the inflammatory response. *Transplant Proc.* 25:2092–94
48. Russell ME, Hancock WW, Wallace AF, Wyner LR, Karnovsky MJ. 1995. Modulation of inflammatory activation pathways in the Lewis-to-F-344 rat cardiac rejection model. *Transplant Proc.* 27:2100–4
49. Fenner F. 1972. Howard Walter Florey. In *The Dictionary of Scientific Biography*, ed. GC Gillispie, 5:41–44. New York: Scribner's

Immunobiology and Pathogenesis of Viral Hepatitis

Luca G. Guidotti[1,2] and Francis V. Chisari[1]

[1]Department of Molecular and Experimental Medicine, Scripps Research Institute, La Jolla, California 92037; email: guidotti@scripps.edu, fchisari@scripps.edu

[2]Immunopathogenesis of Liver Infections Unit, San Raffaele Scientific Institute, Milan 20132, Italy

Annu. Rev. Pathol. Mech. Dis. 2006. 1:23–61

The *Annual Review of Pathology: Mechanisms of Disease* is online at pathmechdis.annualreviews.org

doi: 10.1146/annurev.pathol.1.110304.100230

1553-4006/06/0114-0023$20.00

Key Words

hepatitis B virus, hepatitis C virus, cytotoxic T cells, liver cirrhosis, hepatocellular carcinoma, extrahepatic diseases

Abstract

Among the many viruses that are known to infect the human liver, hepatitis B virus (HBV) and hepatitis C virus (HCV) are unique because of their prodigious capacity to cause persistent infection, cirrhosis, and liver cancer. HBV and HCV are noncytopathic viruses and, thus, immunologically mediated events play an important role in the pathogenesis and outcome of these infections. The adaptive immune response mediates virtually all of the liver disease associated with viral hepatitis. However, it is becoming increasingly clear that antigen-nonspecific inflammatory cells exacerbate cytotoxic T lymphocyte (CTL)-induced immunopathology and that platelets enhance the accumulation of CTLs in the liver. Chronic hepatitis is characterized by an inefficient T cell response unable to completely clear HBV or HCV from the liver, which consequently sustains continuous cycles of low-level cell destruction. Over long periods of time, recurrent immune-mediated liver damage contributes to the development of cirrhosis and hepatocellular carcinoma.

INTRODUCTION

Hepatitis B virus (HBV): prototypic member of the Hepadnaviridae family; a DNA virus that causes hepatitis in humans and chimpanzees

Hepatitis C virus (HCV): member of the Flaviviridae family; an RNA virus that causes hepatitis in humans and chimpanzees

Hepatocellular carcinoma (HCC): malignancy that usually develops as a consequence of persistent liver disease (most frequently during chronic viral hepatitis)

Hepatitis B virus (HBV) and hepatitis C virus (HCV) are noncytopathic, hepatotropic members of the hepadnavirus and flavivirus families, respectively, that are spread by contact with infected blood and body fluids and cause acute and chronic necroinflammatory liver diseases (1–5).

HBV infection in immunocompetent adults results in a self-limited, transient liver disease and viral clearance in more than 95% of adults, whereas more than 90% of neonates exposed to HBV at birth become persistently infected. Persistent HBV infection is associated with varying degrees of chronic liver disease, and it often progresses to the development of cirrhosis and hepatocellular carcinoma (HCC) (1, 3). More than 350 million people are chronically infected by HBV, and approximately one million die from these late complications each year worldwide (1, 3, 5). In contrast to the natural history of HBV, 70%–90% of acute HCV infections become persistent, and more than 170 million people worldwide are currently chronically infected by HCV and experience the same late stage complications of cirrhosis of the liver and HCC (4, 6).

Although a highly effective vaccine against HBV infection has been available for the past 20 years (7), there is no vaccine against HCV. Furthermore, many patients who are persistently infected by HBV or HCV do not respond to currently available therapies (nucleoside analogues, interferon-alpha, and ribavirin) (3–5). Improved understanding of the biology and pathogenesis of these infections is required if we are to develop an HCV vaccine and better treatments for these chronic infections.

A large body of evidence indicates that the outcome of HBV and HCV infections and the pathogenesis of the attendant liver diseases are determined by immune-mediated host-virus interactions. The experimental approaches to HBV and HCV pathogenesis have been difficult because the host range of these viruses is limited to humans and chimpanzees, and because of the lack of cell culture systems and small-animal models that are susceptible to infection. Nonetheless, a great deal of new information pertaining to the pathogenetic mechanisms that may cause liver disease during HBV and HCV infection has been obtained in recent years, thanks to the analysis of the natural history (5, 6) and immunobiology (1, 8) of HBV and HCV in humans and chimpanzees, and infections with related hepadnaviruses [e.g., woodchuck hepatitis virus (WHV) and duck hepatitis virus (DHBV)] (9) or flaviviruses [e.g., bovine viral diarrhea virus (BVDV)] (10) in susceptible species. Additional insight has been gained from multidisciplinary studies of cell lines (11–22) and mouse models that express specific viral genes or replicate the viral life cycles to varying degrees (23–36). To better understand the pathogenesis of these infections, a brief description of the tropism, entry, and replication strategies of these viruses is provided below.

Cell Tropism, Entry, and Replication of Hepatitis B Virus and Hepatitis C Virus

It is widely accepted that the parenchymal cell of the liver, i.e., the hepatocyte, is the primary site of both infections. The mechanisms by which HBV or HCV enter hepatocytes or other susceptible cells are still largely unknown, mostly because of the lack of infectible cell culture systems. Thus, the putative receptors for these viruses have not been identified, even though several studies have suggested that the initial step of HBV infection may involve the interaction of the envelope polypeptides of HBV with a variety of cell membrane proteins [including endonexin II (37), IL-6 (38), annexin V (39), apolipoprotein H (40), transferrin receptor (41), and gp180/carboxypeptidase D in the case of DHBV (42, 43)]. Similarly, binding activity of the E2 glycoprotein of HCV has been demonstrated for CD81 (44, 45), the human scavenger receptor class B type I (SR-B1) (46), the dendritic cell-specific intercellular adhesion molecule-3-grabbing nonintegrin (DC-SIGN) (47, 48), and the liver and lymph node-specific intercellular adhesion molecule-3-grabbing nonintegrin (L-SIGN) (47, 49). Furthermore, antibodies specific for HCV E1 and E2 glycoproteins can block the infection of susceptible cells with pseudotyped lentiviral vectors expressing these envelope proteins (45, 50, 51). The difficulty in demonstrating that HBV or HCV actually uses these proteins to infect hepatocytes, coupled with the notion that most of these putative receptors are expressed in many nonhepatic cell types (such as mononuclear leukocytes), suggests that some of these molecules may act as coreceptors and that one or more unidentified proteins must be involved in the entry of HBV or HCV into the hepatocyte.

Following entry, the life cycles of HBV and HCV are significantly different (see also **Figures 1** and **2** for schemes of the HBV and HCV life cycle). The HBV nucleocapsids are released into the cytoplasm and transported to the nuclear pore. There the relaxed circular viral DNA genome is released into the nucleus, where it is repaired by cellular polymerases into an episomal minichromosome, termed covalently closed circular (ccc) DNA, which represents the viral transcriptional template (5, 9, 52). The cccDNA molecule encodes 4 capped and polyadenylated RNAs that produce the structural and nonstructural viral proteins (5, 9, 52). One of the major HBV transcripts is a 3.5-kb greater-than-genome length RNA that is translated to produce the viral core and polymerase proteins. This transcript also serves as a pregenomic RNA that is encapsidated with the polymerase by the core protein in the cytoplasm of the hepatocyte (5, 9, 52). Viral replication occurs within these capsids by reverse transcription of the pregenomic RNA to produce a single-strand DNA copy that serves as the template for second-strand DNA synthesis that produces a circular double-stranded DNA genome (5, 9, 52). Viral capsids containing double-stranded DNA traffic either back to the nucleus to amplify the viral cccDNA genome or to the endoplasmic reticulum, where they engage the viral envelope proteins, bud into the lumen, and exit the cell as virions that can infect other cells (5, 9, 52).

In contrast to HBV, the HCV genome consists of a 9.6-kb linear, plus-stranded, uncapped RNA molecule that is translated as a single polyprotein precursor of roughly 3000 amino acid residues (53). This large polypeptide is processed by cellular and viral proteases into structural (C, E1, and E2/p7) and nonstructural (NS2, NS3, NS4A, NS4B, NS5A, and NS5B) protein subunits (54–68). Unlike HBV, the HCV life cycle and viral replication is driven by a minus-strand intermediate within a membranous compartment in the cytoplasm of the cell (53). Hence, there is a potentially important difference between HBV and HCV at this level, given that the double-stranded HBV DNA genome is completely sequestered within capsid particles, whereas the double-stranded HCV RNA genome is freely exposed in the cytoplasm of the infected cell (53). As most cell types of the innate immune system recognize incoming viruses by detecting double-stranded RNA (dsRNA) produced during the replication process, it is not surprising that, as we describe below, these two viruses induce very different early innate defense mechanisms.

EARLY INNATE DEFENSE MECHANISMS AND THEIR POTENTIAL CONTRIBUTION TO LIVER DISEASE

The host-virus relationship is a dynamic process in which the virus tries to decrease its visibility, whereas the host attempts to prevent and eradicate infection with minimal collateral damage to itself. Initially, the virus must recognize, bind and enter its target cells, and migrate to the appropriate cellular

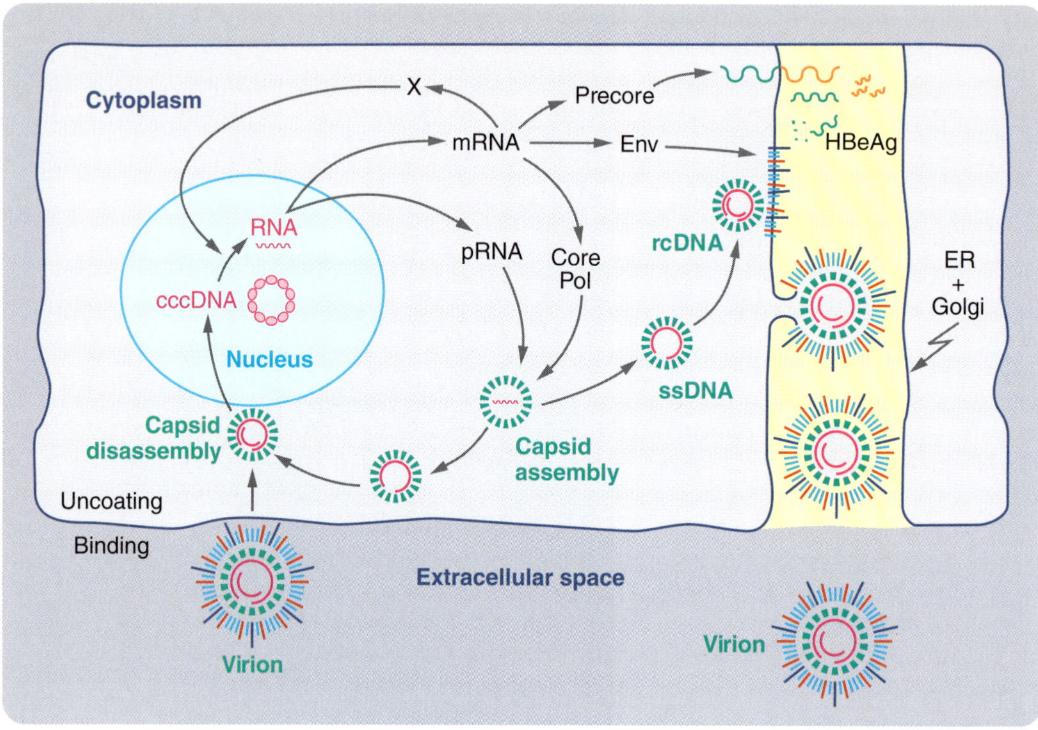

Figure 1

Hepatitis B virus (HBV) life cycle. Entry of the HBV virion from the extracellular space into susceptible cells is a poorly defined process that is presumably receptor-mediated and leads to uncoating and transport of the capsid to the nucleus. Following capsid disassembly, the second strand of the open circular viral genome is completed, and the ends of each strand are ligated. This leads to the production of a covalently closed circular DNA (cccDNA) molecule, which is the transcriptional template of the virus. Pol II-driven transcription results in production of the viral RNAs that are transported out of the nucleus. Once in the cytoplasm, the transcripts are translated into the corresponding proteins as shown. The precore protein contains a leader sequence that transports it into the endoplasmic reticulum (ER) where it is further processed and eventually secreted as HBeAg (*as shown*). The X protein is a transcription factor that does not enter the nucleus; rather it interacts with cellular transcription factors in the cytoplasm that enter the nucleus and activate HBV promoter activity. The envelope proteins (Env) traverse the ER membrane as integral membrane proteins (as shown). The core and polymerase proteins assemble around the pregenomic RNA (pRNA) to form HBV RNA-containing capsids, within which the RNA is reverse transcribed to produce the first single-strand viral DNA (ssDNA, as shown). ssDNA serves as the template for second-strand DNA synthesis, thereby producing capsids containing a partially double-stranded, relaxed circular DNA molecule (rcDNA, as shown). Although the RNA-containing capsid is maturing into a DNA-containing capsid, it migrates bidirectionally within the cytoplasm. One pathway terminates at the ER membrane where it interacts with the envelope proteins that trigger an internal budding reaction. This reaction results in the formation of virions that are transported out of the cell by the default secretory pathway. The second pathway transports the maturing capsid to the nucleus to amplify the pool of cccDNA.

compartment, where its genome is transcribed, translated, and replicated to permit the assembly and export of new virions. Depending on the nature of the infected cells and the infecting virus, early innate defense mechanisms that recognize one or more viral products may be triggered by the infection to limit the extent of viral spread. These mechanisms include (*a*) the induction of apoptosis by the virus (69), (*b*) the production of antiviral cytokines such as interferon (IFN) type I (designated IFN-α/β) by the infected cells (70), and (*c*) the triggering of effector functions of cellular components of the innate immune system [such as natural killer cells (NK) and natural killer T cells (NKT cells), etc.] (71). NK and NKT cells can be rapidly recruited to the site of virus infection and have the potential to recognize infected cells very early [i.e., before major histocompatibility complex (MHC) class I expression is significantly induced on the cell surface] (71). Activated NK and NKT cells may participate in disease pathogenesis both directly (by killing infected cells) and indirectly, by producing soluble factors (i.e., cytokines and chemokines) that have antiviral activity (71–73), recruit inflammatory cells into the infected tissue (71–73), and shape the adaptive immune response (71). Most of what is known about the early innate defense mechanisms in HBV and HCV infection has been learned in experimentally infected chimpanzees, as they can be studied from the onset of infection through the course of the associated disease. On the basis of these studies (see below), it is clear that both HBV and HCV replicate and spread throughout the liver noncytopathically, and that early innate defense mechanisms do not significantly contribute to the control of viremia or to the pathogenesis of liver disease.

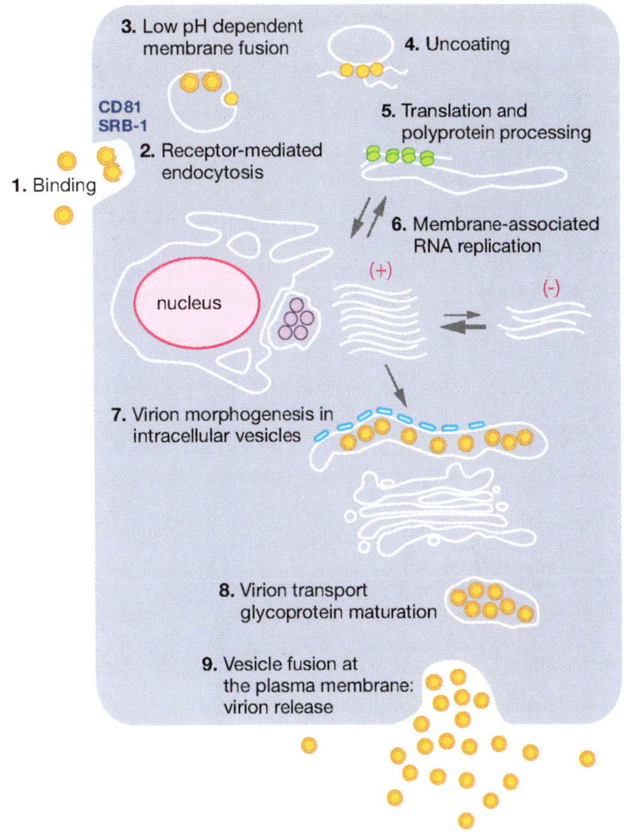

Figure 2

Hepatitis C virus (HCV) life cycle. Like hepatitis B virus (HBV), entry of the HCV virion from the extracellular space into susceptible cells is a poorly defined process that is presumably receptor-mediated and possibly involves CD81 and SRB-1. Similar to other flaviviruses, it is thought that following receptor binding (1) and receptor-mediated endocytosis (2), HCV is released into the cytoplasm (3) where uncoating of the virion can occur (4). This is followed by internal ribosomal entry site (IRES)-mediated translation and polyprotein processing (5), and RNA replication in a specific membrane alteration, the membranous web (6). Packaging and assembly of new virions occurs within intracellular vesicles (7), where maturation (8) precedes vesicle fusion at the plasma membrane and virion release (9).

Is Hepatitis B Virus or Hepatitis C Virus Directly Cytopathic for the Hepatocyte?

One mechanism whereby infected cells can limit the initial viral spread is the induction of apoptosis. The evidence that HBV or HCV can induce apoptosis is contradictory, as both pro- and antiapoptotic effects have been detected in cultured cells and transgenic mouse models expressing different viral products (74, 75). Importantly, however, during the early phase of HBV and HCV infection in chimpanzees (i.e., before virus-specific T cells enter the liver) there is no histological or biochemical evidence of hepatocyte damage (8, 76–80). Furthermore, when cellular immune responses are deficient or pharmacologically suppressed, HBV and HCV can replicate at high levels in the liver of patients [and, in the case of HBV, in transgenic mice as well (36)] in the absence of detectable pathological

IFN: interferon

NK: natural killer

NKT cells: natural killer T cells

consequences (1–5). Collectively, these results indicate that HBV and HCV replicate noncytopathically within the primary hepatocyte in vivo and they suggest that hepatocyte damage during viral hepatitis is an immune-mediated event.

Viral hepatitis: necroinflammatory liver disease commonly caused in humans by one or more of the hepatotropic viruses

Hepatocytes Differentially Sense Hepatitis B and Hepatitis C Viral Infections

Virus replication often results in the rapid induction of IFN-α/β by the infected cell (70). Production of IFN-α/β activates a variety of intracellular antiviral mechanisms that have the potential to minimize pathogenetic processes by limiting viral production and spread (70).

Global gene expression profiling performed on liver RNA obtained at multiple time points after HCV infection in chimpanzees indicates that the expression of many genes known to be stimulated by IFN-α/β is significantly induced as HCV spreads asymptomatically throughout the liver and virus titers increase in the circulation (81–83). This induction is presumably due to the fact that HCV replicates via dsRNA intermediates in the cytoplasm, where it can readily activate the cellular dsRNA-sensing apparatus and initiate the signaling cascade (53). Remarkably, however, HCV manages to replicate within the liver despite induction of these genes, possibly because structural (e.g., E2) and nonstructural proteins of HCV (e.g., NS3 and NS5A) have the potential (at least in vitro) to block IFN-α/β induction and counteract antiviral mechanisms downstream of IFN-α/β-stimulated transcription (84–90), as we discuss later in this review.

In contrast, similar analyses in chimpanzees revealed that HBV acts like a stealth virus early after infection, remaining undetected until the onset of the adaptive immune response several weeks later (91). The relative invisibility of HBV to the innate sensing machinery of the cells likely reflects its replication strategy, which retains the transcriptional template in the nucleus, involves the production of capped and polyadenylated viral mRNAs that resemble the structure of normal cellular transcripts, and sequesters its replicating genome within viral capsid particles in the cytoplasm (5, 9, 52). Thus, whereas spreading of HBV within the liver may be facilitated by the lack of IFN-α/β induction, HCV may achieve similar results by actively counteracting the IFN-α/β response it induces (see below).

Natural Killer Cell and Natural Killer T Cell Responses to Hepatitis B and Hepatitis C Viruses

Although NK and NKT cells have been implicated in the pathogenesis of cytopathic hepatotropic viral infections like murine cytomegalovirus (MCMV) in mice (71), there is little or no evidence that these cells play a pathogenetic role during the early phase of HBV or HCV infection. Indeed, as activated NK cells and NKT cells are a rich source of IFN-γ (71) and as IFN-γ-inducible genes are not detected in the liver of chimpanzees when HBV or HCV initially spreads throughout the liver (76, 77, 81–83, 91), it is reasonable to assume that these cells are not routinely activated early in infection. The observations that (*a*) the interaction of the E2 protein of HCV with CD81 on NK cells inhibits their activation (90) and (*b*) NK cell functions can be deficient in individuals infected with HCV (92) suggest that HCV may directly contribute to evasion of the NK cell response (see below).

It is also unlikely that cells of the innate immune system contribute to the pathogenesis of viral hepatitis during the symptomatic phase of acute or chronic HBV and HCV infections because $CD8^+$ T cell depletion prevents or delays the onset of liver injury and viral clearance in chimpanzees acutely infected by HBV (77) or HCV (93). It is, therefore, assumed from these, and other observations that we describe below, that the adaptive immune response plays a crucial role in the pathogenesis of HBV and HCV infection.

THE ADAPTIVE IMMUNE RESPONSE TO HEPATITIS B AND C VIRUSES AND ITS CONTRIBUTION TO LIVER DISEASE

Virus-specific $CD8^+$ cytotoxic T lymphocytes (CTLs) and $CD4^+$ T-helper cells play key effector and regulatory roles, respectively, in antiviral immunity. Like innate immune cells described above, these T cells participate in viral pathogenesis either directly (by killing infected cells) or indirectly (by producing soluble factors such as cytokines and chemokines) that contribute to the inflammatory process and/or inhibit viral replication (1, 94). Because they can promote the priming, expansion, function and trafficking of cellular immune responses, T cell–derived cytokines and chemokines contribute to immunopathology (1, 94, 95). Conversely, T cell–derived antiviral cytokines can also inhibit viral replication and viral antigen expression noncytopathically, and possibly even purge viruses from viable infected cells (94). The latter effects are likely to contain tissue damage by diminishing the number of infected cells that must be killed to eradicate the infection and/or by reducing the production of antigen and, therefore, the visibility of the infected cell to the cellular immune response. T cell–derived cytokines and chemokines also participate in the shaping of antiviral antibody responses that contribute to viral clearance mainly by blocking virus entry into susceptible cells and by removing infectious virions from the circulation. Neutralizing and non-neutralizing antibodies (Abs) can also promote antiviral and pathogenetic events by activating the complement system, which has the potential to lyse antibody-coated viruses or virus-infected cells (96–98).

The Role of Cytotoxic T Lymphocytes in Hepatitis B and C Viral Pathogenesis

Cytotoxic T lymphocytes (CTLs): components of the adaptive immune response that can recognize virus-infected cells and function in antiviral immunity

Efficient antiviral CTL responses are thought to be primed by viral antigens processed by dendritic cells and other professional antigen processing cells (APCs) in lymphoid organs (99, 100). In contrast, if T cell priming occurs within the liver, the priming is more likely to induce T cell inactivation, tolerance or apoptosis (101, 102). Although $CD4^+$ T-helper cells are normally primed by APCs that have internalized soluble viral antigens produced by other cells, priming of CTLs usually requires the processing of viral proteins that are either endogenously produced within or phagocytosed by professional APCs (99, 100). For viruses like HBV or HCV that do not appreciably infect professional APCs, tissue-derived dendritic cells that have processed apoptotic virus-infected cells and debris are likely to migrate to the regional lymph nodes to allow CTL priming to occur (99, 100). Primed CTLs clonally expand, leave the lymph nodes, migrate to the infected tissue, recognize viral antigen, and perform their effector functions. Whereas virus-specific CTLs in most virus infections can be detected in the infected tissue as early as five to seven days after exposure (103), the initial influx of T cells into the liver of chimpanzees acutely infected with HBV or HCV does not occur until two to three months after infection, despite the fact that circulating virus-specific CTLs can be detected in the peripheral blood as early as two to three weeks post exposure (8, 77, 78). This observation could reflect the absence of processed viral antigen at the surface of infected hepatocytes during active viral replication, an event that may be facilitated by the fact that MHC class I expression is minimal in hepatocytes except in the context of an inflammatory response (104).

Several lines of evidence indicate that the CTL response plays a crucial effector role in the pathogenesis of liver disease during HBV

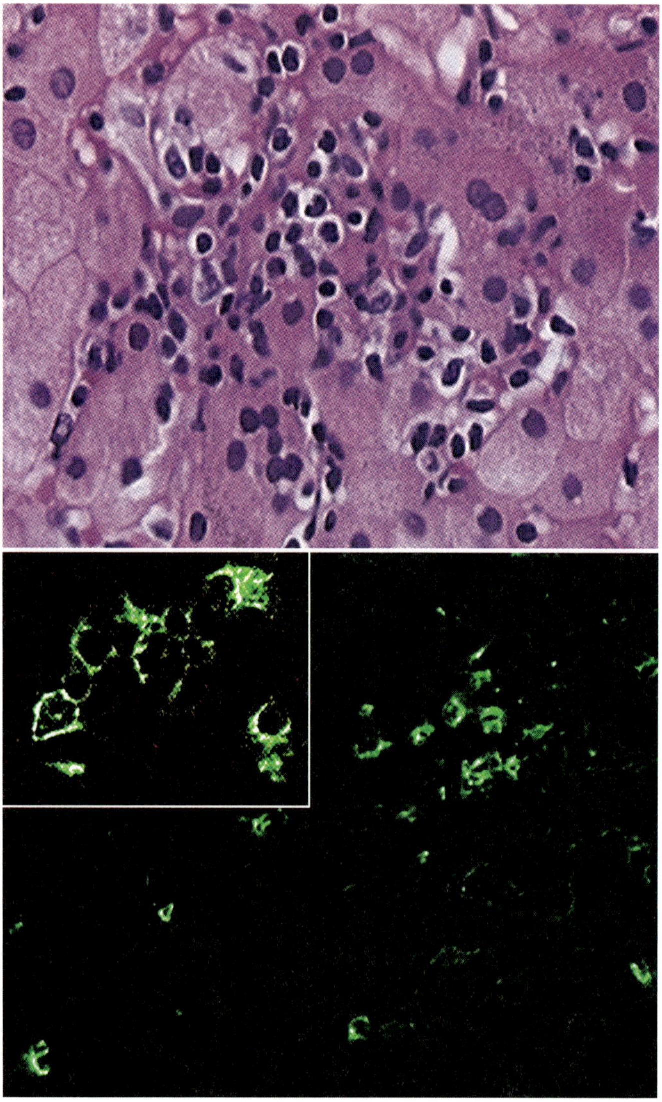

Figure 3

The onset of liver injury coincides with the entry of virus-specific CD8$^+$ T cells into the liver of chimpanzees infected by hepatitis C virus (HCV). By eights weeks after infection, lymphomononuclear necroinflammatory foci are detectable in the liver of an HCV-infected chimpanzee that subsequently cleared the infection (*top*; H&E stain, original magnification X 200). The same liver biopsy was also stained with an anti-human CD8 monoclonal antibody by indirect immunofluorescence (*bottom*). CD8$^+$ T cells were easily detectable within these foci (*inset*; original magnification X 400) and they were also diffusely detectable throughout the liver (original magnification X 200). Following isolation and in vitro expansion, this population of CD8$^+$ T cells was shown to contain HCV-specific cytotoxic T lymphocytes (78).

or HCV infection. First, the beginning of liver injury coincides with the entry of virus-specific CD8$^+$ T cells into the liver of chimpanzees infected by HBV or HCV (8, 76–78) (see also **Figure 3**), and depletion of these cells (but not of CD4$^+$ cells) at the peak of viremia delays the onset of biochemical, histological, and clinical evidence of hepatitis (8, 77). Second, the strong association between the magnitude of virus-specific CTL responses and liver disease severity has been shown not only in infected chimpanzees but also in many studies in patients acutely or chronically infected with HBV or HCV (1, 8). Indeed, patients with acute viral hepatitis who successfully clear HBV or HCV usually develop a relatively severe degree of hepatocyte damage that is associated with a relatively vigorous, multispecific, polyclonal CTL response to several HBV- or HCV-encoded antigens that is usually associated with (1, 8). In contrast, liver cell injury is more contained in chronically infected patients in whom the CTL response is extremely weak and narrowly focused (as always occurs during chronic HBV infection) or possibly unable to recognize infected hepatocytes owing to viral mutational escape (as occurs during chronic HCV infection) (1, 8). Third (see also below), adoptive transfer of HBV-specific CTL lines and clones into immunologically tolerant HBV transgenic mice produces liver disease with hepatocyte necrosis and inflammation that is histologically very similar to acute viral hepatitis in humans (105, 106).

All together, these results indicate that the CTL response is required to induce most (if not all) of the liver disease that is associated with viral hepatitis. Although hepatocellular injury is clearly initiated by the cytopathic activity of virus-specific CTLs, additional functions of these cells are likely at play during HBV and possibly HCV infection. On one side, activated CTLs produce cytokines (such as IFN-γ) that, via the chemokines (e.g., CXCL9 and CXCL10) they locally induce, recruit into the liver large numbers of antigen-nonspecific inflammatory cells that have the potential to amplify the liver damage initiated by the CTLs (107). On the other side and as we mention above, the same cytokines have the potential to induce noncytopathic antiviral mechanisms that contribute to viral clearance (94). Most of the evidence pertaining to these pathogenetic and antiviral mechanisms has been obtained in transgenic mice that replicate HBV at high levels in their liver (36) (see below). Although the absence of small-animal models that replicate HCV has hindered the analysis of HCV pathogenesis, for reasons that are apparent below it is likely that similar antiviral mechanisms are operative during HCV infection as well.

Mechanisms of Cytotoxic T Lymphocyte-Induced Liver Disease and Viral Clearance

As we mention above, passive transfer of virus-specific CTL lines and clones into HBV transgenic mice results in the development of a necroinflammatory liver disease that histologically resembles viral hepatitis in man (105–111). The first step in the disease process is antigen recognition by the CTLs, which rapidly induces hepatocellular apoptosis (105) (see also **Figure 4**, *left*). By transferring HBV-specific CTL clones that are genetically deficient in either FasL or Perforin into the same HBV transgenic mice, it has also

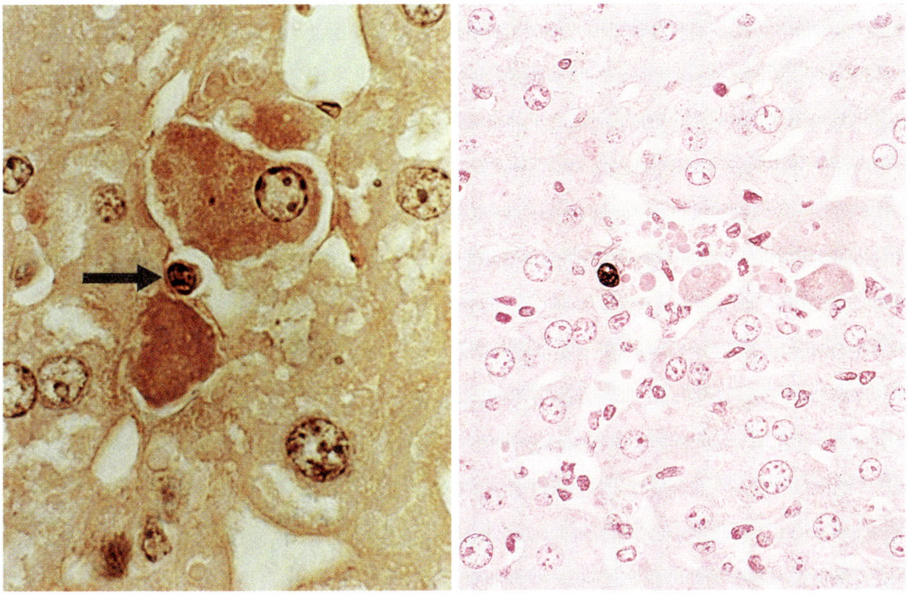

Figure 4

Sequential histopathological manifestations of liver disease after transfer of hepatitis B virus (HBV)-specific cytotoxic T lymphocyte (CTLs) into HBV-transgenic mice. Bromodeoxyuridine (BrdU)-labeled HBsAg-specific CTLs were injected into HBsAg-positive transgenic mice, and their livers were examined immunohistologically with anti-BrdU antibodies 4 h later (*left*). Note that the BrdU-positive CTL (*arrow*) is closely associated with apoptotic hepatocytes in which nuclear chromatin margination and cytoplasmic condensation are evident (indirect immunoperoxidase labeling for BrdU, lightly counterstained with H&E; original magnification X 600). By 24 h after CTL transfer, many host-derived (i.e., BrdU-negative) inflammatory cells are recruited into the liver, thereby contributing to the formation of necroinflammatory foci in which apoptotic hepatocytes and BrdU-labeled CTLs are outnumbered by host-derived mononuclear and polymorphonuclear inflammatory cells (*right*; indirect immunoperoxidase labeling for BrdU, lightly counterstained with H&E, original magnification X 600).

PMNs: polymorphonuclear cells

been shown that both the Perforin and Fas death pathways must be activated simultaneously for virus-specific CTLs to be cytopathic in the liver (109). CTL killing in vivo is an inefficient process that requires direct physical contact between the CTLs and the infected cells. Thus, it is not surprising that in this model the initial apoptotic process affects a small number of hepatocytes (105). As time progresses, however, many host-derived inflammatory cells are recruited into the liver, thereby contributing to the formation of necroinflammatory foci in which apoptotic hepatocytes and virus-specific CTLs are outnumbered by host-derived mononuclear and polymorphonuclear inflammatory cells (105, 107, 108) (see also **Figure 4**, *right*).

The leukocyte recruitment process is a chemokine-dependent event, as blocking the IFN-γ-inducible chemokines CXCL9 and CXCL10 reduces both the migration of antigen-nonspecific mononuclear cells into the liver and the severity of liver disease after CTL injection (107). Importantly, this effect occurs without affecting the migratory or antigen-recognition potential of the virus-specific CTLs (107). The association of reduced liver disease with reduced recruitment of antigen-nonspecific mononuclear cells implies that these cells can amplify the liver damage initiated by the CTLs. Furthermore, as most of the CTL-dependent antiviral activity depends on the IFN-γ that they locally produce after antigen recognition (see Reference 107 and also below), the notion that neutralization of CXCL9 and CXCL10 is associated with maintenance of antiviral effects but diminished tissue damage may have implications for the development of immunotherapeutic approaches for the treatment of chronic HBV infection.

Recent studies also showed that the severity of CTL-induced liver disease in this model is ameliorated by the depletion of Gr-1^+ cells [Gr-1 is an antigen highly expressed by polymorphonuclear neutrophils (PMNs)], which secondarily abolishes the intrahepatic recruitment of all antigen-nonspecific Gr-1^- mononuclear cells (i.e., NK and NKT cells, T and B lymphocytes, monocytes, macrophages, dendritic cells) despite the strong induction of chemokine gene expression (110). Those results suggest that CTL-induced functions in addition to chemokine expression are necessary for mononuclear cell recruitment to occur. These functions likely include the production of matrix metalloproteinases (MMPs) by PMNs (such as MMP-8 and MMP-9) because (*a*) these enzymes are rapidly activated in the liver after CTL transfer and (*b*) inhibition of these enzymes reduces the intrahepatic recruitment of antigen-nonspecific mononuclear cells and much of the attendant liver disease (111). These results are compatible with the observation that PMNs are the first cell type to be recruited into the liver following antigen recognition by the CTLs. According to this hypothesis, the production of MMPs by PMNs (and perhaps other cells) may cleave components of the extracellular matrix or perform yet undefined functions that facilitate the recruitment of mononuclear cells into the liver parenchyma in response to chemoattractants. A cartoon summarizing the results we describe above is provided in **Figure 5**.

Mechanisms related to those we describe above may contribute to the pathogenesis of viral hepatitis in man, where, as in the HBV transgenic mice, the number of HBV or HCV-specific CTLs detected in the liver is outnumbered by recruited, virus-nonspecific T cells (112, 113) and other inflammatory cells (114). Furthermore, the IFN-γ-dependent secondary processes that lead to the intrahepatic recruitment of inflammatory cells during natural infection are likely to be quite similar to those observed in the HBV transgenic mice, regardless of the nature of the cell type that originally produces this cytokine or the virus that infects the liver. Accordingly, it is noteworthy that intrahepatic expression of CXCL9 and CXCL10 is induced during chronic HCV infection in humans and that this is associated

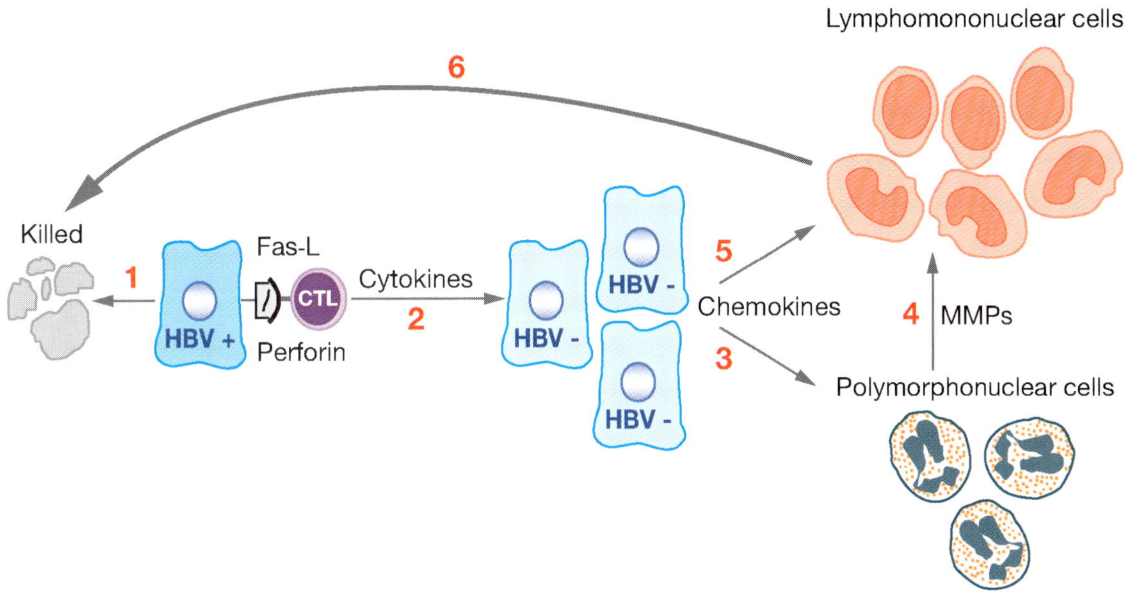

Figure 5

Mechanisms of cytotoxic T-lymphocyte (CTL)-induced liver disease and viral clearance. After antigen recognition, hepatitis B virus (HBV)-specific CTLs kill a small number of hepatocytes (1) via Fas L– and Perforin-mediated pathways and produce antiviral cytokines (2) that inhibit HBV replication noncytopathically in a greater number of cells. The same cytokines can activate parenchymal and nonparenchymal cells of the liver to produce chemokines (3) that recruit antigen-nonspecific polymorphonuclear cells (e.g., neutrophils) into the organ. Production of matrix metalloproteinases by these cells (4) in addition to chemokine induction (5) may contribute to the migration of antigen-nonspecific lymphomononuclear cells (e.g., natural killer cells, T cells, and macrophages) into the liver and the amplification of the liver disease initiated by the CTL (6). MMPs, matrix metalloproteinases.

with increased numbers of liver-infiltrating inflammatory cells and enhanced liver disease (115, 116).

The pathogenetic mechanisms whereby antigen-nonspecific inflammatory cells induce liver damage are not well understood and may involve the local production of proinflammatory and cytotoxic mediators (including TNF-α, proteases such as Perforin, hydrogen peroxide, superoxide anion, and nitric oxide). Furthermore, some of these cell subtypes (in particular NK cells, NKT cells, and T-helper cells), as well as platelets, express Fas-L (117–119), a glycoprotein known to induce apoptosis in Fas-positive cells such as hepatocytes (120).

New studies in our laboratory also demonstrate that platelets play a previously unrecognized role in the pathogenesis of CTL-induced liver disease (236). These studies show that platelets are detectable within intrahepatic necroinflammatory foci following transfer of virus-specific CTLs into HBV transgenic mice or following infection of normal inbred mice with replication-deficient adenoviruses. Selective platelet depletion significantly reduces the intrahepatic accumulation of virus-specific CTLs and the resulting liver damage without impairing CTL effector functions. Furthermore, transfusion of platelets into thrombocytopenic animals restores CTL homing and liver disease severity, but not when platelet activation is inhibited in vivo. Accordingly, platelet activation is required to promote CTL/platelet interactions under flow conditions in vitro. On the basis of these results, one can envision that an initial immune-induced inflammatory response results in changes of the vessel wall that promotes platelet activation, which in turn favors the local accumulation of virus-specific CTLs through specific interactions with activated platelets.

Importantly, the IFN-γ produced by activated CTLs following antigen recognition is also responsible for most of the antiviral potential of the CTLs (94, 106, 121). Indeed, in the HBV transgenic mouse model, IFN-γ prevents the assembly of replication-competent HBV RNA-containing capsids in the hepatocyte (122) in a proteasome- (123) and kinase-dependent (124) manner. During this remarkable process, the viral nucleocapsids disappear from the cytoplasm of the hepatocytes (106, 122), and the viral RNAs are destabilized by a SSB/La-dependent mechanism in the nucleus (125–128), whereas the hepatocytes remain perfectly healthy (106, 125, 129).

This notion that IFN-γ produced by activated CTLs can play a direct role in viral clearance was corroborated by studies in chimpanzees acutely infected with HBV (76, 77). It was shown in these animals that most of the viral DNA disappeared from the liver before the peak of liver disease and concomitant with the initial intrahepatic appearance of IFN-γ (76, 77). Moreover, neither intrahepatic IFN-γ induction nor viral clearance occurred in HBV-infected chimpanzees that were depleted of CTLs at the peak of infection (77). Similarly, CTL-mediated destruction of infected cells is probably not the only way to eliminate HCV as well because (*a*) viral clearance in chimpanzees can occur in the absence of liver disease as long as antiviral CTLs are present and produce IFN-γ (130) and (*b*) IFN-γ has been shown to inhibit replication of HCV replicons in vitro (15, 131–133).

The Role of T-Helper Cells in Hepatitis B and C Virus Pathogenesis

On the basis of their central role as regulators of the immune response in other viral infections (134), it is likely that $CD4^+$ T-helper cells contribute to the control of HBV or HCV infection mainly by facilitating the induction and maintenance of virus-specific $CD8^+$ T cells. In keeping with this, relatively vigorous HBV- or HCV-specific $CD4^+$ T cell responses are always associated with quantitatively and qualitatively significant $CD8^+$ T cell responses in humans and chimpanzees that resolve HBV or HCV infection (1, 8). Although it is thought that most patients who become chronically infected by HBV probably never mount significant $CD4^+$ and $CD8^+$ T cell responses (1), this hypothesis is not certain because of (*a*) the relative rarity of chronic progression in acutely infected adults, and (*b*) the difficulty of identifying acutely infected patients for analysis before they become symptomatic. In contrast, recent observations indicate that virus-specific cellular immune responses can occur during the acute phase of HCV infection in patients or chimpanzees that ultimately become persistently infected (8, 93, 135). Although associated with temporary control of viremia, these $CD4^+$ and $CD8^+$ T cell responses are usually transient in nature (8, 93, 135), functionally defective (8, 93, 135), and associated with virus escape mutations in MHC class I epitopes (8, 93, 135). These results suggest that, when it occurs, the initial priming and expansion of HCV-specific $CD4^+$ and $CD8^+$ T cells does not automatically guarantee clearance of HCV infection. Rather, permanent HCV control appears to require functional $CD4^+$ and $CD8^+$ T cell responses that are sustained over relatively long periods of time (8, 93, 135).

Despite the fact that T-helper cells have been shown to have cytolytic activity in vitro, the role of this process in the pathogenesis of viral hepatitis is entirely unclear. However, recent observations in an acutely HBV-infected chimpanzee that was depleted of $CD4^+$ T cells at the peak of infection fail to support this notion because the liver disease was comparable in this animal and immunologically unmanipulated controls (77).

Collectively, these results indicate that virus-specific $CD4^+$ T helper cells are not likely to directly mediate liver disease during HBV or HCV infection; rather they probably play a crucial immunoregulatory role in viral hepatitis, particularly at the level of CTL induction and/or the establishment or maintenance of a memory cell pool. Recent work in HCV-infected chimpanzees depleted of $CD4^+$ or memory $CD8^+$ T cells corroborated the notions that (*a*) virus-specific CTLs are required to control the virus and (*b*) they depend on $CD4^+$ T cell help (8, 93, 135).

The Role of Antibodies in Hepatitis B and C Virus Pathogenesis

As we mention above, neutralizing antibodies (Abs) can block viral entry into susceptible cells (98). The role of neutralizing Abs in the resolution or prevention of HBV or HCV infection is poorly understood. Evidence that Abs with neutralizing activity emerge following a self-limited HBV infection is supported by the observation that chimpanzees that resolved a previous infection are completely protected from rechallenge (136). Like other infections with noncytopathic viruses such as lymphocytic choriomeningitis virus (LCMV) (137), the appearance of neutralizing Abs is thought to occur relatively late after HBV exposure and, thus, it is unlikely to play a role in the early phase of viral clearance during acute infection (1). The evidence that neutralizing Abs can control long-term noncytopathic infections that are not completely cleared [e.g., LCMV (138)] coupled with the observation that complete viral clearance (viral sterilization) following clinical recovery from HBV infection may never occur (139, 140) suggest that a sustained neutralizing Ab response may prevent the reemergence of HBV in patents that resolved the infection.

Recent work, using infectious pseudotyped viruses bearing HCV envelope glycoproteins, indicates that most patients acutely infected with HCV do not develop neutralizing Abs and, when they do appear, they do not correlate with viral clearance (141), similar to HBV infection. In contrast, using the pseudotyped virus neutralization assay, neutralizing Abs to HCV can be detected in most chronically HCV-infected patients (141, 142). Although this is consistent with the fact that passive transfer of serum from chronically HCV-infected patients can protect chimpanzees challenged with the same virus (143), it also indicates that the antibodies are ineffective at terminating an ongoing infection, presumably because the viruses that originally elicited the antibodies have been counterselected, and the antibodies are not neutralizing for the concurrent quasispecies. Thus, in contrast to chronic HBV infection, neutralizing Abs are present in patients who are chronically infected with HCV, presumably reflecting sensitization to viruses that were counterselected and no longer present.

Neutralizing and nonneutralizing antiviral Abs can also accelerate the removal of virions from the circulation by the interaction of the Fc portion of virus-bound antibodies with Fc receptors present on the surface of phagocytic cells (96, 97). Through the same Fc-dependent interactions, antiviral Abs may facilitate virus-uptake by professional APCs in secondary lymphoid organs and therefore enhance the presentation of viral antigens to T and B cells (144). Finally, antiviral Abs can promote complement activation and induce complement-dependent lytic activities against viruses or virus-infected cells (96, 97). Although complement activation enhances the neutralization function of HCV-specific Abs against pseudotyped viruses in vitro (145), direct experimental evidence that any of these Ab-mediated functions occurs during natural HBV or HCV infection is lacking.

As we describe below in greater depth, in addition to liver injury, HBV and HCV infections are associated with a variety of extrahepatic diseases that can cause a significant increase in morbidity and even mortality (146–149). Deposition of circulating immune complexes (containing mostly IgM, IgG, and HBsAg) is believed to play a pathogenetic role in the development of manifestations such as skin rash, arthritis, arthralgia, glomerulonephritis, polyarteritis nodosa, and papular acrodermatitis that can occur during acute and, especially, chronic HBV infection (147, 148). Similarly, immune complexes have been linked to cryoglobulinemia, glomerulonephritis, porphyria cutanea tarda, and necrotizing cutaneous vasculitis during chronic HCV infection (146, 149).

EVASION OF THE INNATE AND ADAPTIVE IMMUNE RESPONSE

On the basis of the studies summarized above, it is clear that the immune response to HBV or HCV plays a crucial role in viral clearance and liver disease. It is therefore reasonable to assume that viral persistence following these infections requires that innate and/or adaptive immune responses must be either not induced or deficient, or, if present, they must be overwhelmed, counteracted or evaded.

Virus Factors Affecting Innate Immune Responses

As we describe above, because the initial spread of HCV throughout the liver occurs despite the transcriptional activation of both a large number of IFN-inducible genes [including some with known antiviral activity such as 2′5′-oligoadenylate synthetase and MxA (81–83)] and the downstream genes that they themselves induce (81–83), the evidence suggests that HCV-infected hepatocytes readily sense and respond to the infection, but that this response fails to control viral replication. The apparent resistance of HCV to these early innate defense mechanisms has been ascribed to the capacity of the HCV NS3/4A protease to block signaling from toll-like receptor-3 (TLR-3) and a recently discovered dsRNA-binding protein (RIG-I) that triggers IRF-3 activation and IFN-β gene expression (237–240).

In addition, several structural and nonstructural proteins of HCV inhibit nonoverlapping functions of the innate immune response. For example, the E2 and NS5A proteins of HCV have been shown to bind to the kinase domain of dsRNA-dependent protein kinase (PKR) and inhibit interferon regulatory factor (IRF)-1 phosphorylation (84–86). In addition, NS3 has been shown to prevent the phosphorylation, dimerization, nuclear translocation and, therefore, the transactivating function of IRF-3 (87). Although activated IRF-1 and IRF-3 are both known to induce IFN-β gene expression and stimulate expression of genes downstream of IFN-β (150, 151), in view of the ability of E2, NS3, and NS5A to inhibit the activation of IFN-regulated genes one would not expect IFN-regulated genes to be strongly induced in the liver during HCV infection. Nonetheless, genomic analysis of the liver of many HCV-infected chimpanzees has shown a strong correlation between the level of HCV viremia and the intrahepatic expression of a large number of IFN-regulated genes (81–83). Thus, despite its ability to block IFN induction in vitro, HCV strongly induces these antiviral genes in vivo but appears to be resistant to their effects. Although more studies are needed to understand the basis for these apparently contradictory observations, at present we favor the notion that HCV circumvents the IFN signaling cascade by inducing it in either uninfected liver cells or infected cells, but inhibiting the antiviral effector functions of IFN-induced genes downstream of IFN induction. In keeping with this hypothesis, previous reports showed that IFN-α/β induction by Newcastle disease virus (NDV) is completely normal in IRF-1 deficient cells (152, 153). These results indicate that IRF-1 does not mediate the induction of IFN-α/β by viral infection, and they support the notion that, if IRF-1 blockade occurs at all in HCV-infected cells, the effect is likely to be at the target gene level rather than at the level of IFN induction. Furthermore, reports that NDV-induced IFN-α/β mRNA expression is profoundly reduced in IRF-3-deficient cells (154) suggest that IRF-3 is required for IFN induction following viral infection. However, as IFN induced genes are strongly upregulated during HCV infection, the negative impact of NS3 on IRF-3 activation in the liver would appear to be minimal. In summary, much more work must be done before we understand the mechanisms that make it possible for HCV to flourish in the face of active IFN induction in the infected liver. Indeed, the roles of IRF-1 and IRF-3 in this process, if any, remain to be determined.

In contrast to the strong induction of IFN-regulated genes during HCV infection, as we discuss above, early innate defense mechanisms are not induced in the liver during HBV infection (91). Although we do not know the reason for these surprising differences, we suspect that they are due to the different replication strategies of the two viruses as described above. Whatever the reason for these differences, the fact that HBV has not needed to develop evasion or subversion strategies to escape the innate immune response may explain why it is so readily controlled when confronted by the cellular and molecular machinery of the adaptive immune response, and, as we discuss in the next section, why it has evolved mechanisms apparently intended to blunt the induction and impact of that response.

Virus Factors Affecting Adaptive Immune Responses

The HBV precore protein (HBeAg) is a secreted, truncated form of the HBV core protein (HBcAg) that is not required for viral assembly, replication, or infection (155–158). Thanks to its capacity to cross the placenta and induce neonatal tolerance in HBV transgenic mice (159), it has been proposed that the precore protein may perform a similar function in humans and facilitate viral persistence following neonatal infection. Furthermore, the precore protein has been recently shown to inhibit induction of the T cell response to a cross-reactive epitope in HBcAg in adult T cell receptor transgenic mice. This inhibition of the immune response is mediated either by deletion or anergy of HBcAg/HBeAg cross-reactive T cells, depending on their functional avidity for the tolerogenic epitope (160). Thus, the HBV precore protein may contribute to the outcome and pathogenesis of HBV infection by inducing tolerance in HBcAg-specific T cells and reducing their potential to kill cells. In keeping with these observations, clinical evidence indicates that HBeAg-negative variants of HBV are often cleared following neonatal exposure and are usually associated with more severe and even fulminant course of hepatitis when they infect adults (5, 161). The observation that the hepatitis B surface antigen (HBsAg)-specific $CD8^+$ T cell response is blunted and exhibits altered HLA/peptide tetramer-binding properties in patients chronically infected with HBV with high serum-HBsAg titers (162) suggests that HBsAg may function as a high-dose tolerogen during HBV infection. Lastly, it has been shown that the HBV X protein can reduce cellular proteasome activity when it is overexpressed in vitro (163). If this also occurs during natural infection, the X protein may affect HBV pathogenesis by inhibiting antigen processing and presentation, thereby decreasing the visibility of infected hepatocytes to the immune system.

Finally, mutational inactivation of B cell and T cell epitopes facilitate viral persistence in both HBV and HCV infections, although the inactivation plays a more prominent role in HCV infection because of HCV's higher mutation rate (164–170). Although the most convincing evidence of mutational escape from the T cell response has been demonstrated in HCV-infected chimpanzees (169, 170), mutations involving epitope residues that abrogate (168), anergize (165, 171–173), or antagonize (165, 168, 174–176) recognition by the T cell receptor, binding to MHC (168), proteasome-dependent processing (177), and ATP-dependent transport (178) have also been reported in humans infected by HBV or HCV.

Host Factors Affecting Immune Responses

The observation that immune tolerance to HBV is likely responsible for viral persistence in most neonatal HBV infections, coupled with the fact that a vigorous, multispecific, and polyclonal cellular immune response is usually associated with the clearance of HBV and HCV in immunocompetent adults, suggests that host factors play a crucial role in the outcome of these infections (1, 179). This hypothesis is strongly supported by the de novo induction of expression of a large number of T cell, cytokine and cytokine-induced genes in the liver of chimpanzees during the clearance of HBV and HCV (77, 78, 136, 180). The key remaining question is why the T cell response is either quantitatively weak or qualitatively inadequate to terminate infection in adult-onset chronic HBV and HCV infections. The literature suggests that several nonexclusive mechanisms may be responsible. For example, viral persistence has been associated with primary failure to efficiently mount virus-specific CD4 and CD8 T cell responses in both HCV-infected chimpanzees and in a patient who was studied prospectively following accidental needlestick exposure to HCV (8, 78, 130). Failure to induce a cellular immune response could reflect virus-induced deficiencies in antigen presentation (reviewed in Reference 181), genetically determined restriction of the virus-specific T cell repertoire (reviewed in Reference 182) or antigen overload during immunological priming (reviewed in References 183 and 184). Alternatively, the induction of anergy and/or exhaustion of an initially vigorous T cell response as a result of antigen overload and excessive T cell stimulation, the induction of regulatory T cells, and, at least theoretically, the delivery of negative regulatory signals [e.g., via CTL antigen-4 (CTLA-4), B and T lymphocyte attenuator (BTLA), and programmed death 1 (PD1)] to activated T cells by infected hepatocytes could also play a role in the secondary T cell unresponsiveness that has been observed in patients chronically infected with HBV or HCV. In support of this, it has been shown recently that acute HCV infections that progress to chronicity are often characterized by relatively strong virus-specific $CD4^+$ and $CD8^+$ T cell responses that are not sustained over time (185, 186). Excessive antigen-driven T cell stimulation during persistent infection may also negatively influence the capacity of HCV-specific CTLs to produce antiviral cytokines, as has been suggested from a study where the production of IFN-γ by these cells was found to be compromised following in vitro exposure to antigen (130, 187). Finally, the observation that antiviral treatment in patients chronically infected with HBV can rescue virus-specific CTL responses that were not detectable before therapy (188) suggests that those CTL responses were present in these subjects but suppressed. All together, these results indicate that both primary and secondary immunological unresponsiveness to both viruses occur and, presumably, contribute to the establishment of persistent HBV and HCV infection.

THE RESPONSE OF THE LIVER TO IMMUNE-MEDIATED INJURY

The response of the liver to immune-mediated injury includes hepatocellular regeneration and the activation of reparative inflammatory/fibrogenic processes that resemble those of wound-healing (see below). Regenerative mechanisms may also play a direct antiviral role if HBV or HCV genomes do not survive cell division and the daughter cells are protected from reinfection. As HBV or HCV-infected hepatocytes are eliminated during self-limited infection, the secondary regenerative and reparative events also subside until viral clearance is achieved and full anatomical and functional integrity of the organ is restored. In contrast, the inefficient immune response to HBV and HCV in chronically infected patients sets up continuous cycles of low-level liver cell destruction that (over long periods of time) lead to fibrosis, cirrhosis, steatosis, and HCC. The pathogenesis of these secondary events involves virus- and/or host-dependent factors that perturb normal liver repair functions, lipid metabolism, and antiapoptotic and/or growth promoting activities, as we discuss below.

Liver Cell Regeneration

Although mature hepatocytes are terminally differentiated cells, they retain extraordinary regenerative capacity in response to liver injury or other non-inflammatory stimuli (e.g., partial hepatectomy) (189–192). When mature hepatocytes are destroyed by the immune response, other mature hepatocytes are rapidly triggered to divide. Therefore, this process does not appreciably rely on hepatic progenitor cells (oval cells) or more undifferentiated stem cells (189–192). Oval cells (and perhaps stem cells) divide and differentiate into hepatocytes only when the replication capacity of mature hepatocytes has diminished, as may occur during late stage cirrhosis (see References 193 and 194 and also below). Along these lines, oval cell proliferation has been observed in experimental models of hepatocarcinogenesis (195), although their role in HCC is still uncertain (see below). Given that proliferating mature hepatocytes can readily serve as tumor precursors (196) and oval cells do not appear to generate tumors directly (195), it is likely that, if these cells play a role in hepatocyte transformation, they do it indirectly through the generation of hepatocytes.

Studies by Taub (192), Fausto (190, 191), and others (197) have defined the role of many immediate-early gene products in the initial phase of hepatocyte regeneration after partial hepatectomy. Likely, similar factors contribute to the early liver response to immune-mediated injury. In particular, the entry of hepatocytes from a resting G_0-phase into the cell cycle is induced by various cytokines, growth factors and components of the complement system. Examples of these factors include IL-6, tumor necrosis factor (TNF)-α, transforming growth factor (TGF)-α, hepatocyte growth factor (HGF), epidermal growth factor (EGF), insulin, C3a, and C5a (189, 190, 192, 198, 199). These ligands can activate transcription factors including nuclear factor (NF)-κB, signal transducer and activator of transcription 3 (STAT3), activator protein 1 (AP-1), and CCAAT/enhancer-binding protein (C/EBP) that then initiate the cascade of gene expression ultimately responsible for proliferation (200). Furthermore, a number of antiproliferative genes are also induced during the early phase of liver regeneration (197), in keeping with the concept of an autonomous control of cell-cycle entry by the hepatocyte and suggesting that tight regulation of liver cell proliferation originates very early after a regenerative stimulus.

The extent of hepatocyte turnover during viral hepatitis can be substantial. Indeed, a recent study using integrated viral DNA as a genetic marker for infected cells suggested that 100% of the hepatocytes may divide at least once during the resolution of self-limited WHV infection (201). A large amount of liver cell turnover has also been recently detected by the same technique in chronically infected woodchucks (202), and it has been inferred from a previous study that six to twelve complete liver turnovers per year may occur in this model of chronic infection (203). Although the degree of hepatocyte turnover in acute and chronic HBV or HCV infection in humans cannot be precisely measured, it is likely to be directly proportional to the relative severity and duration of liver disease. The fact that mature mouse hepatocytes can replicate at least 70 times in serial transplantation experiments

ECM: extracellular matrix

(204) suggests that, in theory, mature human hepatocytes could cope easily with the recurrent regenerative stimuli that must occur during decades of chronic infection. If the relative regenerative capacity of hepatocytes diminishes over time (perhaps because of telomere shortening), this condition may facilitate the onset of cirrhosis (193, 194). It is important to note, however, that liver cell regeneration is likely to be directly linked to at least one possible mechanism of hepatocyte transformation. Indeed, liver cancer during HBV or HCV infection almost always occurs in the context of long-standing chronic hepatitis in which the coexistence of mitogenic (hepatocyte regeneration) and mutagenic (inflammation) events may favor random DNA damage that may lead to HCC. As we describe in greater details below, liver cancer can also be promoted by two additional mechanisms, both of which involve viral factors: insertional mutagenesis (for HBV) and expression of oncogenic viral proteins (for HBV and HCV) capable of deregulating liver cell growth or DNA repair.

Collectively, the results we summarize above suggest that liver cell regeneration during viral hepatitis contributes not only to the restoration of liver mass after the immune-mediated destruction of hepatocytes, but also to the long-term complications (cirrhosis and HCC) of chronic infections.

Liver Repair in Response to Immune-Mediated Injury

As we briefly mention above, liver repair in response to immune-mediated injury involves the rapid activation of a complex network of inflammatory and fibrogenic processes that resemble those of wound-healing and contribute to maintenance of the structural integrity of the organ (191, 205). Various cell types participate in these reparative mechanisms: Some, such as hepatic stellate cells (HCS), myofibroblasts, fibroblasts and Kupffer cells, reside within the liver, whereas others, such as monocytes, NK cells and T cells, reach the liver from the circulation (191, 205). Liver repair is characterized by deposition of components (e.g., collagen, laminin, fibronectin, and proteoglycans) of the extracellular matrix (ECM) by activated stellate cells, myofibroblasts and fibroblasts (191, 205). Activation of these cells is thought to be regulated by inflammatory mediators including cytokines (e.g., TGF-β, IL-6 and TNF-α), chemokines (e.g,. CCL21), growth factors [e.g., platelet-derived growth factor (PDGF) and insulin-like growth factor (IGF)-binding protein-1] and other stimuli (e.g., reactive oxygen intermediates, lipid peroxides and nitric oxide) that are produced by resident (e.g., fibroblasts and Kupffer cells) and non-resident (e.g., NK cells and T cells) liver cells (191, 205, 206). Although the regulation of this intricate pathway is beyond the scope of our review, it is important to emphasize that the initially beneficial reparative response can become deregulated, thereby facilitating excessive and qualitatively abnormal ECM deposition within the liver (205, 207). This deposition may occur during chronic HBV or HCV infection, when viral persistence and recurrent immune-mediated liver damage drive the pathogenesis of fibrosis and cirrhosis.

Liver Fibrosis and Cirrhosis

Liver fibrosis and cirrhosis are common consequences of chronic liver diseases of viral (e.g., HBV or HCV) and non-viral (e.g., ethanol, iron or copper accumulation, and biliary tract disorders) etiologies (205, 207). They are characterized by an imbalance between fibrogenesis and fibrolysis (205, 207), which results in the excessive intrahepatic deposition of matrix that is qualitatively different in its composition and organization from that of normal liver repair (205, 207). As a result of this process, a dense, reticulated ECM that is relatively resistant to enzymatic degradation is initially deposited around the portal areas of the liver (portal-based fibrosis) during chronic viral hepatitis. As a function of time, the fibrosis progressively expands into the lobules with the formation of septa that can eventually connect portal and central veins (portocentral bridging fibrosis) (205, 207). Liver cirrhosis represents the final phase of fibrosis in which fibrous septa surround nodules of regenerating hepatocytes causing profound architectural distortion of the liver, functional insufficiency, and diversion of venous blood containing intestinal toxins into the systemic circulation (205, 207). Liver fibrosis and cirrhosis are also responsible for the formation of a basal membrane separating hepatocytes from sinusoidal blood (205, 207). This event (often described as capillarization of the hepatic sinusoids) is thought to alter the normal exchange of soluble factors between blood and hepatocytes (205, 207). The rate by which liver fibrosis and cirrhosis (and cancer, see below) progress during chronic HBV or HCV infection is positively influenced by the severity and duration of liver disease. Thus, it is not surprising that factors known to be associated with more severe liver damage (e.g., older age at onset of infection, male gender, alcohol intake, obesity, diabetes, and HIV coinfection) are also implicated in faster progression of these complications (205, 207).

On the basis of the results summarized above, it is clear that the pathogenesis of fibrosis and cirrhosis during chronic viral hepatitis is multifactorial, involving recurrent immune-mediated liver injury, sustained inflammation, and activation of ECM-producing cells.

Liver Cancer

As mentioned above, the pathogenetic mechanisms whereby HBV or HCV causes HCC involve both host and viral factors. As the interval between viral infection and HCC is typically several decades, these viruses are thought to be neither directly nor acutely oncogenic. Almost all cases of HCC take place after many years of chronic hepatitis (1, 208, 209). As described earlier, chronic hepatitis is characterized by sustained liver disease with associated hepatocellular regeneration (i.e., cellular DNA synthesis) and inflammation (i.e., the production of mutagens), which could precipitate random genetic and chromosomal damage and lead to the development of HCC. The pathogenetic relevance of immune-mediated hepatocyte damage in carcinogenesis during chronic HBV or HCV infection is reinforced by the fact that HCC in humans occurs in the context of necrosis, inflammation and regeneration in a variety of persistent liver diseases other than viral hepatitis, including primary biliary cirrhosis (210), glycogen storage disease (211), α1-antitrypsin deficiency (212), hemochromatosis (213), and alcoholism (214). Thus, it appears that chronic liver cell injury is a premalignant state that promotes cellular processes, like enhanced cellular DNA synthesis and production of inflammatory mutagens coupled with compromised cellular detoxification and repair functions, that could be oncogenic. Persistence of these events for a sufficiently long period of time may result in the multiple genetic and chromosomal alterations that are responsible for the development of HCC. In keeping with this hypothesis, HBV transgenic mice that do not spontaneously develop liver injury have been shown to develop HCC after many months of chronic hepatitis mediated by HBV-specific CTLs (215) (see also **Figure 6**). Importantly, the appearance of HCC in this setting occurs despite the absence of cofactors such as random viral integration, X gene expression or genotoxic agents that have been proposed to contribute to the development of HCC in humans (1, 208, 209).

Although the studies we describe suggest that persistent immune-mediated liver cell injury may be sufficient to trigger HCC, other viral factors may also contribute to hepatocarcinogenesis during chronic HBV or HCV infection. Indeed, HBV DNA integration has been reported to occur in the proximity of a variety of procarcinogenic genes

Liver cirrhosis: a chronic degenerative disease in which scar tissue replaces healthy parenchyma, resulting in impaired liver function

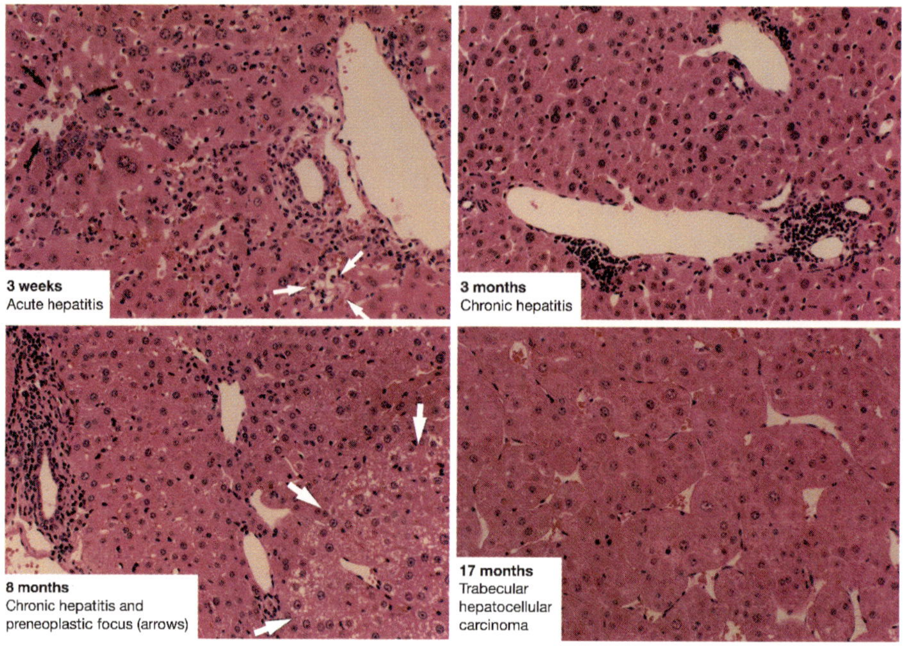

Figure 6

Histopathological features of prolonged chronic immune-mediated hepatitis in hepatits B virus (HBV) transgenic mice (adapted from Reference 215). Three weeks after adoptive transfer of HBV-immune spleen cells, HBV transgenic mice reconstituted with a syngeneic, nontransgenic immune system develop a chronic inflammatory liver disease characterized by a diffuse mononuclear and polymorphonuclear inflammatory infiltrate and focal hepatocellular necrosis and dropout (*arrows; upper left panel*). Three months later, the mice display multiple portal (and intralobular, not shown) inflammatory infiltrates indicative of chronic hepatitis (*upper right panel*). By eight months, the liver disease in these animals is more severe and preneoplastic foci [the edge of one of which is outlined (*arrowheads*)] are detected (*lower left panel*). Eventually, all animals sacrificed 17 months later display well-differentiated hepatocellular carcinoma characterized by trabecular cords composed of several layers of differentiated neoplastic hepatocytes (*lower right panel*). These hepatocytes contain typical abundant eosinophilic cytoplasm and prominent nucleoli and are covered by a thin endothelial lining (H&E stain, original magnification X 200).

(including oncogenes, growth factor receptor genes, and genes regulating telomerase activity or signal transduction pathways) and deregulate their expression. It must be noted, however, that HBV integration should not occur in resting hepatocytes and, therefore, if this process contributes to hepatocarcinogenesis, it is likely to be secondary to procarcinogenic events that trigger hepatocyte turnover (e.g., immune-mediated hepatitis). Moreover, the expression of HBV-derived polypeptides such as the X protein, a C-terminally truncated version of the M-HBs protein, and the full-length L-HBs protein has been linked to the process of malignant transformation of infected hepatocytes. These viral products may contribute to hepatocarcinogenesis by their capacity to activate a variety of cellular promoters (including AP-1 and NF-κB) and interact with several signal transduction pathways [including those related to Janus kinases 1 (Jak1), protein kinase C (PKC), phosphatidylinositol-3 (PI-3), and mitogen-activated protein

(MAP) kinases]. The HBV X protein has also been shown to interact and interfere with numerous transcription factors [including Ca(2+)/cAMP-response element binding protein (CREB), activating transcription factor 3 (ATF)], nuclear factor interleukin-6 (NFIL6), early growth response-1 (Egr1), Ets-1, octamer-binding protein (Oct1), and retinoid x receptor (RXR)], tumor suppressor genes (including p53), and proteins involved in DNA repair functions (including p53 and UVDDB1) (reviewed in Reference 208).

In contrast to HBV, HCV is an RNA virus that does not integrate into the host genome; yet HCV causes chronic hepatitis (i.e., inflammation, liver cell destruction and regeneration) and HCC. It is noteworthy that several proteins encoded by the HCV genome (e.g., the core protein, NS3, and NS5A) have been reported to regulate cell proliferation and viability. The HCV core protein has been shown to activate several major cellular transduction pathways [including those involving extracellular signal-regulated kinases (ERK)/JNK/MAP kinases, NF-κB and STAT-1] to bind proteins involved in cell growth and survival [including tumor necrosis factor-alpha receptor (TNF-αR), lymphotoxin-beta receptor (LT-βR), retinoid X receptor-alpha (RXR-α), and apolipoprotein (apo) A2] and to affect apoptosis. Furthermore, transgenic mice expressing this protein develop HCC (31). NS3 and NS5A can induce a transformed phenotype in fibroblasts by regulating various pathways, including those that involve p53, p21, and Cdk1/2-cyclin complexes (reviewed in Reference 209).

It must be noted that most of the studies pertaining to the potential transforming capacity of HBV or HCV proteins have been done either with transformed cell lines or in transgenic mice that overexpress a specific viral product (reviewed in Reference 209). Although further studies need to be performed in order to understand the relevance of these observations in the context of chronic viral hepatitis and HCC development in humans, it is reasonable to assume that host and viral factors may indeed cooperate in hepatocarcinogenesis (see also **Figure 7**), thereby explaining why the incidence of HCC in chronic HBV or HCV infection is so high, and so much higher than that observed in chronic liver diseases other than viral hepatitis (1, 208, 209).

Liver Steatosis

Liver steatosis is a metabolic disorder characterized by hepatocellular fat accumulation (216), and it is a common histopathological finding in chronic HCV (but not HBV) infection (217). As with HCC, both host and viral factors are thought to predispose and/or contribute to its development. In fact, steatosis in chronically infected patients has been associated with obesity and diabetes as well as with specific genotypes of HCV (217). It is also worth mentioning that recent studies in cell lines and transgenic mice have shown that the core and NS5 proteins of HCV can intracellularly colocalize with lipid droplets and interact with lipid-binding protein such as apoA1 and apoA2 (26, 33, 218, 219). It is believed that such interactions may induce varying degrees of lipid metabolism deregulation, thereby facilitating the occurrence of steatosis (220). Finally, it has also been suggested that the steatotic process may be facilitated by HCV core protein accumulation within mitochondria; this accumulation may subsequently induce oxidative stress and perturb lipid metabolism (30, 33).

EXTRAHEPATIC DISEASES ASSOCIATED WITH HBV OR HCV INFECTION

As we mention above, acute HBV and chronic HBV or HCV infection are also associated with extrahepatic manifestations that affect a variety of organs or tissues, including kidney, blood vessels, skin, and joints. It is

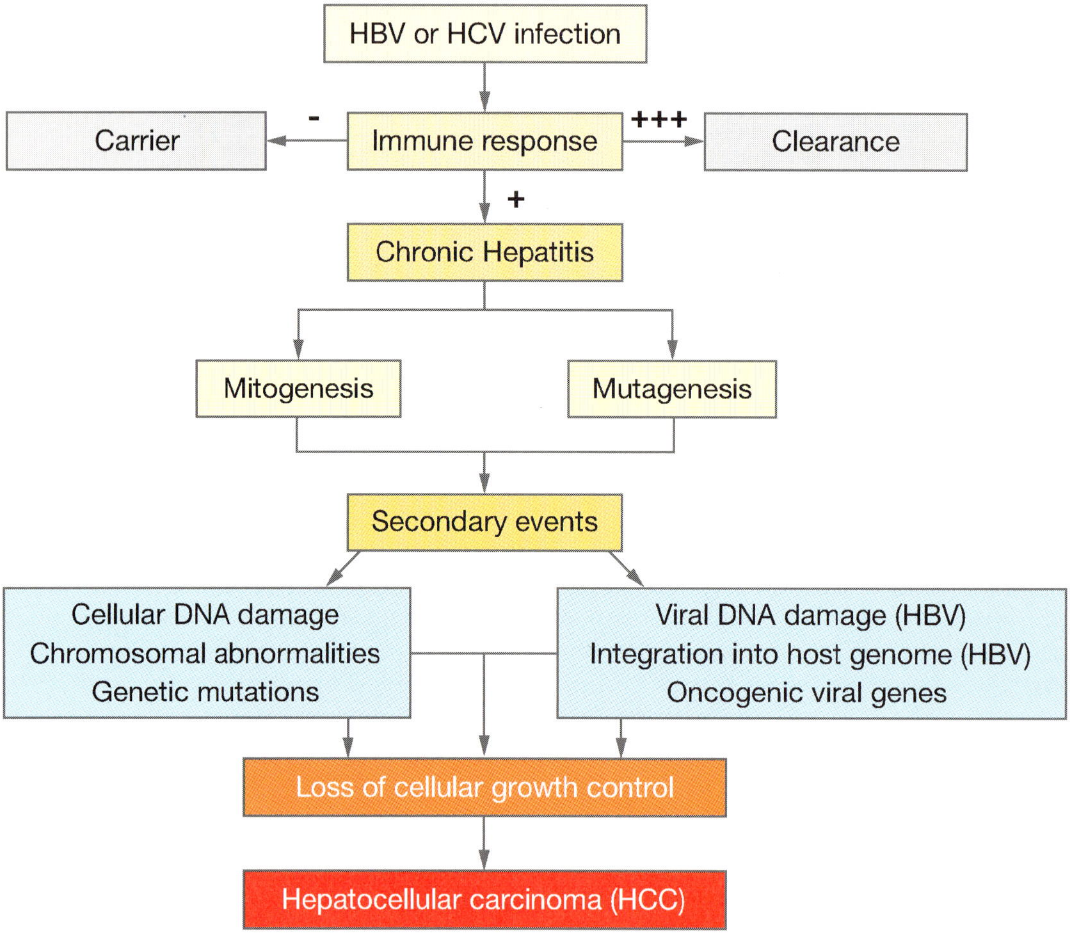

Figure 7

Hepatocarcinogenesis in viral hepatitis. Although a vigorous (+++) immune response to hepatitis B virus (HBV) or hepatitis C virus (HCV) may lead to viral clearance and an absent (–) immune response may lead to the healthy carrier state, an intermediate (+) immune response produces chronic hepatitis. This indolent necroinflammatory and potentially mutagenic liver disease is characterized by chronic liver cell necrosis that stimulates a sustained regenerative response. The collaboration of these mutagenic and mitogenic stimuli has the potential to cause cellular and viral DNA damage, chromosomal abnormalities and genetic mutations that deregulate cellular growth control in a multistep process that leads eventually to hepatocellular carcinoma (HCC).

generally assumed that the main pathogenetic mechanism behind most of these complications involves transient or persistent antigenic stimulation and tissue deposition of circulating antigen-antibody immune complexes. Although a detailed description of all extrahepatic diseases associated with HBV or HCV infection is beyond the scope of this review, a brief summary of some of the most common disorders is provided below.

Extrahepatic Manifestations of Acute Viral Hepatitis

Although acute HCV infection is usually asymptomatic, acute HBV infection is often associated with prodrome of extrahepatic manifestations that are secondary to tissue deposition of immune complexes and resemble serum sickness (reviewed in References 147, 148, and 221). The symptoms may include urticaria, maculopapular rash, and purpura as well as mild, localized or generalized arthritis, frequently involving the small joints of the hands. Skin and joint symptoms usually precede the onset of hepatitis and tend to disappear by the time the patients becomes jaundiced (147, 148, 221). Another fairly common extrahepatic manifestation of acute HBV infection is polyarteritis nodosa (PAN), which also occurs (albeit less frequently) during chronic HBV or HCV infection (147, 148, 221). PAN is a systemic inflammatory disease characterized by vasculitis of small- and medium-sized small arteries caused by immune-complex deposition. PAN can manifest itself as arthritis, glomerulonephritis, neuritis, and skin rashes. The symptoms may include hypertension, renal insufficiency, peripheral neuropathy, myopathy, joint pains, and ischemic myalgias (147, 148, 221). Even though multisystem involvement is typical of PAN, occasionally only one organ or system may be involved (147, 148, 221).

Renal Diseases in Chronic Viral Hepatitis

Epidemiological, clinical and immunological observations indicate that various forms of immune-complex glomerulonephritis are common extrahepatic complications of persistent HBV and HCV infection (reviewed in References 221 and 222). The nature of the viral antigens implicated in these diseases may vary according to the histopathological lesions. For example, HBV-induced membranous nephropathy is mainly characterized by deposits consisting of HBeAg and IgG, although HBsAg and the HCV core protein as well as IgG and C3 are the most abundant components of the immune complexes observed in HBV- or HCV-induced membranoproliferative glomerulonephritis, respectively (221, 222).

Mixed Cryoglobulinemia and B Cell Non-Hodgkins Lymphoma in Chronic Viral Hepatitis

Mixed cryoglobulinemia (MC) is a benign B cell proliferative disorder characterized by polyclonal B cell activation and antibody production that can lead to local or systemic vasculitis secondary to the deposition of circulating immune complexes in small vessels (146). MC is the most common extrahepatic manifestation associated with chronic HCV infection (146, 149, 222) and has also been described in patients chronically infected with HBV (221). MC can be either asymptomatic or evident as relatively mild cutaneous vasculitis or severe vasculitis involving the kidneys and central nervous system. The MC deposits often consist of IgM rheumatoid factors (RF), complement components, polyclonal IgG anti-HCV or anti-HBV antibodies and HCV- or HBV-related antigens and viral nucleic acids (146, 149, 221, 222). Importantly, there is an unusually high prevalence of B cell non-Hodgkin's lymphoma (NHL) in patients chronically infected with HCV, and recent studies demonstrating lymphoma regression following successful antiviral therapy and clearance of HCV support a causative role for HCV in this malignant B cell proliferative disorder (223). The causative mechanism(s) are not well-defined, although persistent antigenic stimulation and polyclonal B cell activation by circulating viral proteins are likely candidates. In keeping with this, binding of the HCV E2 glycoprotein to CD81 on B cells has been shown to induce proliferation and activation of these cells in vitro (224), and low level HCV replication has been reported in primary or transformed B cell lines (including some obtained from HCV-infected NHL) (225). Further studies aimed at understanding how HCV promotes B cell proliferative disorders are certainly warranted.

Porphyria Cutanea Tarda and Lichen Planus in Chronic Viral Hepatitis

Porphyria cutanea tarda (PCT) is an interesting dermatological complication of chronic HBV and HCV infections (146, 149, 221, 222). PCT belongs to a group of disorders (porphyrias) of the heme biosynthesis pathway resulting from decreased activity of uroporphyrinogen decarboxylase (UROD) in the liver. PCT can be either inherited or acquired, and it has been proposed that, in addition to hepatic iron overload, HBV and HCV may be additional factors contributing to PCT disease progression (226). Lichen planus (LP) is a chronic inflammatory disease that affects skin and mucous membranes of squamous cell origin. Various reports suggest that HCV infection is relatively common in patients with LP and that HCV may cause LP, especially the oral form of the disease. A constant feature of LP patients with chronic HCV infection is the presence of polyclonal hypergammaglobulinemia, and immune complexes have been implicated in the pathogenesis of HCV-related LP (227). In addition, evidence for HCV infection of LP lesions (227) and secondary infiltration of virus-specific T cells (228) has been recently provided, suggesting that T cell-mediated immunopathology may also participate in this disorder.

Sjögren's Syndrome and Other Diseases in Chronic Hepatitis C Viral Infection

Sjögren's syndrome (SS) is an autoimmune disease that primarily affects salivary and lachrymal glands and is associated with chronic HCV but not HBV infection (146, 149, 222). Indeed, histological changes typical of SS have been detected in the salivary glands of patients chronically infected with HCV (229). Like LP, it has been proposed that the pathogenesis of SS may involve both tissue deposition of immune complexes as well as T cell-mediated immunopathology (146, 149, 222). In keeping with this, HCV replication has been detected in epithelial cells from salivary glands of patients with SS (230), and a lymphocytic exocrinopathy resembling SS has been described in the salivary and lacrymal glands of transgenic mice that express HCV E1 and E2 (24). Finally, HCV has also been linked to additional diseases such as type II diabetes and autoimmune thyroiditis, although these associations remain a matter of controversy (229). The interesting observation that HCV core transgenic mice are insulin resistant (231) suggests that HCV may contribute to the development of type II diabetes in humans.

CONCLUSION

Thanks to technological advances and model systems that have made it possible to study many of the host-virus interactions that influence these infections, our understanding of the immunobiology and pathogenesis of HBV and HCV infections has greatly improved in recent years. The basic principles of HBV and HCV replication and gene expression have been uncovered, infectious viral genomes have been cloned and sequenced, and all viral gene products have been essentially characterized (9, 232); a variety of animal models have been developed for HBV (233–235), and several cell-culture-adapted HCV replicons have been established (21) that now make it possible to dissect the mysteries of HCV replication and to test the antiviral activity of cellular gene products and candidate drugs.

It is quite clear that both viruses replicate noncytopathically in the hepatocyte, and that most of the clinical syndromes associated with these infections reflect the immune response. It is also apparent that the innate immune response does not contribute significantly to the pathogenesis of liver disease or viral clearance in either infection, whereas the adaptive immune response, especially the virus-specific CTL response, contributes to both. Recent observations reveal, however, that antigen-nonspecific inflammatory cells can enhance

CTL-induced immunopathology in the liver, and that platelets facilitate the intrahepatic accumulation of CTLs. These observations suggest that the host response to these infections is a highly complex but coordinated process. On the basis of these results, it is evident that CTL effector functions play a prominent role in the resolution of HBV and HCV infection, and that viral persistence reflects the failure to induce or maintain these CTL-dependent events. Moreover, according to this scenario, an inefficient T cell response that fails to clear the infections creates a smoldering chronic necroinflammatory process, the end result of which is hepatic fibrosis, cirrhosis and HCC. In addition, these infections are associated with a variety of extrahepatic disorders, which are largely immunological in origin.

In spite of these accomplishments, however, many issues pertaining to the biology, immunobiology and pathogenesis of HBV and HCV infections remain unresolved, some of which are highlighted in the Unresolved Issues/Future Directions section of this review. Future studies aimed at addressing these issues will not only improve our understanding of the host-virus interactions that determine the pathogenesis and outcome of infection, but may also lead to the discovery of new approaches for the prevention and treatment of HBV and HCV infections and their life-threatening complications.

SUMMARY POINTS

1. HBV and HCV replicate noncytopathically in the hepatocyte.
2. The innate immune response does not contribute significantly to the pathogenesis of liver disease or viral clearance in either infection.
3. The adaptive immune response, especially the virus-specific CTL response, plays a major role in both liver disease pathogenesis and viral clearance during HBV or HCV infection.
4. Antigen-nonspecific inflammatory cells enhance CTL-induced immunopathology in the liver.
5. Platelets may facilitate CTL homing within the liver.
6. Viral persistence reflects the failure to induce or maintain CTL-effector functions and/or viral evasion of the immune response.
7. Chronic inflammation contributes to the development of the complications (fibrosis, cirrhosis, and HCC) of persistent HBV or HCV infection.
8. HBV and HCV infections are associated with a variety of extrahepatic disorders, which are mainly immunological in origin.

UNRESOLVED ISSUES/FUTURE DIRECTIONS

These issues have been addressed recently in an "Action Plan for Liver Disease Research," prepared by the NIH with strong input from the scientific community (see the following Web site: **http://www.niddk.nih.gov/fund/divisions/ddn/ldrb/ldrb_action_plan.htm**). The highest priority issues, in our opinion, are as follows:

1. Tissue culture and small-animal models of HBV and HCV infections need to be developed.
2. The biology of viral entry, replication, egress, and spread of HBV and HCV needs to be elucidated.
3. The host factors that control the induction and maintenance of an effective antiviral immune response against both viruses need to be identified.
4. An effective vaccine needs to be developed for the prevention of HCV, and improved antiviral strategies need to be produced for the treatment of chronic HBV and HCV infections.

RELATED RESOURCES

1. Brechot C. 2004. Pathogenesis of hepatitis B virus-related hepatocellular carcinoma: old and new paradigms. *Gastroenterology* 127:S56–61
2. Ganem D, Prince AM. 2004. Hepatitis B virus infection–natural history and clinical consequences. *N. Engl. J. Med.* 350:1118–29
3. Guidotti LG, Chisari FV. 2001. Noncytolytic control of viral infections by the innate and adaptive immune response. *Annu. Rev. Immunol.* 19:65–91
4. Liang TJ, Heller T. 2004. Pathogenesis of hepatitis C-associated hepatocellular carcinoma. *Gastroenterology* 127:S62–71
5. Lindenbach BD, Rice CM. 2003. Molecular biology of flaviviruses. *Adv. Virus Res.* 59:23–61
6. Shoukry NH, Cawthon AG, Walker CM. 2004. Cell-mediated immunity and the outcome of hepatitis C virus infection. *Annu. Rev. Microbiol.* 58:391–424

ACKNOWLEDGMENTS

This work was supported by grants ai20001, ca76403, ca54560, ca108304, ca40489 (to F.V.C.), and ai40696 (to L.G.G.) from the National Institutes of Health. This is manuscript number 17742-mem from the Scripps Research Institute.

LITERATURE CITED

1. Chisari FV, Ferrari C. 1995. Hepatitis B virus immunopathogenesis. *Annu. Rev. Immunol.* 13:29–60
2. Lauer GM, Walker BD. 2001. Hepatitis C virus infection. *N. Engl. J. Med.* 345:41–52
3. Ferrari C, Missale G, Boni C, Urbani S. 2003. Immunopathogenesis of hepatitis B. *J. Hepatol.* 39(Suppl 1):S36–42
4. Pawlotsky JM. 2004. Pathophysiology of hepatitis C virus infection and related liver disease. *Trends Microbiol.* 12:96–102
5. Ganem D, Prince AM. 2004. Hepatitis B virus infection–natural history and clinical consequences. *N. Engl. J. Med.* 350:1118–29
6. Hoofnagle JH. 2002. Course and outcome of hepatitis C. *Hepatology* 36:S21–29

7. Tiollais P, Pourcel C, Dejean A. 1985. The hepatitis B virus. *Nature* 317:489–95
8. Shoukry NH, Cawthon AG, Walker CM. 2004. Cell-mediated immunity and the outcome of hepatitis C virus infection. *Annu. Rev. Microbiol.* 58:391–424
9. Seeger C, Mason WS. 2000. Hepatitis B virus biology. *Microbiol. Mol. Biol. Rev.* 64:51–68
10. Buckwold VE, Beer BE, Donis RO. 2003. Bovine viral diarrhea virus as a surrogate model of hepatitis C virus for the evaluation of antiviral agents. *Antiviral Res.* 60:1–15
11. Moradpour D, Englert C, Wakita T, Wands JR. 1996. Characterization of cell lines allowing tightly regulated expression of hepatitis C virus core protein. *Virology* 222:51–63
12. Sells MA, Chen ML, Acs G. 1987. Production of hepatitis B virus particles in Hep G2 cells transfected with cloned hepatitis B virus DNA. *Proc. Natl. Acad. Sci. USA* 84:1005–9
13. Lohmann V, Korner F, Dobierzewska A, Bartenschlager R. 2001. Mutations in hepatitis C virus RNAs conferring cell culture adaptation. *J. Virol.* 75:1437–49
14. Lohmann V, Korner F, Koch J, Herian U, Theilmann L, Bartenschlager R. 1999. Replication of subgenomic hepatitis C virus RNAs in a hepatoma cell line. *Science* 285:110–13
15. Blight KJ, Kolykhalov AA, Rice CM. 2000. Efficient initiation of HCV RNA replication in cell culture. *Science* 290:1972–75
16. Ikeda M, Yi M, Li K, Lemon SM. 2002. Selectable subgenomic and genome-length dicistronic RNAs derived from an infectious molecular clone of the HCV-N strain of hepatitis C virus replicate efficiently in cultured Huh7 cells. *J. Virol.* 76:2997–3006
17. Lanford RE, Guerra B, Lee H, Averett DR, Pfeiffer B, et al. 2003. Antiviral effect and virus-host interactions in response to alpha interferon, gamma interferon, poly(i)-poly(c), tumor necrosis factor alpha, and ribavirin in hepatitis C virus subgenomic replicons. *J. Virol.* 77:1092–104
18. Kapadia SB, Brideau-Andersen A, Chisari FV. 2003. Interference of hepatitis C virus RNA replication by short interfering RNAs. *Proc. Natl. Acad. Sci. USA* 18:2014–48
19. Pietschmann T, Lohmann V, Kaul A, Krieger N, Rinck G, et al. 2002. Persistent and transient replication of full-length hepatitis C virus genomes in cell culture. *J. Virol.* 76: 4008–21
20. Wieland SF, Vega RG, Muller R, Evans CF, Hilbush B, et al. 2003. Searching for interferon-induced genes that inhibit hepatitis B virus replication in transgenic mouse hepatocytes. *J. Virol.* 77:1227–36
21. Bartenschlager R, Kaul A, Sparacio S. 2003. Replication of the hepatitis C virus in cell culture. *Antiviral Res.* 60:91–102
22. Pasquetto V, Wieland SF, Uprichard SL, Tripodi M, Chisari FV. 2002. Cytokine-sensitive replication of hepatitis B virus in immortalized mouse hepatocyte cultures. *J. Virol.* 76:5646–53
23. Koike K, Moriya K, Ishibashi K, Matsuura Y, Suzuki T, et al. 1995. Expression of hepatitis C virus envelope proteins in transgenic mice. *J. Gen. Virol.* 76(Pt 12):3031–38
24. Koike K, Moriya K, Ishibashi K, Yotsuyanagi H, Shintani Y, et al. 1997. Sialadenitis histologically resembling Sjogren syndrome in mice transgenic for hepatitis C virus envelope genes. *Proc. Natl. Acad. Sci. USA* 94:233–36
25. Pasquinelli C, Shoenberger JM, Chung J, Chang KM, Guidotti LG, et al. 1997. Hepatitis C virus core and E2 protein expression in transgenic mice. *Hepatology* 25:719–27
26. Moriya K, Yotsuyanagi H, Shintani Y, Fujie H, Ishibashi K, et al. 1997. Hepatitis C virus core protein induces hepatic steatosis in transgenic mice. *J. Gen. Virol.* 78(Pt 7):1527–31
27. Honda A, Hatano M, Kohara M, Arai Y, Hartatik T, et al. 2000. HCV-core protein accelerates recovery from the insensitivity of liver cells to Fas-mediated apoptosis induced by an injection of anti-Fas antibody in mice. *J. Hepatol.* 33:440–47

28. Machida K, Tsukiyama-Kohara K, Seike E, Tone S, Shibasaki F, et al. 2001. Inhibition of cytochrome c release in Fas-mediated signaling pathway in transgenic mice induced to express hepatitis C viral proteins. *J. Biol. Chem.* 276:12140–46
29. Disson O, Haouzi D, Desagher S, Loesch K, Hahne M, et al. 2004. Impaired clearance of virus-infected hepatocytes in transgenic mice expressing the hepatitis C virus polyprotein. *Gastroenterology* 126:859–72
30. Okuda M, Li K, Beard MR, Showalter LA, Scholle F, et al. 2002. Mitochondrial injury, oxidative stress, and antioxidant gene expression are induced by hepatitis C virus core protein. *Gastroenterology* 122:366–75
31. Moriya K, Fujie H, Shintani Y, Yotsuyanagi H, Tsutsumi T, et al. 1998. The core protein of hepatitis C virus induces hepatocellular carcinoma in transgenic mice. *Nat. Med.* 4:1065–47
32. Wakita T, Taya C, Katsume A, Kato J, Yonekawa H, et al. 1998. Efficient conditional transgene expression in hepatitis C virus cDNA transgenic mice mediated by the Cre/loxP system. *J. Biol. Chem.* 273:9001–6
33. Lerat H, Honda M, Beard MR, Loesch K, Sun J, et al. 2002. Steatosis and liver cancer in transgenic mice expressing the structural and nonstructural proteins of hepatitis C virus. *Gastroenterology* 122:352–65
34. Larkin J, Clayton M, Sun B, Perchonock CE, Morgan JL, et al. 1999. Hepatitis B virus transgenic mouse model of chronic liver disease. *Nat. Med.* 5:907–12
35. Chisari FV, Pinkert CA, Milich DR, Filippi P, McLachlan A, et al. 1985. A transgenic mouse model of the chronic hepatitis B surface antigen carrier state. *Science* 230:1157–60
36. Guidotti LG, Matzke B, Schaller H, Chisari FV. 1995. High-level hepatitis B virus replication in transgenic mice. *J. Virol.* 69:6158–69
37. Hertogs K, Leenders WPJ, Depla E, DeBruin WCC, Meheus L, et al. 1993. Endonexin II, present on human liver plasma membranes, is a specific binding protein of small hepatitis B virus envelope protein. *Virology* 197:549–57
38. Neurath AR, Strick N, Sproul P. 1992. Search for hepatitis B virus cell receptors reveals binding sites for interleukin 6 on the virus envelope protein. *J. Exp. Med.* 175:461–69
39. Gong ZJ, De Meyer S, van Pelt J, Hertogs K, Depla E, et al. 1999. Transfection of a rat hepatoma cell line with a construct expressing human liver annexin V confers susceptibility to hepatitis B virus infection. *Hepatology* 29:576–84
40. Mehdi H, Kaplan MJ, Anlar FY, Yang X, Bayer R, et al. 1994. Hepatitis B virus surface antigen binds to apolipoprotein H. *J.Virol.* 68:2415–24
41. Franco A, Paroli M, Testa U, Benvenuto R, Peschle C, et al. 1992. Transferrin receptor mediates uptake and presentation of hepatitis B envelope antigen by T lymphocytes. *J. Exp. Med.* 175:1195–205
42. Kuroki K, Eng F, Ishikawa T, Turck C, Harada F, Ganem D. 1995. gp180, a host cell glycoprotein that binds duck hepatitis B virus particles, is encoded by a member of the carboxypeptidase gene family. *J. Biol. Chem.* 270:15022–28
43. Tong S, Li J, Wands JR. 1999. Carboxypeptidase D is an avian hepatitis B virus receptor. *J. Virol.* 73:8696–702
44. Pileri P, Uematsu Y, Campagnoli S, Galli G, Falugi F, et al. 1998. Binding of hepatitis C virus to CD81. *Science* 282:938–41
45. Zhang J, Randall G, Higginbottom A, Monk P, Rice CM, McKeating JA. 2004. CD81 is required for hepatitis C virus glycoprotein-mediated viral infection. *J. Virol.* 78:1448–55
46. Scarselli E, Ansuini H, Cerino R, Roccasecca RM, Acali S, et al. 2002. The human scavenger receptor class B type I is a novel candidate receptor for the hepatitis C virus. *EMBO J.* 21:5017–25

47. Lozach PY, Lortat-Jacob H, de Lacroix de Lavalette A, Staropoli I, Foung S, et al. 2003. DC-SIGN and L-SIGN are high affinity binding receptors for hepatitis C virus glycoprotein E2. *J. Biol. Chem.* 278:20358–66
48. Pohlmann S, Zhang J, Baribaud F, Chen Z, Leslie GJ, et al. 2003. Hepatitis C virus glycoproteins interact with DC-SIGN and DC-SIGNR. *J. Virol.* 77:4070–80
49. Gardner JP, Durso RJ, Arrigale RR, Donovan GP, Maddon PJ, et al. 2003. L-SIGN (CD 209L) is a liver-specific capture receptor for hepatitis C virus. *Proc. Natl. Acad. Sci. USA* 100:4498–503
50. Bartosch B, Dubuisson J, Cosset FL. 2003. Infectious hepatitis C virus pseudo-particles containing functional E1-E2 envelope protein complexes. *J. Exp. Med.* 197:633–42
51. Hsu M, Zhang J, Flint M, Logvinoff C, Cheng-Mayer C, et al. 2003. Hepatitis C virus glycoproteins mediate pH-dependent cell entry of pseudotyped retroviral particles. *Proc. Natl. Acad. Sci. USA* 100:7271–76
52. Summers J. 1988. The replication cycle of hepatitis B viruses. *Cancer* 61:1957–62
53. Moradpour D, Brass V, Bieck E, Friebe P, Gosert R, et al. 2004. Membrane association of the RNA-dependent RNA polymerase is essential for hepatitis C virus RNA replication. *J. Virol.* 78:13278–84
54. Rinck G, Birghan C, Harada T, Meyers G, Thiel HJ, Tautz N. 2001. A cellular J-domain protein modulates polyprotein processing and cytopathogenicity of a pestivirus. *J. Virol.* 75:9470–82
55. Waxman L, Whitney M, Pollok BA, Kuo LC, Darke PL. 2001. Host cell factor requirement for hepatitis C virus enzyme maturation. *Proc. Natl. Acad. Sci. USA* 98:13931–35
56. Reed KE, Rice CM. 2000. Overview of hepatitis C virus genome structure, polyprotein processing, and protein properties. *Curr. Top. Microbiol. Immunol.* 242:55–84
57. Lohmann V, Koch JO, Bartenschlager R. 1996. Processing pathways of the hepatitis C virus proteins. *J. Hepatol.* 24:11–19
58. Tanji Y, Hijikata M, Satoh S, Kaneko T, Shimotohno K. 1995. Hepatitis C virus-encoded nonstructural protein NS4A has versatile functions in viral protein processing. *J. Virol.* 69:1575–81
59. Tanji Y, Hijikata M, Hirowatari Y, Shimotohno K. 1994. Hepatitis C virus polyprotein processing: kinetics and mutagenic analysis of serine proteinase-dependent cleavage. *J. Virol.* 68:8418–22
60. Selby MJ, Glazer E, Masiarz F, Houghton M. 1994. Complex processing and protein:protein interactions in the E2:NS2 region of HCV. *Virology* 204:114–22
61. Mizushima H, Hijikata M, Asabe S, Hirota M, Kimura K, Shimotohno K. 1994. Two hepatitis C virus glycoprotein E2 products with different C termini. *J. Virol.* 68:6215–22
62. Lin C, Lindenbach BD, Pragai BM, McCourt DW, Rice CM. 1994. Processing in the hepatitis C virus E2-NS2 region: identification of p7 and two distinct E2-specific products with different C termini. *J. Virol.* 68:5063–73
63. Failla C, Tomei L, De Francesco R. 1994. Both NS3 and NS4A are required for proteolytic processing of hepatitis C virus nonstructural proteins. *J. Virol.* 68:3753–60
64. Grakoui A, McCourt DW, Wychowski C, Feinstone SM, Rice CM. 1993. A second hepatitis C virus-encoded proteinase. *Proc. Natl. Acad. Sci. USA* 90:10583–87
65. Bartenschlager R, Ahlborn-Laake L, Mous J, Jacobsen H. 1993. Nonstructural protein 3 of the hepatitis C virus encodes a serine-type proteinase required for cleavage at the NS3/4 and NS4/5 junctions. *J. Virol.* 67:3835–44
66. Tomei L, Failla C, Santolini E, De Francesco R, La Monica N. 1993. NS3 is a serine protease required for processing of hepatitis C virus polyprotein. *J. Virol.* 67:4017–26

67. Grakoui A, McCourt DW, Wychowski C, Feinstone SM, Rice CM. 1993. Characterization of the hepatitis C virus-encoded serine proteinase: determination of proteinase-dependent polyprotein cleavage sites. *J. Virol.* 67:2832–43
68. Hijikata M, Kato N, Ootsuyama Y, Nakagawa M, Shimotohno K. 1991. Gene mapping of the putative structural region of the hepatitis C virus genome by in vitro processing analysis. *Proc. Natl. Acad. Sci. USA* 88:5547–51
69. Koyama AH, Irie H, Fukumori T, Hata S, Iida S, et al. 1998. Role of virus-induced apoptosis in a host defense mechanism against virus infection. *J. Med. Invest.* 45:37–45
70. Samuel CE. 2001. Antiviral actions of interferons. *Clin. Microbiol. Rev.* 14:778–809
71. Biron CA, Nguyen KB, Pien GC, Cousens LP, Salazar-Mather TP. 1999. Natural killer cells in antiviral defense: function and regulation by innate cytokines. *Annu. Rev. Immunol.* 17:189–220
72. Kakimi K, Lane TE, Chisari FV, Guidotti LG. 2001. Cutting edge: Inhibition of hepatitis B virus replication by activated NK T cells does not require inflammatory cell recruitment to the liver. *J. Immunol.* 167:6701–5
73. Kakimi K, Guidotti LG, Koezuka Y, Chisari FV. 2000. Natural killer T cell activation inhibits hepatitis B virus replication in vivo. *J. Exp. Med.* 192:921–30
74. Buendia MA. 1998. Hepatitis B viruses and cancerogenesis. *Biomed. Pharmacother.* 52:34–43
75. Bantel H, Schulze-Osthoff K. 2003. Apoptosis in hepatitis C virus infection. *Cell Death Differ.* 10(Suppl 1):S48–58
76. Guidotti LG, Rochford R, Chung J, Shapiro M, Purcell R, Chisari FV. 1999. Viral clearance without destruction of infected cells during acute HBV infection. *Science* 284:825–29
77. **Thimme R, Wieland S, Steiger C, Ghrayeb J, Reimann KA, et al. 2003. CD8(+) T cells mediate viral clearance and disease pathogenesis during acute hepatitis B virus infection. *J. Virol.* 77:68–76**

Viral clearance and liver disease during acute HBV infection in chimpanzees are mediated by $CD8^+$ cells (but not $CD4^+$ cells).

78. Thimme R, Bukh J, Spangenberg HC, Wieland S, Pemberton J, et al. 2002. Viral and immunological determinants of hepatitis C virus clearance, persistence, and disease. *Proc. Natl. Acad. Sci. USA* 99:15661–68
79. Walker CM. 1997. Comparative features of hepatitis C virus infection in humans and chimpanzees. *Springer Semin. Immunopathol.* 19:85–98
80. Lanford RE, Bigger C, Bassett S, Klimpel G. 2001. The chimpanzee model of hepatitis C virus infections. *Ilar. J.* 42:117–26
81. Su AI, Pezacki JP, Wodicka L, Brideau AD, Supekova L, et al. 2002. Genomic analysis of the host response to hepatitis C virus infection. *Proc. Natl. Acad. Sci. USA* 99:15669–74
82. Bigger CB, Brasky KM, Lanford RE. 2001. DNA microarray analysis of chimpanzee liver during acute resolving hepatitis C virus infection. *J. Virol.* 75:7059–66
83. Bigger CB, Guerra B, Brasky KM, Hubbard G, Beard MR, et al. 2004. Intrahepatic gene expression during chronic hepatitis C virus infection in chimpanzees. *J. Virol.* 78:13779–92
84. Gale MJ Jr, Korth MJ, Tang NM, Tan SL, Hopkins DA, et al. 1997. Evidence that hepatitis C virus resistance to interferon is mediated through repression of the PKR protein kinase by the nonstructural 5A protein. *Virology* 230:217–27
85. Taylor DR, Shi ST, Romano PR, Barber GN, Lai MM. 1999. Inhibition of the interferon-inducible protein kinase PKR by HCV E2 protein. *Science* 285:107–10
86. Pflugheber J, Fredericksen B, Sumpter R Jr, Wang C, Ware F, et al. 2002. Regulation of PKR and IRF-1 during hepatitis C virus RNA replication. *Proc. Natl. Acad. Sci. USA* 99:4650–55

87. Foy E, Li K, Wang C, Sumpter R Jr, Ikeda M, et al. 2003. Regulation of interferon regulatory factor-3 by the hepatitis C virus serine protease. *Science* 300:1145–48
88. Marusawa H, Hijikata M, Chiba T, Shimotohno K. 1999. Hepatitis C virus core protein inhibits Fas- and tumor necrosis factor alpha-mediated apoptosis via NF-kappaB activation. *J. Virol.* 73:4713–20
89. Tseng CT, Klimpel GR. 2002. Binding of the hepatitis C virus envelope protein E2 to CD81 inhibits natural killer cell functions. *J. Exp. Med.* 195:43–49
90. Crotta S, Stilla A, Wack A, D'Andrea A, Nuti S, et al. 2002. Inhibition of natural killer cells through engagement of CD81 by the major hepatitis C virus envelope protein. *J. Exp. Med.* 195:35–42
91. Wieland S, Thimme R, Purcell RH, Chisari FV. 2004. Genomic analysis of the host response to hepatitis B virus infection. *Proc. Natl. Acad. Sci. USA* 101:6669–74
92. Ahmad A, Alvarez F. 2004. Role of NK and NKT cells in the immunopathogenesis of HCV-induced hepatitis. *J. Leukoc. Biol.* 76:743–59
93. **Shoukry NH, Grakoui A, Houghton M, Chien DY, Ghrayeb J, et al. 2003. Memory CD8+ T cells are required for protection from persistent hepatitis C virus infection. *J. Exp. Med.* 197:1645–55**

Memory CD8+ T cells are necessary for long-term protection in HCV infection.

94. Guidotti LG, Chisari FV. 2001. Noncytolytic control of viral infections by the innate and adaptive immune response. *Annu. Rev. Immunol.* 19:65–91
95. Bone-Larson CL, Simpson KJ, Colletti LM, Lukacs NW, Chen SC, et al. 2000. The role of chemokines in the immunopathology of the liver. *Immunol. Rev.* 177:8–20
96. Cooper NR, Nemerow GR. 1983. Complement, viruses, and virus-infected cells. *Springer Semin. Immunopathol.* 6:327–47
97. Cooper NR, Nemerow GR. 1984. The role of antibody and complement in the control of viral infections. *J. Invest. Dermatol.* 83:121s–27s
98. Burton DR, Williamson RA, Parren PW. 2000. Antibody and virus: binding and neutralization. *Virology* 270:1–3
99. Steinman RM, Inaba K, Turley S, Pierre P, Mellman I. 1999. Antigen capture, processing, and presentation by dendritic cells: recent cell biological studies. *Hum. Immunol.* 60:562–67
100. Sallusto F, Lanzavecchia A. 1999. Mobilizing dendritic cells for tolerance, priming, and chronic inflammation. *J. Exp. Med.* 189:611–14
101. Bertolino P, McCaughan GW, Bowen DG. 2002. Role of primary intrahepatic T-cell activation in the 'liver tolerance effect'. *Immunol. Cell Biol.* 80:84–92
102. Crispe IN. 2003. Hepatic T cells and liver tolerance. *Nat. Rev. Immunol.* 3:51–62
103. Oldstone MB. 1994. The role of cytotoxic T lymphocytes in infectious disease: history, criteria, and state of the art. *Curr. Top. Microbiol. Immunol.* 189:1–8
104. Pignatelli M, Waters J, Brown D, Lever A, Iwarson S, et al. 1986. HLA class I antigens on the hepatocyte membrane during recovery from acute hepatitis B virus infection and during interferon therapy in chronic hepatitis B virus infection. *Hepatology* 6:349–53
105. Ando K, Guidotti LG, Wirth S, Ishikawa T, Missale G, et al. 1994. Class I-restricted cytotoxic T lymphocytes are directly cytopathic for their target cells in vivo. *J. Immunol.* 152:3245–53
106. Guidotti LG, Ishikawa T, Hobbs MV, Matzke B, Schreiber R, Chisari FV. 1996. Intracellular inactivation of the hepatitis B virus by cytotoxic T lymphocytes. *Immunity* 4:25–36
107. **Kakimi K, Lane TE, Wieland S, Asensio VC, Campbell IL, et al. 2001. Blocking chemokine responsive to gamma-2/interferon (IFN)-gamma inducible protein and**

Antigen nonspecific inflammatory cells amplify CTL-mediated liver damage.

monokine induced by IFN-gamma activity in vivo reduces the pathogenetic but not the antiviral potential of hepatitis B virus-specific cytotoxic T lymphocytes. *J. Exp. Med.* 194:1755–66

108. Ando K, Moriyama T, Guidotti LG, Wirth S, Schreiber RD, et al. 1993. Mechanisms of class I restricted immunopathology. A transgenic mouse model of fulminant hepatitis. *J. Exp. Med.* 178:1541–54
109. Nakamoto Y, Guidotti LG, Pasquetto V, Schreiber RD, Chisari FV. 1997. Differential target cell sensitivity to CTL-activated death pathways in hepatitis B virus transgenic mice. *J. Immunol.* 158:5692–97
110. Sitia G, Isogawa M, Kakimi K, Wieland SF, Chisari FV, Guidotti LG. 2002. Depletion of neutrophils blocks the recruitment of antigen-nonspecific cells into the liver without affecting the antiviral activity of hepatitis B virus-specific cytotoxic T lymphocytes. *Proc. Natl. Acad. Sci. USA* 99:13717–22
111. **Sitia G, Isogawa M, Iannacone M, Campbell IL, Chisari FV, Guidotti LG. 2004. MMPs are required for recruitment of antigen-nonspecific mononuclear cells into the liver by CTLs. *J. Clin. Invest.* 113:1158–67**

MMPs mediate homing of antigen nonspecific inflammatory cells into the liver.

112. Maini MK, Boni C, Lee CK, Larrubia JR, Reignat S, et al. 2000. The role of virus-specific CD8(+) cells in liver damage and viral control during persistent hepatitis B virus infection. *J. Exp. Med.* 191:1269–80
113. Bertoletti A, Maini MK. 2000. Protection or damage: a dual role for the virus-specific cytotoxic T lymphocyte response in hepatitis B and C infection? *Curr. Opin. Immunol.* 12:403–8
114. Ishak KG. 1976. Light microscopic morphology of viral hepatitis. *Am. J. Clin. Pathol.* 65:787–827
115. Shields PL, Morland CM, Salmon M, Qin S, Hubscher SG, Adams DH. 1999. Chemokine and chemokine receptor interactions provide a mechanism for selective T cell recruitment to specific liver compartments within hepatitis C-infected liver. *J. Immunol.* 163:6236–43
116. Prezzi C, Casciaro MA, Francavilla V, Schiaffella E, Finocchi L, et al. 2001. Virus-specific CD8(+) T cells with type 1 or type 2 cytokine profile are related to different disease activity in chronic hepatitis C virus infection. *Eur. J. Immunol.* 31:894–906
117. Smyth MJ, Cretney E, Kelly JM, Westwood JA, Street SE, et al. 2005. Activation of NK cell cytotoxicity. *Mol. Immunol.* 42:501–10
118. Roberts AI, Devadas S, Zhang X, Zhang L, Keegan A, et al. 2003. The role of activation-induced cell death in the differentiation of T-helper-cell subsets. *Immunol. Res.* 28:285–93
119. Ahmad R, Menezes J, Knafo L, Ahmad A. 2001. Activated human platelets express Fas-L and induce apoptosis in Fas-positive tumor cells. *J. Leukoc. Biol.* 69:123–28
120. Ogasawara J, Watanabe-Fukunaga R, Adachi M, Matsuzawa A, Kasugai T, et al. 1993. Lethal effect of the anti-Fas antibody in mice. *Nature* 364:806–9
121. McClary H, Koch R, Chisari FV, Guidotti LG. 2000. Relative sensitivity of hepatitis B virus and other hepatotropic viruses to the antiviral effects of cytokines. *J. Virol.* 74:2255–64
122. Wieland SF, Guidotti LG, Chisari FV. 2000. Intrahepatic induction of alpha/beta interferon eliminates viral RNA-containing capsids in hepatitis B virus transgenic mice. *J. Virol.* 74:4165–73
123. Robek MD, Wieland SF, Chisari FV. 2002. Inhibition of hepatitis B virus replication by interferon requires proteasome activity. *J. Virol.* 76:3570–74
124. Robek MD, Boyd BS, Wieland SF, Chisari FV. 2004. Signal transduction pathways that inhibit hepatitis B virus replication. *Proc. Natl. Acad. Sci. USA* 101:1743–47

125. Tsui LV, Guidotti LG, Ishikawa T, Chisari FV. 1995. Posttranscriptional clearance of hepatitis B virus RNA by cytotoxic T lymphocyte-activated hepatocytes. *Proc. Natl. Acad. Sci. USA* 92:12398–402
126. Heise T, Guidotti LG, Chisari FV. 2001. Characterization of nuclear RNases that cleave hepatitis B virus RNA near the La protein binding site. *J. Virol.* 75:6874–83
127. Heise T, Guidotti LG, Chisari FV. 1999. La autoantigen specifically recognizes a predicted stem-loop in hepatitis B virus RNA. *J. Virol.* 73:5767–76
128. Heise T, Guidotti LG, Cavanaugh VJ, Chisari FV. 1999. Hepatitis B virus RNA-binding proteins associated with cytokine-induced clearance of viral RNA from the liver of transgenic mice. *J. Virol.* 73:474–81
129. Guidotti LG, Ando K, Hobbs MV, Ishikawa T, Runkel L, et al. 1994. Cytotoxic T lymphocytes inhibit hepatitis B virus gene expression by a noncytolytic mechanism in transgenic mice. *Proc. Natl. Acad. Sci. USA* 91:3764–68
130. Thimme R, Oldach D, Chang KM, Steiger C, Ray SC, Chisari FV. 2001. Determinants of viral clearance and persistence during acute hepatitis C virus infection. *J. Exp. Med.* 194:1395–406
131. Cheney IW, Lai VC, Zhong W, Brodhag T, Dempsey S, et al. 2002. Comparative analysis of anti-hepatitis C virus activity and gene expression mediated by alpha, beta, and gamma interferons. *J. Virol.* 76:11148–54
132. Frese M, Pietschmann T, Moradpour D, Haller O, Bartenschlager R. 2001. Interferon-alpha inhibits hepatitis C virus subgenomic RNA replication by an MxA-independent pathway. *J. Gen. Virol.* 82:723–33
133. Frese M, Schwarzle V, Barth K, Krieger N, Lohmann V, et al. 2002. Interferon-gamma inhibits replication of subgenomic and genomic hepatitis C virus RNAs. *Hepatology* 35:694–703
134. Whitmire JK, Asano MS, Murali-Krishna K, Suresh M, Ahmed R. 1998. Long-term CD4 Th1 and Th2 memory following acute lymphocytic choriomeningitis virus infection. *J. Virol.* 72:8281–88
135. Grakoui A, Shoukry NH, Woollard DJ, Han JH, Hanson HL, et al. 2003. HCV persistence and immune evasion in the absence of memory T cell help. *Science* 302:659–62
136. Bassett SE, Guerra B, Brasky K, Miskovsky E, Houghton M, et al. 2001. Protective immune response to hepatitis C virus in chimpanzees rechallenged following clearance of primary infection. *Hepatology* 33:1479–87
137. Ciurea A, Klenerman P, Hunziker L, Horvath E, Senn BM, et al. 2000. Viral persistence in vivo through selection of neutralizing antibody-escape variants. *Proc. Natl. Acad. Sci. USA* 97:2749–54
138. Ciurea A, Klenerman P, Hunziker L, Horvath E, Odermatt B, et al. 1999. Persistence of lymphocytic choriomeningitis virus at very low levels in immune mice. *Proc. Natl. Acad. Sci. USA* 96:11964–69
139. Michalak TI, Pasquinelli C, Guilhot S, Chisari FV. 1994. Hepatitis B virus persistence after recovery from acute viral hepatitis. *J. Clin. Invest.* 93:230–39
140. Rehermann B, Ferrari C, Pasquinelli C, Chisari FV. 1996. The hepatitis B virus persists for decades after patients' recovery from acute viral hepatitis despite active maintenance of a cytotoxic T-lymphocyte response. *Nat. Med.* 2:1104–8
141. Logvinoff C, Major ME, Oldach D, Heyward S, Talal A, et al. 2004. Neutralizing antibody response during acute and chronic hepatitis C virus infection. *Proc. Natl. Acad. Sci. USA* 101:10149–54

The onset of hepatitis coincides with the onset of the CD8$^+$ T cell response in HCV-infected patients.

Control of HCV replication by memory CD8$^+$ T cells requires CD4$^+$ T cell help.

Chimpanzees that previously cleared an HCV infection became infected upon re-challenge, yet mounted significant humoral and cellular immune responses and rapidly cleared the infection.

142. Burioni R, Mancini N, Carletti S, Perotti M, Grieco A, et al. 2004. Cross-reactive pseudovirus-neutralizing anti-envelope antibodies coexist with antibodies devoid of such activity in persistent hepatitis C virus infection. *Virology* 327:242–48
143. Farci P, Shimoda A, Wong D, Cabezon T, De Gioannis D, et al. 1996. Prevention of hepatitis C virus infection in chimpanzees by hyperimmune serum against the hypervariable region 1 of the envelope 2 protein. *Proc. Natl. Acad. Sci. USA* 93:15394–99
144. Bachmann MF, Zinkernagel RM. 1997. Neutralizing antiviral B cell responses. *Annu. Rev. Immunol.* 15:235–70
145. Meyer K, Basu A, Przysiecki CT, Lagging LM, Di Bisceglie AM, et al. 2002. Complement-mediated enhancement of antibody function for neutralization of pseudotype virus containing hepatitis C virus E2 chimeric glycoprotein. *J. Virol.* 76:2150–58
146. Manns MP, Rambusch EG. 1999. Autoimmunity and extrahepatic manifestations in hepatitis C virus infection. *J. Hepatol.* 31(Suppl 1):39–42
147. Amarapurkar DN, Amarapurkar AD. 2002. Extrahepatic manifestations of viral hepatitis. *Ann. Hepatol* 1:192–95
148. Han SH. 2004. Extrahepatic manifestations of chronic hepatitis B. *Clin. Liver Dis.* 8:403–18
149. Agnello V, De Rosa FG. 2004. Extrahepatic disease manifestations of HCV infection: some current issues. *J. Hepatol.* 40:341–52
150. Watanabe N, Sakakibara J, Hovanessian AG, Taniguchi T, Fujita T. 1991. Activation of IFN-beta element by IRF-1 requires a posttranslational event in addition to IRF-1 synthesis. *Nucleic Acids Res.* 19:4421–28
151. Fujita T, Kimura Y, Miyamoto M, Barsoumian EL, Taniguchi T. 1989. Induction of endogenous IFN-alpha and IFN-beta genes by a regulatory transcription factor, IRF-1. *Nature* 337:270–72
152. Matsuyama T, Kimura T, Kitagawa M, Pfeffer K, Kawakami T, et al. 1993. Targeted disruption of IRF-1 or IRF-2 results in abnormal type I IFN gene induction and aberrant lymphocyte development. *Cell* 75:83–97
153. Reis LF, Ruffner H, Stark G, Aguet M, Weissmann C. 1994. Mice devoid of interferon regulatory factor 1 (IRF-1) show normal expression of type I interferon genes. *EMBO J.* 13:4798–806
154. Sato M, Suemori H, Hata N, Asagiri M, Ogasawara K, et al. 2000. Distinct and essential roles of transcription factors IRF-3 and IRF-7 in response to viruses for IFN-alpha/beta gene induction. *Immunity* 13:539–48
155. Tong SP, Brotman B, Li JS, Vitvitski L, Pascal D, et al. 1991. In vitro and in vivo replication capacity of the precore region defective hepatitis B virus variants. *J. Hepatol.* 13 (Suppl 4):S68–73
156. Tong SP, Diot C, Gripon P, Li J, Vitvitski L, et al. 1991. In vitro replication competence of a cloned hepatitis B virus variant with a nonsense mutation in the distal pre-C region. *Virology* 181:733–37
157. Chang C, Enders G, Sprengel R, Peters N, Varmus HE, Ganem D. 1987. Expression of the precore region of an avian hepatitis B virus is not required for viral replication. *J. Virol.* 61:3322–25
158. Chen HS, Kew MC, Hornbuckle WE, Tennant BC, Cote PJ, et al. 1992. The precore gene of the woodchuck hepatitis virus genome is not essential for viral replication in the natural host. *J. Virol.* 66:5682–84
159. Milich DR, Jones JE, Hughes JL, Price J, Raney AK, McLachlan A. 1990. Is a function of the secreted hepatitis B e antigen to induce immunologic tolerance in utero? *Proc. Natl. Acad. Sci. USA* 87:6599–603

160. Chen MT, Billaud JN, Sallberg M, Guidotti LG, Chisari FV, et al. 2004. A function of the hepatitis B virus precore protein is to regulate the immune response to the core antigen. *Proc. Natl. Acad. Sci. USA* 101:14913–18
161. Brunetto MR, Giarin MM, Oliveri F, Chiaberge E, Baldi M, et al. 1991. Wild-type and e antigen-minus hepatitis B viruses and course of chronic hepatitis. *Proc. Natl. Acad. Sci. USA* 88:4186–90
162. Reignat S, Webster GJ, Brown D, Ogg GS, King A, et al. 2002. Escaping high viral load exhaustion: CD8 cells with altered tetramer binding in chronic hepatitis B virus infection. *J. Exp. Med.* 195:1089–101
163. Hu Z, Zhang Z, Doo E, Coux O, Goldberg AL, Liang TJ. 1999. Hepatitis B virus X protein is both a substrate and a potential inhibitor of the proteasome complex. *J. Virol.* 73:7231–40
164. Rehermann B, Pasquinelli C, Mosier SM, Chisari FV. 1995. Hepatitis B virus (HBV) sequence variation of cytotoxic T lymphocyte epitopes is not common in patients with chronic HBV infection. *J. Clin. Invest.* 96:1527–34
165. Bertoletti A, Sette A, Chisari FV, Penna A, Levrero M, et al. 1994. Natural variants of cytotoxic epitopes are T-cell receptor antagonists for antiviral cytotoxic T cells. *Nature* 369:407–10
166. Waters JA, Kennedy M, Voet P, Hauser P, Petre J, et al. 1992. Loss of the common "A" determinant of hepatitis B surface antigen by a vaccine-induced escape mutant. *J. Clin. Invest.* 90:2543–47
167. Carman WF, Zanetti AR, Karayiannis P, Waters J, Manzillo G, et al. 1990. Vaccine-induced escape mutant of hepatitis B virus. *Lancet* 336:325–29
168. Chang KM, Rehermann B, McHutchison JG, Pasquinelli C, Southwood S, et al. 1997. Immunological significance of cytotoxic T lymphocyte epitope variants in patients chronically infected by the hepatitis C virus. *J. Clin. Invest.* 100:2376–85
169. Erickson AL, Kimura Y, Igarashi S, Eichelberger J, Houghton M, et al. 2001. The outcome of hepatitis C virus infection is predicted by escape mutations in epitopes targeted by cytotoxic T lymphocytes. *Immunity* 15:883–95
170. Weiner A, Erickson AL, Kansopon J, Crawford K, Muchmore E, et al. 1995. Persistent hepatitis C virus infection in a chimpanzee is associated with emergence of a cytotoxic T lymphocyte escape variant. *Proc. Natl. Acad. Sci. USA* 92:2755–59
171. Giuggio VM, Bonkovsky HL, Smith J, Rothman AL. 1998. Inefficient recognition of autologous viral sequences by intrahepatic hepatitis C virus-specific cytotoxic T lymphocytes in chronically infected subjects. *Virology* 251:132–40
172. Maini MK, Reignat S, Boni C, Ogg GS, King AS, et al. 2000. T cell receptor usage of virus-specific CD8 cells and recognition of viral mutations during acute and persistent hepatitis B virus infection. *Eur. J. Immunol.* 30:3067–78
173. Ishikawa T, Kono D, Chung J, Fowler P, Theofilopoulos A, et al. 1998. Polyclonality and multispecificity of the CTL response to a single viral epitope. *J. Immunol.* 161:5842–50
174. Tsai SL, Chen YM, Chen MH, Huang CY, Sheen IS, et al. 1998. Hepatitis C virus variants circumventing cytotoxic T lymphocyte activity as a mechanism of chronicity. *Gastroenterology* 115:954–65
175. Kaneko T, Moriyama T, Udaka K, Hiroishi K, Kita H, et al. 1997. Impaired induction of cytotoxic T lymphocytes by antagonism of a weak agonist borne by a variant hepatitis C virus epitope. *Eur. J. Immunol.* 27:1782–87
176. Bertoletti A, Costanzo A, Chisari FV, Levrero M, Artini M, et al. 1994. Cytotoxic T lymphocyte response to a wild type hepatitis B virus epitope in patients chronically infected by variant viruses carrying substitutions within the epitope. *J. Exp. Med.* 180:933–43

177. Seifert U, Liermann H, Racanelli V, Halenius A, Wiese M, et al. 2004. Hepatitis C virus mutation affects proteasomal epitope processing. *J. Clin. Invest.* 114:250–59
178. Selby M, Erickson A, Dong C, Cooper S, Parham P, et al. 1999. Hepatitis C virus envelope glycoprotein E1 originates in the endoplasmic reticulum and requires cytoplasmic processing for presentation by class I MHC molecules. *J. Immunol.* 162:669–76
179. Chisari FV. 2000. Rous-Whipple Award lecture. Viruses, immunity, and cancer: lessons from hepatitis B. *Am. J. Pathol.* 156:1117–32
180. Cooper S, Erickson AL, Adams EJ, Kansopon J, Weiner AJ, et al. 1999. Analysis of a successful immune response against hepatitis C virus. *Immunity* 10:439–49
181. Yewdell JW, Bennink JR. 1999. Mechanisms of viral interference with MHC class I antigen processing and presentation. *Annu. Rev. Cell. Dev. Biol.* 15:579–606
182. Nikolich-Zugich J, Slifka MK, Messaoudi I. 2004. The many important facets of T-cell repertoire diversity. *Nat. Rev. Immunol.* 4:123–32
183. Doherty PC. 1993. Immune exhaustion: driving virus-specific $CD8^+$ T cells to death. *Trends Microbiol.* 1:207–9
184. Schwartz RH. 2003. T cell anergy. *Annu. Rev. Immunol.* 21:305–34
185. Lechner F, Gruener NH, Urbani S, Uggeri J, Santantonio T, et al. 2000. $CD8^+$ T lymphocyte responses are induced during acute hepatitis C virus infection but are not sustained. *Eur. J. Immunol.* 30:2479–87
186. Ulsenheimer A, Gerlach JT, Gruener NH, Jung MC, Schirren CA, et al. 2003. Detection of functionally altered hepatitis C virus-specific CD4 T cells in acute and chronic hepatitis C. *Hepatology* 37:1189–98
187. Lechner F, Wong DK, Dunbar PR, Chapman R, Chung RT, et al. 2000. Analysis of successful immune responses in persons infected with hepatitis C virus. *J. Exp. Med.* 191:1499–12
188. Boni C, Penna A, Ogg GS, Bertoletti A, Pilli M, et al. 2001. Lamivudine treatment can overcome cytotoxic T-cell hyporesponsiveness in chronic hepatitis B: new perspectives for immune therapy. *Hepatology* 33:963–71
189. Michalopoulos GK, DeFrances MC. 1997. Liver regeneration. *Science* 276:60–66
190. Fausto N, Campbell JS. 2003. The role of hepatocytes and oval cells in liver regeneration and repopulation. *Mech. Dev.* 120:117–30
191. Fausto N. 2004. Liver regeneration and repair: hepatocytes, progenitor cells, and stem cells. *Hepatology* 39:1477–87
192. Taub R. 2004. Liver regeneration: from myth to mechanism. *Nat. Rev. Mol. Cell. Biol.* 5:836–47
193. Paradis V, Youssef N, Dargere D, Ba N, Bonvoust F, et al. 2001. Replicative senescence in normal liver, chronic hepatitis C, and hepatocellular carcinomas. *Hum. Pathol.* 32:327–32
194. Wiemann SU, Satyanarayana A, Tsahuridu M, Tillmann HL, Zender L, et al. 2002. Hepatocyte telomere shortening and senescence are general markers of human liver cirrhosis. *FASEB J.* 16:935–42
195. Sell S. 2002. Cellular origin of hepatocellular carcinomas. *Semin. Cell Dev. Biol.* 13:419–24
196. Bralet MP, Pichard V, Ferry N. 2002. Demonstration of direct lineage between hepatocytes and hepatocellular carcinoma in diethylnitrosamine-treated rats. *Hepatology* 36:623–30
197. Su AI, Guidotti LG, Pezacki JP, Chisari FV, Schultz PG. 2002. Gene expression during the priming phase of liver regeneration after partial hepatectomy in mice. *Proc. Natl. Acad. Sci. USA* 99:11181–86

198. Strey CW, Markiewski M, Mastellos D, Tudoran R, Spruce LA, et al. 2003. The proinflammatory mediators C3a and C5a are essential for liver regeneration. *J. Exp. Med.* 198:913–23
199. Markiewski MM, Mastellos D, Tudoran R, DeAngelis RA, Strey CW, et al. 2004. C3a and C3b activation products of the third component of complement (C3) are critical for normal liver recovery after toxic injury. *J. Immunol.* 173:747–54
200. Taub R, Greenbaum LE, Peng Y. 1999. Transcriptional regulatory signals define cytokine-dependent and -independent pathways in liver regeneration. *Semin. Liver Dis.* 19:117–27
201. Summers J, Jilbert AR, Yang W, Aldrich CE, Saputelli J, et al. 2003. Hepatocyte turnover during resolution of a transient hepadnaviral infection. *Proc. Natl. Acad. Sci. USA* 100:11652–59
202. Mason WS, Jilbert AR, Summers J. 2005. Clonal expansion of hepatocytes during chronic woodchuck hepatitis virus infection. *Proc. Natl. Acad. Sci. USA* 102:1139–44
203. Mason WS, Cullen J, Moraleda G, Saputelli J, Aldrich CE, et al. 1998. Lamivudine therapy of WHV-infected woodchucks. *Virology* 245:18–32
204. Overturf K, al-Dhalimy M, Ou CN, Finegold M, Grompe M. 1997. Serial transplantation reveals the stem-cell-like regenerative potential of adult mouse hepatocytes. *Am. J. Pathol.* 151:1273–80
205. Ramadori G, Saile B. 2004. Inflammation, damage repair, immune cells, and liver fibrosis: specific or nonspecific, this is the question. *Gastroenterology* 127:997–1000
206. Bonacchi A, Petrai I, Defranco RM, Lazzeri E, Annunziato F, et al. 2003. The chemokine CCL21 modulates lymphocyte recruitment and fibrosis in chronic hepatitis C. *Gastroenterology* 125:1060–76
207. Marcellin P, Asselah T, Boyer N. 2002. Fibrosis and disease progression in hepatitis C. *Hepatology* 36:S47–56
208. Brechot C. 2004. Pathogenesis of hepatitis B virus-related hepatocellular carcinoma: old and new paradigms. *Gastroenterology* 127:S56–61
209. Liang TJ, Heller T. 2004. Pathogenesis of hepatitis C-associated hepatocellular carcinoma. *Gastroenterology* 127:S62–71
210. Melia WM, Johnson PJ, Neuberger J, Zaman S, Portmann BC, Williams R. 1984. Hepatocellular carcinoma in primary biliary cirrhosis: detection by alpha-fetoprotein estimation. *Gastroenterology* 87:660–63
211. Limmer J, Fleig WE, Leupold D, Bittner R, Ditschuneit H, Beger HG. 1988. Hepatocellular carcinoma in type I glycogen storage disease. *Hepatology* 8:531–37
212. Eriksson S, Carlson J, Velez R. 1986. Risk of cirrhosis and primary liver cancer in alpha 1-antitrypsin deficiency. *N. Engl. J. Med.* 314:736–39
213. Niederau C, Fischer R, Sonnenberg A, Stremmel W, Trampisch HJ, Strohmeyer G. 1985. Survival and causes of death in cirrhotic and in noncirrhotic patients with primary hemochromatosis. *N. Engl. J. Med.* 313:1256–62
214. Lieber CS, Garro A, Leo MA, Mak KM, Worner T. 1986. Alcohol and cancer. *Hepatology* 6:1005–19
215. Nakamoto Y, Guidotti LG, Kuhlen CV, Fowler P, Chisari FV. 1998. Immune pathogenesis of hepatocellular carcinoma. *J. Exp. Med.* 188:341–50
216. Browning JD, Horton JD. 2004. Molecular mediators of hepatic steatosis and liver injury. *J. Clin. Invest.* 114:147–52
217. Dev A, Patel K, McHutchison JG. 2004. Hepatitis C and steatosis. *Clin. Liver Dis.* 8:881–92, ix

A significant amount of hepatocyte turnover and clonal expansion of hepatocytes may occur during chronic hepadnaviral infection.

218. Barba G, Harper F, Harada T, Kohara M, Goulinet S, et al. 1997. Hepatitis C virus core protein shows a cytoplasmic localization and associates to cellular lipid storage droplets. *Proc. Natl. Acad. Sci. USA* 94:1200–5
219. Shi ST, Polyak SJ, Tu H, Taylor DR, Gretch DR, Lai MM. 2002. Hepatitis C virus NS5A colocalizes with the core protein on lipid droplets and interacts with apolipoproteins. *Virology* 292:198–210
220. Lai MM. 2002. Hepatitis C virus proteins: direct link to hepatic oxidative stress, steatosis, carcinogenesis and more. *Gastroenterology* 122:568–71
221. Trepo C, Guillevin L. 2001. Polyarteritis nodosa and extrahepatic manifestations of HBV infection: the case against autoimmune intervention in pathogenesis. *J. Autoimmun.* 16:269–74
222. Mehta S, Levey JM, Bonkovsky HL. 2001. Extrahepatic manifestations of infection with hepatitis C virus. *Clin. Liver Dis.* 5:979–1008
223. Hermine O, Lefrere F, Bronowicki JP, Mariette X, Jondeau K, et al. 2002. Regression of splenic lymphoma with villous lymphocytes after treatment of hepatitis C virus infection. *N. Engl. J. Med.* 347:89–94
224. Zuckerman E. 2003. Expansion of $CD5^+$ B-cell overexpressing CD81 in HCV infection: towards better understanding the link between HCV infection, B-cell activation and lymphoproliferation. *J. Hepatol.* 38:674–76
225. Lerat H, Rumin S, Habersetzer F, Berby F, Trabaud MA, et al. 1998. In vivo tropism of hepatitis C virus genomic sequences in hematopoietic cells: influence of viral load, viral genotype, and cell phenotype. *Blood* 91:3841–49
226. Fargion S, Fracanzani AL. 2003. Prevalence of hepatitis C virus infection in porphyria cutanea tarda. *J. Hepatol.* 39:635–38
227. Nagao Y, Sata M. 2004. Hepatitis C virus and lichen planus. *J. Gastroenterol. Hepatol.* 19:1101–13
228. Pilli M, Penna A, Zerbini A, Vescovi P, Manfredi M, et al. 2002. Oral lichen planus pathogenesis: A role for the HCV-specific cellular immune response. *Hepatology* 36:1446–52
229. Haddad J, Deny P, Munz-Gotheil C, Ambrosini JC, Trinchet JC, et al. 1992. Lymphocytic sialadenitis of Sjogren's syndrome associated with chronic hepatitis C virus liver disease. *Lancet* 339:321–23
230. Arrieta JJ, Rodriguez-Inigo E, Ortiz-Movilla N, Bartolome J, Pardo M, et al. 2001. In situ detection of hepatitis C virus RNA in salivary glands. *Am. J. Pathol.* 158:259–64
231. Shintani Y, Fujie H, Miyoshi H, Tsutsumi T, Tsukamoto K, et al. 2004. Hepatitis C virus infection and diabetes: direct involvement of the virus in the development of insulin resistance. *Gastroenterology* 126:840–48
232. Lindenbach BD, Rice CM. 2003. Molecular biology of flaviviruses. *Adv. Virus Res.* 59:23–61
233. Chisari FV. 1996. Hepatitis B virus transgenic mice: models of viral immunobiology and pathogenesis. *Curr. Top. Microbiol. Immunol.* 206:149–73
234. Tennant BC, Gerin JL. 2001. The woodchuck model of hepatitis B virus infection. *Ilar J.* 42:89–102
235. Schultz U, Grgacic E, Nassal M. 2004. Duck hepatitis B virus: an invaluable model system for HBV infection. *Adv. Virus Res.* 63:1–70
236. Iannacone M, Sitia G, Isogawa M, Marchese P, Castro MG, et al. 2005. Platelets mediate cytotoxic T lymphocyte-induced liver damage. *Nat. Med.* 11:1167–69

237. Li K, Foy E, Ferreon JC, Nakamura M, Ferreon AC, et al. 2005. Immune evasion by hepatitis C virus NS3/4A protease-mediated cleavage of the Toll-like receptor 3 adaptor protein TRIF. *Proc. Natl. Acad. Sci. USA* 102(8):2992–97
238. Yoneyama M, Kikuchi M, Natsukawa T, Shinobu N, Imaizumi T, et al. 2004. The RNA helicase RIG-I has an essential function in double-stranded RNA-induced innate antiviral responses. *Nat. Immunol.* 7:730–37
239. Foy E, Li K, Sumpter R Jr, Loo YM, Johnson CL, et al. 2005. Control of antiviral defenses through hepatitis C virus disruption of retinoic acid-inducible gene-I signaling. *Proc. Natl. Acad. Sci. USA* 102(8):2986–91
240. Sumpter R Jr, Loo YM, Foy E, Li K, Yoneyama M, et al. 2005. Regulating intracellular antiviral defense and permissiveness to hepatitis C virus RNA replication through a cellular RNA helicase, RIG-I. *J. Virol.* 79(5):2689–99

The Pathogenesis of *Helicobacter pylori*–Induced Gastro-Duodenal Diseases

John C. Atherton

Wolfson Digestive Diseases Centre and Institute of Infections, Immunity, and Inflammation, University of Nottingham, Nottingham NG7 2UH, United Kingdom; email: john.atherton@nottingham.ac.uk

Annu. Rev. Pathol. Mech. Dis. 2006. 1:63–96

First published online as a Review in Advance on October 3, 2005

The *Annual Review of Pathology: Mechanisms of Disease* is online at pathmechdis.annualreviews.org

doi: 10.1146/annurev.pathol.1.110304.100125

1553-4006/06/0114-0063$20.00

Key Words

Helicobacter pylori, gastric adenocarcinoma, duodenal ulcer, gastric ulcer, gastric MALT lymphoma, reflux esophagitis

Abstract

Helicobacter pylori is the main cause of peptic ulceration, distal gastric adenocarcinoma, and gastric lymphoma. Only 15% of those colonized develop disease, and pathogenesis depends upon strain virulence, host genetic susceptibility, and environmental cofactors. Virulence factors include the cag pathogenicity island, which induces proinflammatory, pro-proliferative epithelial cell signaling; the cytotoxin VacA, which causes epithelial damage; and an adhesin, BabA. Host genetic polymorphisms that lead to high-level pro-inflammatory cytokine release in response to infection increase cancer risk. Pathogenesis is dependent upon inflammation, a Th-1 acquired immune response and hormonal changes including hypergastrinaemia. Antral-predominant inflammation leads to increased acid production from the uninflamed corpus and predisposes to duodenal ulceration; corpus-predominant gastritis leads to hypochlorhydria and predisposes to gastric ulceration and adenocarcinoma. Falling prevalence of *H. pylori* in developed countries has led to a falling incidence of associated diseases. However, whether there are disadvantages of an *H. pylori*-free stomach, for example increased risk of esosphageal adenocarcinoma, remains unclear.

DISEASES CAUSED BY *HELICOBACTER PYLORI*

Helicobacter pylori colonizes more than half the world's population and is the main cause of peptic ulceration, gastric adenocarcinoma, and gastric lymphoma. Approximately 80% of peptic ulcer cases are caused by *H. pylori*; most of the rest are caused by nonsteroidal anti-inflammatory drugs (NSAIDs). When *H. pylori* is the etiological factor, its treatment heals ulcers and prevents their recurrence. Gastric adenocarcinoma is the second highest cause of cancer deaths worldwide. The nearly one million deaths per year are due to a combination of high incidence, aggressive disease course, and lack of effective treatment options. *H. pylori* causes distal but not proximal gastric adenocarcinoma, distal being the much more common form. *H. pylori* also causes B cell mucosa-associated lymphoid tissue (MALT) lymphoma of the stomach. These lymphomas can undergo high-grade transformation but, remarkably, when low-grade, usually resolve following *H. pylori* treatment. Finally, *H. pylori* infection is negatively associated with more severe forms of reflux esophagitis and its sequelae Barrett's esophagus and esophageal adenocarcinoma. There is much argument about whether this negative association is causal.

There has been recent interest in whether *H. pylori* may cause or be a risk factor for human diseases outside the upper gastrointestinal tract. These include idiopathic thrombocytopenic purpura [which appears to improve with *H. pylori* treatment (1, 2)], various skin diseases, liver diseases (although these have been associated more commonly with Helicobacters other than *H. pylori*), and cardiovascular and cerebrovascular disease (3, 4). Although interesting and potentially important, the causality of these associations is unproven, so the various theories on pathogenesis of these diseases are not discussed further.

NATURAL HISTORY OF *HELICOBACTER PYLORI* INFECTION

H. pylori colonization usually occurs in childhood, but infection persists lifelong in the absence of treatment. In the rare cases where colonization first occurs in adults, it can cause a profound gastritis with hypochlohydria, epigastric discomfort, and nausea (5, 6). Whether childhood colonization causes symptoms or changes in gastric acidity is unknown. *H. pylori* persistence is central to pathogenesis; ulcers occur mainly in mid- or late adulthood after many years of infection and inflammation, and gastric adenocarcinoma occurs in late adulthood after an even longer period of chronic inflammation and epithelial damage.

Colonization of and Persistence in the Gastric Niche

H. pylori is the only human bacterium to persistently inhabit the gastric mucus (**Figures 1** and **2**) (7). Elucidation of its complete genome sequence has allowed construction in silico of its metabolic pathways and other aspects of its biology (8, 9) and postgenomic techniques using whole genome strategies and microarray technology (for example, see Reference 10) have speeded experimentation. This and other work show that factors important for colonization include motility (**Figure 1**), environmental sensing, chemotaxis (11), iron acquisition (12), and acid resistance. Acid resistance is crucial in the gastric niche, and more than 300 genes are acid-regulated or acid-affected (13, 14). One of these genes encodes the most abundant protein of *H. pylori*, urease, which hydrolyzes urea to ammonia and carbon dioxide. This leads to a rise in cytoplasmic pH, which buffers the periplasm and allows survival in acidic conditions. Urea entry into the cytoplasm is regulated by a unique acid-gated urea channel (UreI), allowing instantaneous

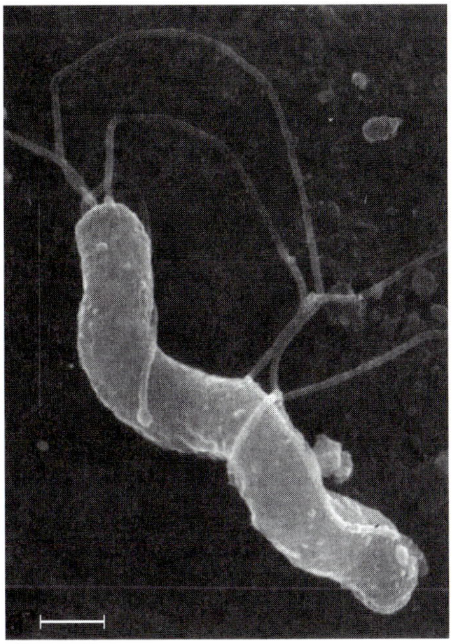

Figure 1

Electron micrograph of *Helicobacter pylori*. Bar is 0.5 μm. The spiral shape and multiple flagella confer corkscrew motility in the gastric mucus. (Image kindly donated by Lucinda J. Thompson, Department of Microbiology and Immunology, Stanford, CA, USA. Pictures taken at the School of Microbiology and Immunology, University of New South Wales, NSW, Australia.)

adaptation to acid challenge (15). The presence of *H. pylori* urease in the stomach forms the basis for the most widely used biopsy-based test (the biopsy urease test) and the most widely used noninvasive test (the urea breath test) (16).

H. pylori only inhabits gastric-type mucus and so cannot colonize the duodenum or esophagus unless these have undergone gastric metaplasia. The bacteria are found over mucus-secreting cells and not deep in gastric glands (**Figure 2**). This localization correlates with the expression by epithelial cells of Trefoil factor 1, to which *H. pylori* binds strongly and specifically (17). Other factors potentially contributing to *H. pylori*'s absence from gastric glands include the presence of growth-suppressing O-glycans (18) and of human β-defensins. *H. pylori* organisms are distributed through the mucus layer; this distribution is maintained by the mucus pH gradient, disruption of which leads to uncontrolled spread of the bacteria in an animal model (19). A small subset of *H. pylori* organisms adhere to the gastric mucosa, and this is important in pathogenesis as adhesion triggers expression of many new bacterial genes, including some encoding virulence factors (20). A few bacteria may also become intracellular; this is commonly seen in cell culture systems, but the extent of its occurrence and its importance in vivo remains controversial. In cultured epithelial cells, *H. pylori* enters by a zipper-like mechanism (21) and survives in multivesicular vacuoles (22). It can also survive in vitro in monocytes (23) and neutrophils (24) but the relevance of this in vivo remains unclear.

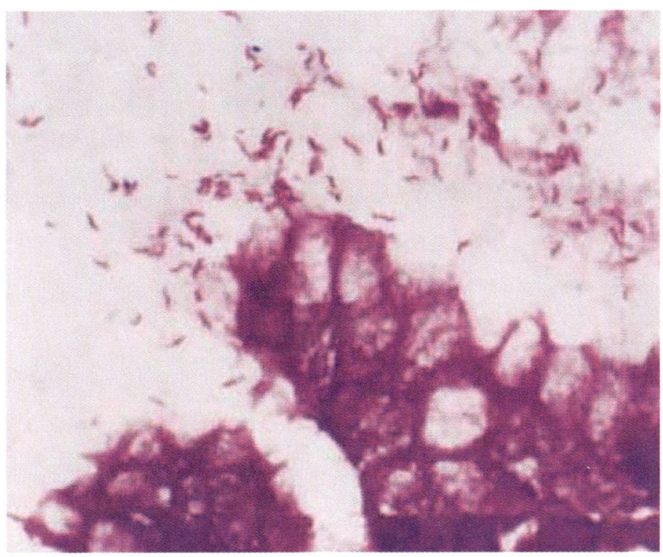

Figure 2

Light micrograph of *Helicobacter pylori* in association with the gastric mucosa. Note that most bacteria are free-swimming in the mucus, but a proportion is closely associated with the epithelial surface. This close association is essential for pathogenesis. (Image kindly donated by Marjorie M. Walker, Department of Histopathology, Imperial College, London, UK.)

Helicobacter pylori–Induced Inflammation and Evasion of the Immune Response

All strains of *H. pylori* induce a marked immune response with local neutrophil, lymphocyte and other inflammatory cell infiltration, and both local and systemic antibody production and cell-mediated responses. This is important in pathogenesis but ineffective at clearing the infection. Many *H. pylori* proteins, particularly urease (25, 26) and a bacterioferritin named HP-NAP (*H. pylori* neutrophil-activating protein) (27, 28), contribute to the genesis of inflammation. However, inflammation is more intense and disease more likely if the *H. pylori* strain expresses specific virulence factors.

Although *H. pylori* does cause inflammation, the bacteria has both minimized the extent to which it provokes an inflammatory response and developed mechanisms for evading it. It has evolved its lipopolysaccharide and flagellin to minimize recognition by the innate immune system's toll-like receptors (TLR4 and 5, respectively) (29–31). It has also evolved to interfere with local immune responses; for example, it inhibits nitric oxide production by macrophages (32) and downregulates chemokine receptors on neutrophils (33). *H. pylori* also directly blocks immune cell products that kill bacteria; for example, it produces enzymes, such as methionine sulfoxide reductase, that combat bacteriocidal oxidative stress (34). Finally, there is increasing evidence that the organism influences the acquired immune response to render it ineffective in *H. pylori* clearance; this point is discussed later.

Adaptation and Genetic Diversity

H. pylori strains acquire DNA through horizontal acquisition from other strains more frequently than do any other bacterial species. This leads to immense genetic diversity (35). Strains adapt within individual stomachs by exchange, loss, and gain of DNA (36); one study has estimated a mean of 60 small DNA imports per year (37). This genetic variation likely allows adaptation to different niches, including perhaps different gastric microenvironments and different individual human hosts (38). Adaptation and generation of diversity also appears important for persistence: In an animal model, mutations that block genetic adaptation lead to a polarized T helper (Th)-1-type response rather than a Th2 response, which in turn leads to early clearance of infection (39).

PATHOGENESIS: WHY DO ONLY SOME INFECTIONS RESULT IN DISEASE?

All strains of *H. pylori* persist lifelong and all cause gastric inflammation. However, only 15% of infections result in peptic ulceration and only 0.5%–2% in gastric adenocarcinoma. Who develops disease depends upon three factors: (*a*) the virulence of the infecting *H. pylori* strain, (*b*) the type and extent of the host immune response to infection, and (*c*) modulating cofactors such as smoking and diet. *H. pylori* virulence factors may damage epithelial cells directly or stimulate them to produce proinflammatory cytokines, thus inducing inflammation. Infections causing high-level inflammation increase the risk of all *H. pylori*–induced diseases. Which disease develops depends upon the type and distribution of inflammation in the stomach. The determinants of the distribution of inflammation in the stomach are unclear, but host genetics have a proven role, and environmental and strain factors may also be important. People with *H. pylori*–induced duodenal ulcers are less likely than others to develop gastric adenocarcinoma later in life (40), implying that *H. pylori* infection predisposes an individual to one or another of these diseases, but not usually to both.

Bacterial Virulence Factors

The cytotoxin-associated gene pathogenicity island and cytotoxin-associated gene A. The name of the cytotoxin-associated gene (*cag*) pathogenicity island (PAI) is misleading because (*a*) the vacuolating cytotoxin gene, *vacA*, is on a different part of the *H. pylori* genome, and (*b*) both the expression and toxin activity of VacA are independent of the *cag* PAI. PAIs are large sections of DNA that are acquired by bacterial species and render them pathogenic. The *cag* PAI, which contains approximately 30 genes, was acquired by *H. pylori* distantly in its evolution from an unknown source and inserted into its glutamate racemase gene (41). Strains may either possess the whole PAI (*cag*+), lack it entirely (*cag*-), or have parts of it deleted; these latter strains are usually phenotypically similar to *cag*- strains (42). Proportions of *cag*+, *cag*−, and intermediate strains vary in different countries, but in all countries *cag*+ strains predominate and in many, such as Japan and China, they are virtually ubiquitous. In large disease association studies, one of the PAI genes, *cagA*, or, alternatively, a serological response to the CagA protein, has been used as a marker of the *cag* PAI. *cagA*+ strains are more commonly associated with both peptic ulceration and gastric adenocarcinoma than *cagA*- strains, which are rarely, if ever, disease-associated (43–46). The high prevalence of *cagA*+ strains in countries like Japan may contribute to the high incidence of *H. pylori*–associated diseases, such as gastric adenocarcinoma, in these countries.

Genes in the *cag* PAI encode proteins that comprise a type IV secretion system (T4SS) used for translocating bacterial products directly into the host cell cytoplasm (41). The T4SS can be visualized microscopically as a sheathed, rigid needle linking *H. pylori* to the epithelial cell (47, 48). The protein CagA is translocated through this needle into epithelial cells (29, 49–52), where it is phosphorylated on tyrosine residues by host cell Src family kinases and stimulates cell-signaling pathways (53, 54) (**Figure 3**). The most obvious effect in vitro is stimulation of cell-shape change such that the cell elongates and develops long processes. This has been termed the hummingbird phenotype (49, 69). These and other non-*cag*-dependent (49, 70) cytoskeletal changes may be important in forming close interactions between bacteria and cells (49, 71). Interestingly, one study has shown that hummingbird changes are dependent upon CagA-induced activation of the hepatocyte growth factor receptor c-Met, which is an oncogene (56). A second major effect of CagA is stimulation of transcription factors involved in multiple cell functions, including cellular proliferation, through activation of c-Fos and c-Jun (62, 65). Unregulated CagA signaling can lead to apoptosis (67), but activated (phosphorylated) CagA inhibits the Src kinase that phosphorylates it, thus creating a negative-feedback loop and perhaps minimizing such uncontrolled effects (54, 67). In vivo, *cag*+ *H. pylori* is associated with epithelial proliferation, but it is unclear whether it is predominantly pro- (72) or anti-apoptotic (73). It is important to determine which is the case; a disrupted balance in favor of apoptosis may affect epithelial restitution and ulcer healing, whereas uncontrolled proliferation may predispose to carcinogenesis. A final function of CagA, which is not dependant upon its tyrosine phosphorylation, is to disrupt apical junctional complexes between epithelial cells, resulting in loss of barrier function (55). This may benefit the bacteria by allowing nutrient transfer and could also be pathogenic through destroying the epithelial cell barrier.

Most strains express the CagA protein, but the protein differs in structure between strains. Firstly, the CagA protein may have between zero and five active tyrosine phosphorylation sites; more sites lead to higher levels of CagA phosphorylation in epithelial cells and more profound cytoskeletal change (59, 74). Strains with more sites are more commonly isolated from people with precancerous gastric changes (e.g., atrophy and intestinal metaplasia) and with gastric cancer (74–76).

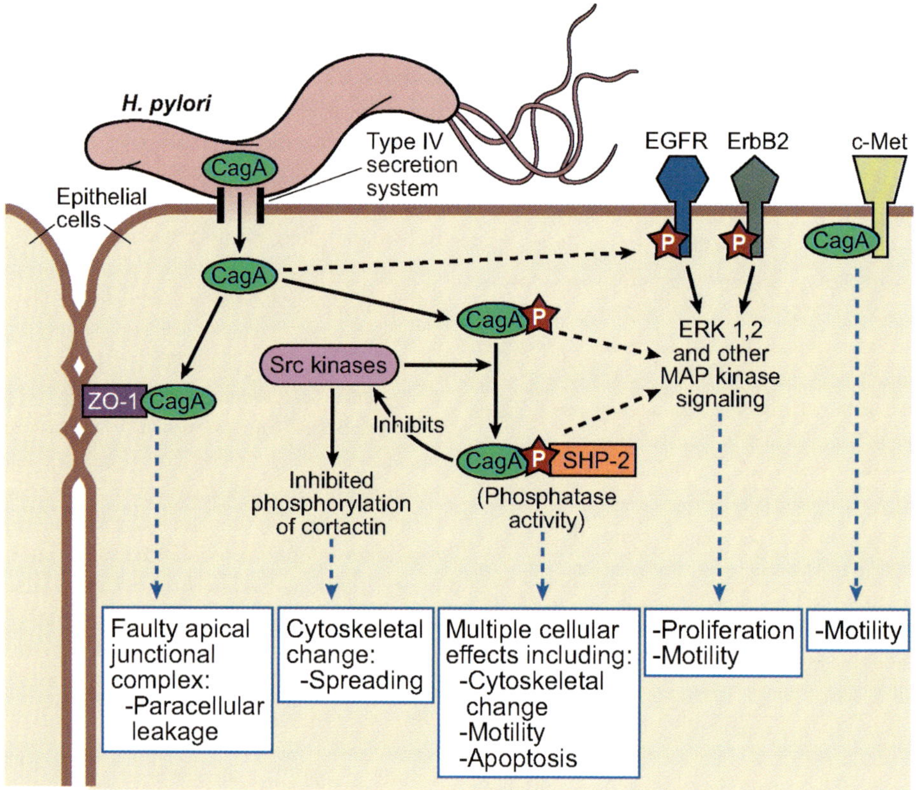

Figure 3

CagA signaling and effects in epithelial cells. The green oval is the CagA protein. Red Ps represent tyrosine phosphorylation. Dashed black lines show activation where precise pathways are unclear. Dashed blue lines and blue boxes show end effects of CagA on the epithelial cell. CagA is translocated through a bacterial type IV secretion system directly into the epithelial cytoplasm, where it is phosphorylated on tyrosine residues by host cell Src kinases. Phosphorylated CagA binds to and activates SHP-2 phosphatase (Src homology 2–containing protein-tyrosine phosphatase-2), which leads to widespread dephosphorylation of host proteins and multiple cellular effects. These effects are downregulated, however, by inhibition by phosphorylated CagA of the Src kinases that activated it. Other effects of Src kinases are also downregulated, leading to cytoskeletal changes. CagA binds to the zona occludens 1 protein (ZO-1), affecting junctional complexes and epithelial integrity. It transactivates the epidermal growth factor receptor (EGFR) and similar receptors leading to extracellular signal-regulated protein kinase (ERK) signaling and ultimately to activator protein-1 (AP-1)–mediated pro-proliferative effects. ERK and JNK (c-Jun N-terminal kinase) MAP (mitogen-activated protein) kinase pathways are also activated by phosphorylated CagA. Finally, CagA associates with the c-Met receptor as an adaptor protein and this is necessary for epithelial cell motility. Effects differ somewhat between different cell lines, and it is not clear which effects are most pertinent in vivo (53–68).

Secondly, CagA from East Asian strains has a different binding site for the signaling protein SHP-2 (see **Figure 3**) and binds this protein more avidly, thus inducing higher levels of cytoskeletal change. Such strains are associated with higher levels of inflammation and atrophy and are more likely to be isolated from patients with gastric cancer (77).

The main neutrophil-attracting chemokine in *H. pylori* gastritis is interleukin (IL)-8, and *cag*+ strains induce higher levels of IL-8 production in epithelial cells than *cag*– strains. This effect is dependent upon expression of at least mainly intact *cag*-encoded T4SS, but is not dependent upon CagA translocation and phosphorylation (66, 78). Contact between the *cag*-encoded T4SS and epithelial cells allows soluble components of the bacterial peptidoglycan cell wall, known as muramyl dipeptides, to enter the cell; these peptides are detected by Nod1, part of the cell's system for recognizing intracellular bacteria (79). This detection then stimulates signaling through nuclear factor κB (NFκB) activation and nuclear translocation (79–81), which in turn leads to transcription of various genes, including those encoding IL-8, human β-defensin 2 (82), anti-apoptotic factors (83), and matrix metalloproteinases 7 and 9 (81, 84). The importance of the *cag* PAI for inflammation and disease has been demonstrated in the Mongolian gerbil model. *H. pylori*–infected gerbils develop gastric ulcers, precancerous gastric changes, and ultimately, in some cases, gastric adenocarcinoma. Infection with an isogenic mutant strain unable to make the T4SS results in none of these effects (85).

In summary, the *cag* PAI is needed for disease, but not all *cag*+ strains are disease-associated. The *cag*-encoded T4SS induces inflammation independently of CagA, and this inflammation is necessary for disease. Strains that deliver more active CagA are more commonly associated with precancerous changes and cancer. Unfortunately, however, this association between strain pathogenicity and disease is complicated by the fact that strains can evolve to change their pathogenicity. The size and importance of this effect is undetermined, but individual examples have been found of strains losing the *cag* PAI or gaining or losing CagA tyrosine phosphorylation sites within individual stomachs (86, 87). Such evolution could potentially benefit *H. pylori* by allowing adaption to a changing gastric niche. However, the implications for pathogenesis remain unclear.

The vacuolating cytotoxin. Unlike the *cag* PAI, the vacuolating cytotoxin gene, *vacA*, is present in all strains. However, it is polymorphic, varying most markedly in two regions termed the mid- and signal regions (88, 89) (**Figure 4**). The main signal region types are s1 and s2, and the mid-region types are m1 and m2. The *vacA* gene may comprise any combination of signal and mid-region types, although the s2/m1 combination is rare (89, 90). The importance of type-s2 *vacA* is that its product is virtually nontoxic (89, 91) and among s1-type *vacA*, s1/m1 is toxic for a wider range of cells than s1/m2 (91, 92). In observational studies in humans, *vacA* s2-type strains are rarely associated with disease (93–96). Although both *vacA* s1/m1- and s1/m2-type strains may be disease-associated, where both are common, patients with gastric adenocarcinoma usually have the s1/m1-type of *vacA* (97–99). In Japan, s1/m1-type *vacA* is ubiquitous, perhaps contributing to the high incidence of gastric adenocarcinoma. In the few instances where strains are nontoxic in Japan, this is owing usually to inactivating mutations in s1/m1-type *vacA* rather than the occurrence of other types (100).

vacA is translated into a pre-protoxin, which is an autotransporter that undergoes N- and C-terminal cleavage during bacterial secretion (101) (**Figure 4**). The mature secreted toxin comprises two subunits, which remain associated. Both are required for toxin activity, and the larger p58 subunit mediates binding of the toxin to the epithelial cell. Studies of the toxin and its effects on cells have concentrated on in vitro effects of the most active (and most disease-associated) s1/m1 form. VacA can be transferred to epithelial cells either by secretion or by contact-dependent transfer, which may be a more efficient method (102). It can bind to several epithelial cell receptors: (*a*) receptor protein tyrosine phosphatase (RPTP) β and α (103–105), (*b*) the epidermal growth factor receptor (EGFR) (106), and (*c*) a glycosylphosphatidylinositol (GPI)-anchored protein associated with lipid rafts (107, 108). In vitro, VacA is internalized by endocytosis (108). Both internalization and subsequent effects are dependent upon acid

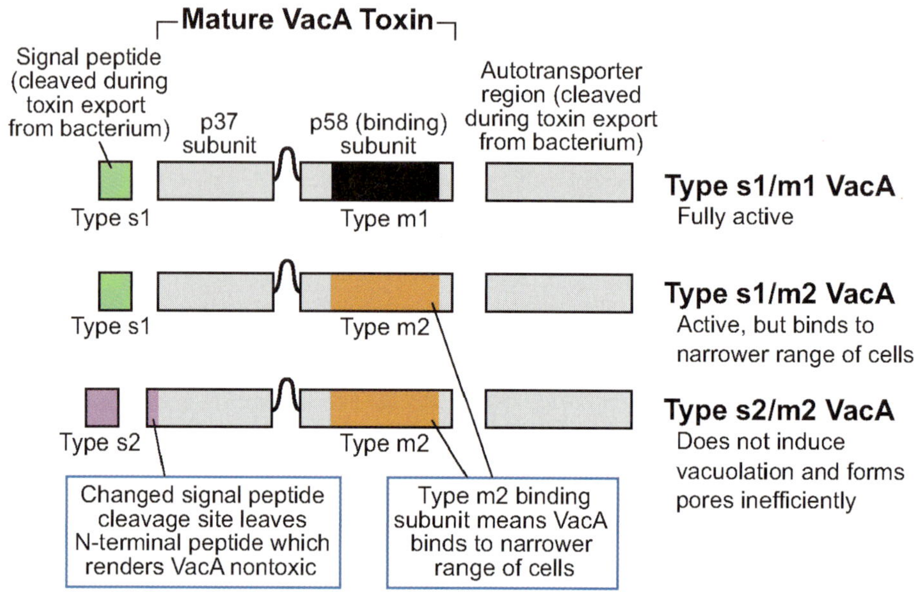

Figure 4

Polymorphism in the vacuolating cytotoxin protein, VacA, between *Helicobacter pylori* strains. The *vacA* gene varies most markedly in the signal region (encoding the signal peptide), which may be type s1 or s2, and in the mid-region (encoding part of the p58 binding subunit), which may be type m1 or m2. Three types of toxin are commonly found: s1/m1, s1/m2, and s2/m2 (the s2/m1 combination occurs but is rare).

activation of VacA, making the toxin particularly well suited to the stomach (109, 110).

VacA is a pore-forming toxin (111), and this action underlies many of its other effects, including vacuolation (112) (**Figure 5**). VacA forms hexameric pores, which are selective to anions and small neutral molecules, including urea. This urea permease activity may be an important aid to acid survival through providing a substrate for urease (113). When surface pores are endocytosed, they become processed into late-endosomal compartments (114), which then undergo osmotic swelling to become large acidic vacuoles. Whereas this vacuolation is the most obvious effect of VacA in vitro, is not marked in vivo. This fact has led to interest in other VacA functions. One important effect may be increased paracellular permeability and potential nutrient acquisition (115). Such a role would fit well with the

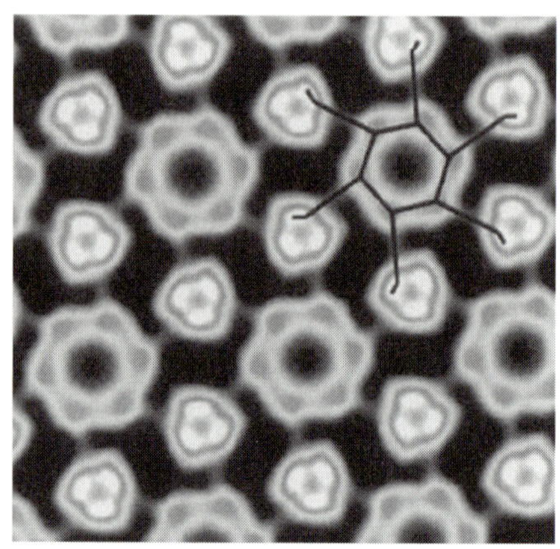

Figure 5

Atomic force microscopy image of the vacuolating cytotoxin, VacA, on an artificial lipid membrane. The "flowers" represent anion-selective membrane pores. The line drawing in the top right corner shows a VacA hexamer with a diameter of 28 nm. (Reproduced with permission from Reference 111. Copyright 1999 National Academy of Sciences USA.)

expression of *vacA* in nutrient-depleted conditions such as iron starvation (116). Another interesting effect of VacA is induction of apoptosis (117, 118) at least partly through a novel mechanism of toxin-induced pore formation in mitochondria that allows cytochrome c release (119, 120). However, high concentrations are needed for this effect; consequently, there is some doubt about its importance in vivo (120). More subtle effects include interference with cell signaling, as VacA stimulates p38 and ERK1/2 MAP kinases (121).

VacA causes epithelial damage in mouse models both when given orally as a single agent (101) and when delivered by a toxigenic strain of *H. pylori* during gastric infection (122). Interestingly, mice null for the VacA receptor RPTPβ do not develop ulcers (123) and work in vitro shows that, although cells lacking this receptor can still take up VacA and undergo vacuolation, both cell signaling and detachment from a basement membrane are blocked (123). Although VacA is not needed for proinflammatory signaling by epithelial cells, it may induce cytokine release from other cell types [for example, mast cells (124)]. However, recent interest has focused more on the immunosuppressive rather than the immunostimulatory effects of VacA. In vitro, VacA can interfere with antigen presentation, which occurs in compartments that are similar to late endosomes (125). More surprisingly, it can specifically inhibit T cell activation and proliferation (126–128). This observation has led to speculation that VacA may help prevent clearance of highly host-interactive (*cag*+) *H. pylori* strains. In support of this (or at least some gain of function for possessing both the *cag* PAI and an active form of VacA), possession of the *cag* PAI and expression of an active s1 form of the cytotoxin are closely associated features of *H. pylori* strains.

Some forms of VacA are nontoxic and less often associated with disease (**Figure 4**). The s2 form has a short N-terminal peptide extension on the mature protein. This extension blocks vacuolating activity (91, 129), leads to slower, less effective pore formation (130), and does not cause apoptosis (118). The s1/m1 form is fully active, but the sl/m2 form binds to and vacuolates a narrow range of epithelial cell types; this activity is a direct consequence of changes in the binding subunit encoded by the *vacA* m region (91, 92). Less active forms of *vacA* are maintained in the *H. pylori* population, but their benefit to *H. pylori* is unclear. Interestingly, *H. pylori* can evolve through recombination to change its toxicity (131), potentially allowing adaptation and changing levels of host interaction. However, the frequency with which this recombination occurs and its importance in pathogenesis remain undefined.

***Helicobacter pylori* adhesion and blood group antigen-binding adhesin A.** Although most *H. pylori* organisms are freeliving in gastric mucus, a small proportion adhere to epithelial cells. Adhesion is, at least in part through binding to blood group antigens, expressed on gastric epithelial cells. The most important of these antigens is Lewis b (132). Lewis b expression in the stomach is associated with higher *H. pylori* density; in stomachs not expressing Lewis b, expression of other blood group antigens such as Lewis x and Lewis a also increase bacterial density, but to a lesser extent (133). Transgenic mice expressing human Lewis b develop gastritis and gastric ulcer, whereas wild-type mice do not, confirming the importance of both Lewis b and bacterial-epithelial adhesion for disease (134). Lewis x binding is mediated by the *H. pylori* sialic-acid-binding adhesin, SabA (135), but research has concentrated on Lewis b binding through the blood group antigen-binding adhesin (BabA) (136). Strains possessing the gene *babA2*, which encodes active BabA, are associated with increased epithelial proliferation and inflammation and also increased risk for duodenal ulcer, gastric atrophy, intestinal metaplasia, and gastric adenocarcinoma (137–139). Lewis b binding can change by mutation through several mechanisms. For example, *babA2* can be lost during experimental infection in Macaque monkeys (140). In vitro, if *babA2* is disrupted, bacteria can regain the Lewis b binding phenotype by recombining a nonexpressed homolog, *babA1*, into another locus, *babB*, where it is then expressed (141, 142). There is good evidence that binding of *H. pylori* has evolved in specific human populations to adapt to that population: In indigenous South American populations, which are blood group O, *H. pylori* strains have evolved BabA to bind blood group O antigens best (38).

Outer inflammatory protein A. Outer inflammatory protein A (OipA) is an outer membrane protein of *H. pylori* that contributes to the induction of IL-8 production by epithelial cells (143). It is present in all strains, but variable numbers of dinucleotide repeats in its 5′ region mean that an active protein may or may not be produced because of a common mutational adaption system in bacteria known as slipped strand mispairing (143). "On" status is associated in vivo with increased bacterial density, increased IL-8 levels in the gastric mucosa, increased neutrophil infiltration and duodenal ulceration, but not with atrophy (143).

Induced-by-contact-with-epithelium gene A and *Helicobacter pylori* methylases. Contact of *H. pylori* with epithelium induces transcription of the induced-by-contact-with-epithelium gene (*iceA1*), and presence of this gene rather than a distant homologue, *iceA2*, has been associated with duodenal ulceration (DU) and gastric adenocarcinoma (144, 145). The role of *iceA1* in pathogenesis is not obvious, as it does not usually encode a functional protein and has homology with a restriction endonuclease gene in other bacteria. As restriction endonucleases act as bacterial defense agents that break down foreign bacterial DNA, they are not usually associated with pathogenesis. Consequently, disease associations with the *iceA* genes may be chance findings. However, an alternative possibility is that expression of the methylase *hpy1M*, which accompanies *iceA1* (all restriction enzymes are associated with a specific methylase to protect self-DNA from the restriction enzyme activity), may be important. Methylases have a demonstrated role in virulence in *Salmonella typhimurium* (146). In *H. pylori*, the presence of *iceA1* leads to higher expression of its cognate methylase gene, *hpyIM*, than does the presence of *iceA2* (147). Another *H. pylori* methylase gene, *hpyIIIM*, can also be differentially transcribed depending upon the gene in the immediate upstream locus (148). However, in this case, methylase function is lost via the replacement of *hpyIIIM* by the *H. pylori* restriction endonuclease replacing gene A (*hrg)*; this genotype has been weakly associated with cancer in Asian populations (148, 149). Further studies are needed to confirm whether methylation has a direct role in *H. pylori* virulence.

Host Genetic Polymorphisms and *Helicobacter pylori*–Induced Disease

Polymorphisms in human cytokine genes affect the level of cytokine production by cells after contact with *H. pylori*. Specific polymorphisms in the *IL-1β* gene and the IL-1 receptor-antagonist gene (*IL-1RN*) lead to increased gastric mucosal levels of IL-1β in individuals infected with *H. pylori* (150, 151) and increased levels of inflammation (150–154). The polymorphisms also increase the risk of gastric atrophy, achlorhydria, intestinal metaplasia (151, 152, 154, 155), and distal gastric adenocarcinoma (46, 153, 155–158). The effect of these polymorphisms on duodenal ulcer risk is uncertain; one report showed an increased risk with proinflammatory polymorphisms (159), but another showed a reduced risk (152). Such a reduced risk would be logical for people with an atrophic, hypochlorhydric stomach. Although polymorphisms affecting IL-1β levels are best studied, others also appear important. Tumor necrosis factor α (*TNFa*) polymorphisms have not been demonstrated to affect gastric mucosal levels of TNFα (151), but they have been shown to affect gastric inflammation and cancer risk in some (153, 157) but not all (151, 158) studies. Polymorphisms affecting the immunosuppressive cytokine IL-10 affect mucosal levels and may lead to colonization by more virulent *H. pylori* strains (151); they also increase gastric cancer risk (157). IL-1β, TNFα, and *H. pylori* all induce IL-8 secretion by epithelial cells; an IL-8 polymorphism causing increased IL-8 production in vitro has been associated with an enhanced risk of gastric adenocarcinoma and gastric ulcer in a Japanese population (160).

Carriage of multiple proinflammatory polymorphisms increases the level of gastric inflammation associated with *H. pylori* infection and the risk of atrophy, intestinal metaplasia, and gastric carcinoma (153, 157). As expected, infection with *H. pylori* strains possessing known virulence factors further increases these risks (46, 154). Individuals with both multiple proinflammatory cytokine polymorphisms and the most virulent *H. pylori* strains can have up to fiftyfold increased risk of gastric cancer as compared with individuals lacking these factors.

Importance of the Immune Response in Pathogenesis

H. pylori–induced inflammation is central to the pathogenesis of all *H. pylori*–associated diseases. It is increased by proinflammatory cytokine polymorphisms and by bacterial virulence factors such as the *cag* PAI and OipA. It is also modulated by T helper cells, which control the type of response and its cytokine profile. Acquired immune responses to micro-organisms can be predominantly Th-1 (mainly cell mediated) or Th-2 (mainly antibody dependent). *H. pylori* stimulates both responses, although gastric mucosal cytokine profiles suggest that the Th-1 response predominates (**Figure 6**) (161, 162). The Th-1 response is important in the pathogenesis of *H. pylori*–induced disease. Mice either genetically prone to or manipulated to have a Th-1 response (for example, IL-4 null mice) develop more intense *H. pylori* gastritis (163, 164). T cell transfer experiments show that Th-1 cells are directly responsible (163). Mice genetically manipulated to have a Th-1 response develop inflammation, epithelial apoptosis, and disruption of cell organization in gastric glands even in the absence of *H. pylori* (165). In contrast, mice deficient in T cell responses do not show these changes. Even infusion of the Th-1 cytokine interferon-γ (IFN-γ) alone induces gastric inflammation and atrophy, although effects are enhanced with helicobacter coinfection (166). In addition,

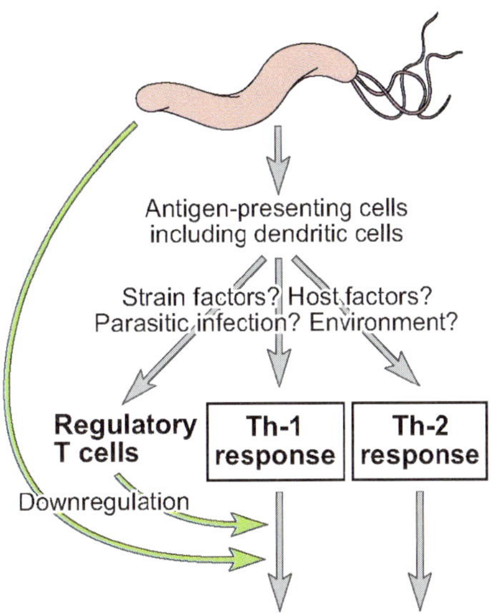

	Th-1	Th-2
H. pylori density	Low	High
Gastritis	Severe	Mild
Atrophy and cancer risk	High	Low

Figure 6

The central role of the T helper (Th)-cell response to *Helicobacter pylori* infection. Th-1, Th-2, and regulatory T cells are activated, but the balance of the response varies between people owing to unknown factors. Studies in animal models and supportive data in humans (*see text*) show that a strong Th-1 response increases severity of gastritis and cancer risk. Both *H. pylori* and the host downregulate this Th-1 response. This potentially benefits *H. pylori* by allowing more dense colonization and benefits the host by downregulating mucosal inflammation.

IFN-γ–deficient mice have less inflammation and less atrophy when infected with helicobacter (164, 167, 168), a result that further confirms the importance of IFN-γ.

H. pylori appears to induce a Th-1 response by interaction with dendritic cells. In vitro, *H. pylori* coculture with dendritic cells induces maturation and activation of high-level IL-12 production, characteristic of a Th-1 response. This effect is at least partially dependent upon the presence of the *cag* PAI (169, 170). Once matured, dendritic cells are also resistant to *H. pylori*–induced apoptosis; this resistance potentially allows these cells to fulfil their T helper–directing function (171).

An unregulated Th-1 response is potentially deleterious to *H. pylori*, as bacterial density is reduced (163, 172–174). *H. pylori* appears to have adapted to downregulate the Th-1 response it induces, possibly to avoid clearance. *H. pylori* strains expressing Lewis antigens on their lipopolysaccharide bind the dendritic cell-specific intracellular adhesion molecule-3 (ICAM3)-grabbing nonintegrin (DCSIGN) lectin on gastric dendritic cells and thus block Th-1 cell development. Interestingly, Lewis-negative variants do not bind DCSIGN; these strains induce a strong Th-1 response, which suggests rapid adaption of *H. pylori* to modulate the T helper–cell balance (175). *H. pylori* also activates Cox-2 in mononuclear cells, which reduces Th-1 polarization (176). Regulatory T cells may downregulate the Th-1 response: T-memory-cells from *H. pylori*–infected people proliferate and produce IFN-γ less effectively than those from *H. pylori*–uninfected people; this phenomenon is dependent upon regulatory T cell activity, as depletion of regulatory T cells abolishes the effect and addition of regulatory T cells induces it (177). Finally, the Th-1 response can be downregulated by external factors. The *Helicobacter felis*–infected mouse model has been immunologically manipulated by experimental helminth coinfection; this leads to increased *H. pylori* density, but reduced Th-1 cytokine levels and no gastric atrophy (172). It has been suggested that the high incidence in Africa of parasitic infections, which suppress Th-1 responses, may explain the so-called African enigma—the low incidence of *H. pylori*–associated disease in Africa despite high *H. pylori* prevalence.

The Role of Hormonal Changes and Acid Homeostasis in the Pathogenesis of Ulcers and Gastric Adenocarcinoma

***Helicobacter pylori*–induced hormonal changes and their importance in disease.** *H. pylori* infection is associated with reduced numbers of somatostatin-producing D cells in the stomach and reduced somatostatin production (178–180). This may be partly due to suppression of somatostatin release by inflammatory mediators, including nitric oxide (181). Hypergastrinemia develops because gastrin production from G cells is released from its usual negative feedback by somatostatin; a direct stimulatory action of cytokines on G cells may also contribute (**Figure 7**) (179). In a mouse model, the Th-1 cytokine IFN-γ induces hypergastrinemia and reduces somatostatin levels (182). The gastritis induced in this model is reversed by administering the somatostatin analogue octreotide, implying that Th-1 responses drive inflammation through hormonal changes. Direct evidence of the importance of hypergastrinemia in disease comes from the gastrin-overexpressing INS-GAS mouse model. These mice have increased acid secretion, but in later life develop reduced acid secretion, gastric atrophy, and gastric adenocarcinoma (183). These phenomena occur even in the absence of helicobacter infection, although its presence considerably speeds the process. In the *H. pylori*–infected gerbil model, the course of hypergastrinemia development correlates with epithelial cell proliferation, which may underlie the rapid progression to atrophy (184). Hypergastrinemia has a number of other potentially prooncogenic effects such as upregulation of the Cox-2 gene through MAP kinase stimulation (185) and upregulation of expression of the Reg protein, which is involved in gastric atrophy (186).

Recent research suggests further hormonal effects of *H. pylori* through altering the production of leptin by chief and parietal cells and the production of ghrelin in oxyntic glands. Leptin and ghrelin have local effects on gastric acid production. More importantly, however, leptin has a satiety-signaling effect, whereas ghrelin provides a signal to increase food intake and reduce physical activity. Gastric leptin levels drop and ghrelin levels increase after *H. pylori* treatment (187–189); if these changes reflect long-term effects of *H. pylori*, the result of colonization may be a thinner body habitus. This hypothesis is extremely speculative, as long-term effects of *H. pylori* on leptin, ghrelin, and their effects are unknown; however, research in this area is important, as there are potential implications for obesity-related diseases (7).

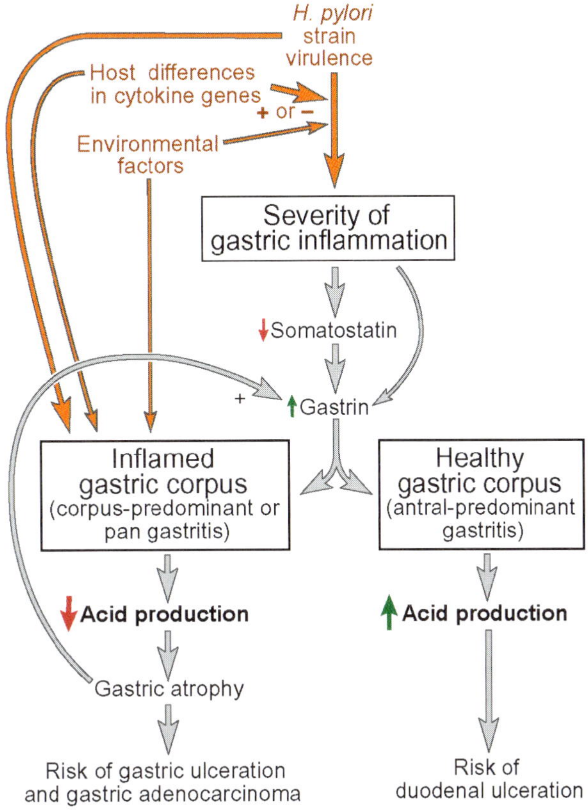

Figure 7

The key factors underlying *Helicobacter pylori*–associated disease (*boxed*) and the external effects modulating them (*orange*). *H. pylori* induces inflammation, but strain, host, and environmental factors may modulate its severity. High-level inflammation increases the risk of all *H. pylori*–associated diseases. The effects of the resultant hypergastrinemia differ according to whether the gastric corpus is inflamed. Host cytokine polymorphisms affect the pattern of inflammation in the stomach but environmental and strain determinants may also contribute. Research has concentrated on factors that influence inflammation in the corpus and so increase gastric cancer risk. Relatively little is known about factors that lead to a lack of inflammation in the corpus and affect duodenal ulcer risk.

Pathogenesis of duodenal ulceration. DU is associated with dense *H. pylori* infection and severe inflammation (190), but only when inflammation occurs in an antral-predominant pattern. The reason some people develop this pattern of inflammation remains unclear, but the hormonal changes associated with antral-predominant inflammation that lead to DU have been studied (**Figure 7**). In people who develop antral-predominant inflammation, *H. pylori*–induced hypergastrinemia leads to an increased maximal acid output, which indicates an increased parietal cell mass (191). The gastric corpus, which contains the parietal cells, is relatively uninflamed, which allows high-level acid production. Hypergastrinemia and the increased acid production it causes are sufficient to cause DU even without *H. pylori*, as occurs in Zollinger-Ellison syndrome (where excess gastrin is produced by a gastrinoma). However, in *H. pylori* infection the bacterium appears to play a further role in ulcerogenesis: Gastric hyperchlorhydria leads to an increased acid load in the duodenum, which subsequently develops protective gastric metaplasia (192, 193). Although *H. pylori* cannot colonize the normal duodenum, it can colonize this gastric metaplastic tissue, and the resulting local inflammation and damage further predispose to DU (193).

Pathogenesis of gastric ulceration. The epidemiology of prepyloric and pyloric ulceration is similar to that of DU, but that of *H. pylori*–induced ulceration elsewhere in the stomach is more similar to that of gastric adenocarcinoma. Unlike DU, gastric ulceration (GU) is associated with a pan-gastritic inflammation pattern and reduced or normal acid production. The pathogenesis of GU is poorly understood, but GUs arise most commonly at the transitional zone between antrum and corpus on the lesser gastric curve. This area in particular can be densely colonized by *H. pylori* and become heavily inflamed (194); it is likely that the heavy inflammation and epithelial damage at this site lead directly to ulceration.

Pathogenesis of gastric adenocarcinoma. Gastric adenocarcinoma is associated with pan-gastritis or corpus-predominant gastritis (**Figure 7**). Autoimmune gastritis also has this pattern of inflammation and is an independent risk factor for distal gastric adenocarcinoma. Why *H. pylori*–induced inflammation has a pan-gastritic or corpus-predominant pattern in some people when it is antral-predominant in others is unknown. One possibility is that, like autoimmune gastritis, it may be caused by immune effectors with specificity for the gastric proton pump ATPase. In support of this, T cells have been identified that cross-react between *H. pylori* proteins and the ATPase (195). Pan-gastritis is associated with reduced acid secretion, despite hypergastrinemia (196) (**Figure 7**). This association is due partly to a loss of gastric glands (atrophy). However, *H. pylori* treatment increases acid production rapidly in some people with pan-gastritis and hypochlorhydria (although not usually to normal levels) (196). This result implies a direct suppressive effect of *H. pylori*–induced inflammatory mediators or products. IL-1β is a known acid suppressant; it, TNFα (197), and, in a recent report, the Th-1 cytokines IFN-γ and IL-12 (198) suppress acid production in isolated rabbit parietal cells. Acid suppression by auto-antibodies against the proton pump, increased cytokine production in the gastric corpus, or a combination of these factors further increase hypergastrinemia and so may accelerate development of gastric atrophy and intestinal metaplasia. Proton pump inhibitors (PPIs), drugs used for the profound suppression of acid, both induce a pan-gastritic or corpus-predominant pattern of inflammation and speed atrophy and intestinal metaplasia when used in *H. pylori*–infected people (199). However, there is no evidence so far that use of these drugs has increased gastric cancer incidence. Once acid production is reduced, other bacteria may colonize the stomach and cause further inflammation that may contribute to hypergastrinemia; interestingly, in a mouse model, PPI-induced hypergastrinemia could be reversed fully by treatment with antibiotics (200).

Adenocarcinoma can arise in the atrophic stomach regardless of whether the atrophy is induced by *H. pylori* or by autoimmune mechanisms. This implies that the role of *H. pylori* is principally in inducing atrophy, which is then in itself a precancerous state. This is supported by a large *H. pylori* eradication study, in which *H. pylori* eradication appeared to prevent later cancer development in patients that did not have atrophy and intestinal metaplasia, but not in patients who already had these premalignant conditions (201). Also, *H. pylori* density is much reduced in the atrophic stomach, so direct *H. pylori*–induced effects there should also be reduced.

Carcinogenesis in the environment of gastric atrophy is likely owing to reactive oxygen and nitrogen species secondary to the accompanying inflammation, and possibly partly caused by overgrowth of other bacteria in the now achlorhydric stomach (200). In a mouse model, mutations in epithelial cell DNA are characteristic of such oxidative damage (202), and inducible nitric oxide synthase–deficient mice are less likely to develop cancer following *H. pylori* infection and chemical carcinogen challenge than normal mice (203). Also, chemoprevention trials using antioxidants in patients with atrophy or intestinal metaplasia show some regression of these conditions (204), and high ascorbic acid levels, which are antioxidant, are associated with lower levels of gastric cancer development in humans (205).

Other mechanisms of carcinogenesis have also been either demonstrated or implied in the atrophic stomach. Parietal cells express the Sonic hedgehog protein, which is the main organizer of cell polarity in gastric pits. Sonic hedgehog expression is lost in atrophy and intestinal metaplasia (206), and mice engineered to have parietal cell ablation develop epithelial disorganisation and amplification of epithelial progenitors. This disruption potentially exposes stem cells to mutagenic agents (207). The intestinal metaplasia that develops in the atrophic stomach comprises a widespread metaplastic cell lineage in both rodents and man and can be recognized by its expression of Trefoil factor 2 (208). The contention that carcinoma develops directly from intestinal metaplasia is supported by a transgenic mouse model expressing the Cdx-2 protein. These mice develop extensive intestinal metaplasia in the stomach and malignant changes within the intestinal metaplastic epithelium (209). A startling and important recent finding is that the metaplastic and neoplastic cells arising in the stomach of the *H. pylori*–infected mouse appear to be derived from bone marrow; this finding has important implications for carcinogenesis in the stomach and elsewhere (210).

Although cancer can arise in the atrophic stomach without *H. pylori*, there is some evidence that direct interaction of *H. pylori* with the epithelium may confer an additive or alternative risk. Firstly, the less common diffuse type of gastric adenocarcinoma, which is not addressed in the studies mentioned above and often affects younger adults (211), can arise directly in inflamed nonatrophic mucosa. Secondly, in animal models such as the hypergastrinemic INS-GAS mouse, carcinogenesis is speeded by helicobacter infection. Thirdly, human trials have shown that *H. pylori* treatment in patients with atrophy and intestinal metaplasia may slow the progression of changes, if not halt them (204, 212). Finally, recent reports suggest that *H. pylori* may survive and express virulence factors intracellularly in metaplastic, dysplastic, and neoplastic epithelial cells in vivo, although these reports need further confirmation (213).

Following the theory that direct oncogenic effects of *H. pylori* do contribute to

HELICOBACTER PYLORI AND GASTRIC LYMPHOMA

The uninfected stomach has no mucosa-associated lymphoid tissue (MALT), so its acquisition depends upon infection with helicobacter species, usually *H. pylori*. The risk factors for its transformation into low-grade extranodal B cell lymphoma of MALT (MALT lymphoma) are poorly defined: *cag*+ strains do not increase risk markedly (237–240), but low-grade MALT lymphomas do usually arise in the context of a pan-gastritic inflammation pattern (241). In vitro, proliferation of clonal B cells is driven by the presence of non-neoplastic T cells, whose effects in turn are dependant upon the presence of *H. pylori* (242). *H. pylori* also appears to act through direct antigen stimulation of tumor cells (243). In humans, remarkably, eradication of *H. pylori* frequently leads to regression of these low-grade lymphomas (244, 245). The natural history of MALT lymphomas is that they are only very slowly progressive, but they sometimes undergo high-grade transformation to diffuse large-cell B cell lymphomas. These lymphomas have mutations consistent with oxidative damage and are more commonly associated with *cag*+ *H. pylori* strain infection and a more inflamed stomach (238, 239). High-grade lymphomas rarely regress following *H. pylori* treatment. Recently, a subgroup of low-grade B cell MALT lymphomas (approximately 25%) have been found to have a translocation from chromosome 11 to 18 (246, 247). This causes a specific fusion between the activator protein-12 (*AP-12*) and *MALT-1* genes that creates a new gene (248) whose product stimulates NFκB signaling (249). This is known to be anti-apoptotic and so promotes cell survival. T(11;18)+ lymphomas are relatively locally invasive but rarely undergo high-grade transformation; most importantly, they are unresponsive to *H. pylori* treatment (250, 251). Like t(11;18)+ lymphomas at other sites in the body, these lymphomas arise in association with a neutrophil infiltrate, and, as expected from this fact, they are usually associated with *cag*+ *H. pylori* infection (252).

carcinogenesis in vivo, several potential mechanisms exist. As described earlier, CagA signaling is strongly pro-proliferative, and this effect may not be balanced by increased apoptosis: Although *H. pylori* has proapoptotic effects on cells (214, 215), it also has anti-apoptotic effects including NFκB activation, reduction in p27 levels (216), and downregulation of the TNF-related apoptosis-inducing ligand (TRAIL) system (217). Whether proliferation and anti-apoptotic effects have a direct role in epithelial transformation is unclear, but they do appear important in the pathogenesis of gastric atrophy: Fas-deficient mice, which have impaired apoptosis, develop extensive and severe atrophy (217). Other direct effects of *H. pylori* on gastric epithelial cells that have potential carcinogenic importance are its stimulation of reactive oxygen species (ROS) and oxidative damage (218) and its impairment of DNA mismatch repair (219). However, *H. pylori* also downregulates the oxidative damage it causes by inducing enzymes that scavenge ROS (220), and the host minimizes ROS-induced DNA damage by expressing the oxidative repair proteins Ape-1 and Rel-1 (221). That *H. pylori* needs to protect itself against oxidative damage suggests that the generation of ROS may be a host defense system for inhibiting *H. pylori* metabolism or otherwise damaging *H. pylori* (222, 223).

Protection by *Helicobacter pylori* against severe gastro-esophageal reflux and its complications. The incidence of gastro-esophageal reflux disease (GERD) and its complications, Barrett's esophagus (intestinal metaplasia in the esophagus), and esophageal adenocarcinoma, is rising rapidly in developed countries. Over the same time period, the incidences of gastric adenocarcinoma and peptic ulceration are falling, mimicking the falling prevalence of *H. pylori* infection (224). Epidemiological observations support a link between *H. pylori* and protection against severe GERD. Reflux esophagitis is rare in countries where *H. pylori* infection is common, such as China and Japan. Many association studies have shown that people with complicated reflux disease, including esophageal adenocarcinoma, are less likely than others to have *H. pylori* infection (225, 226). More recently, a case control study nested in a cohort established in 1964 has shown that *H. pylori*–positive subjects are less likely than *H. pylori*–negative subjects to develop esophageal adenocarcinoma (odds ratio 0.37) (227).

If the negative association between *H. pylori* and GERD complications is causal, the most likely mechanism is through effects of *H. pylori* on gastric acid secretion. Although some *H. pylori*–infected individuals have increased acid secretion, a reduction is more common, and thus, at a population level, absence of *H. pylori* should lead to higher mean acid secretion. In patients with GERD, the refluxate would on average be more acidic, which would increase damage caused and thereby increase the population risk of complications, including esophageal adenocarcinoma. Support for this idea comes from studies showing that *cag*+ *H. pylori* infection, which has more profound effects on acid secretion, is associated with less severe esophagitis and a larger reduction in both Barrett's esophagus and esophageal cancer risk (228–230) [although not all reports confirm this observation (227)]. Further support comes from the greater reduction in risk seen in people with corpus-predominant gastritis, atrophy, intestinal metaplasia, and low acid secretion (225, 231, 232). Evidence from intervention studies is less clearcut; after *H. pylori* treatment, some people show a reduction, some show no effect, and some show an increase in reflux symptoms and GERD endoscopic severity. However, such heterogeneity between studies may be predicted, as effects of *H. pylori* treatment on acid secretion would be expected to differ between individuals and populations depending upon pretreatment gastric inflammation pattern, acid secretion, parietal cell mass, and presence and level of gastric atrophy.

HELICOBACTER PYLORI/HUMAN COEVOLUTION: IMPLICATIONS FOR DISEASE AND ITS MANAGEMENT

H. pylori has colonized humans for at least 2500 years, and likely since we first evolved (7, 37); other mammals have their own specialized indigenous gastric helicobacters, implying differential evolution of these bacteria to suit different niches. *H. pylori* has adapted to persist, and this adaptation involved manipulation of both human acquired immunity and gastric physiology. Human gastric physiology has also likely evolved to coexist with *H. pylori*. In many developing countries (probably representing the history of humanity) *H. pylori* is ubiquitous and gastric acid secretion is, on average, reduced. One could regard the acid production in the modern *H. pylori*–free stomach as abnormally high, or at least new for humans. This could contribute to complications of GERD.

That humans have not evolved to clear *H. pylori* infection has led to speculation that the bacterium may confer some benefit. If so, this would most likely be in childhood, as this is when *H. pylori* is usually acquired. Several studies have addressed whether *H. pylori* may protect against other infections, and a negative association has been shown with gastroenteritis (233). Mechanisms and even causality are unclear, but an intriguing possibility is that an increased acid barrier in some people may protect against bacterial infections. As in the INS-GAS hypergastrinemic mouse (234), perhaps *H. pylori*+ children in previous generations had increased acid production, which protected them from infectious disease; reduced acid secretion and its complications in postreproductive adulthood would be evolutionarily neutral.

Whether *H. pylori* confers evolutionary benefit to humans, it is unlikely to confer evolutionary disadvantages. Gastric adenocarcinoma occurs after human reproductive years and DU is a disease of the late nineteenth and twentieth centuries (235, 236). Why duodenal ulcers arose at this time is unclear. However, as *H. pylori* infection is likely to have been ubiquitous before this point, and *H. pylori* virulence and human genetics are unlikely to have changed during the timescale, environmental changes are the most likely cause. One possibility is that the modern stomach produces more acid because it is healthier, possibly owing to increased nutrition, lack of gastric irritants, or perhaps *H. pylori* infection at a later age. The increase in acid production may subsequently predispose humans to antral-predominant infection/inflammation and DU. The advent of smoking may also have been a contributory factor.

The future burden of *H. pylori*–associated diseases is unclear. In many developed countries *H. pylori* prevalence is falling. This reduction is mirrored by a fall in incidence of peptic ulceration and gastric adenocarcinoma with a concomitant rise in reflux esophagitis and its complications, including esophageal adenocarcinoma (224). However, on the basis of current trends, esophageal adenocarcinoma is unlikely to approach previous levels of gastric adenocarcinoma in mankind's *H. pylori*–ubiquitous history. In developing countries, *H. pylori*–associated diseases remain major medical problems, and worldwide, the burden of these problems is increasing because of an aging world population. With modernization, *H. pylori* prevalence in developing countries is likely to decrease eventually, but whether, before that, we will see an increase in ulcer incidence as occurred in developed countries in the past century is unclear. Vaccination is the main hope for rapid intervention, and perhaps prevention of the considerable morbidity from peptic ulceration and the nearly one million deaths per year from gastric cancer. Vaccine research is ongoing, but an effective vaccine has still not been developed. Preventing *H. pylori* infection is likely to do more good than harm, but research is needed before intervention to ensure that this is the case.

SUMMARY POINTS

1. *H. pylori* infection causes peptic ulceration, gastric adenocarcinoma, and gastric lymphoma. It may protect against complications of gastro-esophageal reflux disease.
2. Pathogenesis depends upon persistent infection over decades.
3. Which infections result in disease depends upon bacterial virulence, host genetic susceptibility, and environmental factors.
4. Strains possessing the *cag* PAI are more pro-inflammatory, more pro-proliferative, and more likely to cause disease.
5. The vacuolating cytotoxin VacA causes epithelial damage, and *H. pylori* strains expressing more active forms of VacA are more likely to cause disease.
6. Host proinflammatory cytokine polymorphisms predispose *H. pylori*–infected people to gastric adenocarcinoma.
7. *H. pylori* induces gastric atrophy, which may progress to adenocarcinoma even if *H. pylori* is treated.
8. *H. pylori* and humans have co-evolved and co-adapted. The absence of *H. pylori* changes human gastric physiology.

FUTURE DIRECTIONS/UNRESOLVED ISSUES

1. How does *H. pylori* persist throughout human life?
2. What are the mechanisms underlying gastric carcinogenesis?
3. Can an effective human vaccine be developed?
4. Are there adverse consequences for an *H. pylori*–free human population?

RELATED RESOURCES

1. Atherton JC. 2004. Understanding *Helicobacter pylori*. In: *Molecular Insights Into Gastroenterology*, ed. D Adams, TT MacDonald, pp. 51–60. London: BMJ Publishing Group
2. Isaacson PG, Du MQ. 2004. Timeline - MALT lymphoma: from morphology to molecules. *Nat. Rev. Cancer* 4(8):644–53
3. Merrell DS, Falkow S. 2004. Frontal and stealth attack strategies in microbial pathogenesis. *Nature* 430(6996):250–56
4. Peek RM Jr, Blaser MJ. 1999. *Helicobacter pylori* strain-specific genotypes and modulation of the gastric epithelial cell cycle. *Cancer Res.* 59(24):6124–31

ACKNOWLEDGMENTS

I would like to thank Miss Emma Bradley for all her help with the preparation of this manuscript.

LITERATURE CITED

1. Franchini M, Veneri D. 2004. Helicobacter pylori infection and immune thrombocytopenic purpura: an update. *Helicobacter* 9:342–46
2. Jackson S, Beck PL, Pineo GF, Poon MC. 2005. Helicobacter pylori eradication: novel therapy for immune thrombocytopenic purpura? A review of the literature. *Am. J. Hematol.* 78:142–50
3. Pellicano R, Fagoonee S, Rizzetto M, Ponzetto A. 2003. Helicobacter pylori and coronary heart disease: Which directions for future studies? *Crit. Rev. Microbiol.* 29:351–59
4. Gasbarrini A, Carloni E, Gasbarrini G, Chisholm SA. 2004. Helicobacter pylori and extragastric diseases - other Helicobacters. *Helicobacter* 9:57–66
5. Morris A, Nicholson G. 1987. Ingestion of Campylobacter-Pyloridis causes gastritis and raised fasting gastric Ph. *Am. J. Gastroenterol.* 82:192–99
6. Graham DY, Alpert LC, Smith JL, Yoshimura HH. 1988. Iatrogenic Campylobacter-Pylori infection is a cause of epidemic achlorhydria. *Am. J. Gastroenterol.* 83:974–80
7. Blaser MJ, Atherton JC. 2004. Helicobacter pylori persistence: biology and disease. *J. Clin. Invest.* 113:321–33
8. **Tomb JF, White O, Kerlavage AR, Clayton RA, Sutton GG, et al. 1997. The complete genome sequence of the gastric pathogen Helicobacter pylori. *Nature* 388:539–47**

Publication of the complete genome sequence of *H. pylori* provided immediate insights into its biology and has revolutionized research methods.

9. Alm RA, Ling LSL, Moir DT, King BL, Brown ED, et al. 1999. Genomic-sequence comparison of two unrelated isolates of the human gastric pathogen Helicobacter pylori. *Nature* 397:176–80
10. Kavermann H, Burns BP, Angermuller K, Odenbreit S, Fischer W, et al. 2003. Identification and characterization of Helicobacter pylori genes essential for gastric colonization. *J. Exp. Med.* 197:813–22
11. Terry K, Williams SM, Connolly L, Ottemann KM. 2005. Chemotaxis plays multiple roles during Helicobacter pylori animal infection. *Infect. Immun.* 73:803–11
12. Waidner B, Greiner S, Odenbreit S, Kavermann H, Velayudhan J, et al. 2002. Essential role of ferritin Pfr in Helicobacter pylori iron metabolism and gastric colonization. *Infect. Immun.* 70:3923–29
13. Wen Y, Marcus EA, Matrubutham U, Gleeson MA, Scott DR, et al. 2003. Acid-adaptive genes of Helicobacter pylori. *Infect. Immun.* 71:5921–39
14. McGowan CC, Necheva AS, Forsyth MH, Cover TL, Blaser MJ. 2003. Promoter analysis of Helicobacter pylori genes with enhanced expression at low pH. *Mol. Microbiol.* 48:1225–39
15. **Weeks DL, Eskandari S, Scott DR, Sachs G. 2000. A H+-gated urea channel: the link between Helicobacter pylori urease and gastric colonization. *Science* 287:482–85**

Explained how *H. pylori* could survive sudden acid exposure in the stomach.

16. Atherton JC, Blaser MJ. 2004. Chapter 154: Helicobacter pylori infections. In *Harrison's Principals of Internal Medicine*, ed. DL Kasper, E Braunwald, AS Fauci, SL HAuser, DL Longo, JL Jameson, pp. 886–89 . New York: McGraw-Hill. 16th ed.
17. Clyne M, Dillon P, Daly S, O'Kennedy R, May FEB, et al. 2004. Helicobacter pylori interacts with the human single-domain trefoil protein TFF1. *Proc. Natl. Acad. Sci. USA* 101:7409–14
18. Kawakubo M, Ito Y, Okimura Y, Kobayashi M, Sakura K, et al. 2004. Natural antibiotic function of a human gastric mucin against Helicobacter pylori infection. *Science* 305:1003–6

19. Schreiber S, Konradt M, Groll C, Scheid P, Hanauer G, et al. 2004. The spatial orientation of Helicobacter pylori in the gastric mucus. *Proc. Natl. Acad. Sci. USA* 101:5024–29
20. Kim N, Marcus EA, Wen Y, Weeks DL, Scott DR, et al. 2004. Genes of Helicobacter pylori regulated by attachment to AGS cells. *Infect. Immun.* 72:2358–68
21. Kwok T, Backert S, Schwarz H, Berger J, Meyer TF. 2002. Specific entry of Helicobacter pylori into cultured gastric epithelial cells via a zipper-like mechanism. *Infect. Immun.* 70:2108–20
22. Amieva MR, Salama NR, Tompkins LS, Falkow S. 2002. Helicobacter pylori enter and survive within multivesicular vacuoles of epithelial cells. *Cell. Microbiol.* 4:677–90
23. Rittig MG, Shaw B, Letley DP, Thomas RJ, Argent RH, et al. 2003. Helicobacter pylori-induced homotypic phagosome fusion in human monocytes is independent of the bacterial vacA and cag status. *Cell. Microbiol.* 5:887–99
24. Odenbreit S, Gebert B, Puls J, Fischer W, Haas R. 2001. Interaction of Helicobacter pylori with professional phagocytes: role of the cag pathogenicity island and translocation, phosphorylation and processing of CagA. *Cell. Microbiol.* 3:21–31
25. Ohta T, Shibata H, Kawamori T, Iimuro M, Sugimura T, et al. 2001. Marked reduction of Helicobacter pylori-induced gastritis by urease inhibitors, acetohydroxamic acid and flurofamide, in Mongolian gerbils. *Biochem. Biophys. Res. Commun.* 285:728–33
26. Harris PR, Ernst PB, Kawabata S, Kiyono H, Graham MF, et al. 1998. Recombinant Helicobacter pylori urease activates primary mucosal macrophages. *J. Infect. Dis.* 178:1516–20
27. Satin B, Del Giudice G, Della Bianca V, Dusi S, Laudanna C, et al. 2000. The neutrophil-activating protein (HP-NAP) of Helicobacter pylori is a protective antigen and a major virulence factor. *J. Exp. Med.* 191:1467–76
28. Tonello F, Dundon WG, Satin B, Molinari M, Tognon G, et al. 1999. The Helicobacter pylori neutrophil-activating protein is an iron-binding protein with dodecameric structure. *Mol. Microbiol.* 34:238–46
29. Backhed F, Rokbi B, Torstensson E, Zhao Y, Nilsson C, et al. 2003. Gastric mucosal recognition of Helicobacter pylori is independent of Toll-like receptor 4. *J. Infect. Dis.* 187:829–36
30. Smith MF, Mitchell A, Li GL, Ding S, Fitzmaurice AM, et al. 2003. Toll-like receptor (TLR) 2 and TLR5, but not TLR4, are required for Helicobacter pylori-induced NF-kappa B activation and chemokine expression by epithelial cells. *J. Biol. Chem.* 278:32552–60
31. Gewirtz AT, Yu Y, Krishna US, Israel DA, Lyons SL, et al. 2004. Helicobacter pylori flagellin evades toll-like receptor 5-mediated innate immunity. *J. Infect. Dis.* 189:1914–20
32. Gobert AP, McGee D, Akhtar M, Mendz GL, Newton JC, et al. 2001. Helicobacter pylori arginase inhibits nitric oxide production by eukaryotic cells: a strategy for bacterial survival. *Gut* 49:429
33. Schmausser B, Andrulis M, Endrich S, Lee SK, Josenhans C, et al. 2004. Expression and subcellular distribution of toll-like receptors TLR4, TLR5 and TLR9 on the gastric epithelium in Helicobacter pylori infection. *Clin. Exp. Immunol.* 136:521–26
34. Alamuri P, Maier RJ. 2004. Methionine sulphoxide reductase is an important antioxidant enzyme in the gastric pathogen Helicobacter pylori. *Mol. Microbiol.* 53:1397–406
35. Suerbaum S, Smith JM, Bapumia K, Morelli G, Smith NH, et al. 1998. Free recombination within Helicobacter pylori. *Proc. Natl. Acad. Sci. USA* 95:12619–24

Shows that *H. pylori* strains recombine more frequently than any other bacterial species, allowing maintenance of enormous genetic diversity.

36. Israel DA, Salama N, Krishna U, Rieger UM, Atherton JC, et al. 2001. Helicobacter pylori genetic diversity within the gastric niche of a single human host. *Proc. Natl. Acad. Sci. USA* 98:14625–30
37. Falush D, Kraft C, Taylor NS, Correa P, Fox JG, et al. 2001. Recombination and mutation during long-term gastric colonization by Helicobacter pylori: estimates of clock rates, recombination size, and minimal age. *Proc. Natl. Acad. Sci. USA* 98:15056–61
38. Aspholm-Hurtig M, Dailide G, Lahmann M, Kalia A, Ilver D, et al. 2004. Functional adaptation of BabA, the H. pylori ABO blood group antigen binding adhesin. *Science* 305:519–22
39. Robinson K, Loughlin MF, Potter R, Jenks PJ. 2005. Host adaptation and immune modulation are mediated by homologous recombination in Helicobacter pylori. *J. Infect. Dis.* 191:579–87
40. Hansson LE, Nyren O, Hsing AW, Bergstrom R, Josefsson S, et al. 1996. The risk of stomach cancer in patients with gastric or duodenal ulcer disease. *New Engl. J. Med.* 335:242–49
41. **Censini S, Lange C, Xiang ZY, Crabtree JE, Ghiara P, et al. 1996. cag, a pathogenicity island of Helicobacter pylori, encodes type I-specific and disease-associated virulence factors. *Proc. Natl. Acad. Sci. USA* 93:14648–53**

Characterized the *cag* pathogenicity island, now recognized as the most important *H. pylori* virulence factor.

42. Nilsson C, Sillen A, Eriksson L, Strand ML, Enroth H, et al. 2003. Correlation between cag pathogenicity island composition and Helicobacter pylori-associated gastroduodenal disease. *Infect. Immun.* 71:6573–81
43. Crabtree JE, Taylor JD, Wyatt JI, Heatley RV, Shallcross TM, et al. 1991. Mucosal Iga recognition of Helicobacter pylori 120-kDa protein, peptic ulceration, and gastric pathology. *Lancet* 338:332–35
44. Nomura AMY, Perez-Perez GI, Lee J, Stemmermann G, Blaser MJ. 2002. Relation between Helicobacter pylori cagA status and risk of peptic ulcer disease. *Am. J. Epidemiol.* 155:1054–59
45. Blaser MJ, Perezperez GI, Kleanthous H, Cover TL, Peek RM, et al. 1995. Infection with Helicobacter pylori strains possessing caga is associated with an increased risk of developing adenocarcinoma of the stomach. *Cancer Res.* 55:2111–15
46. Figueiredo C, Machado JC, Pharoah P, Seruca R, Sousa S, et al. 2002. Helicobacter pylori and interleukin 1 genotyping: an opportunity to identify high-risk individuals for gastric carcinoma. *J. Natl. Cancer Inst.* 94:1680–87
47. Rohde M, Puls J, Buhrdorf R, Fischer W, Haas R. 2003. A novel sheathed surface organelle of the Helicobacter pylori cag type IV secretion system. *Mol. Microbiol.* 49:219–34
48. Tanaka J, Suzuki T, Mimuro H, Sasakawa C. 2003. Structural definition on the surface of Helicobacter pylori type IV secretion apparatus. *Cell. Microbiol.* 5:395–404
49. Segal ED, Cha J, Lo J, Falkow S, Tompkins LS. 1999. Altered states: involvement of phosphorylated CagA in the induction of host cellular growth changes by Helicobacter pylori. *Proc. Natl. Acad. Sci. USA* 96:14559–64
50. Asahi M, Azuma T, Ito S, Ito Y, Suto H, et al. 2000. Helicobacter pylori CagA protein can be tyrosine phosphorylated in gastric epithelial cells. *J. Exp. Med.* 191:593–602
51. **Odenbreit S, Puls J, Sedlmaier B, Gerland E, Fischer W, et al. 2000. Translocation of Helicobacter pylori CagA into gastric epithelial cells by type IV secretion. *Science* 287:1497–500**

Shows how the CagA protein is translocated into epithelial cells where it stimulates specific signaling pathways.

52. Stein M, Rappuoli R, Covacci A. 2000. Tyrosine phosphorylation of the Helicobacter pylori CagA antigen after cag-driven host cell translocation. *Proc. Natl. Acad. Sci. USA* 97:1263–68

53. Stein M, Bagnoli F, Halenbeck R, Rappuoli R, Fantl WJ, et al. 2002. c-Src/Lyn kinases activate Helicobacter pylori CagA through tyrosine phosphorylation of the EPIYA motifs. *Mol. Microbiol.* 43:971–80
54. Selbach M, Moese S, Hauck CR, Meyer TF, Backert S. 2002. Src is the kinase of the Helicobacter pylori CagA protein in vitro and in vivo. *J. Biol. Chem.* 277:6775–78
55. Amieva MR, Vogelmann R, Covacci A, Tompkins LS, Nelson WJ, et al. 2003. Disruption of the epithelial apical-junctional complex by Helicobacter pylori CagA. *Science* 300:1430–34
56. Churin Y, Al-Ghoul L, Kepp O, Meyer TE, Birchmeier W, et al. 2003. Helicobacter pylori CagA protein targets the c-Met receptor and enhances the motogenic response. *J. Cell. Biol.* 161:249–55
57. El-Etr SH, Mueller A, Tompkins LS, Falkow S, Merrell DS. 2004. Phosphorylation-independent effects of CagA during interaction between Helicobacter pylori and T84 polarized monolayers. *J. Infect. Dis.* 190:1516–23
58. Higashi H, Nakaya A, Tsutsumi R, Yokoyama K, Fujii Y, et al. 2004. Helicobacter pylori CagA induces Ras-independent morphogenetic response through SHP-2 recruitment and activation. *J. Biol. Chem.* 279:17205–16
59. Higashi H, Tsutsumi R, Fujita A, Yamazaki S, Asaka M, et al. 2002. Biological activity of the Helicobacter pylori virulence factor CagA is determined by variation in the tyrosine phosphorylation sites. *Proc. Natl. Acad. Sci. USA* 99:14428–33
60. Hirata Y, Maeda S, Mitsuno Y, Tateishi K, Yanai A, et al. 2002. Helicobacter pylori CagA protein activates serum response element-driven transcription independently of tyrosine phosphorylation. *Gastroenterology* 123:1962–71
61. Keates S, Sougioultzis S, Keates AC, Zhao DZ, Peek RM, et al. 2001. cag plus Helicobacter pylori induce transactivation of the epidermal growth factor receptor in AGS gastric epithelial cells. *J. Biol. Chem.* 276:48127–34
62. Meyer-ter-Vehn T, Covacci A, Kist M, Pahl HL. 2000. Helicobacter pylori activates mitogen-activated protein kinase cascades and induces expression of the proto-oncogenes c-fos and c-jun. *J. Biol. Chem.* 275:16064–72
63. Mitsuno Y, Maeda S, Yoshida H, Hirata Y, Ogura K, et al. 2002. Helicobacter pylori activates the proto-oncogene c-fos through SRE transactivation. *Biochem. Biophys. Res. Commun.* 291:868–74
64. Mimuro H, Suzuki T, Tanaka J, Asahi M, Haas R, et al. 2002. Grb2 is a key mediator of Helicobacter pylori CagA protein activities. *Mol. Cell.* 10:745–55
65. Naumann M, Wessler S, Bartsch C, Wieland B, Covacci A, et al. 1999. Activation of activator protein 1 and stress response kinases in epithelial cells colonized by Helicobacter pylori encoding the cag pathogenicity island. *J. Biol. Chem.* 274:31655–62
66. Selbach M, Moese S, Meyer TF, Backert S. 2002. Functional analysis of the Helicobacter pylori cag pathogenicity island reveals both VirD4-CagA-dependent and VirD4-CagA-independent mechanisms. *Infect. Immun.* 70:665–71
67. Tsutsumi R, Higashi H, Higuchi M, Okada M, Hatakeyama M. 2003. Attenuation of Helicobacter pylori CagA-SHP-2 signaling by interaction betwwen CagA and C-terminal Src kinase. *J. Biol. Chem.* 278:3664–70
68. Yamazaki S, Yamakawa A, Ito Y, Ohtani M, Higashi H, et al. 2003. The CagA protein of Helicobacter pylori is translocated into epithelial cells and binds to SHP-2 in human gastric mucosa. *J. Infect. Dis.* 187:334–37

69. Moese S, Selbach M, Kwok T, Brinkmann V, Konig W, et al. 2004. Helicobacter pylori induces AGS cell motility and elongation via independent signaling pathways. *Infect. Immun.* 72:3646–9
70. Bebb JR, Letley DP, Rhead JL, Atherton JC. 2003. Helicobacter pylori supernatants cause epithelial cytoskeletal disruption that is bacterial strain and epithelial cell line dependent but not toxin VacA dependent. *Infect. Immun.* 71:3623–27
71. Segal ED, Falkow S, Tompkins LS. 1996. Helicobacter pylori attachment to gastric cells induces cytoskeletal rearrangements and tyrosine phosphorylation of host cell proteins. *Proc. Natl. Acad. Sci. USA* 93:1259–64
72. Moss SF, Sordillo EM, Abdalla AM, Makarov V, Hanzely Z, et al. 2001. Increased gastric epithelial cell apoptosis associated with colonization with cagA plus Helicobacter pylori strains. *Cancer Res.* 61:1406–11
73. Peek RM Jr, Moss SF, Tham KT, Perez-Perez GI, Wang S, et al. 1997. Helicobacter pylori cagA+ strains and dissociation of gastric epithelial cell proliferation from apoptosis. *J. Natl. Cancer Inst.* 89:863–68
74. Argent RH, Kidd M, Owen RJ, Thomas RJ, Limb MC, et al. 2004. Determinants and consequences of different levels of CagA phosphorylation for clinical isolates of Helicobacter pylori. *Gastroenterology* 127:514–23
75. Yamaoka Y, El-Zimaity HM, Gutierrez O, Figura N, Kim JG, et al. 1999. Relationship between the cagA 3' repeat region of Helicobacter pylori, gastric histology, and susceptibility to low pH. *Gastroenterology* 117:342–49
76. Azuma T, Yamakawa A, Yamazaki S, Fukuta K, Ohtani M, et al. 2002. Correlation between variation of the 3' region of the cagA gene in Helicobacter pylori and disease outcome in Japan. *J. Infect. Dis.* 186:1621–30
77. Azuma T, Yamazaki S, Yamakawa A, Ohtani M, Muramatsu A, et al. 2004. Association between diversity in the Src homology 2 domain-containing tyrosine phosphatase binding site of Helicobacter pylori CagA protein and gastric atrophy and cancer. *J. Infect. Dis.* 189:820–27
78. Fischer W, Puls J, Buhrdorf R, Gebert B, Odenbreit S, et al. 2001. Systematic mutagenesis of the Helicobacter pylori cag pathogenicity island: essential genes for CagA translocation in host cells and induction of interleukin-8. *Mol. Microbiol.* 42:1337–48
79. Viala J, Chaput C, Boneca IG, Cardona A, Girardin SE, et al. 2004. Nod1 responds to peptidoglycan delivered by the Helicobacter pylori cag pathogenicity island. *Nat. Immun.* 5:1166–74
80. Maeda S, Yoshida H, Ogura K, Mitsuno Y, Hirata Y, et al. 2000. H. pylori activates NF-kappa B through a signaling pathway involving I kappa B kinases, NF-kappa B-inducing kinase, TRAF2, and TRAF6 in gastric cancer cells. *Gastroenterology* 119:97–108
81. Mori N, Sato H, Hayashibara T, Senba M, Geleziunas R, et al. 2003. Helicobacter pylori induces matrix metalloproteinase-9 through activation of nuclear factor kappaB. *Gastroenterology* 124:983–92
82. Wada A, Ogushi K, Kimura T, Hojo H, Mori N, et al. 2001. Helicobacter pylori-mediated transcriptional regulation of the human beta-defensin 2 gene requires NF-kappa B. *Cell. Microbiol.* 3:115–23
83. Yanai A, Hirata Y, Mitsuno Y, Maeda S, Shibata W, et al. 2003. Helicobacter pylori induces antiapoptosis through nuclear factor-kappa B activation. *J. Infect. Dis.* 188:1741–51

84. Bebb JR, Letley DP, Thomas RJ, Aviles F, Collins HM, et al. 2003. Helicobacter pylori upregulates matrilysin (MMP-7) in epithelial cells in vivo and in vitro in a Cag dependent manner. *Gut* 52:1408–13
85. Ogura K, Maeda S, Nakao M, Watanabe T, Tada M, et al. 2000. Virulence factors of Helicobacter pylori responsible for gastric diseases in Mongolian gerbil. *J. Exp. Med.* 192:1601–10
86. Kersulyte D, Chalkauskas H, Berg DE. 1999. Emergence of recombinant strains of Helicobacter pylori during human infection. *Mol. Microbiol.* 31:31–43
87. Aras RA, Lee Y, Kim SK, Israel D, Peek RM, et al. 2003. Natural variation in populations of persistently colonizing bacteria affect human host cell phenotype. *J. Infect. Dis.* 188:486–96
88. Cover TL, Tummuru MK, Cao P, Thompson SA, Blaser MJ. 1994. Divergence of genetic sequences for the vacuolating cytotoxin among Helicobacter pylori strains. *J. Biol. Chem.* 269:10566–73
89. **Atherton JC, Cao P, Peek RM, Tummuru MKR, Blaser MJ, et al. 1995. Mosaicism in vacuolating cytotoxin alleles of Helicobacter pylori—association of specific vacA types with cytotoxin production and peptic ulceration. *J. Biol. Chem.* 270:17771–77**

Describes genetic variation in the vacuolating cytotoxin gene, *vacA*; this underlies differential toxicity of *H. pylori* strains.

90. Letley DP, Lastovica A, Louw JA, Hawkey CJ, Atherton JC. 1999. Allelic diversity of the Helicobacter pylori vacuolating cytotoxin gene in South Africa: rarity of the vacA s1a genotype and natural occurrence of an s2/m1 allele. *J. Clin. Microbiol.* 37:1203–5
91. Letley DP, Rhead JL, Twells RJ, Dove B, Atherton JC. 2003. Determinants of non-toxicity in the gastric pathogen Helicobacter pylori. *J. Biol. Chem.* 278:26734–41
92. Pagliaccia C, de Bernard M, Lupetti P, Ji X, Burroni D, et al. 1998. The m2 form of the Helicobacter pylori cytotoxin has cell type-specific vacuolating activity. *Proc. Natl. Acad. Sci. USA* 95:10212–17
93. Atherton JC, Cao P, Peek RM Jr, Tummuru MK, Blaser MJ, et al. 1995. Mosaicism in vacuolating cytotoxin alleles of Helicobacter pylori. Association of specific vacA types with cytotoxin production and peptic ulceration. *J. Biol. Chem.* 270:17771–77
94. Atherton JC, Peek RM Jr, Tham KT, Cover TL, Blaser MJ. 1997. Clinical and pathological importance of heterogeneity in vacA, the vacuolating cytotoxin gene of Helicobacter pylori. *Gastroenterology* 112:92–99
95. Atherton JC, Cover TL, Papini E, Telford JL. 2001. Vacuolating cytotoxin. In *Helicobacter Pylori: Physiology and Genetics*, ed. HLT Mobley, GL Mendz, SL Hazell, pp. 97–110. Washington: ASM Press.
96. van Doorn LJ, Figueiredo C, Sanna R, Pena S, Midolo P, et al. 1998. Expanding allelic diversity of Helicobacter pylori vacA. *J. Clin. Microbiol.* 36:2597–603
97. Kidd M, Lastovica AJ, Atherton JC, Louw JA. 1999. Heterogeneity in the Helicobacter pylori vacA and cagA genes: association with gastroduodenal disease in South Africa? *Gut* 45:499–502
98. Miehlke S, Kirsch C, Agha-Amiri K, Gunther T, Lehn N, et al. 2000. The Helicobacter pylori vacA s1, m1 genotype and cagA is associated with gastric carcinoma in Germany. *Int. J. Cancer* 87:322–27
99. Figueiredo C, Van Doorn LJ, Nogueira C, Soares JM, Pinho C, et al. 2001. Helicobacter pylori genotypes are associated with clinical outcome in Portuguese patients and show a high prevalence of infections with multiple strains. *Scand. J. Gastroenterol.* 36:128–35

100. Ito Y, Azuma T, Ito S, Suto H, Miyaji H, et al. 1998. Full-length sequence analysis of the vacA gene from cytotoxic and noncytotoxic Helicobacter pylori. *J. Infect. Dis.* 178:1391–98
101. Telford JL, Ghiara P, Dellorco M, Comanducci M, Burroni D, et al. 1994. Gene structure of the Helicobacter pylori cytotoxin and evidence of its key role in gastric disease. *J. Exp. Med.* 179:1653–58
102. Ilver D, Barone S, Mercati D, Lupetti P, Telford JL. 2004. Helicobacter pylori toxin VacA is transferred to host cells via a novel contact-dependent mechanism. *Cell. Microbiol.* 6:167–74
103. Yahiro K, Wada A, Nakayama M, Kimura T, Ogushi K, et al. 2003. Protein-tyrosine phosphatase alpha, RPTP alpha, is a Helicobacter pylori VacA receptor. *J. Biol. Chem.* 278:19183–89
104. Yahiro K, Niidome T, Kimura M, Hatakeyama T, Aoyagi H, et al. 1999. Activation of Helicobacter pylori VacA toxin by alkaline or acid conditions increases its binding to a 250-kDa receptor protein-tyrosine phosphatase beta. *J. Biol. Chem.* 274:36693–99
105. Padilla PI, Wada A, Yahiro K, Kimura M, Niidome T, et al. 2000. Morphologic differentiation of HL-60 cells is associated with appearance of RPTPbeta and induction of Helicobacter pylori VacA sensitivity. *J. Biol. Chem.* 275:15200–6
106. Seto K, Hayashi-Kuwabara Y, Yoneta T, Suda H, Tamaki H. 1998. Vacuolation induced by cytotoxin from Helicobacter pylori is mediated by the EGF receptor in HeLa cells. *FEBS Lett.* 431:347–50
107. Schraw W, Li Y, McClain MS, van der Goot FG, Cover TL. 2002. Association of Helicobacter pylori vacuolating toxin (VacA) with lipid rafts. *J. Biol. Chem.* 277:34642–50
108. Kuo CH, Wang WC. 2003. Binding and internalization of Helicobacter pylori VacA via cellular lipid rafts in epithelial cells. *Biochem. Biophys. Res. Commun.* 303:640–44
109. McClain MS, Schraw W, Ricci V, Boquet P, Cover TL. 2000. Acid activation of Helicobacter pylori vacuolating cytotoxin (VacA) results in toxin internalization by eukaryotic cells. *Mol. Microbiol.* 37:433–42
110. Ricci V, Sommi P, Fiocca R, Necchi V, Romano M, et al. 2002. Extracellular pH modulates Helicobacter pylori-induced vacuolation and VacA toxin internalization in human gastric epithelial cells. *Biochem. Biophys. Res. Commun.* 292:167–74
111. Czajkowsky DM, Iwamoto H, Cover TL, Shao ZF. 1999. The vacuolating toxin from Helicobacter pylori forms hexameric pores in lipid bilayers at low pH. *Proc. Natl. Acad. Sci. USA* 96:2001–6
112. Szabo I, Brutsche S, Tombola F, Moschioni M, Satin B, et al. 1999. Formation of anion-selective channels in the cell plasma membrane by the toxin VacA of Helicobacter pylori is required for its biological activity. *EMBO J.* 18:5517–27
113. Tombola F, Morbiato L, Del Giudice G, Rappuoli R, Zoratti M, et al. 2001. The Helicobacter pylori VacA toxin is a urea permease that promotes urea diffusion across epithelia. *J. Clin. Invest.* 108:929–37
114. Papini E, Debernard M, Milia E, Bugnoli M, Zerial M, et al. 1994. Cellular vacuoles induced by Helicobacter pylori originate from late endosomal compartments. *Proc. Natl. Acad. Sci. USA* 91:9720–24
115. Papini E, Satin B, Norais N, de Bernard M, Telford JL, et al. 1998. Selective increase of the permeability of polarized epithelial cell monolayers by Helicobacter pylori vacuolating toxin. *J. Clin. Invest.* 102:813–20
116. Merrell DS, Thompson LJ, Kim CC, Mitchell H, Tompkins LS, et al. 2003. Growth phase-dependent response of Helicobacter pylori to iron starvation. *Infect. Immun.* 71:6510–25

117. Kuck D, Kolmerer B, Iking-Konert C, Krammer PH, Stremmel W, et al. 2001. Vacuolating cytotoxin of Helicobacter pylori induces apoptosis in the human gastric epithelial cell line AGS. *Infect. Immun.* 69:5080–87
118. Cover TL, Krishna US, Israel DA, Peek RM Jr. 2003. Induction of gastric epithelial cell apoptosis by Helicobacter pylori vacuolating cytotoxin. *Cancer Res.* 63:951–57
119. Galmiche A, Rassow J, Doye A, Cagnol S, Chambard JC, et al. 2000. The N-terminal 34 kDa fragment of Helicobacter pylori vacuolating cytotoxin targets mitochondria and induces cytochrome c release. *EMBO J.* 19:6361–70
120. Willhite DC, Cover TL, Blanke SR. 2003. Cellular vacuolation and mitochondrial cytochrome c release are independent outcomes of Helicobacter pylori vacuolating cytotoxin activity that are each dependent on membrane channel formation. *J. Biol. Chem.* 278:48204–9
121. Nakayama M, Kimura M, Wada A, Yahiro K, Ogushi K, et al. 2004. Helicobacter pylori VacA activates the p38/activating transcription factor 2-mediated signal pathway in AZ-521 cells. *J. Biol. Chem.* 279:7024–28
122. Marchetti M, Arico B, Burroni D, Figura N, Rappuoli R, et al. 1995. Development of a mouse model of Helicobacter pylori infection that mimics human disease. *Science* 267:1655–58
123. Fujikawa A, Shirasaka D, Yamamoto S, Ota H, Yahiro K, et al. 2003. Mice deficient in protein tyrosine phosphatase receptor type Z are resistant to gastric ulcer induction by VacA of Helicobacter pylori. *Nat. Genet.* 33:375–81
124. de Bernard M, Cappon A, Pancotto L, Ruggiero P, Rivera J, et al. 2005. The Helicobacter pylori VacA cytotoxin activates RBL-2H3 cells by inducing cytosolic calcium oscillations. *Cell. Microbiol.* 7:191–98
125. Molinari M, Salio M, Galli C, Norais N, Rappuoli R, et al. 1998. Selective inhibition of Ii-dependent antigen presentation by Helicobacter pylori toxin VacA. *J. Exp. Med.* 187:135–40
126. Gebert B, Fischer W, Weiss E, Hoffmann R, Haas R. 2003. Helicobacter pylori vacuolating cytotoxin inhibits T lymphocyte activation. *Science* 301:1099–102
127. Boncristiano M, Paccani SR, Barone S, Ulivieri C, Patrussi L, et al. 2003. The Helicobacter pylori vacuolating toxin inhibits T cell activation by two independent mechanisms. *J. Exp. Med.* 198:1887–97
128. Sundrud MS, Torres VJ, Unutmaz D, Cover TL. 2004. Inhibition of primary human T cell proliferation by Helicobacter pylori vacuolating toxin (VacA) is independent of VacA effects on IL-2 secretion. *Proc. Natl. Acad. Sci. USA* 101:7727–32
129. Letley DP, Atherton JC. 2000. Natural diversity in the N terminus of the mature vacuolating cytotoxin of Helicobacter pylori determines cytotoxin activity. *J. Bacteriol.* 182:3278–80
130. McClain MS, Cao P, Iwamoto H, Vinion-Dubiel AD, Szabo G, et al. 2001. A 12-amino-acid segment, present in type s2 but not type s1 Helicobacter pylori VacA proteins, abolishes cytotoxin activity and alters membrane channel formation. *J. Bacteriol.* 183:6499–508
131. Aviles-Jimenez F, Letley DP, Gonzalez-Valencia G, Salama N, Torres J, et al. 2004. Evolution of the Helicobacter pylori vacuolating cytotoxin in a human stomach. *J. Bacteriol.* 186:5182–85
132. Boren T, Falk P, Roth KA, Larson G, Normark S. 1993. Attachment of Helicobacter pylori to human gastric epithelium mediated by blood-group antigens. *Science* 262:1892–95

133. Sheu BS, Sheu SM, Yang HB, Huang AH, Wu JJ. 2005. Host gastric Lewis expression determines the bacterial density of Helicobacter pylori in babA2 genopositive infection. *Gut* 52:927–32
134. Guruge JL, Falk PG, Lorenz RG, Dans M, Wirth HP, et al. 1998. Epithelial attachment alters the outcome of Helicobacter pylori infection. *Proc. Natl. Acad. Sci. USA* 95:3925–30
135. Mahdavi J, Sonden B, Hurtig M, Olfat FO, Forsberg L, et al. 2002. Helicobacter pylori SabA adhesin in persistent infection and chronic inflammation. *Science* 297:573–78
136. Ilver D, Arnqvist A, Ogren J, Frick IM, Kersulyte D, et al. 1998. Helicobacter pylori adhesin binding fucosylated histo-blood group antigens revealed by retagging. *Science* 279:373–77
137. Gerhard M, Lehn N, Neumayer N, Boren T, Rad R, et al. 1999. Clinical relevance of the Helicobacter pylori gene for blood-group antigen-binding adhesin. *Proc. Natl. Acad. Sci. USA* 96:12778–83
138. Prinz C, Schoniger M, Rad R, Becker I, Keiditsch E, et al. 2001. Key importance of the Helicobacter pylori adherence factor blood group antigen binding adhesin during chronic gastric inflammation. *Cancer Res.* 61:1903–9
139. Yu J, Leung WK, Go MYY, Chan MCW, To KF, et al. 2002. Relationship between Helicobacter pylori babA2 status with gastric epithelial cell turnover and premalignant gastric lesions. *Gut* 51:480–84
140. Solnick JV, Hansen LM, Salama NR, Boonjakuakul JK, Syvanen M. 2004. Modification of Helicobacter pylori outer membrane protein expression during experimental infection of rhesus macaques. *Proc. Natl. Acad. Sci. USA* 101:2106–11
141. Backstrom A, Lundberg C, Kersulyte D, Berg DE, Boren T, et al. 2004. Metastability of Helicobacter pylori bab adhesin genes and dynamics in Lewis b antigen binding. *Proc. Natl. Acad. Sci. USA* 101:16923–28
142. Hennig EE, Mernaugh R, Edl J, Cao P, Cover TL. 2004. Heterogeneity among Helicobacter pylori strains in expression of the outer membrane protein BabA. *Infect. Immun.* 72:3429–35
143. Yamaoka Y, Kwon DH, Graham DY. 2000. A M-r 34,000 proinflammatory outer membrane protein (oipA) of Helicobacter pylori. *Proc. Natl. Acad. Sci. USA* 97:7533–38
144. Peek RM, Thompson SA, Donahue JP, Tham KT, Atherton JC, et al. 1998. Adherence to gastric epithelial cells induces expression of a Helicobacter pylori gene, iceA, that is associated with clinical outcome. *Proc. Assoc. Am. Physicians* 110:531–44
145. Kidd M, Peek RM, Lastovica AJ, Israel DA, Kummer AF, et al. 2001. Analysis of iceA genotypes in South African Helicobacter pylori strains and relationship to clinically significant disease. *Gut* 49:629–35
146. Heithoff DM, Sinsheimer RL, Low DA, Mahan MJ. 1999. An essential role for DNA adenine methylation in bacterial virulence. *Science* 284:967–70
147. Xu Q, Blaser MJ. 2001. Promoters of the CATG-specific methyltransferase gene hpyIM differ between iceA1 and iceA2 Helicobacter pylori strains. *J. Bacteriol.* 183:3875–84
148. Ando T, Aras RA, Kusugami K, Blaser MJ, Wassenaar TM. 2003. Evolutionary history of hrgA, which replaces the restriction gene hpyIIIR in the hpyIII locus of Helicobacter pylori. *J. Bacteriol.* 185:295–301
149. Ando T, Wassenaar TM, Peek RM, Aras RA, Tschumi AI, et al. 2002. A Helicobacter pylori restriction endonuclease-replacing gene, hrgA, is associated with gastric cancer in Asian strains. *Cancer Res.* 62:2385–89

150. Hwang IR, Kodama T, Kikuchi S, Sakai K, Peterson LE, et al. 2002. Effect of interleukin 1 polymorphisms on gastric mucosal interleukin 1 beta production in Helicobacter pylori infection. *Gastroenterology* 123:1793–803
151. Rad R, Dossumbekova A, Neu B, Lang R, Bauer S, et al. 2004. Cytokine gene polymorphisms influence mucosal cytokine expression, gastric inflammation, and host specific colonisation during Helicobacter pylori infection. *Gut* 53:1082–89
152. Furuta T, El-Omar EM, Xiao F, Shirai N, Takashima M, et al. 2002. Interleukin 1 beta polymorphisms increase risk of hypochlorhydria and atrophic gastritis and reduce risk of duodenal ulcer recurrence in Japan. *Gastroenterology* 123:95–105
153. Machado JC, Figueiredo C, Canedo P, Nabais S, Alves CC, et al. 2003. A proinflammatory genetic profile increases the risk of chronic atrophic gastritis and gastric carcinoma. *Gastroenterology* 125:364–71
154. Rad R, Prinz C, Neu B, Neuhofer M, Zeitner M, et al. 2003. Synergistic effect of Helicobacter pylori virulence factors and interleukin-1 polymorphisms for the development of severe histological changes in the gastric mucosa. *J. Infect. Dis.* 188:272–81
155. El-Omar EM, Carrington M, Chow WH, McColl KEL, Bream JH, et al. 2000. Interleukin-1 polymorphisms associated with increased risk of gastric cancer. *Nature* 404:398–402

The first description of human cytokine polymorphisms affecting gastric cancer risk in *H. pylori*-infected people.

156. Machado JC, Pharoah P, Sousa S, Carvalho R, Oliveira C, et al. 2001. Interleukin 1B and interleukin 1RN polymorphisms are associated with increased risk of gastric carcinoma. *Gastroenterology* 121:823–29
157. El-Omar EM, Rabkin CS, Gammon MD, Vaughan TL, Risch HA, et al. 2003. Increased risk of noncardia gastric cancer associated with proinflammatory cytokine gene polymorphisms. *Gastroenterology* 124:1193–201
158. Garza-Gonzalez E, Bosques-Padilla FJ, El-Omar E, Hold G, Tijerina-Menchaca R, et al. 2005. Role of the polymorphic IL-1B, IL-1RN and TNF-A genes in distal gastric cancer in Mexico. *Int. J. Cancer* 114:237–41
159. Hsu PI, Li CN, Tseng HH, Lai KH, Hsu PN, et al. 2004. The Interleukin-1 RN polymorphism and Helicobacter pylori infection in the development of duodenal ulcer. *Helicobacter* 9:605–13
160. Ohyauchi M, Imatani A, Yonechi M, Asano N, Miura A, et al. 2005. The polymorphism interleukin 8–2251 A/T influences the susceptibility of Helicobacter pylori related gastric diseases in the Japanese population. *Gut* 54:330–35
161. Bamford KB, Fan X, Crowe SE, Leary JF, Gourley WK, et al. 1998. Lymphocytes in the human gastric mucosa during Helicobacter pylori have a T helper cell 1 phenotype. *Gastroenterology* 114:482–92
162. D'Elios MM, Manghetti M, De Carli M, Costa F, Baldari CT, et al. 1997. T helper 1 effector cells specific for Helicobacter pylori in the gastric antrum of patients with peptic ulcer disease. *J. Immunol.* 158:962–67
163. Mohammadi M, Nedrud J, Redline R, Lycke N, Czinn SJ. 1997. Murine CD4 T-cell response to Helicobacter infection: TH1 cells enhance gastritis and TH2 cells reduce bacterial load. *Gastroenterology* 113:1848–57
164. Smythies LE, Waites KB, Lindsey JR, Harris PR, Ghiara P, et al. 2000. Helicobacter pylori-induced mucosal inflammation is Th1 mediated and exacerbated in IL-4, but not IFN-gamma, gene-deficient mice. *J. Immunol.* 165:1022–29
165. Yamori M, Yoshida M, Watanabe T, Shirai Y, Iizuka T, et al. 2004. Antigenic activation of Th1 cells in the gastric mucosa enhances dysregulated apoptosis and turnover of the epithelial cells. *Biochem. Biophys. Res. Commun.* 316:1015–21

166. Cui G, Houghton J, Finkel N, Carlson J, Wang TC. 2003. IFN-gamma infusion induces gastric atrophy, metaplasia and dysplasia in the absence of *Helicobacter pylori* infection - a role for the immune response in *Helicobacter* disease. *Gastroenterology* 2003:A19
167. Mohammadi M, Czinn S, Redline R, Nedrud J. 1996. Helicobacter-specific cell-mediated immune responses display a predominant Th1 phenotype and promote a delayed-type hypersensitivity response in the stomachs of mice. *J. Immunol.* 156:4729–38
168. Obonyo M, Guiney DG, Harwood J, Fierer J, Cole SP. 2002. Role of gamma interferon in Helicobacter pylori induction of inflammatory mediators during murine infection. *Infect. Immun.* 70:3295–99
169. Guiney DG, Hasegawa P, Cole SP. 2003. Helicobacter pylori preferentially induces interleukin 12 (IL-12) rather than IL-6 or IL-10 in human dendritic cells. *Infect. Immun.* 71:4163–66
170. Kranzer K, Eckhardt A, Aigner M, Knoll G, Deml L, et al. 2004. Induction of maturation and cytokine release of human dendritic cells by Helicobacter pylori. *Infect. Immun.* 72:4416–23
171. Galgani M, Busiello I, Censini S, Zappacosta S, Racioppi L, et al. 2004. Helicobacter pylori induces aptosis of human monocytes but not monocyte-derived dendritic cells: role of the cag pathogenicity island. *Infect. Immun.* 72:4480–85
172. Fox JG, Beck P, Dangler CA, Whary MT, Wang TC, et al. 2000. Concurrent enteric helminth infection modulates inflammation and gastric immune responses and reduces helicobacter-induced gastric atrophy. *Nat. Med.* 6:536–42

This animal study raises the interesting hypothesis that parasite modulation of the immune response may affect disease risk.

173. Foryst-Ludwig A, Naumann M. 2000. p21-activated kinase 1 activates the nuclear factor kappa B (NF-kappa B)-inducing kinase-Ikappa B kinases NF-kappa B pathway and proinflammatory cytokines in Helicobacter pylori infection. *J. Biol. Chem.* 275:39779–85
174. Girardin SE, Boneca IG, Carneiro LAM, Antignac A, Jehanno M, et al. 2003. Nod1 detects a unique muropeptide from Gram-negative bacterial peptidoglycan. *Science* 300:1584–87
175. Bergman MP, Engering A, Smits HH, van Vliet SJ, van Bodegraven AA, et al. 2004. Helicobacter pylori modulates the T helper cell 1/T helper cell 2 balance through phase-variable interaction between lipopolysaccharide and DC-SIGN. *J. Exp. Med.* 200:979–90
176. Meyer F, Ramanujam KS, Gobert AP, James SP, Wilson KT. 2003. Cutting edge: cyclooxygenase-2 activation suppresses Th1 polarization in response to Helicobacter pylori. *J. Immunol.* 171:3913–17
177. Lundgren A, Suri-Payer E, Enarsson K, Svennerholm AM, Lundin BS. 2003. Helicobacter pylon-specific CD4(+) CD25(high) regulatory T cells suppress memory T-cell responses to H. pylori in infected individuals. *Infect. Immun.* 71:1755–62
178. Moss SF, Legon S, Bishop AE, Polak JM, Calam J. 1992. Effect of Helicobacter pylori on gastric somatostatin in duodenal-ulcer disease. *Lancet* 340:930–2
179. Beales I, Calam J, Post L, Srinivasan S, Yamada T, et al. 1997. Effect of transforming growth factor alpha and interleukin 8 on somatostatin release from canine fundic D cells. *Gastroenterology* 112:136–43
180. Odum L, Petersen HD, Andersen IB, Hansen BF, Rehfeld JF, et al. 1994. Gastrin and somatostatin in Helicobacter pylori infected antral mucosa. *Gut* 35:615–18
181. Arebi N, Healey ZV, Bliss PW, Ghatei M, Van Noorden S, et al. 2002. Nitric oxide regulates the release of somatostatin from cultured gastric rabbit primary D-cells. *Gastroenterology* 123:566–76
182. Zavros Y, Rathinavelu S, Kao JY, Todisco A, Del Valle J, et al. 2003. Treatment of Helicobacter gastritis with IL-4 requires somatostatin. *Proc. Natl. Acad. Sci. USA* 100:12944–49

The hypergastrinemic mouse described here is an important model of gastric carcinogenesis and underlines the key role of gastrin.

183. Wang TC, Dangler CA, Chen D, Goldenring JR, Koh T, et al. 2000. Synergistic interaction between hypergastrinemia and Helicobacter infection in a mouse model of gastric cancer. *Gastroenterology* 118:36–47

184. Peek RM, Wirth HP, Moss SF, Yang MQ, Abdalla AM, et al. 2000. Helicobacter pylori alters gastric epithelial cell cycle events and gastrin secretion in Mongolian gerbils. *Gastroenterology* 118:48–59

185. Guo YS, Cheng JZ, Jin GF, Gutkind JS, Hellmich MR, et al. 2002. Gastrin stimulates cyclooxygenase-2 expression in intestinal epithelial cells through multiple signaling pathways - evidence for involvement of Erk5 kinase and transactivation of the epidermal growth factor receptor. *J. Biol. Chem.* 277:48755–63

186. Fukui H, Franceschi F, Penland RL, Sakai T, Sepulveda AR, et al. 2003. Effects of Helicobacter pylori infection on the link between regenerating gene expression and serum gastrin levels in Mongolian gerbils. *Lab. Invest.* 83:1777–86

187. Azuma T, Suto H, Ito Y, Ohtani M, Dojo M, et al. 2001. Gastric leptin and Helicobacter pylori infection. *Gut* 49:324–29

188. Breidert M, Miehlke S, Glasow A, Orban Z, Stolte M, et al. 1999. Leptin and its receptor in normal human gastric mucosa and in Helicobacter pylori-associated gastritis. *Scand. J. Gastroenterol.* 34:954–61

189. Nwokolo CU, Freshwater DA, O'Hare P, Randeva HS. 2003. Plasma ghrelin following cure of Helicobacter pylori. *Gut* 52:637–40

190. Atherton JC, Tham KT, Peek RM, Cover TL, Blaser MJ. 1996. Density of Helicobacter pylori infection in vivo as assessed by quantitative culture and histology. *J. Infect. Dis.* 174:552–56

191. Gillen D, El-Omar EM, Wirz AA, Ardill JES, McColl KEL. 1998. The acid response to gastrin distinguishes duodenal ulcer patients from Helicobacter pylori–infected healthy subjects. *Gastroenterology* 114:50–57

192. Hamlet A, Olbe L. 1996. The influence of Helicobacter pylori infection on postprandial duodenal acid load and duodenal bulb pH in humans. *Gastroenterology* 111:391–400

193. Khulusi S, Badve S, Patel P, Lloyd R, Marrero JM, et al. 1996. Pathogenesis of gastric metaplasia of the human duodenum: role of Helicobacter pylori, gastric acid, and ulceration. *Gastroenterology* 110:452–58

194. Van Zanten S, Dixon MF, Lee A. 1999. The gastric transitional zones: neglected links between gastroduodenal pathology and Helicobacter ecology. *Gastroenterology* 116:1217–29

195. Amedei A, Bergman MP, Appelmelk BJ, Azzurri A, Benagiano M, et al. 2003. Molecular mimicry between Helicobacter pylori antigens and H+, K+-adenosine triphosphatase in human gastric autoimmunity. *J. Exp. Med.* 198:1147–56

196. ElOmar EM, Oien K, ElNujumi A, Gillen D, Wirz A, et al. 1997. Helicobacter pylori infection and chronic gastric acid hyposecretion. *Gastroenterology* 113:15–24

197. Beales ILP, Calam J. 1998. Interleukin 1 beta and tumour necrosis factor alpha inhibit acid secretion in cultured rabbit parietal cells by multiple pathways. *Gut* 42:227–34

198. Padol IT, Hunt RH. 2004. Effect of Th1 cytokines on acid secretion in pharmacologically characterised mouse gastric glands. *Gut* 53:1075–81

199. Kuipers EJ, Uyterlinde AM, Pena AS, Hazenberg HJA, Bloemena E, et al. 1995. Increase of Helicobacter pylori-associated corpus gastritis during acid suppressive therapy-implications for long-term safety. *Am. J. Gastroenterol.* 90:1401–6

200. Zavros Y, Rieder G, Ferguson A, Samuelson LC, Merchant JL. 2002. Hypergastrinemia in response to gastric inflammation suppresses somatostatin. *Am. J. Physiol. Gastrointest. Liver Physiol.* 282:G175–G83
201. Wong BCY, Lam SK, Wong WM, Chen JS, Zheng TT, et al. 2004. Helicobacter pylori eradication to prevent gastric cancer in a high-risk region of China - a randomized controlled trial. *JAMA* 291:187–94
202. Touati E, Michel V, Thiberge JM, Wuscher N, Huerre M, et al. 2003. Chronic Helicobacter pylori infections induce gastric mutations in mice. *Gastroenterology* 124:1408–19
203. Nam KT, Oh SY, Ahn B, Kim YB, Jang DD, et al. 2004. Decreased Helicobacter pylori associated gastric carcinogenesis in mice lacking inducible nitric oxide synthase. *Gut* 53:1250–55
204. Correa P, Fontham ETH, Bravo JC, Bravo LE, Ruiz B, et al. 2000. Chemoprevention of gastric dysplasia: randomized trial of antioxidant supplements and anti-Helicobacter pylori therapy. *J. Natl. Cancer Inst.* 92:1881–88
205. You WC, Zhang L, Gail MH, Chang YS, Liu WD, et al. 2000. Gastric cancer: Helicobacter pylori, serum vitamin C, and other risk factors. *J. Natl. Cancer Inst.* 92:1607–12
206. Dimmler A, Brabletz T, Hlubek F, Hafner M, Rau T, et al. 2003. Transcription of sonic hedgehog, a potential factor for gastric morphogenesis and gastric mucosa maintenance, is up-regulated in acidic conditions. *Lab. Invest.* 83:1829–37
207. Syder AJ, Oh JD, Guruge JL, O'Donnell D, Karlsson M, et al. 2003. The impact of parietal cells on Helicobacter pylori tropism and host pathology: an analysis using gnotobiotic normal and transgenic mice. *Proc. Natl. Acad. Sci. USA* 100:3467–72
208. Nomura S, Baxter T, Yamaguchi H, Leys C, Vartapetian AB, et al. 2004. Spasmolytic polypeptide expressing metaplasia to preneoplasia in H-felis-infected mice. *Gastroenterology* 127:582–94
209. Mutoh H, Sakurai S, Satoh K, Tamada K, Kita H, et al. 2004. Development of gastric carcinoma from intestinal metaplasia in CDx2-transgenic mice. *Cancer Res.* 64:7740–47
210. Houghton J, Stoicov C, Nomura S, Rogers AB, Carlson J, et al. 2004. Gastric cancer originating from bone marrow-derived cells. *Science* 306:1568–71

That gastric cancer may develop from bone marrow-derived gastric stem cells is changing our views on carcinogenesis.

211. Lauren P. 1965. 2 Histological main types of gastric carcinoma-diffuse and so-called intestinal-type carcinoma—an attempt at a histo-clinical classification. *Acta Pathol. Microbiol. Scand.* 64:31–49
212. Leung WK, Lin SR, Ching JYL, To KF, Ng EKW, et al. 2004. Factors predicting progression of gastric intestinal metaplasia: results of a randomised trial on Helicobacter pylori eradication. *Gut* 53:1244–49
213. Semino-Mora C, Doi SQ, Marty A, Simko V, Carlstedt I, et al. 2003. Intracellular and interstitial expression of Helicobacter pylori virulence genes in gastric precancerous intestinal metaplasia and adenocarcinoma. *J. Infect. Dis.* 187:1165–77
214. Wagner S, Beil W, Westermann J, Logan RPH, Bock CT, et al. 1997. Regulation of gastric epithelial cell growth by Helicobacter pylori: evidence for a major role of apoptosis. *Gastroenterology* 113:1836–47
215. Ashktorab H, Frank S, Khaled AR, Durum SK, Kifle B, et al. 2004. Bax translocation and mitochondrial fragmentation induced by Helicobacter pylori. *Gut* 53:805–13
216. Eguchi H, Carpentier S, Kim SS, Moss SF. 2004. p27(kip1) regulates the apoptotic response of gastric epithelial cells to Helicobacter pylori. *Gut* 53:797–804
217. Jones NL, Day AS, Jennings H, Shannon PT, Galindo-Mata E, et al. 2002. Enhanced disease severity in Helicobacter pylori-infected mice deficient in Fas signaling. *Infect. Immun.* 70:2591–97

218. Obst B, Wagner S, Sewing KF, Beil W. 2000. Helicobacter pylori causes DNA damage in gastric epithelial cells. *Carcinogenesis* 21:1111–15
219. Kim JJ, Tao H, Carloni E, Leung WK, Graham DY, et al. 2002. Helicobacter pylori impairs DNA mismatch repair in gastric epithelial cells. *Gastroenterology* 123:542–53
220. Smoot DT, Elliott TB, Verspaget HW, Jones D, Allen CR, et al. 2000. Influence of Helicobacter pylori on reactive oxygen-induced gastric epithelial cell injury. *Carcinogenesis* 21:2091–95
221. Ding SZ, O'Hara AM, Denning TL, Dirden-Kramer B, Mifflin RC, et al. 2004. Helicobacter pylori and H2O2 increase AP endonuclease-1/redox factor-1 expression in human gastric epithelial cells. *Gastroenterology* 127:845–58
222. Nagata K, Yu H, Nishikawa M, Kashiba M, Nakamura A, et al. 1998. Helicobacter pylori generates superoxide radicals and modulates nitric oxide metabolism. *J. Biol. Chem.* 273:14071–73
223. O'Rourke EJ, Chevalier C, Pinto AV, Thiberge JM, Ielpi L, et al. 2003. Pathogen DNA as target for host-generated oxidative stress: role for repair of bacterial DNA damage in Helicobacter pylori colonization. *Proc. Natl. Acad. Sci. USA* 100:2789–94
224. el-Serag HB, Sonnenberg A. 1998. Opposing time trends of peptic ulcer and reflux disease. *Gut* 43:327–33
225. Yamaji Y, Mitsushima T, Ikuma H, Okamoto M, Yoshida H, et al. 2001. Inverse background of Helicobacter pylori antibody and pepsinogen in reflux oesophagitis compared with gastric cancer: analysis of 5732 Japanese subjects. *Gut* 49:335–40
226. Ye WM, Held M, Lagergren J, Engstrand L, Blot WJ, et al. 2004. Helicobacter pylori infection and gastric atrophy: risk of adenocarcinoma and squamous-cell carcinoma of the esophagus and adenocarcinoma of the gastric cardia. *J. Natl. Cancer Inst.* 96:388–96
227. de Martel C, Llosa AE, Farr SM, Friedman GD, Vogelman JH, et al. 2005. Helicobacter pylori infection and the risk of development of esophageal adenocarcinoma. *J. Infect. Dis.* 191:761–67
228. Warburton-Timms VJ, Charlett A, Valori RM, Uff JS, Shepherd NA, et al. 2001. The significance of cagA(+) Helicobacter pylori in reflux oesophagitis. *Gut* 49:341–46
229. Chow WH, Blaser MJ, Blot WJ, Gammon MD, Vaughan TL, et al. 1998. An inverse relation between cagA+ strains of Helicobacter pylori infection and risk of esophageal and gastric cardia adenocarcinoma. *Cancer Res.* 58:588–90
230. Vaezi MF, Falk GW, Peek RM, Vicari JJ, Goldblum JR, et al. 2000. CagA-positive strains of Helicobacter pylori may protect against Barrett's esophagus. *Am. J. Gastroenterol.* 95:2206–11
231. El-Serag HB, Sonnenberg A, Jamal MM, Inadomi JM, Crooks LA, et al. 1999. Corpus gastritis is protective against reflux oesophagitis. *Gut* 45:181–85
232. Koike T, Ohara S, Sekine H, Iijima K, Abe Y, et al. 2001. Helicobacter pylori infection prevents erosive reflux oesophagitis by decreasing gastric acid secretion. *Gut* 49:330–34
233. Rothenbacher D, Blaser MJ, Bode G, Brenner H. 2000. Inverse relationship between gastric colonization of Helicobacter pylori and diarrheal illnesses in children: results of a population-based cross-sectional study. *J. Infect. Dis.* 182:1446–49
234. Wang G, Ge ZM, Rasko A, Taylor DE. 2000. Lewis antigens in Helicobacter pylori: biosynthesis and phase variation. *Mol. Microbiol.* 36:1187–96
235. Baron JH, Sonnenberg A. 2001. Period- and cohort-age contours of deaths from gastric and duodenal ulcer in New York 1804–1998. *Am. J. Gastroenterol.* 96:2887–91
236. Susser S. 1962. Civilisation and peptic ulcer. *Lancet* 1:115–18

237. deJong D, vanderHulst RWM, Pals G, vanDijk WC, vanderEnde A, et al. 1996. Gastric non-Hodgkin lymphomas of mucosa-associated lymphoid tissue are not associated with more aggressive Helicobacter pylori strains as identified by CagA. *Am. J. Clin. Pathol.* 106:670–75

238. Peng HZ, Ranaldi R, Diss TC, Isaacson PG, Bearzi I, et al. 1998. High frequency of CagA+ Helicobacter pylori infection in high-grade gastric MALT B-cell lymphomas. *J. Pathol.* 185:409–12

239. Delchier JC, Lamarque D, Levy M, Tkoub EM, Copie-Bergman C, et al. 2001. Helicobacter pylori and gastric lymphoma: high seroprevalence of CagA in diffuse large B-cell lymphoma but not in low-grade lymphoma of mucosa-associated lymphoid tissue type. *Am. J. Gastroenterol.* 96:2324–28

240. Lehours P, Menard A, Dupouy S, Bergey B, Richy F, et al. 2004. Evaluation of the association of nine Helicobacter pylori virulence factors with strains involved in low-grade gastric mucosa-associated lymphoid tissue lymphoma. *Infect. Immun.* 72:880–88

241. Miehlke S, Yu J, Schuppler M, Frings C, Kirsch C, et al. 2001. Helicobacter pylori vacA, iceA, and cagA status and pattern of gastritis in patients with malignant and benign gastroduodenal disease. *Am. J. Gastroenterol.* 96:1008–13

242. Hussell T, Isaacson PG, Crabtree JE, Spencer J. 1993. The response of cells from low-grade B-cell gastric lymphomas of mucosa-associated lymphoid-tissue to Helicobacter pylori. *Lancet* 342:571–74

243. Du M, Diss TC, Xu C, Peng H, Isaacson PG, et al. 1996. Ongoing mutation in MALT lymphoma immunoglobulin gene suggests that antigen stimulation plays a role in the clonal expansion. *Leukemia* 10:1190–97

244. Wotherspoon AC, Doglioni C, Diss TC, Pan LX, Moschini A, et al. 1993. Regression of primary low-grade B-cell gastric lymphoma of mucosa-associated lymphoid-tissue type after eradication of Helicobacter pylori. *Lancet* 342:575–77

Proved that these lymphomas are *H. pylori* driven, and led to effective treatment by *H. pylori* eradication.

245. Fischbach W, Goebeler-Kolve ME, Dragosics B, Greiner A, Stolte M. 2004. Long term outcome of patients with gastric marginal zone B cell lymphoma of mucosa associated lymphoid tissue (MALT) following exclusive Helicobacter pylori eradication therapy: experience from a large prospective series. *Gut* 53:34–37

246. Ott G, Katzenberger T, Greiner A, Kalla J, Rosenwald A, et al. 1997. The t(11;18)(q21;q21) chromosome translocation is a frequent and specific aberration in low-grade but not high-grade malignant non-Hodgkin's lymphomas of the mucosa-associated lymphoid tissue (MALT-) type. *Cancer Res.* 57:3944–48

247. Auer IA, Gascoyne RD, Connors JM, Cotter FE, Greiner TC, et al. 1997. t(11;18)(q21;q21) is the most common translocation in MALT lymphomas. *Ann. Oncol.* 8:979–85

248. Dierlamm J, Baens M, Wlodarska I, Stefanova-Ouzounova M, Hernandez JM, et al. 1999. The apoptosis inhibitor gene API2 and a novel 18q gene, MLT, are recurrently rearranged in the t(11;18)(q21;q21) associated with mucosa-associated lymphoid tissue lymphomas. *Blood* 93:3601–9

249. Lucas PC, Yonezumi M, Inohara N, McAllister-Lucas LM, Abazeed ME, et al. 2001. Bcl10 and MALT1, independent targets of chromosomal translocation in MALT lymphoma, cooperate in a novel NF-kappa B signaling pathway. *J. Biol. Chem.* 276:19012–19

250. Liu HX, Ruskon-Fourmestraux A, Lavergne-Slove A, Ye HT, Molina T, et al. 2001. Resistance of t(11;18) positive gastric mucosa-associated lymphoid tissue lymphoma to Helicobacter pylori eradication therapy. *Lancet* 357:39–40

251. Liu HX, Ye HT, Ruskone-Fourmestraux A, de Jong D, Pileri S, et al. 2001. t(11;18) is a marker for all stage gastric MALT lymphomas that will not respond to H. pylori eradication. *Blood* 98:767A
252. Ye HT, Liu HX, Attygalle A, Wotherspoon AC, Nicholson AG, et al. 2003. Variable frequencies of t(11;18)(q21;q21) in MALT lymphomas of different sites: significant association with CagA strains of H. pylori in gastric MALT lymphoma. *Blood* 102:1012–18

Molecular Pathology of Malignant Gliomas

David N. Louis

Molecular Pathology Unit, Department of Pathology and Cancer Center, Massachusetts General Hospital and Harvard Medical School, Boston, Massachusetts 02114; email: dlouis@partners.org

Annu. Rev. Pathol. Mech. Dis. 2006. 1:97–117

First published online as a Review in Advance on October 3, 2005

The *Annual Review of Pathology: Mechanisms of Disease* is online at pathmechdis.annualreviews.org

doi: 10.1146/annurev.pathol.1.110304.100043

1553-4006/06/0114-0097$20.00

Key Words

astrocytoma, glioblastoma, oligodendroglioma, genetics, pathology

Abstract

Malignant gliomas, the most common type of primary brain tumor, are a spectrum of tumors of varying differentiation and malignancy grades. These tumors may arise from neural stem cells and appear to contain tumor stem cells. Early genetic events differ between astrocytic and oligodendroglial tumors, but all tumors have an initially invasive phenotype, which complicates therapy. Progression-associated genetic alterations are common to different tumor types, targeting growth-promoting and cell cycle control pathways and resulting in focal hypoxia, necrosis, and angiogenesis. Knowledge of malignant glioma genetics has already impacted clinical management of these tumors, and researchers hope that further knowledge of the molecular pathology of malignant gliomas will result in novel therapies.

Glioma: a tumor with cells displaying glial differentiation

Astrocytoma: a glial tumor with cells histologically resembling astrocytes

Oligodendrogliomas: a glial tumor with cells histologically resembling oligodendrocytes

Glioblastoma: the most malignant form of astrocytoma (WHO grade IV)

INTRODUCTION

Malignant gliomas are the most common primary brain tumors in adults (see Sidebar). Over the past 20 years, genetic, cell biological, and animal modeling studies have implicated a number of molecules in the formation and progression of malignant gliomas (1–3). This review focuses on recent advances that provide insight into the molecular pathology of malignant gliomas, i.e., the interface of the clinical, microscopic, and molecular aspects of malignant gliomas.

Malignant gliomas constitute a spectrum of clinicopathological entities (4), from low- to high-grade malignancies; but nearly all low-grade tumors eventually progress to high-grade malignancy. These tumors can be envisaged as progressing through a set of developmental steps: transformation from a cell of origin, acquisition of invasive properties, activation of cellular proliferative signals and abrogation of cell cycle control, upregulation of angiogenesis, and further clonal evolution. This review covers topics that follow these biological steps and concludes with a discussion of the emerging area of molecular diagnosis of malignant gliomas.

CELLS OF ORIGIN

The cells of origin for malignant gliomas remain enigmatic. Most glioma classifications made over the past 80 years have postulated that astrocytomas arise from astrocytes, and oligodendrogliomas from oligodendrocytes (5). However, there is no evidence that most brain cells undergo division normally during adult life, which would be a requirement if neoplasms arose from mature brain cells. Glial cells could undergo neoplastic events during reactive proliferation, but no epidemiological evidence convincingly links processes likely to evoke reactive proliferation, such as trauma, with the development of glial brain tumors (6). Furthermore, for neuronal tumors such as medulloblastomas, invoking the mature neuron as a cell of origin is difficult, given its terminally differentiated status after fetal life. A possible resolution to this problem is based on the idea of a "window of neoplastic vulnerability," implying that oncogenic events may occur in still-proliferating fetal cells (7). In this theory, neuronal tumors such as medulloblastomas are uncommon and occur early in life because they undergo oncogenic events during a short period early in embryonic and fetal life, when neuronal cells are still actively dividing. Thus, glial tumors are more common and arise later in life, because glial proliferation occurs later, during a longer period in gestational and postnatal life.

Recent work in both animal models and primary gliomas suggests the more likely possibility that malignant gliomas arise from neural progenitor cells (**Figure 1**) (see Differentiation and Tumor Phenotype, below). Neuroectodermal stem cells that reside in adult mammalian brains have proliferative potential, are migratory, and can pursue diverse paths of differentiation—all these features are intrinsic to glioma cells and likely characteristics of neoplastic cells of origin. Thus, there is a large possibility that the endogenous adult neuroectodermal stem cells are cells of origin for primary brain tumors. Differential targeting of oncogenic events to specific cell types can be accomplished by restricting the expression of a viral receptor to either progenitor cells or maturing astrocytes, followed by the introduction of oncogenes in specific viral vectors (8). This approach is enabled by the generation of transgenic mice that selectively express the viral receptor in either nestin-expressing or GFAP-expressing cells; the nestin-expressing cells form during an earlier stage in neuroectodermal cell development. In these studies, glial progenitor cells are more permissive to oncogenic transformation than are more mature astrocytic cells. For instance, overexpressing oncogenic Ras and Akt in progenitor cells, which mimicks the elevated activity of these signaling pathways found in human glioblastomas, results in mouse brain tumors that are histologically similar to their human counterparts, but targeting more mature astrocytic progenitors is not equally oncogenic (8). Targeting platelet-derived growth factor (PDGF)-B expression to progenitor cells results in tumors identical to human oligodendrogliomas (9). In addition, oncogenic events such as *CDNK2A/p16* deletion can drive more mature astrocytic cells to cells that have a progenitor phenotype, with multipotent differentiation potential (10). Furthermore, malignant gliomas likely contain tumor stem cells, a relatively primitive population responsible for populating and repopulating the tumors as they develop and progress (11–13); such tumor stem cells may be transformed variants of normal neural progenitor cells. The existence of these tumor stem cells may have major therapeutic implications as well because therapies that do not ablate the tumor stem cells will ultimately prove ineffective in eradicating the tumor.

CLINICOPATHOLOGICAL ASPECTS OF MALIGNANT GLIOMAS

Malignant gliomas are the most common primary brain tumor, accounting for the great majority of adult neuro-oncology cases. Nearly all are diffusely infiltrating tumors that affect the cerebral hemispheres of adults. In general, malignant gliomas are not curable tumors, despite aggressive therapy that includes surgery, chemotherapy, and radiation.

Traditional pathological approaches divide the adult diffuse gliomas into astrocytomas, oligodendrogliomas, and mixed oligoastrocytomas. These distinctions are based on light microscopic similarities between normal glial cells (astrocytes and oligodendrocytes) and tumor cells, as well as protein expression similarities using immunohistochemistry (e.g., glial fibrillary acidic protein). Traditional pathological approaches also grade these malignant gliomas into three degrees of malignancy: World Health Organization (WHO) grade II, grade III (anaplastic), and grade IV (reserved for glioblastoma, the most malignant form of astrocytoma). Grade II lesions are associated with a survival period between 5 and 15 years; grade III tumors with survival times often less than 3 years, and grade IV tumors with extremely poor prognoses of approximately 1 year. Younger adults, patients whose tumors can be extensively removed, and patients who have good functional status prior to surgery have better prognoses. In addition, oligodendroglial tumors tend to have better prognoses and be more chemosensitive than astrocytomas.

NEOPLASTIC TRANSFORMATION

In many epithelial malignancies, genetic changes in the progression from normal to hyperplastic to benign to malignant cells can be identified. For diffuse gliomas, however, the first identifiable step is a low-grade malignancy [World Health Organization (WHO) grade II astrocytoma, oligodendroglioma, or oligoastrocytoma]. The earliest events in glial neoplastic transformation remain unclear. Nonetheless, the genetic events most common in grade II gliomas differ between the two major types, astrocytoma and oligodendroglioma. Oligoastrocytomas have genetic features of either astrocytoma or oligodendroglioma.

Astrocytoma

p53, the tumor suppressor encoded by the *TP53* gene on chromosome 17p, plays an integral role in a number of cellular processes, including cell cycle arrest, response to DNA damage, apoptosis, angiogenesis, and differentiation. In grade II astrocytomas, inactivating *TP53* mutations are found in more than 50% of tumors (14). *TP53* mutation frequencies may also vary with race, as they are more common in astrocytomas from nonwhite individuals (15). Mutation studies complemented by functional studies and mouse modeling have recapitulated the role of p53 inactivation in the early stages of astrocytoma formation. For instance, cortical astrocytes from mice without functional p53 appear immortalized when grown in vitro and rapidly acquire a transformed phenotype. Cortical astrocytes from mice with one functional copy of *TP53* behave more like wild-type astrocytes and show signs of immortalization and transformation only after they have lost the

PDGF: platelet-derived growth factor

World Health Organization grade (WHO): an estimate of malignancy from II to IV for malignant gliomas

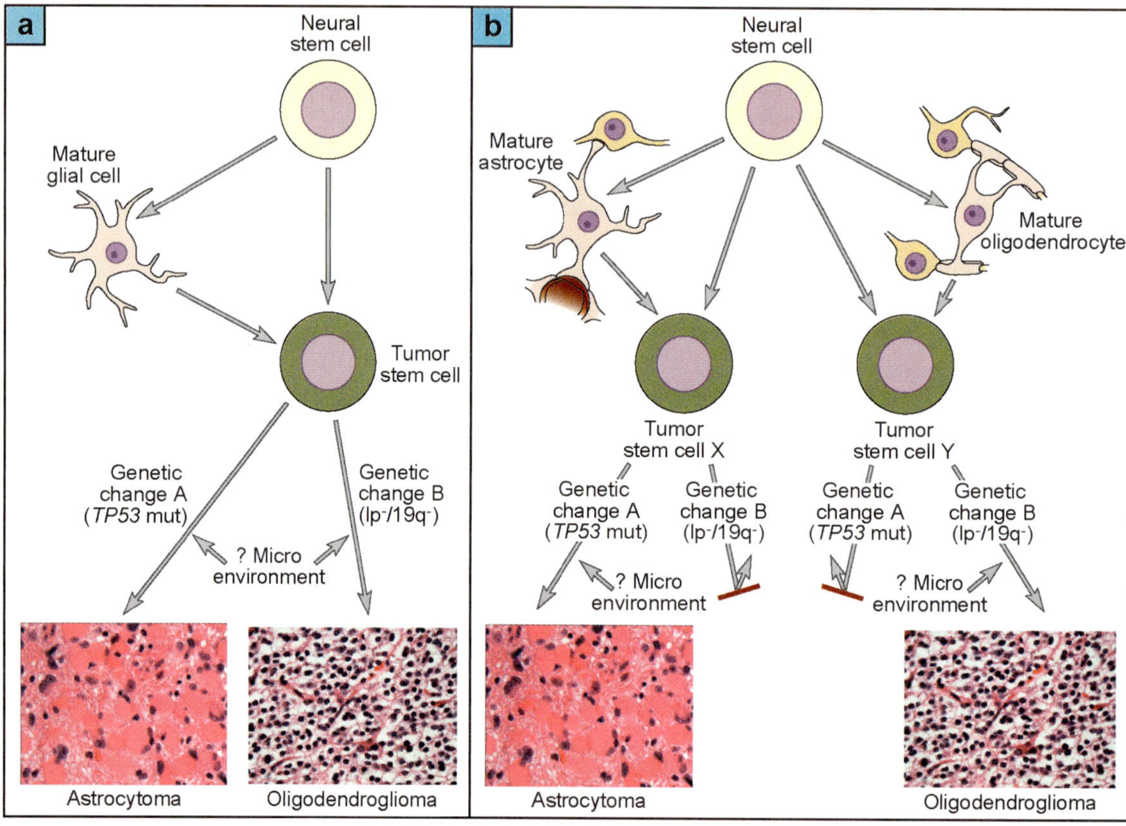

Figure 1

Stem cells and tumor differentiation. (*a*) A single type of tumor stem cell can arise either from a neural stem cell or from a mature glial cell. The end phenotype of astrocytoma or oligodendroglioma depends upon the activation of particular cellular pathways, either as a result of undergoing one set of genetic changes (e.g., *TP53* mutation) or another (e.g., 1p and 19q loss), possibly influenced by the tumor micro-environment. (*b*) Possible different types of tumor stem cells for various tumor types. In this model, one tumor stem cell (X) is permissive for neoplastic transformation only in the setting of particular genetic changes (e.g., *TP53* mutation), perhaps partially as a result of micro-environmental factors; other genetic changes (e.g., 1p and 19q loss) are lethal, hence the restriction to an astrocytic phenotype. Another stem cell (Y), perhaps influenced by micro-environmental factors, undergoes tumorigenesis only in the setting of other genetic changes (e.g., 1p and 19q loss), yielding an oligodendroglial tumor.

Oligoastrocytoma: a glial tumor with some cells histologically resembling astrocytes and others histologically resembling oligodendrocytes

functional *TP53* copy (16). Mouse models have also demonstrated that p53 inactivation contributes to astrocytoma tumorigenesis (17). Thus, the abrogation of astrocytic p53 function appears to facilitate some events integral to neoplastic transformation, setting the stage for further malignant progression. In addition (see **Figure 3**), in higher-grade astrocytomas, the p53 pathway may be deregulated by alterations of other components, including amplification of *MDM2* or *MDM4* and 9p deletions that result in loss of the ARF product of the *CDKN2A* gene (18, 19).

Many growth factors and their receptors are overexpressed in astrocytomas, including PDGF, fibroblast growth factors (FGFs), vascular endothelial growth factor (VEGF), and epidermal growth factor receptor (EGFR). PDGF ligands and receptors, found in the majority of cases, are expressed approximately equally in all grades of astrocytoma, which suggests that such overexpression is also important in the initial stages of astrocytoma formation (20). Tumors often overexpress cognate PDGF ligands and receptors in an autocrine stimulatory fashion. Loss of chromosome 17p in the *TP53* gene is closely correlated with PDGFα-receptor overexpression, implying that *TP53* mutations have an oncogenic effect only in the presence of PDGFα-receptor overexpression (21). This interdependence is highlighted by observations that mouse astrocytes without functional p53 transform only in the presence of specific growth factors (16). Less common genomic alterations associated with grade II astrocytomas include loss of chromosome arm 22q (22) and gain of chromosome arm 7q (23). The use of comparative genomic hybridization and array-comparative genomic hybridization has identified a number of other chromosomal arms that display copy number gains or loss in grade II astrocytomas, but these are less commonly affected (24).

Oligodendroglioma

Allelic loss in oligodendrogliomas occur preferentially on chromosomes 1p and 19q, affecting 40%–80% of these tumor types (25). These losses are closely associated; oligodendroglial tumors with 1p loss usually also have 19q loss, which suggests that the two putative tumor suppressor genes located in these chromosomal segments may be involved in biologically distinct pathways that are linked in some functional manner. Because of the frequent loss of these loci in low-grade as well as anaplastic oligodendrogliomas and oligoastrocytomas, the 1p and 19q tumor suppressors are probably important early in oligodendroglial tumorigenesis. These genes have not yet been identified, but have been the subject of extensive searches. The 19q gene most likely maps to a relatively small area of 19q13.3, but there remains substantial concern that this region may harbor the 19q glioma gene associated with astrocytoma progression (26–28). For 1p, the mapping has been less focused, primarily because small deletions are rare and because the short arm of chromosome 1 is quite large and probably contains multiple tumor suppressor genes (25, 29). Identification of the relevant genes will presumably shed light on the relationship between 1p and 19q loss, as well as on the associations between 1p and 19q loss and therapeutic sensitivity and survival (see Molecular Diagnostics, below).

VEGF: vascular endothelial growth factor

EGFR: epidermal growth factor receptor

Oligoastrocytoma

The molecular changes of the oligodendroglial and astrocytic components in oligoastrocytomas are similar despite their histological differences (30). Oligoastrocytomas, in most cases, have genetic changes typical of astrocytomas, i.e., *TP53* mutations, or oligodendrogliomas, i.e., 1p and 19q loss (31). Because the histological diagnosis of oligoastrocytoma varies somewhat from institution to institution, different reports cite different frequencies of these events in oligoastrocytomas. In general, approximately one third of oligoastrocytomas has an astrocytoma genotype and one third has an oligodendroglioma genotype.

DIFFERENTIATION AND TUMOR PHENOTYPE

The factors governing glioma cell differentiation, and therefore tumor phenotype, are unclear. The most compelling evidence addressing these factors has come from mouse glioma modeling. Mouse modeling studies show a telling histological difference between tumors arising in glial progenitor cells versus maturing astrocytes, as well as between progenitor cells undergoing different tumorigenic events (8). For example, whereas overexpression of Ras and Akt in progenitor cells yields astrocytic tumors such as glioblastomas, overexpression of PDGF-B in the same cell type produces tumors histologically similar to oligodendrogliomas (9). Thus, transformation of glial progenitor cells can result in tumors that have phenotypic properties of astrocytomas or oligodendrogliomas (9). As mentioned above, however, it is possible that more mature cells can be driven, as a result of oncogenic events, toward a less differentiated, pleuripotent cell type that can subsequently differentiate along highly divergent pathways, including neuronal (10).

The occurrence of oligoastrocytomas provides further evidence, both in humans and in the animal models, for cells of origin and pathways of differentiation. As mentioned above, the phenotypically distinct regions in oligoastrocytomas have similar genetic alterations (30); these are clonal lesions with marked phenotypic diversity. The mouse models provide intriguing corollary data because the neoplastic transformation of maturing astrocytes using viral oncogenes can drive these cells toward both oligodendroglial and astrocytic phenotypes in the same tumor, creating genetically engineered murine oligoastrocytomas (9).

Recent mouse modeling of gliomas has generated a preponderance of oligodendroglial tumors—despite the attempt to generate astrocytomas (32). Interestingly, they have been generated by using different oncogenes, targeting different cells, and using different transgenic technologies. A tempting explanation for these combined findings is that oligodendroglioma represents a common phenotypic pathway for glial neoplasia, at least in the mouse. In this sense, the "soil" may be of more importance than the "seed"; either the cells undergoing the oncogenic hits are inherently restricted in their phenotypic repertoire or the cerebral environment restricts the transformed cells.

Most genetically engineered murine gliomas and most human malignant glial tumors do not display overt neuronal differentiation. Nonetheless, as more sensitive neuronal markers are becoming available, more "gliomas" are being shown to express both neuronal and glial markers. It is likely that most "gliomas" will prove to be more heterogeneous tumors, particularly if they have developed from pleuripotent progenitor cells. The predominance of the glial phenotype may reflect a relative restriction of transformed postnatal progenitor cells to glial differentiation or that the brain environment or the intrinsic cellular programs operative in proliferating precursor cells favor glial differentiation. Regardless of the exact mechanism, the activation or inactivation of specific protein pathways, perhaps associated with the micro-environment, governs the eventual phenotype of neoplasms arising from particular precursor cells.

An understanding of glioma phenotype must also take into account the observations (see above) that astrocytic tumors are associated with *TP53* mutations, and oligodendrogliomas with 1p and 19q loss. It is possible that astrocytomas and oligodendrogliomas arise from the same cells of origin, but different genetic events drive differentiation along different lines; i.e., *TP53* mutation drives or allows astrocytic differentiation and 1p and 19q loss drives or allows oligodendroglial differentiation (**Figure 1*a***). Alternatively, astrocytomas and oligodendrogliomas may arise from different cells of origin that are oncogenically permissive only for particular events; i.e., disruption of the p53 pathway is only oncogenic as an initiating event in particular precursor cells, and oncogenesis in such precursor cells necessitates astrocytic differentiation (**Figure 1*b***). Note that oligodendroglial tumors with 1p and 19q loss preferentially affect particular areas of the brain, raising the possibility that oncogenesis in specific precursor cell populations in different brain regions must proceed along distinct genetic pathways to reach the common phenotypic endpoint of oligodendroglioma (33).

INVASION

Gliomas have a remarkable tendency to infiltrate the surrounding brain, which confounds therapeutic attempts at local control

(**Figure 2**). These invasive abilities are often apparent in low-grade as well as high-grade tumors, implying that the invasive phenotype is acquired early in tumorigenesis. The patterns of brain invasion in gliomas are the stereotypic so-called secondary structures of Scherer that are seen in histological evaluation. For instance, there is preferential invasion along white-matter tracts: Many gliomas cross the corpus callosum to form butterfly lesions; other gliomas remain confined to the white matter, stopping abruptly at the gray-white-matter junction. Other characteristic migratory patterns include preferential growth around neurons in the gray matter (perineuronal satellitosis), perivascular growth, and subpial spread.

These behaviors imply that glioma cells have either a tropism for particular sites or a restricted ability to invade in the potential regions between specific cell combinations. Explanations of glioma invasion must take

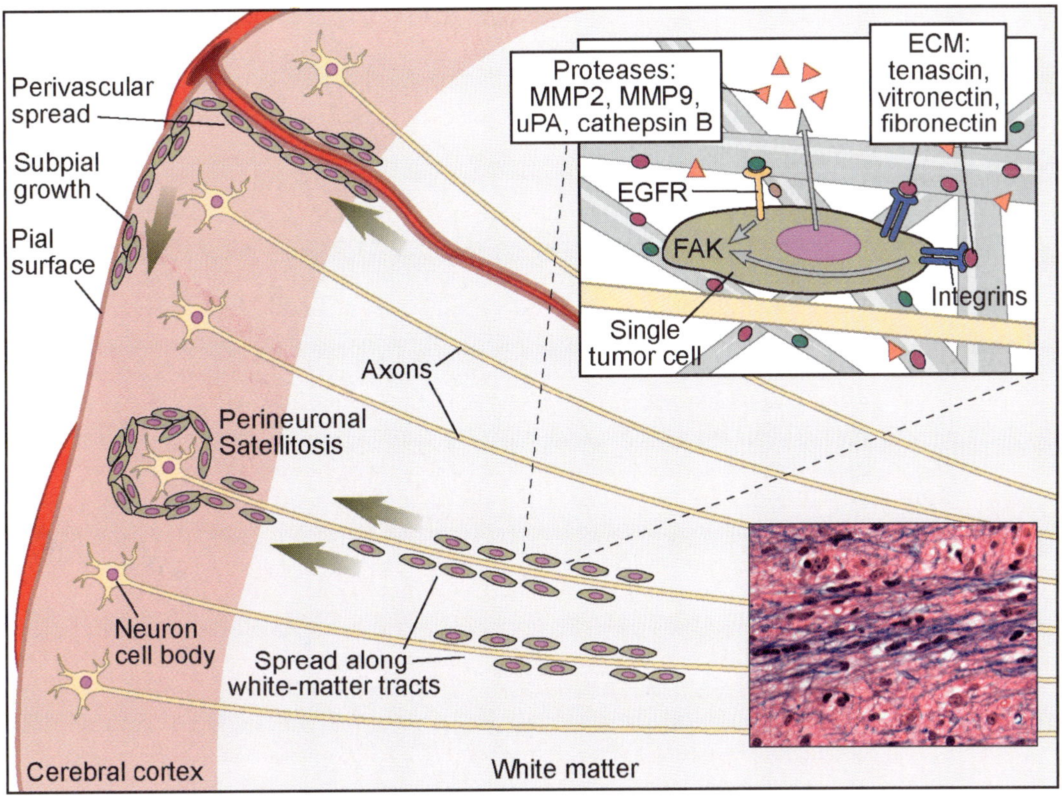

Figure 2

Invasion. Malignant glioma cells show preferential invasion along white-matter tracts, around neurons and blood vessels, and in the subpial region. The photomicrograph (*lower right corner*; Luxol fast blue H&E stain, 400X) illustrates individual elongated, hyperchromatic tumor nuclei oriented along myelinated axons (which stain bright blue with the Luxol fast blue stain). The inset at the top right illustrates molecular events relating to the invasion of single cells: elaboration of proteases such as matrix metalloproteinases MMP2 and MMP9, urokinase-type plasminogen activator (uPA), and cathepsin B; expression of integrins that interact with extracellular matrix (ECM) components such as tenascin, vitronectin, and fibronectin that are themselves expressed by tumor cells; and activation of focal adhesion kinase (FAK)-mediated cellular signaling pathways via epidermal growth factor receptor (EGFR) or integrin signaling (*see text*).

MMP: matrix metalloproteinase

FAK: focal adhesion kinase

these predilections into account. Moreover, glioma invasion must be viewed as a combination of the ability to migrate and the ability to modulate the extracellular space. Unfortunately, investigations of glioma invasion have been hampered by a paucity of representative experimental models. Most invasion models are in vitro systems, with some focusing on migration and others on invasion. Most follow-up studies have involved correlations with expression in primary tumors and only some in vitro findings have been confirmed in xenograft models.

Invasion of glioma cells into the brain most likely reflects a dynamic interplay between cell-cell adhesion, remodeling of the extracellular matrix, and cell motility (34). But invasion into brain parenchyma is biologically distinct from invasion of carcinomas into adjacent tissues in that the extracellular matrix of the brain is distinct from the extracellular matrix of most organs. In general, the extracellular matrix of the brain is ill-defined and scant. The matrix consists primarily of hyaluronic acid, except in two areas: around blood vessels and at the pial surface (glia limitans). At these sites, there is well-defined and more traditional basal lamina that includes collagens. Glioma cells preferentially involve the perivascular and subpial spaces—places at which basal lamina is well-defined—but they also involve perineuronal and white-matter locations—places at which the extracellular matrix is ill-defined. Furthermore, glioma cells elaborate many extracellular matrix substances, such as tenascin and vitronectin (35). Some malignant gliomas even feature extensive reticulin-rich pericellular networks and others are frankly desmoplastic. Therefore, an understanding of glioma invasion must acknowledge the particular anatomy of the brain as well as extracellular matrix alterations brought about by glioma growth.

Investigations into astrocytoma invasion have highlighted the complex nature of cell-cell and cell-extracellular matrix interactions (34, 36). Proteases are elaborated by glioma cells—including cysteine, serine, and metalloproteinases—and appear to play a significant role. These selective proteases degrade the extracellular environment in order to facilitate migration, but it is also likely that protease action remodels the environment in a manner that facilitates tumor cell growth. A number of proteases have been implicated, but most studies have focused on matrix metalloproteinases MMP2 and MMP9, the serine protease urokinase-type plasminogen activator and its receptor, and the cysteine protease cathepsin B (36). Expression of these proteases increases with glioma grade, and interference with the function of these proteases in vitro results in decreased invasive and/or migratory properties.

Researchers have also studied interactions between glioma cell surface molecules and extracellular matrix molecules. Most malignant gliomas express a variety of integrin receptors that mediate interactions with molecules in the extracellular space. The integrin heterodimers that have been most clearly implicated in glioma migration and invasion are $\alpha_2\beta_1$, $\alpha_5\beta_1$, $\alpha_6\beta_1$, and $\alpha_v\beta_3$, which interact with tenascin, fibronectin, laminin, and vitronectin, respectively (35). Activation of these integrins through interaction with extracellular ligands results in alterations of the cellular cytoskeleton, promoting locomotion. Attention has also focused on focal adhesion kinase (FAK) as a significant intermediate signaling molecule in glioma migration. FAK is a cytoplasmic tyrosine kinase expressed in high-grade gliomas and activated by EGFR and integrins such as $\alpha v\beta 3$ and $\alpha v\beta 5$. FAK subsequently signals through different pathways that affect proliferation, survival, and migration (37).

Many of the growth factors expressed in astrocytomas, such as FGF, EGF, and VEGF, also stimulate migration. Significantly, those glioblastomas with *EGFR* gene amplification do not demonstrate uniform distribution of the amplified cells within the tumor (38). Rather, *EGFR*-amplified cells are preferentially located at the infiltrating edges of these tumors. Given that *EGFR* gene amplicons are found on double-minute chromosomes, which must be maintained by positive selection during cell division, *EGFR* amplification likely confers a greater selective advantage at the infiltrating edge. Gene expression profiling data further supports the notion that EGFR signaling contributes to glioma cell invasion. Overexpression of the vIII EGFR mutant (a constitutively active EGFR variant missing most of the extracellular domain; see Tumor Progression, below) results in upregulated expression of multiple genes associated with invasion, including metalloproteinases (MMP1 and MMP13) and collagens (39). Furthermore, in glioma invasion model systems, inhibition of EGFR appears to inhibit invasion (40). It is likely that other growth factor pathways also influence invasion. For example, activation of insulin-like growth factor binding protein 2 upregulates MMP2 activity and increases invasion in glioblastoma (41). The invasive phenotype may also relate to other genetic alterations, such as loss of 1p and 19q in oligodendrogliomas. Those oligodendrogliomas with 1p and 19q loss are more likely to be bilateral tumors with ill-defined radiographic borders, features consistent with a more invasive phenotype (33, 42).

The potential clinical benefits of understanding the biological basis of glioma invasion cannot be overstated. Nearly all recurrences of malignant gliomas occur at or near the original treatment site, presumably representing an expansion of tumor cell groups that had already infiltrated the adjacent brain by the time of initial surgery. Most current therapies such as surgery and radiotherapy effectively target the tumor center, but fail to affect infiltrating tumor cells. Other novel treatment approaches such as antiangiogenic therapy may find glioma invasion an insurmountable hurdle: In experimental models, antiangiogenic therapy of tumor xenografts decreases the main tumor but increases the number of peritumoral, satellite tumors (43). Thus, understanding the molecular basis of glioma invasion is a high priority in glioma research (44).

TUMOR PROGRESSION

The known molecular changes underlying malignant progression are similar among the different types of glioma. The progression from WHO grade II to anaplastic, WHO grade III diffuse glioma is associated with a marked increase in clinical aggressiveness (see Sidebar). At a histological level, grade III tumors have increased cellularity and mitotic activity that is usually identifiable by light microscopy, as well as proliferative indices substantially above those of grade II tumors. At a molecular level, many genetic alterations target cell cycle regulatory genes. Most of these abnormalities converge on the critical cell cycle regulatory complex that includes the p16, cyclin-dependent kinase (cdk) 4, cdk6, cyclin D1, and retinoblastoma (Rb) proteins. The simplest schema (see **Figure 3**) suggests that p16 inhibits the cdk/cyclin D complexes, which prevents these complexes from phosphorylating pRb and thus ensures that pRb maintains its brake on the cell cycle. Individual components in this pathway are altered in as many as 50% of anaplastic astrocytomas and in nearly all glioblastomas and are common in higher-grade oligodendroglial tumors as well.

Chromosome 9p loss occurs in approximately 50% of anaplastic astrocytomas and glioblastomas, with 9p deletions affecting primarily the region of the *CDKN2A* gene that encodes the p16 and ARF proteins. The *CDKN2A* gene is inactivated by either homozygous deletion or, less commonly, point mutations or hypermethylation, thereby affecting p16 and ARF expression. In oligodendroglial tumors, hypermethylation of the gene is particularly common (45). The role of p16 in glioma progression has been confirmed in mouse glioma models overexpressing either PDGF or EGFR, in which the presence of a p16 null background is sufficient

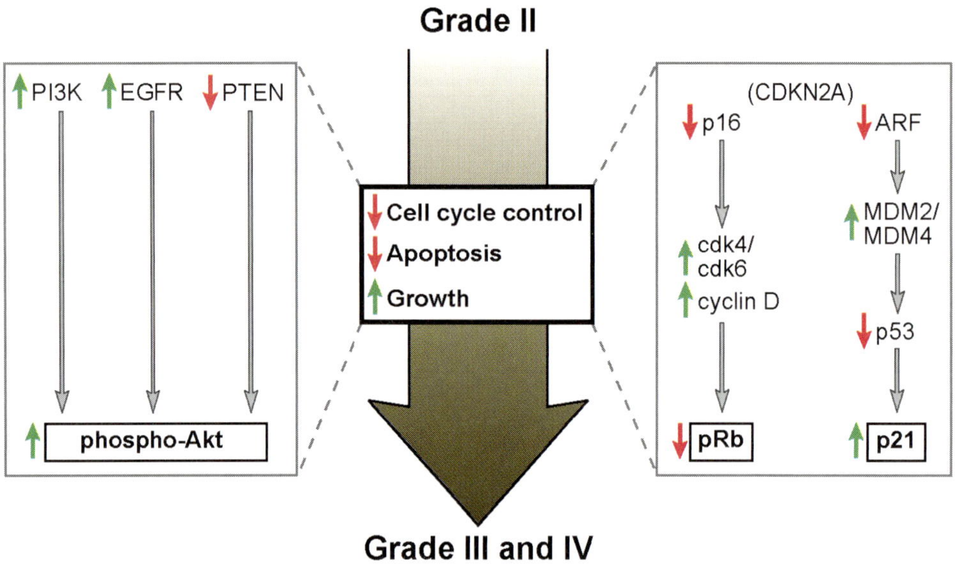

Figure 3

In nearly all cases progression from grade II to grade III and IV malignant glioma is associated with genetic changes that activate the growth signaling pathways that include the epidermal growth factor receptor (EGFR), PTEN, and Akt and that inactivate the cell cycle control pathways that feature p53 and the retinoblastoma protein. Upward arrow, upregulation; downward arrow, downregulation. cdk, cyclin-dependent kinase.

to change the resulting phenotype from low grade to anaplastic (9, 32, 46). Loss of chromosome 13q occurs in one third to one half of high-grade astrocytomas, with the *RB* gene preferentially targeted by chromosome loss and inactivating mutations. *RB* and *CDKN2A* alterations in primary gliomas are inversely correlated, rarely occurring in the same tumor. Inactivation of pRb in mouse astrocytes leads to anaplastic astrocytomas (47). Amplification of the *CDK4* gene, located on chromosome 12q13–14, provides an alternative to subvert cell cycle control and facilitates progression to glioblastoma in 15% of malignant gliomas. *CDK4* amplification, *CDK6* amplification, and cyclin D1 overexpression appear to represent alternative events to *CDKN2A* deletions and *RB* alterations because these genetic changes rarely occur in the same tumors.

Chromosome 10 loss is a frequent finding (60%–95%) in glioblastomas but far less common in anaplastic astrocytomas. At least two tumor suppressor loci are present on the long arm of chromosome 10, and there may be a third locus on the short arm. The *PTEN* gene at 10q23.3 has been implicated as one of these genes, with *PTEN* mutations identified in approximately 20% of glioblastomas and downstream activation of Akt in the vast majority of glioblastomas (8). *PTEN* alterations and chromosome 10 loss also characterize progression in oligodendrogliomas (48–50). PTEN functions as a protein tyrosine phosphatase and has 3′ phosphoinositol phosphatase activity; in addition, PTEN has an amino-terminal domain with homologies to tensin and auxilin. Thus, PTEN may regulate cell migration and cell proliferation via affecting FAK and control of the Akt serine/threonine kinase, respectively. Indeed, introduction of wild-type PTEN into glioma cells with mutant PTEN leads to growth suppression, and alterations in the PTEN pathway facilitate glioma formation in mouse models (8, 47). Data definitively implicating other chromosome 10 genes in glioma progression is lacking. Allelic losses have been found at other loci in high-grade astrocytomas, particularly on 19q (in up to 40% of anaplastic astrocytomas and glioblastomas), indicating a progression-associated glial tumor suppressor gene on chromosome 19q. This tumor suppressor gene maps to 19q13.3, but is yet to be identified (26).

EGFR is a transmembrane receptor tyrosine kinase whose ligands include epidermal growth factor and transforming growth factor alpha (TGFα). The *EGFR* gene is the most frequently amplified oncogene in astrocytic tumors, amplified in approximately 40% of all glioblastoma but in few anaplastic astrocytomas. Glioblastomas with *EGFR* gene amplification display overexpression of EGFR at both the mRNA and protein levels, which suggests that activation of this growth signal pathway is integral to malignant progression. The downstream targets of EGFR activation in glioblastomas include the Shc-Grb2-Ras pathway, which involves EGFR in a cascade that facilitates mitogenesis, decreases apoptosis, and upregulates angiogenesis. Approximately one third of glioblastomas with *EGFR* gene amplification also have specific *EGFR* deletions (the vIII mutant), which produce truncated molecules similar to the v-ErbB oncogene (34). Such truncated EGFR receptors are capable of conferring dramatically enhanced tumorigenicity to glioblastoma cells. Significantly, transgenic overexpression of ErbB in glial cells results in gliomas (32) as does overexpression of downstream Ras in progenitor cells (8).

In summary, deregulation of cell cycle control as well as activation of the EGFR-mediated signaling pathway appear to underlie the progression from grade II malignant gliomas to their high-grade counterparts, including glioblastoma. The similarity of the genetic events in astrocytic, oligodendroglial, and oligoastrocytic gliomas suggests that these changes are not cell specific, but rather affect generic cell control mechanisms necessary to oncogenesis. At the most basic level, many of the alterations can be divided into two large groups: those that result in deregulation of Akt-mTOR signaling and those that result in deregulation of the p53-Rb cell cycle control/apoptosis cascade (**Figure 3**). Although these two sets of alterations have diverse manifestations, it is nonetheless helpful to consider the bulk of changes as relating to these two pathways.

NECROSIS/HYPOXIA

Necrosis is a central feature of the highest-grade malignant gliomas. No histological feature is more powerful in predicting poor behavior (4). The biological correlates of this observation are that by the time necrosis occurs in astrocytomas, the tumor cells have achieved a highly malignant state, or the presence of necrosis encourages outgrowth of highly malignant cells. In all likelihood, there is a vicious cycle involving necrosis-induced hypoxia and various angiogenic and growth factors that combine to foster the highly malignant state of glioblastoma (**Figure 4**).

Necrosis can arise because of a number of different factors. In the setting of rapidly dividing cells with high metabolic demands, small regions of necrosis may develop in areas where metabolic demands exceed supply. Larger necroses, however, may arise from vascular thrombosis secondary to coagulation abnormalities, which are common in patients with malignant gliomas. One possible molecular culprit is tissue factor, which is expressed by the neoplastic cells and can act as a local procoagulant (51). Many necrotic zones in glioblastomas have small, adjacent thrombosed vessels—but these could be secondarily thrombotic as well.

Another intriguing, recently suggested possibility is that in response to hypoxia, small clones of tumor cells acquire molecular characteristics that encourage more active migration, thus clearing a central region more susceptible to necrosis. This hypothesis is based on work showing that glioblastoma tumor cells surrounding necrotic

Figure 4

Necrosis/hypoxia and angiogenesis. An intriguing hypothesis links tumor hypoxia, necrosis, and angiogenesis. (*a*) Localized hypoxia appears to upregulate migration-associated genes, (*b*) leading to migration of tumor cells away from a central hypoxic center (*see photomicrograph inset*; H&E, 200X). (*c*) Necrosis then ensues in the central region (*see photomicrograph inset*; H&E, 200X), sometimes in association with vascular thrombosis, and a palisade of densely packed tumor cells develops. These palisading cells express abundant angiogenic factors such as vascular endothelial growth factor (VEGF), which leads to (*d*) adjacent angiogenesis that includes so-called glomerloid microvascular proliferation (*see photomicrograph inset*; H&E, 200X). Another consequence of hypoxia may be clonal selection of malignant cells that are able to survive selection pressures (*see text*).

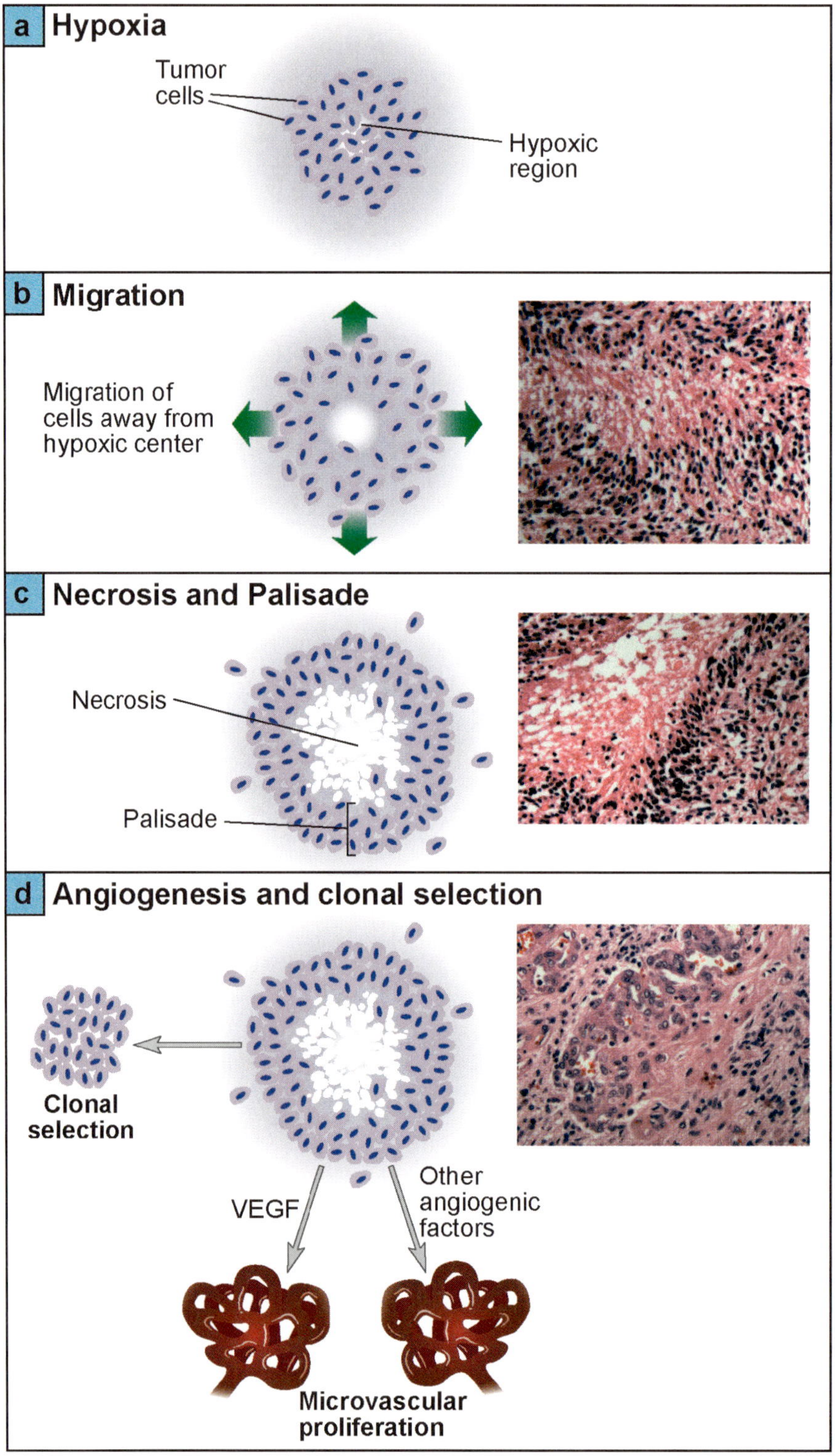

centers (often as so-called pseudopalisades) are less proliferative and more apoptotic than adjacent cells (51, 52). These perinecrotic cells also express hypoxia-inducible genes, such as hypoxia-inducible factor 1 alpha (HIF1α) (52), and in vitro studies have demonstrated that hypoxia increases cellular migration and gelatinase activity. Morphometric analysis of the central necrotic zones of pseudopalisades in glioblastomas demonstrate abnormal and sometimes thrombosed vessels in more than half, suggesting that an initial vaso-occlusive event initiated the hypoxia/necrosis cycle. It is also possible that the endothelial cells of small vessels are driven toward apoptosis and vascular regression as a result of angiopoietin-2 expression (53, 54).

Hypoxia may have a number of other sequelae as well (55, 56). For example, hypoxic cell death may lead to the release of growth factors from the dying cells, and some growth factors may remain intact within the necrotic zones. More importantly, hypoxia may allow the emergence of resistant, and thus highly malignant, clones of tumor cells. Hypoxia may select for those apoptosis-resistant tumor cells bearing inactivated p53 (55). Thus, hypoxia may facilitate angiogenesis, release of growth factors, and emergence of highly malignant clones. We have evaluated this possibility recently with expression profiling of pseudopalisading cells from perinecrotic regions of glioblastomas. When selected molecules that are preferentially expressed in palisading cells are used as prognostic markers in glioblastomas, they correlate with shorter patient survival (76). This supports the notion that these perinecrotic regions are zones in which more malignant clones are actively selected. The selection of more aggressive clones may imply an increased metabolic demand, which may facilitate more regions of hypoxia or necrosis, completing the vicious cycle. In addition, the interactions between hypoxia, necrosis, upregulation of growth factors, and selection of malignant clones begins to provide a simple explanation for the marked histological heterogeneity noted in glioblastomas—and a possible explanation for the marked resistance to conventional cytotoxic therapies seen in clinical patients with glioblastoma.

ANGIOGENESIS

Vascular proliferation is a hallmark of glioblastoma and occurs in two pathologically discernible forms: a diffuse increase in vascular density provided by more densely arrayed small vessels and the unusual complex form of angiogenesis most commonly known as microvascular proliferation (**Figure 4**). The diffuse increase in capillaries is not an obvious feature in H&E-stained tissue sections but is apparent when using immunohistochemistry for vascular markers such as Factor VIII–related antigen or CD31. For example, there is a correlation between astrocytoma tumor grade and microvessel density, as assessed by Factor VIII–related antigen immunohistochemistry (57). However, as with other histological features of malignant gliomas, there can be substantial intratumoral heterogeneity.

The most characteristic form of vascular proliferation, however, is microvascular proliferation in the form of so-called glomeruloid vessels (named after their resemblance to renal glomeruli). These vascular formations are unique to high-grade gliomas and are often used to grade gliomas; for example, nearly all diffuse astrocytic tumors with microvascular proliferation are classified as glioblastomas, and nearly all oligodendroglial tumors with microvascular proliferation are classified as anaplastic oligodendrogliomas. Glomeruloid vessels are complex structures composed of both proliferating endothelial and smooth muscle cells (58), hence the movement to avoid using the older, less accurate term endothelial proliferation (4). The structures are clearly proliferative, and it is not unusual to see mitotic figures within glomeruloid vessels in glioblastomas.

Microvascular proliferation is distributed irregularly in glioblastomas. Most notably, the glomeruloid vessels form semicircular

Table 1 Molecular diagnostic subtypes of malignant glioma

Histological diagnosis	Genetic changes	Clinicopathological correlates
Anaplastic oligodendroglioma	1p and 19q loss	Improved tx sensitivity Longer survival
Oligodendroglioma	1p and 19q loss	Improved tx sensitivity Longer survival
Glioblastoma	*TP53* mutation	Giant cell phenotype Younger age Secondary glioblastoma
Glioblastoma	*EGFR* amplification	Small cell phenotype Older age Primary glioblastoma

garlands that hug regions of necrosis. Less commonly, however, microvascular proliferation can be found primarily at the invading edge of glioblastomas, presumably because angiogenic molecules are expressed by migrating glioma cells in certain tumors.

The biological underpinnings of vascular proliferation in malignant gliomas are complex, with many angiogenic growth factors and their receptors occuring in glioblastomas (34). For example, VEGF and PDGF are expressed by tumor cells whereas their tyrosine kinase receptors, VEGF receptors 1 and 2 and PDGFβ-receptor, are expressed on endothelial cells. VEGF and its receptors, in particular, appear to play a major role in glioblastoma angiogenesis (59, 60). VEGF and its receptors, which cause vascular permeability, may also be responsible for breakdown of the blood-brain barrier and tumoral edema in glioblastoma. VEGF is secreted by tumor cells and bound by the VEGF receptors on endothelial cells. VEGF is a downstream target of a number of the activated signaling pathways in glioblastomas, e.g., via EGFR and Akt. As discussed above (see Necrosis below), VEGF is upregulated by tumor cells surrounding regions of necrosis, perhaps as a result of necrosis-induced hypoxia because hypoxia can stimulate VEGF production.

MOLECULAR DIAGNOSTICS

Although glioma classification has been rooted in microscopic examination for the past 80 years, a molecular diagnostic classification has made significant inroads clinically in the past 5 years (**Table 1**) (3, 5). For anaplastic oligodendrogliomas, the therapeutic relevance of molecular subtyping is already apparent (49, 50, 61). Although no clinical or pathological feature correctly predicts therapeutic response, allelic loss of chromosome 1p is a powerful predictor of a patient's response to PCV (procarbazine, CCNU, and vincristine) chemotherapy, and combined loss of 1p and 19q are strong correlates of longer survival (49, 50, 61). 1p status also appears to be predictive of chemotherapeutic response to temozolamide (62, 63). Anaplastic and grade II oligodendrogliomas can be divided genetically into therapeutically and prognostically relevant subgroups (50). Patients whose tumors have combined but isolated loss of 1p and 19q have marked and durable responses associated with long survival (**Table 1**). Other tumors with chromosome 1p alterations also respond to chemotherapy, but with shorter duration of response and patient survival. Tumors lacking 1p loss are associated with more aggressive behavior.

These results suggest that genetic analysis can be used to tailor therapy at the time of diagnosis. For example, patients with large bifrontal tumors having combined 1p and 19q loss may opt for chemotherapy, but may withhold radiation until recurrence, thus avoiding the potentially incapacitating effects of extensive, early radiation to the brain in long-surviving patients. On the other hand, patients whose tumors have chromosome 1p intact in the face of other genetic events such as *EGFR* gene amplification may opt to forego PCV chemotherapy in favor of radiation and a novel therapy, thus avoiding the myelotoxic effects of PCV. Chromosome 1p status also appears to have prognostic importance in lower-grade (WHO grade II) oligodendrogliomas (63–66). This work has sparked considerable interest in molecular markers for glioma management and has prompted diagnostic 1p and 19q testing at many institutions around the world (25).

For glioblastomas, genetic subsets have been defined on the basis of mutually exclusive gene alterations: e.g., frank *EGFR* amplification vs *TP53* mutation and 17p loss (67, 68). Experimental data also support this distinction by showing that p53-deficient cells are not transformed when cultured in the presence of EGF, whereas they are transformed in the presence of other growth factors (16). Glioblastomas with *TP53* mutations may therefore not be expected to select for cells with *EGFR* gene amplification if EGFR overexpression does not produce a growth advantage in such cells (38).

Those glioblastomas with *EGFR* amplification often occur in older patients and may have a small cell histological appearance (69), which makes them difficult to distinguish from anaplastic oligodendroglioma—a distinction of clinical importance because the two tumor types are treated differently and have markedly different prognoses. Assessment of *EGFR*, 1p, and 19q status can thus be diagnostically helpful in solving such diagnostic challenges (25, 69).

The genetic pathway involving *TP53* mutations may involve progression from a lower-grade astrocytic lesion. Glioblastomas arising from a lower-grade astrocytoma have been termed secondary glioblastoma (3–5); however, true secondary glioblastomas are uncommon, accounting for only approximately 5% of cases (70). Furthermore, although earlier reports had stressed close correlations between the presence of *TP53* mutation and secondary glioblastoma, population-based studies have shown *TP53* mutations in many primary glioblastomas as well (70). The *TP53* mutational spectrum may differ between primary and secondary glioblastomas, with mutations distributed relatively evenly throughout exons 4 through 8 in primary glioblastomas, but with the majority of mutations affecting the hotspot codons 248 and 273 in secondary glioblastomas (70). Younger age at initial diagnosis has been an important prognostic parameter among patients with glioblastoma, with younger patients faring better than older patients. In turn, glioblastomas lacking chromosome 17p occur in patients younger than those characterized by *EGFR* gene amplification (67). The predominance of tumors with 17p loss in a younger population of astrocytoma patients may therefore reflect the age-based difference in prognosis. The data suggest that genetic analysis may explain the clinical observations concerning age differences in astrocytic tumors (71). *TP53* mutations are also more common in those glioblastomas with a giant cell phenotype (72).

Chromosome 7 changes have also been widely noted (24, 73) and correlate with prognosis, with gains being associated with shorter survival times in anaplastic astrocytomas (73). 1p status may also be significant: In a small series of nonoligodendroglial high-grade gliomas, such as glioblastoma, that had shown either remarkable therapeutic responses or long survivals, we found 1p loss in all cases (74); in addition, glioblastomas with 1p and 19q loss may follow less aggressive courses (75).

The genetic heterogeneity of glioblastomas thus raises the possibility that new approaches to astrocytoma classification can also be based on objective biological parameters. At the present time, molecular diagnostic testing is recommended for patients diagnosed with anaplastic oligodendrogliomas, for small cell malignant tumors in which the differential diagnosis is anaplastic oligodendroglioma versus small cell glioblastoma, as well as for patients with grade II oligodendrogliomas for whom therapeutic decisions may be influenced by additional knowledge of probable tumor behavior (25). Such observations further suggest that molecular analyses may eventually guide therapeutic decisions for other types of malignant glioma.

CONCLUSIONS

In the past two decades researchers have witnessed many new approaches to the study of malignant gliomas. Molecular genetic, cell biological, mouse modeling, and translational research efforts have begun to piece together a picture of malignant glioma biology that begins to explain the clinical and microscopic features long observed by oncologists and pathologists. The next challenge will be to complete the puzzle. Once we are able to amalgamate our knowledge of the molecular pathology of malignant gliomas into a coherent framework, we can begin to develop more informed and unified approaches to therapy and diagnosis.

SUMMARY POINTS

1. Malignant gliomas constitute a spectrum of related brain tumors, with differentiation primarily along either astrocytic or oligodendroglial lines and with clinical courses that range from indolent to highly malignant.
2. Malignant gliomas most likely contain populations of tumor stem cells that may differentiate along astrocytic, oligodendroglial, and possibly neuronal lines. It remains unclear if such tumor stem cells arise from transformation of adult neural progenitor cells or transformation of mature glial cells, although the former possibility seems more likely.
3. Diffuse invasion into the surrounding brain is a cardinal feature of the common malignant gliomas that affect the cerebral hemispheres of adults, essentially preventing surgical cure and complicating the delivery of therapeutic agents. Invasion studies have been hampered by the paucity of representative experimental models, but current data point to an interplay between extracellular matrix components (elaborated primarily by the tumor cells), proteases (e.g., metalloproteinases), cell surface receptors (e.g., integrins, EGFR), and signal transduction pathways linked to migration (e.g., FAK).
4. *TP53* mutations are common in those malignant gliomas with an astrocytic phenotype, whereas allelic loss of chromosome arms 1p and 19q are common in those with an oligodendroglial phenotype.
5. Progression from WHO grade II malignant gliomas, whether astrocytic or oligodendroglial, to higher-grade tumors involves similar genetic events, including disruption of the p16-pRb cell cycle control pathway, inactivation of tumor suppressor genes on chromosome 10 (most clearly *PTEN*), and amplification of the *EGFR* gene.
6. Regions of necrosis and microvascular proliferation characterize high-grade malignant gliomas. Evidence suggests that the necrotic regions may initially represent a migratory response to local hypoxia (perhaps brought about by coagulopathic events), followed by frank necrosis. The cells that palisade around the necrosis elaborate angiogenic (e.g., VEGF) and other growth factors, contributing to the marked angiogenesis in these tumors (including the so-called glomeruloid blood vessels).

7. Molecular diagnostic applications have begun to develop from translational studies of glioma genetics. Clinical testing is now used to determine 1p and 19q status in patients with high-grade oligodendrogliomas to estimate response to therapies and potentially to avoid other toxic therapies. Clinical testing for 1p and 19q status may also be relevant in patients with grade II oligodendrogliomas and, coupled with *EGFR* status, may be useful in the pathological differential diagnosis between anaplastic oligodendroglioma and small cell glioblastoma.

UNRESOLVED ISSUES/FUTURE DIRECTIONS

1. Further research into the cell of origin for malignant gliomas would provide the basis for a better understanding of the precise events underlying glial tumorigenesis.
2. Discovering the basic mechanisms underlying glioma cell invasion into brain parenchyma will require improved experimental models of glioma invasion. The invasive nature of glioma cells is perhaps the largest obstacle to effective therapy, making this issue of paramount importance.
3. Early detection of the molecular events that govern the progression from low- to high-grade malignant glioma would be of use if targeted therapies could interrupt molecular pathways promoting malignant progression.
4. The pathological classification of malignant gliomas remains subjective. Molecular classifications have the potential to be more reproducible and accurate and dovetail with molecularly targeted therapies.

ACKNOWLEDGMENTS

The author thanks Dr. Catherine Nutt for helpful discussions concerning the text and figures.

LITERATURE CITED

1. Maher EA, Furnari FB, Bachoo RM, Rowitch DH, Louis DM, et al. 2001. Malignant glioma: genetics and biology of a grave matter. *Genes Dev.* 15:1311–33
2. Holland EC. 2001. Gliomagenesis: genetic alterations and mouse models. *Nat. Rev. Genet.* 2:120–29
3. Louis DN, Pomeroy SL, Cairncross JG. 2002. Focus on CNS neoplasia. *Cancer Cell* 1:125–28
4. **Kleihues P, Cavenee WK. 2000. *World Health Organization Classification of Tumours of the Nervous System*. Lyon: WHO/IARC**
5. Louis DN, Holland EC, Cairncross JG. 2001. Glioma classification: a molecular reappraisal. *Am. J. Pathol.* 159:779–86
6. Davis FG, Preston-Martin S. 1998. Epidemiology: incidence and survival. In *Russell and Rubinstein's Pathology of Tumors of the Nervous System*, ed. DD Bigner, RE McLendon, JM Bruner, pp. 5–45. London: Arnold

A rich source of clinical, pathological, and biological information on all types of human brain tumors.

7. Russell DS, Rubinstein LJ. 1989. *Pathology of Tumours of the Nervous System*. Baltimore: Williams & Wilkins
8. **Holland EC, Celestino J, Dai CK, Schaefer L, Sawaya RE, Fuller GN. 2000. Combined activation of Ras and Akt in neural progenitors induces glioblastoma formation in mice. *Nat. Genet.* 25:55–57**
9. Dai C, Celestino JC, Okada Y, Louis DN, Fuller GN, Holland EC. 2001. PDGF autocrine stimulation dedifferentiates cultured astrocytes and induces oligodendrogliomas and oligoastrocytomas from neural progenitors and astrocytes in vivo. *Genes Dev.* 15:1913–25
10. Bachoo RM, Maher EA, Ligon KL, Sharpless NE, Chan SS, et al. 2002. Epidermal growth factor receptor and Ink4a/Arf: covergent mechanisms governing terminal differentiation and transformation along the neural stem cell to astrocyte axis. *Cancer Cell* 1:269–77
11. **Galli R, Binda E, Orfanelli U, Cipelletti B, Gritti A, et al. 2004. Isolation and characterization of tumorigenic, stem-like neural precursors from human glioblastoma. *Cancer Res.* 64:7011–21**
12. **Singh SK, Hawkins C, Clarke ID, Squire JA, Bayani J, et al. 2004. Identification of human brain tumour initiating cells. *Nature* 432:396–401**
13. Singh SK, Clarke ID, Terasaki M, Bonn VE, Hawkins C, et al. 2003. Identification of a cancer stem cell in human brain tumors. *Cancer Res.* 63:5821–28
14. Okamoto Y, Di Patre PL, Burkhard C, Horstmann S, Jourde B, et al. 2004. Population-based study on incidence, survival rates, and genetic alterations of low-grade diffuse astrocytomas and oligodendrogliomas. *Acta Neuropathol.* 108:49–56
15. Chen PC, Aldape K, Wiencke JK, Kelsey KT, Miike R, et al. 2001. Ethnicity delineates different genetic pathways in malignant glioma. *Cancer Res.* 61:3949–54
16. Bogler O, Huang H-JS, Cavenee WK. 1995. Loss of wild-type p53 bestows a growth advantage on primary cortical astrocytes and facilitates their in vitro transformation. Cancer Res. 55:2746–51
17. Reilly KM, Loisel DA, Bronson RT, McLaughlin ME, Jacks T. 2000. Nf1;Trp53 mutant mice develop glioblastoma with evidence of strain- specific effects. *Nat. Genet.* 26:109–13
18. Ichimura K, Schmidt EE, Goike HM, Collins VP. 1996. Human glioblastomas with no alterations of the CDKN2 (p16^{INK4A}, MTS1) and CDK4 genes have frequent mutations of the retinoblastoma gene. *Oncogene* 13:1065–72
19. Ichimura K, Bolin MB, Goike HM, Schmidt EE, Moshref A, Collins VP. 2000. Deregulation of the p14ARF/MDM2/p53 pathway is a prerequisite for human astrocytic gliomas with G1-S transition control gene abnormalities. *Cancer Res.* 60:417–24
20. Hermanson M, Funa K, Hartman M, Claesson-Welsh L, Heldin CH, et al. 1992. Platelet-derived growth factor and its receptors in human glioma tissue: expression of messenger RNA and protein suggests the presence of autocrine and paracrine loops. *Cancer Res.* 52:3213–19
21. Hermanson M, Funa K, Koopmann J, Maintz D, Waha A, et al. 1996. Association of loss of heterozygosity on chromosome 17p with high platelet-derived growth factor α receptor expression in human malignant gliomas. *Cancer Res.* 56:164–71
22. Ino Y, Silver JS, Blazejewski L, Nishikawa R, Matsutani M, et al. 1999. Common regions of deletion on chromosome 22q12.3–13.1 and 22q13.2 in human astrocytomas appear related to malignancy grade. *J. Neuropathol. Exp. Neurol.* 58:881–85
23. Schrock E, Blume C, Meffert MC, du Manoir S, Bersch W, et al. 1996. Recurrent gain of chromosome arm 7q in low-grade astrocytic tumors studied by comparative genomic hybridization. *Genes Chromosomes Cancer* 15:199–205

The first report of a transgenic malignant glioma model based on molecular alterations found in human glioblastomas that recapitulates glioblastoma histopathology.

References 11 and 12 demonstrate the presence of tumor stem cells in glioblastomas.

24. Hirose Y, Aldape KD, Chang S, Lamborn K, Berger MS, Feuerstein BG. 2003. Grade II astrocytomas are subgrouped by chromosome aberrations. *Cancer Genet. Cytogenet.* 142:1–7
25. Reifenberger G, Louis DN. 2003. Oligodendroglioma: toward molecular definitions in diagnostic neuro-oncology. *J. Neuropathol. Exp. Neurol.* 62:111–26
26. Hartmann C, Johnk L, Kitange G, Wu Y, Ashworth LK, et al. 2002. Transcript map of the 3.7-Mb D19S112-D19S246 candidate tumor suppressor region on the long arm of chromosome 19. *Cancer Res.* 62:4100–8
27. Smith JS, Tachibana I, Pohl U, Lee HK, Thanarajasingam U, et al. 2000. A transcript map of the chromosome 19 q-arm tumor suppressor region. *Genomics* 64:44–50
28. Smith JS, Alderete B, Minn Y, Borell TJ, Perry A, et al. 1999. Localization of common deletion regions on 1p and 19q in human gliomas and their association with histological subtype. *Oncogene* 18:4144–52
29. Felsberg J, Erkwoh A, Sabel MC, Kirsch L, Fimmers R, et al. 2004. Oligodendroglial tumors: refinement of candidate regions on chromosome arm 1p and correlation of 1p/19q status with survival. *Brain Pathol.* 14:121–30
30. Kraus JA, Koopmann J, Kaskel P, Brandner S, Schramm J, et al. 1995. Shared allelic losses on chromosomes 1p and 19q suggest a common origin of oligodendroglioma and oligoastrocytoma. *J. Neuropathol. Exp. Neurol.* 54:91–95
31. Maintz D, Fiedler K, Koopmann J, Rollbrocker B, Nechev S, et al. 1997. Molecular genetic evidence for subtypes of oligoastrocytomas. *J. Neuropathol. Exp. Neurol.* 56:1098–104
32. Weiss WA, Israel M, Cobbs C, Holland E, James CD, et al. 2002. Neuropathology of genetically engineered mice: consensus report and recommendations from an international forum. *Oncogene* 21:7453–63
33. Zlatescu MC, TehraniYazdi AR, Sasaki H, Megyesi JF, Betensky RA, et al. 2001. Tumor location and growth pattern correlate with genetic signature in oligodendroglial neoplasms. *Cancer Res.* 61:6713–15
34. Cavenee WK, Furnari FB, Nagane M, Huang H-JS, Newcombe EW, et al. 2000. Diffuse astrocytomas. In *Pathology and Genetics of Tumours of the Nervous System*, ed. P Kleihues, WK Cavenee, pp. 10–21. Lyon: IARC
35. Uhm JH, Gladson CL, Rao JS. 1999. The role of integrins in the malignant phenotype of gliomas. *Front. Biosci.* 4:D188–99
36. Rao JS. 2003. Molecular mechanisms of glioma invasiveness: the role of proteases. *Nat. Rev. Cancer* 3:489–501
37. Natarajan M, Hecker TP, Gladson CL. 2003. FAK signaling in anaplastic astrocytoma and glioblastoma tumors. *Cancer J.* 9:126–33
38. Okada Y, Hurwitz EE, Esposito JM, Brower MA, Nutt CL, Louis DN. 2003. Selection pressures of TP53 mutation and microenvironmental location influence EGFR gene amplification in human glioblastomas. *Cancer Res.* 63:413–16
39. Lal A, Glazer CA, Martinson HM, Friedman HS, Archer GE, et al. 2002. Mutant epidermal growth factor receptor up-regulates molecular effectors of tumor invasion. *Cancer Res.* 62:3335–39
40. Penar PL, Khoshyomn S, Bhushan A, Tritton TR. 1997. Inhibition of epidermal growth factor receptor-associated tyrosine kinase blocks glioblastoma invasion of the brain. *Neurosurgery* 41:141–51
41. Wang H, Wang HM, Shen WP, Huang H, Hu LM, et al. 2003. Insulin-like growth factor binding protein 2 enhances glioblastoma invasion by activating invasion-enhancing genes. *Cancer Res.* 63:4315–21

42. Megyesi JF, Kachur E, Lee DH, Zlatescu MC, Betensky RA, et al. 2004. Imaging correlates of molecular signatures in oligodendrogliomas. *Clin. Cancer Res.* 10:4303–6
43. Lamszus K, Kunkel P, Westphal M. 2003. Invasion as limitation to anti-angiogenic glioma therapy. *Acta Neurochir. Suppl.* 88:169–77
44. Louis DN, Posner JB, Jacobs T, Kaplan R. 2000. Report of the Brain Tumor Progress Review Group. **http://prg.nci.nih.gov/brain/finalreport.html**
45. Wolter M, Reifenberger J, Blaschke B, Ichimura K, Schmidt EE, et al. 2001. Oligodendroglial tumors frequently demonstrate hypermethylation of the CDKN2A (MTS1, p16INK4a), p14ARF, and CDKN2B (MTS2, p15INK4b) tumor suppressor genes. *J. Neuropathol. Exp. Neurol.* 60:1170–80
46. Weiss WA, Burns MJ, Hackett C, Aldape K, Hill JR, et al. 2003. Genetic determinants of malignancy in a mouse model for oligodendroglioma. *Cancer Res.* 63:1589–95
47. Xiao A, Wu H, Pandolfi PP, Louis DN, Van Dyke T. 2002. Astrocyte inactivation of the pRb pathway predisposes mice to malignant astrocytoma development that is accelerated by PTEN mutation. *Cancer Cell* 1:157–68
48. Sasaki H, Zlatescu MC, Betensky RA, Ino Y, Cairncross JG, Louis DN. 2001. PTEN is a target of chromosome 10q loss in anaplastic oligodendrogliomas and PTEN alterations are associated with poor prognosis. *Am. J. Pathol.* 159:359–67
49. **Cairncross JG, Ueki K, Zlatescu MC, Lisle DK, Finkelstein DM, et al. 1998. Specific chromosomal losses predict chemotherapeutic response and survival in patients with anaplastic oligodendrogliomas. *J. Natl. Cancer Inst.* 90:1473–79**

The first report that malignant gliomas (anaplastic oligodendrogliomas) can be genetically subtyped into clinically relevant groups that have therapeutic and prognostic implications.

50. Ino Y, Betensky RA, Zlatescu MC, Sasaki H, Macdonald DR, et al. 2001. Molecular subtypes of anaplastic oligodendroglioma: implications for patient management at diagnosis. *Clin. Cancer Res.* 7:839–45
51. Brat DJ, Van Meir EG. 2004. Vaso-occlusive and prothrombotic mechanisms associated with tumor hypoxia, necrosis, and accelerated growth in glioblastoma. *Lab. Invest.* 84:397–405
52. **Brat DJ, Castellano-Sanchez AA, Hunter SB, Pecot M, Cohen C, et al. 2004. Pseudopalisades in glioblastoma are hypoxic, express extracellular matrix proteases, and are formed by an actively migrating cell population. *Cancer Res.* 64:920–27**

A detailed study proposing the hypothesis that focal hypoxia can lead to local migration, necrosis, and palisading.

53. Holash J, Maisonpierre PC, Compton D, Boland P, Alexander CR, et al. 1999. Vessel cooption, regression, and growth in tumors mediated by angiopoietins and VEGF. *Science* 284:1994–98
54. Zagzag D, Hooper A, Friedlander DR, Chan W, Holash J, et al. 1999. In situ expression of angiopoietins in astrocytomas identifies angiopoietin-2 as an early marker of tumor angiogenesis. *Exp. Neurol.* 159:391–400
55. Graeber TG, Osmanian C, Jacks T, Housman DE, Koch CJ, et al. 1996. Hypoxia-mediated selection of cells with diminished apoptotic potential in solid tumors. *Nature* 379:88–91
56. Kinzler KW, Vogelstein B. 1996. Life (and death) in a malignant tumor. *Nature* 379:19–20
57. Leon SP, Folkerth RD, Black PM. 1996. Microvessel density is a prognostic indicator for patients with astroglial brain tumors. *Cancer* 77:362–72
58. Haddad SF, Moore SA, Schelper RL, Goeken JA. 1992. Vascular smooth muscle hyperplasia underlies the formation of glomeruloid vascular structures of glioblastoma multiforme. *J. Neuropathol. Exp. Neurol.* 51:488–92
59. Plate KH, Breier G, Weich HA, Risau W. 1992. Vascular endothelial growth factor is a potential tumour angiogenesis factor in human gliomas in vivo. *Nature* 359:845–48
60. Brat DJ, Van Meir EG. 2001. Glomeruloid microvascular proliferation orchestrated by VPF/VEGF: a new world of angiogenesis research. *Am. J. Pathol.* 158:789–96

61. Smith JS, Perry A, Borell TJ, Lee HK, O'Fallon J, et al. 2000. Alterations of chromosome arms 1p and 19q as predictors of survival in oligodendrogliomas, astrocytomas, and mixed oligoastrocytomas. *J. Clin. Oncol.* 18:636–45
62. Chahlavi A, Kanner A, Peereboom D, Staugaitis SM, Elson P, Barnett G. 2003. Impact of chromosome 1p status in response of oligodendroglioma to temozolomide: preliminary results. *J. Neurooncol.* 61:267–73
63. **Hoang-Xuan K, Capelle L, Kujas M, Taillibert S, Duffau H, et al. 2004. Temozolomide as initial treatment for adults with low-grade oligodendrogliomas or oligoastrocytomas and correlation with chromosome 1p deletions. *J. Clin. Oncol.* 22:3133–38**
64. Sasaki H, Zlatescu MC, Betensky RA, Johnk LB, Cutone AN, et al. 2002. Histopathological-molecular genetic correlations in referral pathologist-diagnosed low-grade "oligodendroglioma." *J. Neuropathol. Exp. Neurol.* 61:58–63
65. van den Bent MJ, Looijenga LHJ, Langenberg K, Dinjens W, Graveland W, et al. 2003. Chromosomal anomalies in oligodendroglial tumors are correlated with clinical features. *Cancer* 97:1276–84
66. Bauman GS, Ino Y, Ueki K, Zlatescu MC, Fisher BJ, et al. 2000. Allelic loss of chromosome 1p and radiotherapy plus chemotherapy in patients with oligodendrogliomas. *Int. J. Radiat. Oncol. Biol. Phys.* 48:825–30
67. **von Deimling A, von Ammon K, Schoenfeld D, Wiestler OD, Seizinger BR, Louis DN. 1993. Subsets of glioblastoma multiforme defined by molecular genetic analysis. *Brain Pathol.* 3:19–26**
68. Watanabe K, Tachibana O, Sata K, Yonekawa Y, Kleihues P, Ohgaki H. 1996. Overexpression of the EGF receptor and p53 mutations are mutually exclusive in the evolution of primary and secondary glioblastomas. *Brain Pathol.* 6:217–23
69. Burger PC, Pearl DK, Aldape K, Yates AJ, Scheithauer BW, et al. 2001. Small cell architecture–a histological equivalent of EGFR amplification in glioblastoma multiforme? *J. Neuropathol. Exp. Neurol.* 60:1099–104
70. **Ohgaki H, Dessen P, Jourde B, Horstmann S, Nishikawa T, et al. 2004. Genetic pathways to glioblastoma: a population-based study. *Cancer Res.* 64:6892–99**
71. Simmons ML, Lamborn KR, Takahashi M, Chen P, Israel MA, et al. 2001. Analysis of complex relationships between age, p53, epidermal growth factor receptor, and survival in glioblastoma patients. *Cancer Res.* 61:1122–28
72. Meyer-Puttlitz B, Hayashi Y, Waha A, Rollbrocker B, Bostrom J, et al. 1997. Molecular genetic analysis of giant cell glioblastomas. *Am. J. Pathol.* 151:853–57
73. Kunwar S, Mohapatra G, Bollen A, Lamborn KR, Prados M, Feuerstein BG. 2001. Genetic subgroups of anaplastic astrocytomas correlate with patient age and survival. *Cancer Res.* 61:7683–88
74. Ino Y, Zlatescu MC, Sasaki H, Macdonald DR, Stemmer-Rachamimov AO, et al. 2000. Long patient survival and therapeutic responses in histologically disparate high grade gliomas with chromosome 1p loss. *J. Neurosurg.* 92:983–90
75. Schmidt MC, Antweiler S, Urban N, Mueller W, Kuklik A, et al. 2002. Impact of genotype and morphology on the prognosis of glioblastoma. *J. Neuropathol. Exp. Neurol.* 61:321–28
76. Dong S, Nutt CL, Betensky RA, Stemmer-Rachamimov AO, Denko NC, et al. 2006. Histology-based expression profiling yields novel prognostic markers in human glioblastoma. *J. Neuropathol. Exp. Neurol.* In press

A study documenting correlations between molecular subtypes and clinical outcome in low-grade oligodendrogliomas.

The initial demonstration that malignant gliomas (glioblastomas) can be subtyped on the basis of molecular genetic alterations.

A comprehensive, population-based catalogue of genetic changes found in glioblastomas.

Tumor Stroma and Regulation of Cancer Development

Thea D. Tlsty[1] and Lisa M. Coussens[1,2]

[1]Department of Pathology and Comprehensive Cancer Center, [2]Cancer Research Institute, University of California, San Francisco, San Francisco, California 94115; email: ttlsty@itsa.ucsf.edu, coussens@cc.ucsf.edu

Annu. Rev. Pathol. Mech. Dis. 2006. 1:119–50

First published online as a Review in Advance on October 11, 2005

The *Annual Review of Pathology: Mechanisms of Disease* is online at pathmechdis.annualreviews.org

doi: 10.1146/annurev.pathol.1.110304.100224

1553-4006/06/0114-0119$20.00

Key Words

inflammation, angiogenesis, fibroblast, microenvironment, immune cells, protease

Abstract

In the past 25 years, a majority of cancer studies have focused on examining functional consequences of activating and/or inactivating mutations in critical genes implicated in cell cycle control. These studies have taught us a great deal about the functions of oncogenes and tumor suppressor genes and the signaling pathways regulating cell proliferation and/or cell death. However, such studies have largely ignored the fact that cancers are heterogeneous cellular entities whose growth is dependent upon reciprocal interactions between genetically altered "initiated" cells and the dynamic microenvironment in which they live. This review highlights the aspects of cancer development that, like organogenesis during embryonic development and tissue repair in adult mammals, are regulated by interactions between epithelial cells, activated stromal cells, and soluble and insoluble components of the extracellular matrix.

CANCER: A CHRONIC DISEASE INVOLVING MULTIPLE TISSUE COMPARTMENTS

ECM: extracellular matrix

Angiogenesis: growth of new blood vessels from preexisting vascular beds

Acute: a pathologic or physiologic event of severe and or short duration

Chronic: pathologic or physiologic condition that persists over a long period

Microenvironment: local area including all cellular and noncellular components

What is cancer? Are cancers merely homogeneous masses of aneuploid cells with heightened migratory capabilities? If they were, their therapeutic elimination would have been possible years ago. Instead, cancers are heterogeneous multicellular entities containing cells of multiple lineages whose interactions with one another, the extracellular matrix (ECM), and soluble molecules in their vicinity are dynamic and favor cell proliferation, movement, differentiation, and ECM metabolism, while simultaneously restricting cell death, stationary polarized growth, and ECM stability. Thus, when referring to a "cancer cell" or a discrete property of "cancer," one should articulate which type of cell is being discussed, e.g., a mutated epithelial cell versus a vascular, inflammatory, or other activated stromal cell. Also important is the appreciation that angiogenesis, cell migration, and matrix and tissue remodeling are not unique properties of cancerous growths but instead are regulated programs normally utilized during development and in adult tissues responding to acute tissue stress. What then is unique about cancer as a chronic disease? Why is cancer disadvantageous to the organism harboring it, and what lessons can we learn from development or normal wound repair to aid in eradication of cancerous tissues? This review compares and contrasts the important regulatory programs and molecules implicated in maintaining cell and tissue homeostasis during development and following acute stress as compared with their roles in malignancy.

Cancer Cells and the Extracellular Matrix

All cancers contain a diverse population of cells, including those harboring genetic mutations typically referred to as "tumor" or "cancer" cells as well as other cell types that are activated and/or recruited to the local microenvironment, e.g., fibroblasts, innate and adaptive immune cells, and cells that line blood and lymphatic vessels. Reciprocal interactions between these responding "normal" cells, their mediators, structural components of the ECM, and genetically altered neoplastic cells regulate all aspects of tumorigenicity (1–3).

A functional link between inflammation and cancer has long been recognized. Innate immune cells, including granulocytes, dendritic cells, macrophages, natural killer cells, and mast cells, are prominent components of premalignant and malignant tissues (**Figures 1–3**) and contribute functionally to cancer development largely due to their release of potent soluble mediators that regulate cell proliferation, migration, angiogenesis, tissue remodeling, metabolism, and genomic integrity. Individuals suffering from chronic inflammatory disorders harbor a greatly increased risk for cancer development, owing primarily to the progrowth environment generated by activated inflammatory cells (**Figure 4**).

Fibroblasts are important cells in any context. They are primarily responsible for the synthesis, deposition, and remodeling of the ECM, as well as for the production of many soluble paracrine growth factors that regulate cell proliferation, morphology, survival, and death. Historically, fibroblasts were thought to be passive participants in neoplastic programming of tissues; however, recent data indicate that they exert an active role (2) and, in combination with inflammatory cells, can promote neoplastic programming of tissues (4).

Blood vessels are essential for maintaining tissue homeostasis and are activated during all tissue repair and growth processes as well as during cancer development. Tumor angiogenesis, the growth of new vessels from preexisting vascular beds (**Figure 5**), is regulated in part by local changes in the relative balance between soluble and insoluble molecules that elicit either pro- or antiangiogenic effects

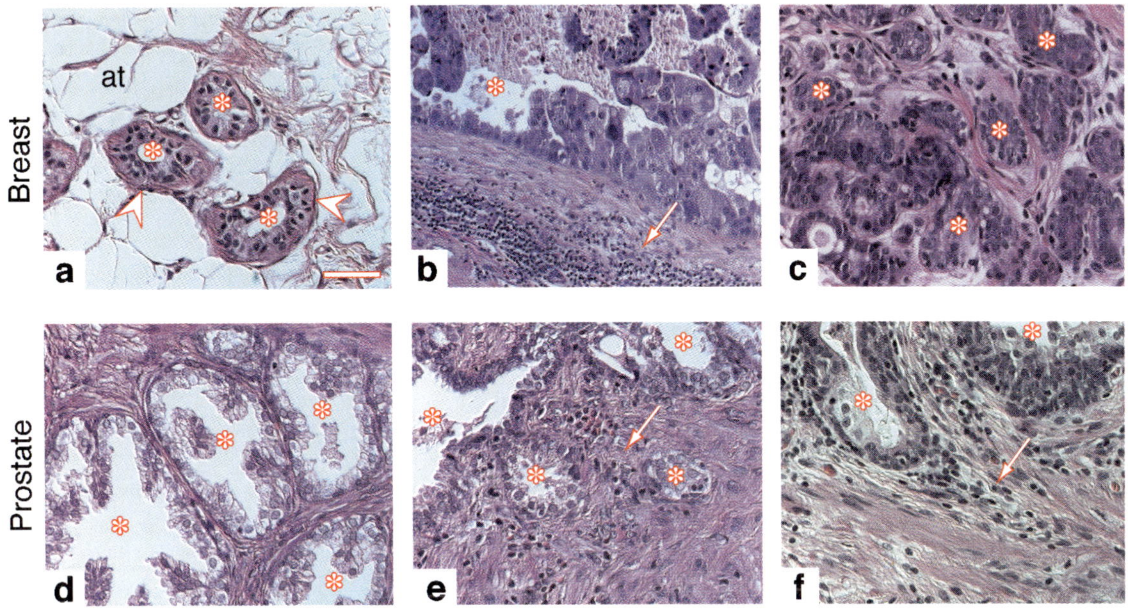

Figure 1

Stromal responses in breast and prostate carcinogenesis. (*a*) Normal mammary gland (*) from a nonpregnant woman of reproductive age showing a duct system, lined by epithelial cells and underlying myoepithelial cells (*arrowheads*). Ducts are surrounded by dense fibrous interlobular adipose tissue (at). (*b*) Ductal carcinoma in situ disorganization of ductal epithelium (*) stromal infiltration of inflammatory cells (*arrow*) in dense collagenous stroma are evident. (*c*) Mammary carcinoma in which ductal epithelial cells (*) form aberrant glandular structures and grow in cords without gland formation, surrounded by dense collagen bundles produced by activated fibroblasts. (*d*) Adult male prostate (benign nodular hyperplasia) with pseudostratified and columnar glandular epithelium with poorly stained foamy cytoplasm. (*e*) Prostatic intraepithelial neoplasia. Premalignant lesion consisting of closely packed irregular accini (*) lined by multiple layers of cuboidal epithelial cells adjacent to dense collagenous stroma and infiltrating inflammatory cells (*arrow*). (*f*) Invasive front of a prostatic adenocarcinoma in which rudiments of prostate gland are present (*) amid dense collagenous stroma infiltrated with diverse inflammatory cells (*arrow*). Bar: 50 μm (*a*, *d*); 100 μm (*b*, *c*, *e*, *f*).

on endothelial and perivascular cell proliferation, differentiation, migration, and/or tube formation.

The three-dimensional organization and architecture of the ECM or stroma surrounding the cells in any tissue are dynamic. The metabolism of ECM molecules—synthesis balanced by degradation—is an important aspect of tissue homeostasis and determines how cells respond to acute and chronic stress. Inappropriate synthesis or degradation of any ECM molecule can alter cell physiology and cause disease. Ultrastructural studies, immunohistochemistry, and biochemical analysis have each contributed to the appreciation that the stroma is altered at critical steps during the neoplastic process (5, 6). Early studies documented a change in the expression of proteins with acquired expression of α-smooth muscle actin, vimentin, smooth muscle myosin, calponin, tenascin, and desmin (5, 7). These proteins are often expressed as a response to wound healing or inflammation (8) and produce many new proteins that reflect a program of mesenchymal cell differentiation. During cancer development, these proteins and other ECM molecules embedded in the neoplastic tissue favor cell

Stroma: cells and connective tissue that provides contextual framework for an organ or tissue

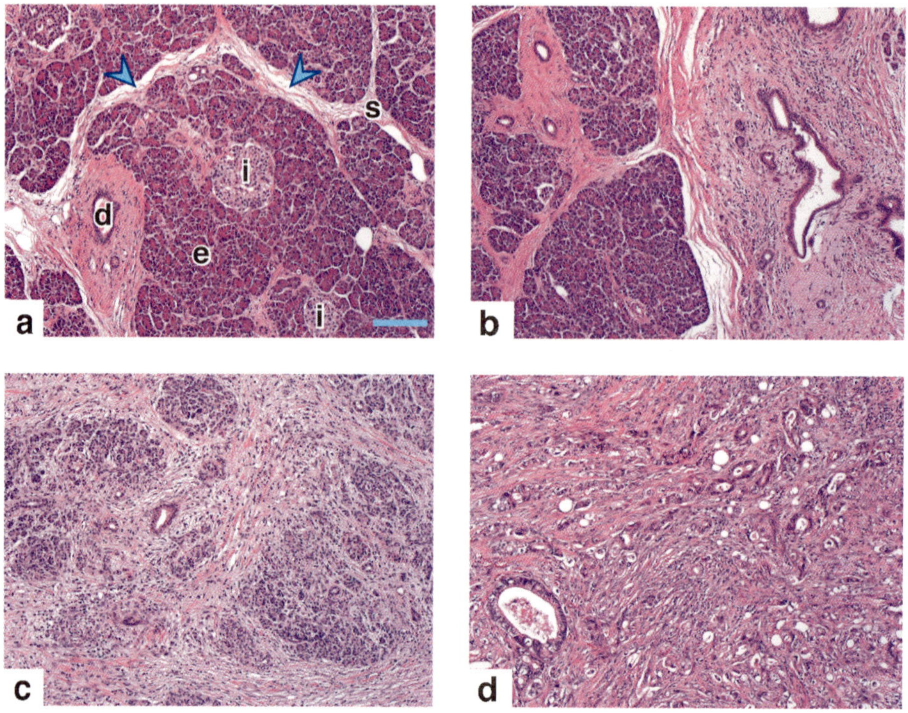

Figure 2

Inflammation and cancer in the human pancreas. H&E of human (*a*) normal pancreas, (*b*) early pancreatitis, (*c*) advanced pancreatitis, and (*d*) pancreatic ductal adenocarcinoma. The pancreas is a highly lobulated gland invested by a thin loose collagenous capsule (*arrowhead*) that extends as septa (s) between lobules. Exocrine acini (e) are densely packed, drain into ducts (d), and surround endocrine islets of Langerhans (i). Hereditary pancreatitis is characterized by a robust desmoplastic response thought to enhance neoplastic risk. Bar: 400 μm (*a–d*).

proliferation, inflammation, angiogenesis, and migration of cells into ectopic tissue compartments. Cancer development is like embryogenesis and adult wound repair in that it is also well-organized and follows highly regulated multistage events. All the cells and molecules comprising a tumor interact and engage in highly regulated reciprocal dialogues favoring malignancy.

THE ORIGINS OF CANCER

Initiation

The current predominant view of cancer is that of a disease involving irreversible genomic change—changes encompassing single mutations in specific genes, or alteration, amplification, or loss of large regions of the genome (9). Dominant gain-of-function and recessive loss-of-function alterations in critical gatekeeper genes, e.g., oncogenes and tumor suppressor genes, have been identified in virtually every form of human cancer and are believed to be at the root of the initiation of neoplastic growth. The sheer number of genes identified in the past 25 years harboring such alterations might suggest that random genetic mutations underlie cancer development. In reality, although a large diversity of mutated genes exist in cancer cells (9, 10), the overall neoplastic risk likely is influenced by a

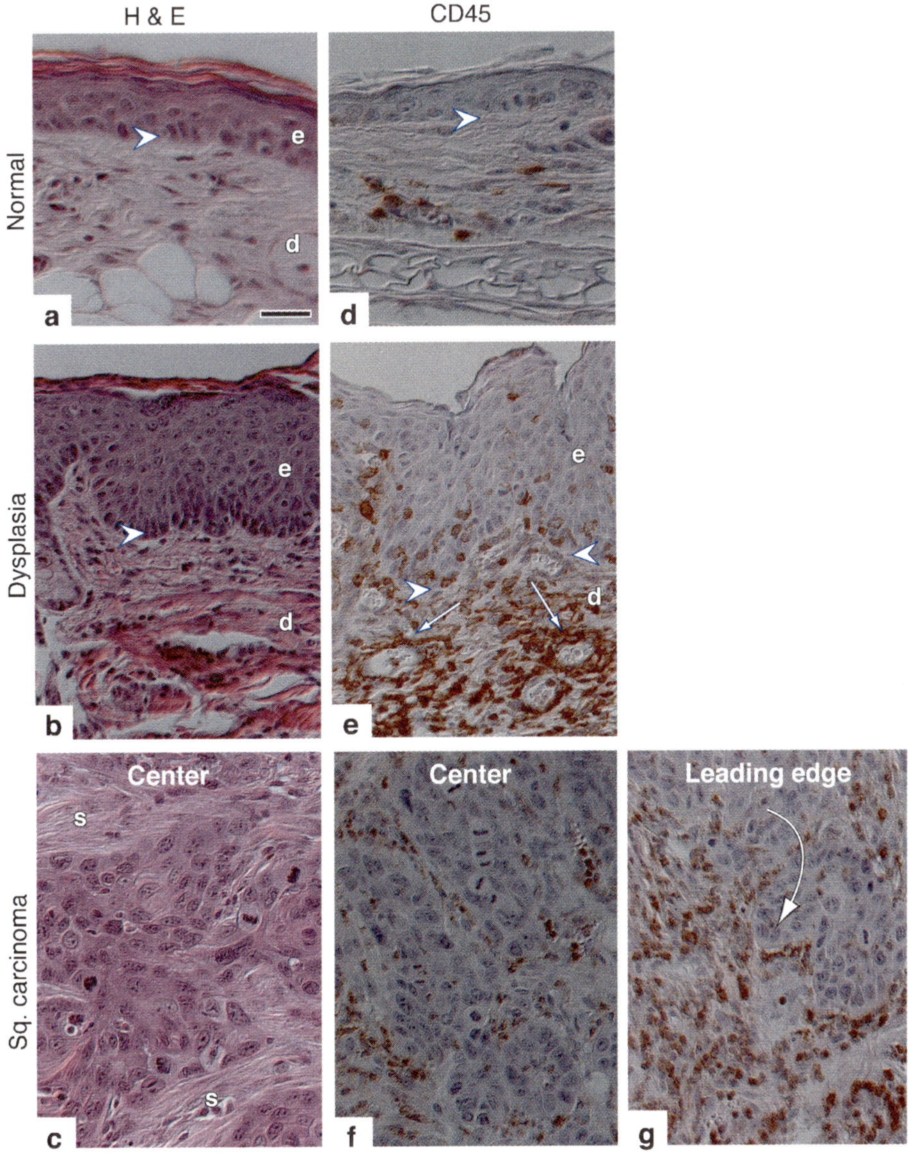

Figure 3

Malignant progression in K14-HPV16 (keratin 14-human papillomavirus type 16) transgenic mice. Skin from normal and transgenic animals stained with H&E (*a–c*) and immunostaining for CD45/leukocyte common antigen (*d–g*). (*a*) Normal ear skin demonstrating the normally thin, four-layered murine epidermis (e) composed of basal, spinous, granular, and corneum cells juxtaposed to the skin basement membrane (*arrowhead*) atop collagen-rich dermal matrix (d) containing few nucleated cells. (*b*) Dysplastic epidermis in which keratinocytes fail to terminally differentiate, basal and spinous layers are expanded, and cellularity in dermal compartment is increased. (*c*) Nests of fully malignant epithelial cells within a squamous cell carcinoma, growing amid dense stromal (s) matrix. (*d–g*) Immunostaining for CD45 (*brown staining*) in normal and neoplastic skin reveals an incremental increase in the presence of leukocytes most prominently infiltrating the dermal compartment in dysplastic skin around angiogenic blood vessels (*arrows*) (*e*) and at the leading edge (*curved arrow*) of an SCC (*g*) as compared with the tumor center (*f*). Bar: 50 μm (*a*, *d*), 100 μm (*b*, *c*, *e–g*).

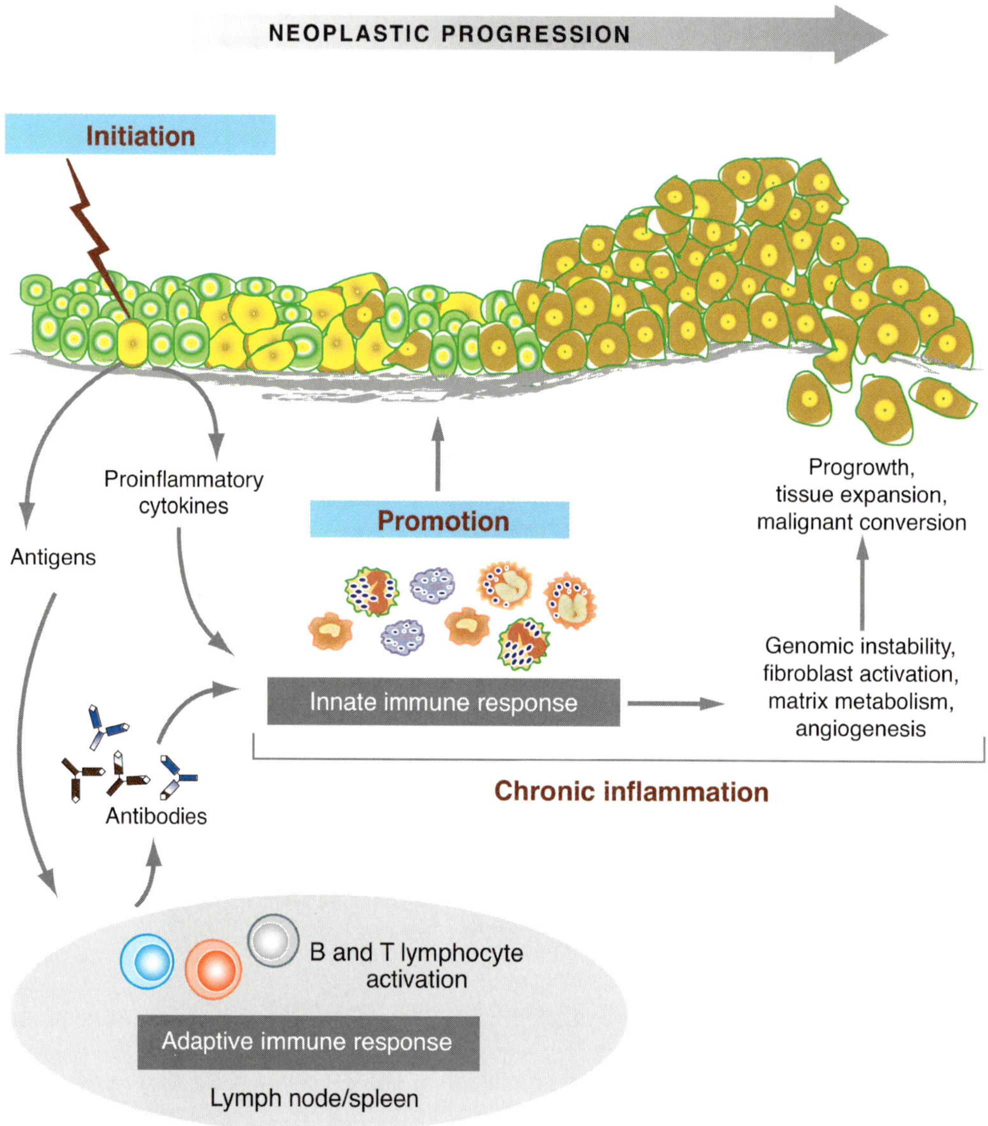

Figure 4

Model for role of innate and adaptive immune cells during inflammation-associated cancer development. Antigens present in early neoplastic tissues are transported to lymphoid organs by dendritic cells that activate adaptive immune responses, e.g., B and T lymphocytes, resulting in chronic activation of innate immune cells in neoplastic tissues. Activated innate immune cells promote tumor development via the modulation of gene expression programs in initiated neoplastic cells, culminating in altered cell cycle progression and enhanced survival. Inflammatory cells positively influence tissue remodeling and development of angiogenic vasculature by production of proangiogenic mediators and production of extracellular proteases. Tissues in which these pathways are chronically engaged exhibit enhanced risk of tumor development.

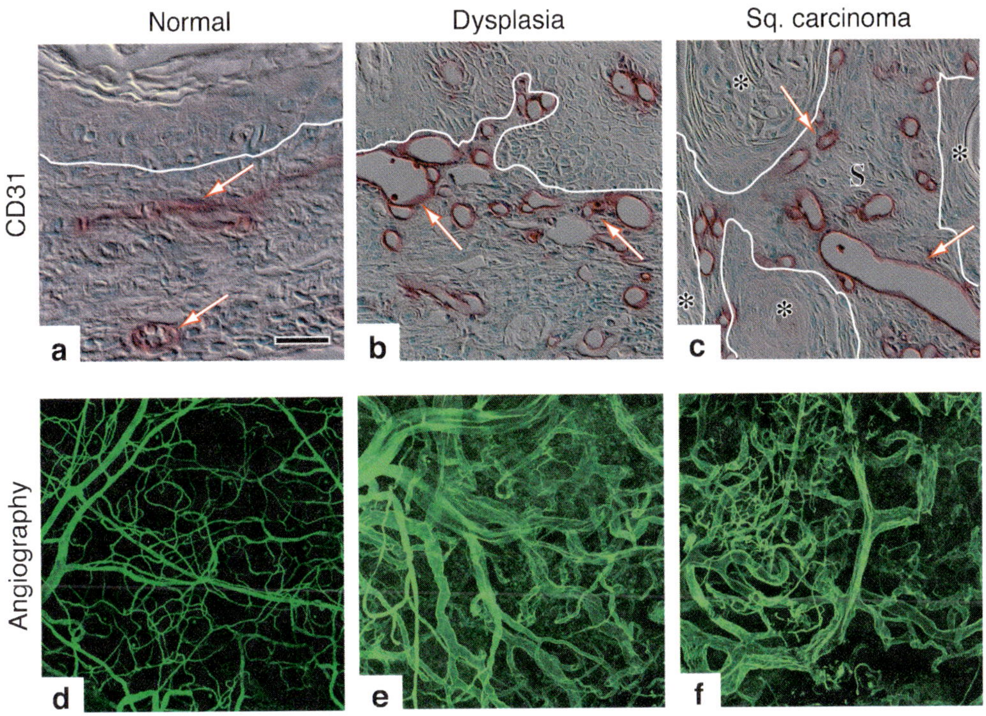

Figure 5

Angiogenesis during cancer development. (*a–c*) Immunoreactivity of CD31-positive endothelial cells in tissue sections reveals vascular (hematogenous and lymphatic) architecture in (*a*) normal mouse skin, (*b*) skin from HPV16 transgenic mice with dysplasia, and (*c*) in a squamous cell carcinoma. In normal skin, vessels are located deep in the dermal compartment (*arrows*). As neoplastic skin develops, vessels density and branching increases at sites where nascent vessels are juxtaposed to skin basement membrane (*arrows*). Stromal vascular structures in carcinomas are prominent (*arrows*) where their dilated nature is obvious. (*d–f*) Fluorescent angiography (220, 221) and whole-mount confocal microscopy of (*d*) normal mouse skin, (*e*) skin from HPV16 transgenic mice with dysplasia, and (*f*) a squamous cell carcinoma reveal three-dimensional organization and architecture of hematogenous vasculature. In premalignant and malignant tissue, angiogenic activation of blood vessels results in highly branched, dilated, and tortuous networks. The black line indicates skin basement membrane (*a*, *b*) and epithelial-stromal interfaces (*c*). Bar: 100 μm (*a–c*); 200 μm (*d–f*).

much lower number of critical physiological pathways that are either chronically enabled or disabled (11). Thus, genomic alterations affecting intrinsic cellular programs, e.g., cell cycle check-point control, programmed cell death, differentiation, metabolism, and cell adhesion, in combination with those affecting extrinsic programs, such as the immune response, matrix metabolism, tissue oxygenation, and vascular status, underlie human cancer development.

Inflammation as a Promoting Force in Cancer Development

Rous was the first to recognize that cancers develop from "subthreshold neoplastic states" (12, 13) caused by inherited mutations (14) or following somatic mutation of critical genes following viral or chemical carcinogen exposure (10, 15). "Initiation," as it is now known, is irreversible and persists in otherwise normal tissue indefinitely until nonspecific stimulation (now referred to as "promotion") occurs,

TGFβ: transforming growth factor β

NSAIDs: nonsteroidal anti-inflammatory drugs

COX-2: cycloygenase-2

typically following exposure of initiated cells to chemical irritants, such as phorbol esters, or from exposure to factors released at sites of chronic inflammation (16–22). In fact, Virchow hypothesized in 1863 (23) that cancer originates at sites of chronic inflammation, in part based on his hypothesis that some classes of irritants (promoters) enhance cell proliferation largely because of the tissue injury and ensuing inflammation that they cause. When tissues are wounded or exposed to a chemical irritant, damaged cells are removed by induction of cell death pathways, while cell proliferation is enhanced to facilitate tissue regeneration or wound healing, thus maintaining homeostasis. Proliferation and inflammation subside after the insulting agent is removed or the repair completed. By contrast, sustained proliferation of initiated cells in environments rich in inflammatory cells, growth/survival factors, activated stroma, and DNA damage–promoting agents potentiates and/or promotes neoplastic risk (17, 20, 22, 24).

Clinical and experimental studies linking inflammation and cancer. Clinical and experimental data indicate that innate immune cells, e.g., granulocytes (neutrophils, basophils, and eosinophils), dendritic cells, macrophages, natural killer cells, and mast cells, play a promoting role during cancer development (17). Many clinical studies have reported the abundance of innate immune cells, in particular mast cells and macrophages, in human tumor samples and correlated their presence with either angiogenesis or a clinical outcome (25–32).

How do inflammatory cells get coopted during neoplastic development? A plausible hypothesis is that many malignancies arise from areas of infection and inflammation simply as part of the normal host response (**Table 1**). Indeed, there is a growing body of evidence that many malignancies, e.g., gastric, cervical, and colon, are associated with bacterial or viral infections (24) or initiated by inherited mutations in genes encoding proteins that regulate tissue homeostasis (33, 34). In fact, more than 15% of malignancies worldwide are attributed to infections, corresponding to ~1.2 million cases per year (35). Population-based studies show that chronic inflammatory conditions predispose humans to certain cancers (**Table 1**) (20–22). Most notably, those patients with chronic *Helicobacter pylori* infection exhibit a 75% increased risk for gastric cancer, the second most common type of cancer globally (35, 36). In addition, experimental studies demonstrate that transforming growth factor β1 (TGFβ1)–deficient mice develop colon cancer and that this cancer is essentially eliminated by maintaining the mice in germ-free environments (37). Other clinical examples of the association between chronic inflammation and increased cancer risk are inflammatory bowel syndrome and colon cancer (20), chronic pancreatitis and pancreatic adenocarcinoma (19), and chronic hepatitis and hepatocellular carcinoma (20) (**Table 1**). Population-based studies examining the effect of various anti-inflammatory compounds, e.g., aspirin, nonsteroidal anti-inflammatory drugs (NSAIDs), and cycloygenase-2 (COX-2) inhibitors, have also concluded that chronic inflammation enhances cancer risk (38–41). These studies have revealed that long-term use of these compounds reduces colon cancer risk by ~50%, gastric and esophageal cancer risk by ~40%, and breast cancer by ~20% (24, 38, 41–46). However, other data show an increased risk of pancreatic cancer and non-Hodgkin's lymphoma among long-term aspirin users (47, 48). Thus, clinical data largely indicate a promoting role for inflammation in neoplastic progression and suggest that the elucidation of the mechanisms by which inflammatory cells participate in carcinogenesis may lead to the development of novel therapeutic agents against human cancer.

The availability of immune-competent mouse models of de novo carcinogenesis has facilitated mechanistic evaluation of the links between chronic inflammation, premalignant progression, tumor growth, and metastasis

Table 1 Chronic inflammatory conditions associated with neoplastic pathologies[a]

Pathologic condition	Associated neoplasm(s)	Etiologic agent
Asbestosis, silicosis	Mesothelioma, Lung carcinoma	Asbestos fibers, silica particles
Bronchitis	Lung carcinoma	Silica, asbestos, smoking (nitrosamines, peroxides)
Cystitis, bladder inflammation	Bladder carcinoma	Chronic indwelling, urinary catheters
Gingivitis, *lichen planus*	Oral squamous cell carcinoma	
Inflammatory bowel disease, Crohn's disease, chronic ulcerative colitis	Colorectal carcinoma	
Lichen sclerosis	Vulvar squamous cell carcinoma	
Chronic pancreatitis, hereditary pancreatitis	Pancreatic carcinoma	Alcholism, mutation in trypsinogen gene
Reflux esophagitis, Barrett's esophagus	Esophageal carcinoma	Gastric acids
Sialadenitis	Salivary gland carcinoma	
Sjögren syndrome, Hashimoto's thyroiditis	MALT[b] lymphoma	
Prostatitis	Prostate carcinoma	
Cancers associated with infectious agents		
Opisthorchis, cholangitis	Cholangiosarcoma, colon carcinoma	Liver flukes (*Opisthorchis viverrini*), bile acids
Chronic cholecystitis	Gall bladder cancer	Bacteria, gall bladder stones
Gastritis/ulcers	Gastric adenocarcinoma, MALT	*Helicobacter pylori*
Hepatitis	Hepatocellular carcinoma	Hepatitis B and/or C virus
Mononucleosis	B-cell non-Hodgkin's lymphoma, Burkitts lymphoma	Epstein-Barr virus
AIDS	Non-Hodgkin's lymphoma, squamous cell carcinoma, Kaposi's sarcoma	Human immunodeficiency virus, human herpesvirus type 8
Osteomyelitis	Carcinoma in draining sinuses	Bacterial infection
Pelvic inflammatory disease, chronic cervicitis	Ovarian carcinoma, cervical/anal carcinoma	Gonnorrhea, chlamydia, human papillomavirus
Chronic cystitis	Bladder, liver, rectal carcinoma, follicular lymphoma of the spleen	Schistosomiasis

[a]Modified from References 17–20, 22, and 23.

[b]MALT, mucosa-associated lymphoid tissue.

formation (17, 23, 24, 49–53). Utilizing a transgenic mouse model of multistage epithelial carcinogenesis in which the early region genes of the human papillomavirus type 16 (HPV16) were expressed under control of the human keratin 14 (K14) promotor (K14-HPV16) mice (54, 55), researchers reported that despite transgene-driven oncogene expression in skin keratinocytes, absence of mast cells or inability to recruit innate immune cells to premalignant skin is sufficient to attenuate neoplastic progression (**Figures 3** and 4) (50, 56, 57). Other studies have reported similar tumor-promoting roles for innate immune cells in the modulation of oncogene expression (58, 59). For example, secretion of the proinflammatory chemokine CXCL-8 by xenografted tumor cells is required for RasV12-dependent tumor-associated inflammation, onset of tumor vascularization, and tumor growth (59). Antibody-mediated depletion of granulocytes attenuates

HPV16: human papillomavirus type 16

K14: keratin 14

TNF: tumor necrosis factor

angiogenesis of RasV12-expressing tumors, suggesting that the recruitment of granulocytes by neoplastic cells facilitates tumor outgrowth (59). Several groups have reported that immature myeloid suppressor $GR1^+CD11b^+$ cells accumulate in the peripheral blood of cancer patients (60, 61) as well as in tumors and lymphoid organs of tumor-bearing animals (62, 63). Myeloid suppressor cells were initially identified as cells that indirectly enhance tumorigenesis by suppressing tumor-specific adaptive immune responses (61, 62, 64). However, myeloid suppressor cells also directly promote tumor growth by contributing to tumor-associated angiogenesis (63).

Macrophage infiltration is a key process during wound healing and similarly, tumor-associated macrophage (TAM) recruitment in human and animal models of cancer development are now known to be determinants of neoplastic progression (65). TAMs have been documented in precursor lesions of cutaneous melanoma, squamous and cervical carcinoma, and mammary adenocarcinoma (49, 58, 66, 67). Precursor lesions containing high numbers of TAMs may subvert normal macrophage-associated developmental processes and aid in the invasion of neoplastic cells into surrounding stroma (67) or in the direct remodeling of stroma, rendering it suitable for appropriate angiogenic and/or lymphangiogenic responses (68, 69). The biological effect of TAMs, however, depends on the local levels of chemokines, such as MCP-1, and the number of macrophages in the area (70). Studies using MCP-1-expressing tumor cells indicate that low concentrations of MCP-1 elicit modest macrophage recruitment and enhance angiogenesis and tumor growth in melanoma xenograft models (70). By contrast, high levels of MCP-1 induce more extensive macrophage infiltration, resulting in robust angiogenic responses and enhanced tumor growth but eventually tumor regression as well (70). Other studies suggest that fully malignant neoplastic cells can divert antitumor macrophage responses and suppress differentiation of mature tumor-antigen-presenting dendritic cells, thereby evading host adaptive immune response (67). Taken together, these data indicate that antitumor leukocyte responses depend upon the robustness of infiltration and relative inhibition of their antitumor activity. The data support the concept that oncogene expression in initiated cells is not sufficient for full neoplastic progression and underscore the role of inflammation as an important component of the host response involved in promoting cancer development.

Inflammation-derived mediators. What inflammatory cell–derived mediators enhance cancer risk and influence tumor development? The inflammatory component of a developing neoplasm includes a diverse population of leukocytes (**Figure 3**), all of which are variably loaded with an assorted array of chemokines, cytokines, cytotoxic mediators including reactive oxygen species, serine-, cysteine- and metallo-proteases, membrane-perforating agents, and soluble mediators of cell killing and cell proliferation, such as tumor necrosis factor (TNF), interleukins, and interferons (49–52, 63, 71–73). Individually, all of these molecules are known mediators of inflammation and evoke innate immune cell recruitment and/or activation, tissue remodeling, and angiogenesis. Together they create a microenvironment favoring cell proliferation, genomic instability, and expansion of cell populations into ectopic tissue microenvironments, i.e., malignant conversion and cancer development.

Leukocytes and other phagocytic cells can induce DNA damage in proliferating cells through their generation of reactive oxygen and nitrogen species, which normally are produced by these cells to fight infection and can react to form peroxynitrite, a mutagenic agent (74). Repeated tissue damage and regeneration of tissue in the presence of such highly reactive nitrogen and oxygen species damages DNA in proliferating cells, and can thus cause permanent genomic alterations, e.g., point mutations, deletions, or rearrangements that promote neoplastic growth.

Several studies have provided molecular-level insight into which intracellular signaling pathways are coopted in initiated cells at risk for cancer development. The proinflammatory transcription factor nuclear factor κB (NFκB), a mediator of cell survival, proliferation, and growth arrest, has been identified as an important molecule linking chronic inflammation and cancer (51, 52, 75). Specific deletion of IKKβ—a key inhibitor of NFκB—in myeloid cells decreased carcinoma growth in a mouse model of colitis-associated cancer through reduced production of tumor-promoting paracrine factors (51). In addition, examination of a mouse model of inflammation-associated hepatocellular carcinogenesis similarly implicated activation of hepatocyte NFκB via production of inflammatory cell–derived TNF (52). These two mouse models reveal that the NFκB pathway acts in two ways to promote tumors: (*a*) by preventing death of cells with malignant potential and (*b*) by stimulating production of proinflammatory cytokines in cells of myeloid and lymphoid origin in tumor masses. These proinflammatory cytokines then signal to initiated and/or otherwise damaged epithelial cells and promote their proliferation and overall cell survival; thus, inflammatory cells in these contexts modulate gene expression and proliferation of neoplastic cells by paracrine regulation of NFκB.

In addition to influencing proliferation and survival of neoplastic cells, tumor-infiltrating inflammatory cells also regulate cancer development by affecting angiogenesis. A reduction in the extent of infiltration of inflammatory cells in mouse carcinogenesis models correlates with attenuated angiogenesis and reduced tumor growth (50, 57, 59). One mechanism by which inflammatory cells regulate angiogenesis is the production of proangiogenic mediators such as vascular endothelial growth factor (VEGF)-A (32, 76).

Tumor-infiltrating leukocytes also indirectly contribute to tumor development by producing extracellular proteases (49, 63, 71, 77–79). Matrix metalloproteinases (MMPs) are a large family of proteolytic enzymes that play key roles in cancer progression (80). MMPs regulate tumor development by remodeling ECM components as well as non-ECM substrates such as cytokines, growth factors, and cell-cell and cell-matrix adhesion molecules, thus contributing to angiogenesis, inflammation, and proliferation (80, 81).

NFκB: nuclear factor κB

VEGF: vascular endothelial growth factor

MMPs: matrix metalloproteinases

Several mechanistic studies have reported that inflammatory cell–derived MMPs functionally contribute to neoplastic progression (49, 63, 71, 81). For example, tumor incidence and growth in the K14-HPV16 mouse model of de novo epithelial carcinogenesis are reduced in the absence of MMP-9 (49). Neoplastic development is partially restored by reconstitution of MMP-9-deficient/K14-HPV16 mice by adoptive transfer of wild-type bone marrow–derived cells, indicating that inflammatory cells functionally contribute to de novo carcinogenesis, at least in part, by their deposition of MMP-9 into the neoplastic microenvironment (49, 82). Moreover, induction of cervical carcinoma in K14-HPV16 mice is markedly reduced when mice are systemically treated with an amino-bisphosphonate that acts on MMP-9-expressing macrophages (53). These data indicate that ECM remodeling and/or increased bioavailability of growth factors that are normally sequestered within the ECM are regulated by inflammatory cells present in the tumor microenvironment. Thus, inflammatory cells create an environment permissive for tumor growth.

Immune cells can also suppress cancer development. The immune system plays dual roles in tumor development and progression (83). In addition to the above studies indicating that immune cells can promote tumor development, other studies have reported that adaptive immune cells, e.g., B and T lymphocytes, may inhibit later stages of cancer development by affecting growth and/or dissemination of primary tumors. Studies supporting this concept, also known as the immune-surveillance theory, have shown that infiltration of tumors by subsets of T lymphocytes can be beneficial and retard tumor growth (84–88). Based on the idea that a tumor can be a recognizable target for the adaptive immune system, several groups have attempted to activate adaptive immune cells to elicit antitumor immune responses (89). This topic is beyond the scope of the present article, but we refer readers to various excellent reviews (83, 90–94).

Alternatively, other groups have examined the role of adaptive immune cells during the early stages of cancer development, e.g., during premalignancy, and found that failure to appropriately activate/educate adaptive immune cells results in failed recruitment of innate immune cells into local neoplastic microenvironments (56, 57). As a consequence, tissue remodeling and angiogenic programs necessary for progression to the malignant states remain quiescent, resulting in attenuated tumor development (**Figure 4**). Taken together, these studies indicate that each stage of cancer development is regulated uniquely and that whereas activation of adaptive immune cells at the tumor stage may be beneficial for minimizing or eradicating malignant cells, activation during earlier stages elicits opposing effects.

Targeting inflammation and chemoprevention. It is now accepted that chronic inflammation fosters tumor development through diverse molecules and pathways. However, it is still unclear which pathways are key for activating inflammation in at-risk tissues and which are involved in maintaining chronic inflammatory states often associated with developing neoplasms. Furthermore, depending on the (pre)malignant states of the epithelial cells and/or level of inflammatory response, the contribution of immune cells to malignancy can be suppressive or enhancing. Thus, although undoubtedly complex, the identification of the major mediators and pathways responsible for triggering inflammatory cell infiltration into damaged tissue or their accumulation in premalignant tissues may provide therapeutic opportunities for the prevention and treatment of cancer. The efficacy of NSAIDS and COX-2 inhibitors (24, 41) in chemoprevention argues for anti-inflammatory therapy at the earliest stages of neoplastic progression. Alternatively, should future anticancer strategies focus on regulating NFκB activation, TNF-bioavailability, or metalloproteinase activity? In answering this question, it is important to point out that all organs are endowed with unique cell death and damage-response pathways that naturally invoke acute activation of innate immune cells. In skin, for example, keratinocyte cell death is by terminal differentiation (95). Inhibiting NFκB in keratinocytes promotes squamous cell carcinogenesis by reducing growth arrest and terminal differentiation of initiated keratinocytes (96) that proliferate in microenvironments in which growth factors, matrix remodeling enzymes, and reactive oxygen species produced by infiltrating inflammatory cells contribute to angiogenesis and keratinocyte DNA damage (17). By contrast, blockade of TNF attenuates skin tumor formation (97). The therapeutic regulation of TNF, however, must also be carefully considered, as this factor too possesses opposing activities that are cell type- and environment-dependent (98). Phase I clinical trials of TNF antagonists are currently underway in patients with advanced cancer; these experiments may help us understand the complexities of these responses (97, 98). Similarly, expression and activity of MMPs vary by organ and in response to damage (80), and although elimination or attenuation of MMP activity clearly evokes a survival advantage in immune-competent mouse models of cancer development, the efficacy of metalloprotease inhibitors in human clinical trials has been disappointing at best (99). So, what lessons can we learn from these failures? We must give special consideration to understanding the stage of tumor progression at which cytostatic agents targeting inflammatory mediators are likely to work alone, and when a combination with standard debulking or cytotoxic therapy may be advantageous. Mouse models that more closely mimic human cancers are rapidly becoming available and must be applied in a way that also recapitulates the current therapeutic approach to the corresponding human disease.

Fibroblasts in Cancer: Phenotypes In Vivo and In Vitro

As the predominant cell in stroma, the fibroblast is responsible for the elaboration of most connective tissue components in the ECM, including collagens and structural proteoglycans, as well as various classes of proteolytic enzymes, their inhibitors, and various growth factors (8). Each organ has specialized requirements, and hence fibroblasts from different organs demonstrate organ-specific variations in the classes of biologically active molecules that they express (100). Furthermore, in response to varying physiologic signals, be they normal or pathologic, stromal fibroblasts change their phenotype and function (100).

Pathologists were the first to observe that fibroblasts in tumors were unique and underwent dynamic changes accompanying tumor progression (101, 102). In tumors, fibroblasts have been referred to as myofibroblasts, peritumoral fibroblasts, reactive stromal cells, and carcinoma-associated fibroblasts (CAFs). They typically exhibit a higher proliferative index, as compared with fibroblasts in normal tissues, often express α-smooth muscle actin, and are commonly surrounded by dense accumulations of fibrillar collagens (8, 103). This phenotype—common to several types of human cancer, e.g., breast, prostate (**Figure 1**), pancreatic (**Figure 2**), colon, and lung—is termed desmoplasia and is associated with the recruitment of inflammatory cells and activation of angiogenic programs.

CAFs isolated from malignant tissues exhibit altered phenotypes, most notably the enhanced production of collagens, hyaluronate, and epithelial growth factors (104, 105), disorganized patterns of growth, and enhanced proliferation (5, 106). Such phenotypes aid in tumor progression. Intriguingly, some of these phenotypes have also been detected in fibroblasts taken from distal, nontumorigenic sites in patients with cancer. Schor and coworkers (107, 108) found altered invasive properties of dermal fibroblasts from patients with cancer or with hereditary predispositions to cancer. Schor and colleagues (108) postulated that fibroblast abnormalities may influence the development of epithelial tumors and that hereditary defects may affect stromal-epithelial interactions and promote tumor formation. These important studies established that CAFs display altered phenotypes and raised the question of their possible functional significance in tumorigenesis.

CAFs: carcinoma-associated fibroblasts

Desmoplasia: hyperplasia of fibroblasts and disproportionate formation of fibrous connective tissue, mainly collagens, especially in the stroma of a carcinoma

Fibroblasts as a promoting force in cancer development. Tissue recombination experiments using fibroblasts and epithelial cells isolated from disparate sites have been instructive in analyzing the role of stromal fibroblasts in carcinogenesis (109). Early studies by Chung and coworkers (110–112) measured stromal effects on tumor progression by analyzing recombinant grafts containing tumorigenic epithelial cells with murine fibroblasts that were either normal, immortalized, transformed by viral or chemical carcinogens, or tumor associated. Depending on the characteristics of the epithelial tumor cell, fibroblasts exerted either a positive or negative effect on tumor development and progression (110–112). Taken together, these studies demonstrated that tumorigenic epithelial cells within recombinant grafts respond to fibroblast-derived signals and that the response depends on the types of gene mutated in adjacent epithelial cells.

In an alternative approach, using human tissues, Tlsty and coworkers (109) examined the effect of fibroblasts on nontumorigenic epithelial cells. These studies determined that CAFs send signals that either initiate abnormal epithelial growth or enhance the progression of nontumorigenic cells to tumorigenic states. The combination of normal human prostatic epithelial cells with CAFs (obtained from prostatic adenocarcinoma) demonstrated an interaction that limited growth potential of the epithelial cells while reinstating their ability to form ductal structures resembling prostatic intraepithelial neoplasia. However, when CAFs were grafted with immortalized human prostatic epithelial cells, the resulting interaction resulted in tumors that often exceeded 5 grams (wet weight), surpassing the weight of control grafts by 500 fold (109). Remarkably, isolation of pure human epithelial cell populations from these tumors and subsequent grafting into animals demonstrated that the epithelial cells were then able to form tumors (i.e., contributing activity from CAFs was no longer necessary), as their transformation was accompanied by nonrandom chromosomal changes (109). Histological examination of these tumors demonstrated their malignant nature, e.g., enhanced cell proliferation, decreased cell death, angiogenesis, and genomic instability. Therefore, through a transient interaction, oncogenic signals from CAFs can stimulate nontumorigenic cells toward a malignant state, thus establishing an active role for fibroblasts in tumorigenic processes.

The stroma can acquire oncogenic activity by a variety of processes. The previous studies obtained fibroblasts from existing tumors and demonstrated their ability to stimulate oncogenesis. Can stroma develop oncogenic signals in the absence of a tumor? If stromal cells could acquire the properties that stimulate tumor initiation and progression through independent means, it would provide considerable insights into the risk factors for tumorigenicity. Recent experiments suggest that this is a possible mechanism of tumor generation and have begun to identify the processes involved.

Exposure to carcinogens. Decades ago, using skin (113) and bladder (114, 115) tissues, investigators observed enhanced tumor formation when carcinogen-treated stroma was heterotypically grafted with untreated epithelial cells. More recently, the effects of carcinogen treatment on stromal cells was examined in murine mammary tissues (116). Here, irradiation of epithelial cell–free mammary stroma (cleared fat pads) facilitated tumor progression of transformed epithelial cells that were subsequently introduced into treated stroma. In the irradiated stroma, mammary epithelial cells developed tumors faster and more often and reached a greater size than the same cells transplanted into unirradiated stroma. These data indicate that carcinogens can affect neoplastic processes not only by inducing genetic changes in epithelial cells but also by altering stromal cells such that they stimulate tumor progression.

Direct induction of fibroblasts by tumorigenic cells. Although the origin of fibroblasts in tumor stroma has been extensively debated, in vitro studies by Ronnov-Jessen and coworkers (117) provided evidence that the conversion of fibroblasts, but not of vascular smooth muscle cells or pericytes, constitutes the major source of myofibroblasts in mammary tissues. Isolation of each of these cell types and subsequent coculture with mammary tumor cells demonstrated that the majority of phenotypic and biochemical changes associated with desmoplasia were present in cocultures with fibroblasts and to a much lesser degree in cocultures with vascular smooth muscle cells. The finding that normal fibroblasts, placed in association with tumor cells, readily convert to α-smooth muscle actin–expressing cells suggests that factors elaborated from tumor cells modulate reprogramming. For example, TGFβ, often produced by tumor cells and present in a latent form in the ECM, induces α-smooth muscle actin and collagen production in cultured fibroblasts (118) and is a potential mediator of desmoplastic responses in tumors.

Wound healing. As discussed above, stroma at sites of wound healing and tumor growth share many characteristics (101, 119). Indeed, experimental evidence indicates that wounding can exert a tumor-promoting effect, and TGFβ has been postulated as a mediator of this effect (120). In Rous sarcoma virus–infected chickens, wounding leads to tumor formation (121). Subcutaneous injection of TGFβ substitutes for the wounding event, demonstrating the role of this molecule in altering the tissue microenvironment. The increased incidence of tumor formation at the sites of scar tissue (122) and in areas of chronic damage is also consistent with the idea that stromal changes accompanying wounding enhance tumorigenicity. The inflammatory response is present in both wound healing and carcinogenesis and may provide a common mechanistic link between the two.

Aging or induction of senescence. Age is a well-known risk factor for tumorigenesis, yet the mechanism underlying risk is uncertain, although accumulated genetic damage is likely involved. However, fibroblasts may play an important role as well. Increased collagen production and altered expression of MMPs are part of a gene expression program activated when fibroblasts enter senescence and when tissues age (123). This expression program can be activated either by prolonged growth of fibroblasts in culture, by aberrant expression of oncogenes (124), or merely by aging of the organism. Age-related alterations in fibroblasts may generate a microenvironment conducive to tumorigenicity (2, 125). Notably, chemically transformed rat hepatocytes demonstrate a greater tumorigenic potential when transplanted into older animals as compared with younger animals (126). Future studies will determine if aging fibroblasts contribute to alterations of stromal-epithelial interactions that modulate carcinogenesis.

Hormone imbalance. Extensive epidemiological data implicate hormonal imbalance in the generation of some forms of cancer (127–129), and experimental manipulation of hormone levels in animals verifies this observation (130). In the Noble rat model, exposure to hormones dramatically altered stromal-epithelial interactions and generated adenocarcinomas (131). Critical regulators, such as TGFβ, insulin-like growth factor-1, and VEGF, are altered upon administration of oncogenic doses of sex hormones, indicating that such alterations in these paracrine regulators of stromal-epithelial interactions can function as etiologic agents (131, 132).

Congenital or acquired mutations that alter stromal-epithelial signals. Fibroblasts containing inherited mutations that predispose to various cancers harbor abnormal phenotypes (2). If these mutations encode functional proteins involved in stromal-epithelial interactions or their regulation, these mutations may result in altering aspects of tissue specificity in the resulting tumor spectra. Such a situation has been postulated for juvenile polyposis of the colon (133, 134). In these polyps, deletions on chromosomes 10 and 18 have been detected in stromal cells, but not in epithelial cells, suggesting that inherited mutations in stromal cells may predispose one to carcinogenic conditions.

In addition to inherited mutations, acquired mutations in fibroblasts may contribute to carcinogenesis. New molecular tools have provided the means with which to examine tumor components individually. The combination of tissue microdissection (using laser capture microscopy) and the polymerase chain reaction has provided evidence that fibroblasts can acquire mutations independently from those in epithelial cells (135). Examination of fibroblast and epithelial cells from patients with ductal carcinoma in situ or infiltrating ductal carcinoma of the breast uncovered a group of mutations that can occur either in one cell type or both types. The high frequency of fibroblasts with acquired mutations whose proximity in the tissue is distal to carcinomatous tissue, in contrast to their absence in normal mammary tissue, suggests that in some cases, stromal alterations may precede mutations in epithelial cells that are at risk for neoplastic progression.

Targeting fibroblasts for chemoprevention. Taken together, fibroblast alterations have tremendous potential to influence oncogenic processes. These alterations may be easily detectable prior to disease formation (136) or may arise in a concomitant time frame. Equally remarkable is the realization that the initial stimuli only need be applied in a transient manner to trigger formation of the lesion. In the examples described above, the need for altered fibroblasts to contribute oncogenic signals for the generation of a tumorigenic lesion was transient, i.e., the interaction of human CAF with epithelial cells (109), the single administration of a carcinogen administered to the stroma (116), or the rapid expression of MMPs (137). In each example, the transformed cell ultimately becomes independent of the fibroblast signals through alterations in its phenotype. In addition, fibroblast alterations may provide a gene expression signature that helps to predict the clinical course of disease (100). Further investigation of these processes will provide opportunities for the identification of novel targets for prevention and therapy. Because the fibroblast population does not seem to exhibit the extreme genomic changes that are so rampant in malignant epithelial cells, they may be a tractable target for therapy.

Tumor-Associated Angiogenesis

When any tissue expands or a primary tumor develops, growing beyond ~2–4 mm^3, influx of oxygen and nutrients and efflux of waste products must be ensured (138). To meet the metabolic needs of a rapidly growing tumor mass, development of a new blood vasculature is required and accomplished by activation of preexisting vascular beds, e.g., angiogenesis (138). During angiogenesis, a well-orchestrated series of events occurs, encompassing endothelial cell proliferation as well as directional migration of endothelial cells through remodeled basement membrane and perivascular stroma toward angiogenic stimuli (expanding populations of neoplastic cells) (139–141). Once endothelial cells display a proliferative and migratory phenotype, recruitment of perivascular support cells enables stabilization of nascent vessels, functional lumen formation, and appropriate blood flow. Activation of proangiogenic molecular and cellular programs in neoplasms is regulated at many levels and controlled by a diverse assortment of positively and negatively acting soluble and insoluble mediators whose balanced equilibrium is kept tightly in check under homeostatic conditions (142). However, under conditions of tissue stress, such as those that occur during the onset of incipient neoplasia, this balance is rapidly upset, favoring the proangiogenic program (139, 141, 143, 144). Whereas these cellular and molecular programs are common to physiological angiogenesis and appropriately turn on and off, tumor-associated angiogenic vasculature (**Figure 5**) is distinctly tortuous, chaotic in organization, and inherently unstable and leaky (145, 146). Thus, manipulating the stability of the tumor vasculature may constitute a viable anticancer therapeutic strategy (147), one that seeks to inhibit proliferation or migration of vascular endothelial cells.

Extracellular proteases and angiogenesis. MMPs are a family of at least 25 highly homologous, secreted or plasma membrane–associated zinc-binding proteinases (80, 148). MMPs can be produced by virtually all cell types, regulate many developmental processes, and participate in a variety of pathological conditions, including cancer, autoimmune diseases, and periodontitis (148). MMPs have been implicated as mediators of tumor angiogenesis at several discrete stages. This conclusion is based on MMP activity toward effector substrates that regulate angiogenesis by positive and negative mechanisms as well as the observation that natural and synthetic inhibitors of MMP activity diminish tumor angiogenesis (80).

Previously, MMPs were thought to facilitate neoplastic progression by merely degrading ECM structural components, thereby allowing a cleared path for migrating neoplastic or endothelial cells. Indeed, cleavage of collagen type I is required for endothelial cell invasion of the ECM and vessel formation (149). Several proangiogenic polypeptide growth factors, most notably VEGF, basic fibroblast growth factor, and TNF, are highly expressed in developing tumors, as they are during physiologic wound healing; however, their bioavailability is limited, as they are either sequestered to ECM molecules or tethered to cells via membrane-spanning or anchorage domains (150). MMPs (and other extracellular proteases) regulate release of these factors, rendering them available for interaction with cognate receptors on vascular cells and thus activating the development of tumor-associated vasculature (80, 150). For example, MMP-9 targets the proangiogenic growth factor VEGF (77) by an indirect mechanism that targets an ECM VEGF-sequestering molecule. Both MMP-2 and MMP-9 activate latent TGFβ residing in the matrix (151), leading to the differential regulation of the proliferation of endothelial and perivascular cells and stabilization of nascent vessels (147, 152). In addition, several MMPs activate components of the plasma clotting system, such as fibrinogen and plasminogen, also implicated as regulators of angiogenesis (153–156). MMPs also modulate immune responses by processing (i.e., activating as well as inactivating) chemokines, a property important for resolution of acute inflammation and linked to progression of premalignant tissues (78, 157).

Whereas remodeling of some soluble or insoluble matrix molecules confers a proangiogeneic phenotype, remodeling of others confers antiangiogenic properties (158). Embedded within some ECM molecules are bioactive cryptic protein fragments released by proteolytic cleavage (80, 159). The first example of the release of a bioactive ECM fragment was the isolation of angiostatin from the urine of mice with Lewis lung cell carcinoma (160). Angiostatin, a plasminogen cleavage product containing kringle regions 1–4, inhibits endothelial cell proliferation, is believed responsible for maintaining Lewis lung cell metastases in a dormant state, and has demonstrated efficacy in limiting tumor burden in transgenic mice predisposed to pancreatic islet cell carcinogenesis (161). Several MMPs, including MMP-2, -7, -9, and -12, can generate angiostatin (159, 162). Another ECM fragment possessing antiangiogenic properties is endostatin, a 20-kDa NC1 fragment of type XVIII collagen (153). Endostatin is produced by cleavage of collagen type XVIII by MMP-3, -7, -9, -12, -13, and -20 (163) and acts by retarding endothelial cell proliferation (153, 160). Restin, by contrast, is a 22-kDa NC1fragment of type XV collagen that inhibits migration, but not proliferation, of endothelial cells in vitro and suppresses tumor-induced angiogenesis in renal xenograft carcinoma models (164). All three chains of type IV collagen ($\alpha1$, $\alpha2$, and $\alpha3$) are potent inhibitors of angiogenesis and tumor growth (159, 165–168). The 24-kDa NC1 fragment of the $\alpha1$ chain of type IV collagen, also termed arrestin, inhibits growth of human tumor xenografts in nude mice by significantly inhibiting growth factor–mediated angiogenesis (165). Furthermore, the antiangiogenic activity of arrestin is mediated by binding to endothelial $\alpha1\beta1$ integrins (165). Likewise, canstatin, the 24-kDa NC1 fragment of the $\alpha2$ chain of type IV collagen, suppresses growth of human tumor xenografts in nude mice by inhibiting angiogenesis (166). In vitro studies indicate that canstatin specifically inhibits proliferation, migration, and tube formation of endothelial cells (166). Lastly, the 24-kDa NC1 fragment of the $\alpha3$ chain of type IV collagen, termed tumstatin, acts as an angiogenesis inhibitor, blocking both endothelial cell proliferation and functional lumen formation

(167–170). Studies using transgenic mouse models also indicate that tumstatin is generated by MMP-9 and suppresses angiogenesis via $\alpha v\beta 3$ integrin interactions (171). Taken together, these studies indicate that protease-generated cleavage products of the ECM, basement membrane proteins, and other soluble molecules act as suppressors or activators of pathological angiogenesis in tissue-dependent and stage-dependent manners and implicate MMPs as important mediators of tumor-associated angiogenesis through both protumor and antitumor mechanisms.

Extracellular Matrix Molecules and Cancer Progression

The function of normal organs is determined by reciprocal communication between cells in an epithelial layer and their surrounding stroma (172), and the same organizational principles apply to cancer. The progression from a hyperproliferative state to malignancy can be characterized by increasingly abnormal communications between all cell types comprising the tumor mass (**Figures 1–3**) (2, 173). Thus, if disruptive stresses in the tumor microenvironment contribute to cancer development, therapeutic strategies aimed at restoring normal communication between different cell types within a tumor may be effective in combating neoplastic disease.

The three-dimensional ECM surrounding cells contains a mixture of fibrillar proteins, glycoproteins, proteoglycans, cytokines, and growth factors (174). The ECM provides both the structural support and contextual information for cells to determine the correct response to a given set of stimuli (175–177). Composition of ECM varies considerably both between and within different tissues, and ECM changes temporally as an adaptation to varying signals during normal developmental processes and during pathological processes such as those that occur in cancer. Epithelial cells can initiate incorrect stromal signaling, resulting in stromal cell production of growth factors that, in turn, stimulate inappropriate proliferation of neighboring epithelial cells (101). Alternatively, an aberrant matrix component produced by stromal cells in response to a local stress can be perceived by neighboring epithelial cells as a signal to proliferate or to enter a new developmental pathway (2, 3, 101, 178).

ECM supports cell adhesion and transmits signals through cell-surface adhesion receptors (179). The ECM of most tissues contains various types of fibrillar and nonfibrillar collagens, noncollagenous glycoproteins, and proteoglycans (180). By contrast, basement membranes are specialized forms of ECM, involved in separating tissue compartments and providing a scaffold on which some cell types, epithelial cells for example, adhere and exhibit polarized and/or differentiated growth (159). ECM remodeling may be essential for maintaining tissue integrity and involves a tightly regulated balance between ECM synthesis and ECM remodeling (159, 180, 181). During wound healing, pericellular ECM molecules in the immediate area of tissue damage are remodeled predominantly by MMPs secreted by epithelial cells, activated fibroblasts, or inflammatory cells (159, 180). In turn, fibroblasts and vascular cells synthesize the appropriate amounts of ECM components (type I collagen, fibronectin, etc.) important for tissue repair (159, 180). By contrast, in fibrotic environments (i.e., liver cirrhosis, renal and lung fibrosis, and scleroderma), the balance between ECM synthesis, accumulation, and degradation is shifted, which favors synthesis and accumulation, resulting in fibrosis, a phenotype that also can be caused by increased synthesis of ECM components independent of the degradative enzymes that remodel ECM (182, 183). A shift in favor of ECM remodeling is seen in degenerative pathologies such as arthritis (184) and tumor development (80, 150, 185). However, it is also clear that some fibrotic and inflammatory conditions increase cancer risk (17) and that some familial cancer syndromes result from gene defects that produce stromal changes before epithelial changes ever occur

(173, 186, 187). For example, a study by Moinfar and colleagues (135) examined genetic alterations in tumor-associated stroma from several independent cases of mammary carcinoma and found chromosomal rearrangements not present in the malignant carcinoma cells. These results indicate that characteristic mutations affecting stromal cells may have contributed to the formation of the epithelial tumors. Under normal homeostatic conditions, these misinterpretations are corrected by either cell cycle arrest or induction of cell death/differentiation programs; however, if the abnormal signal persists, cellular behavior can become increasingly abnormal, creating an evolving, interdependent, heterogeneous tissue (also known as a tumor) defined by its ability to grow and its unresponsiveness to normal physiological controls.

Matrix metabolism and collagen. Solid tumor growth cannot be sustained unless the tumor efficiently coopts fibroblasts, inflammatory cells, and vascular cells to help reset the balance between ECM remodeling (degradation) and ECM synthesis (181). In soft tissues, type I collagen accounts for 80%–90% of all collagenous proteins (188). It belongs to a family of 21 ECM proteins (188) that play a dominant role in maintaining the structural integrity of organs and tissues (189) as well as a more specialized role in regulating cell polarity, migration, survival, and phenotype. Proteins in this family also provide diffusible signaling molecules following breakdown (174). Within this family of molecules, types I, II, III, V, and XI collagens are included in the group of fibril-forming collagens on the basis of their structural and functional features (189).

Under normal homeostatic conditions, fibrillar collagens have a relatively slow metabolic turnover; however, under conditions of tissue remodeling, interstitial collagen metabolism is increased. Recent studies on human prostate, ovarian, lung, breast, and skin malignancies have shown a relationship between increased synthesis of type I collagen, increased collagen content in neoplastic tissues, and increased serum levels of type I collagen degradation products (190–195). These retrospective studies examining interstitial collagen status, in combination with in vitro studies demonstrating a functional relationship between collagenase-specific cleavage of type I collagen and growth factor–induced angiogenesis (149), suggest that type I collagen remodeling is an integral component of neoplastic stroma and may represent a potential target for anticancer therapeutic targeting.

When developing neoplasms undergo malignant conversion and acquire the capacity to invade normal tissue, increased architectural disorder at the invasive front of the neoplastic mass is characteristic (**Figures 1–3**) (185). Increased production of matrix remodeling enzymes and synthesis of many matrix components, most notably type I collagen, occur at this site (50, 185, 196, 197). Multiple cell types contribute to the maintenance of appropriate ECM composition at the invasive front, similar to that observed during wound healing. Activated fibroblasts migrate to premalignant tissue, in which they synthesize new matrix components, e.g., collagen type I and fibronectin, in response to a variety of factors including TFGβ, platelet-derived growth factor, interleukin-1α, interleukin-1β, and mast cell tryptase (17).

ECM composition is dynamic during development wound healing and in neoplastic states, and the architecture and form that ECM molecules assume are of critical importance for appropriate cellular responses. The architecture of tumor-associated ECM is fundamentally different from that of preexisting stroma (**Figures 1–3**) (198). Whereas preexisting collagen fibers in dermal stroma are readily identified by their parallel orientation with respect to the epithelium (188), newly synthesized peritumoral stroma (i.e., type I collagen) is characterized by its loosely woven morphology and nonplanar orientation (181). Increased collagen synthesis in the periphery of benign tumors results in tight encapsulation of malignant cells that can limit neoplastic cell expansion (181). However, invading and metastasizing cancers acquire a capacity to orchestrate stromal responses in favor of malignant progression (i.e., invasion and metastasis) (181), suggesting that initial stromal responses may limit neoplastic propensity but are subsequently redirected to enhance neoplastic progression.

In ocular melanoma, for example, type I collagen is deposited as curved sheets around and in between tumor cell nests in which vascular structures are present (198–201). When type I collagen fibrils assume this arc-loop network, an efficient fluid-conducting meshwork is formed, which is closely apposed to hematogenous vasculature (202). Because vasculature in developing neoplasms is inherently leaky (203), these meshworks may efficiently allow for drainage of plasma and erythrocytes in some tumors while contributing to high interstitial pressure characteristics in others (204).

TARGETING THE TUMOR MICROENVIRONMENT: CLINICAL IMPLICATIONS

An important challenge remains to investigate novel anticancer therapies aimed at targeting both malignant tumor cells and the contexts in which they live. This review has examined facets of inflammation, angiogenesis, and fibroblast and extracellular matrix biology associated with neoplastic programming of tissues. As stated above, the efficacy of NSAIDS and COX-2 inhibitors (24, 41) in chemoprevention argues for the use of anti-inflammatory therapy at the earliest stages of neoplastic progression. Functional roles for extracellular proteases in early neoplastic progression and invasion, malignant conversion, and some metastatic events have clearly been demonstrated and prompted the first clinical testing of noncytotoxic biologic therapeutics. Unfortunately, results with metalloprotease inhibitors thus far have not been encouraging (99). The requirement for efficient vascularization of tumors and discovery of potent pro- and antiangiogenic molecules have produced a diverse array of angiogenesis inhibitors currently undergoing clinical evaluation (141, 147, 205–207). Some of these have demonstrated efficacy and have been approved for limited use in patients (208, 208a).

Fibrotic breast disease can also predispose one to breast cancer (122, 191, 195), and environmentally induced fibrotic disorders can increase incidence of lung and skin cancer (185, 209–212), underscoring the importance of developing therapeutic modalities that target tumor microenvironments. Therefore, future therapeutic strategies may consist of approaches targeting collagen synthesis with pharmacologic inhibitors such as Halofuginone. Halofuginone, which inhibits type I collagen synthesis by blocking TGFβ-mediated phosphorylation and activation of Smad3, has demonstrated efficacy in reducing fibrosis in scleroderma and liver disease (213–215). This inhibitor was recently approved as a therapeutic for scleroderma (215a) and is currently in clinical trials for treatment of various types of solid tumors (215b). Because remodeling of collagen fibrils is also involved in the alignment and formation of endothelial tubular structures (149, 216), inhibition of collagen synthesis may limit tumor-associated angiogenesis (217, 218). Furthermore, collagen type I is an important binding protein for a wide variety of mitogenic and morphogenic growth factors (219); therefore, disturbing the balance of regulated collagen metabolism may alter the bioavailability of these factors and subsequently inhibit neoplastic programming. The body of literature supporting these approaches suggests that we are at the dawn of a new era in cancer therapeutics. Thus, we are optimistic about the development of efficacious noncytotoxic chemopreventatives that would block neoplastic programming of tissues before life-threatening primary and/or metastatic diseases emerge.

SUMMARY POINTS

1. Malignant tumors are composed of several dynamic component parts.
2. As an oncogenic agent, stromal cells can provoke tumorigenicity in adjacent cells in the absence of preexisting neoplastic cells.
3. Chronic inflammatory disorders enhance overall risk for cancer development.
4. Biological processes can contribute opposite effects at different stages of carcinogenesis.
5. Stromal targets for therapy have advantages over epithelial targets.
6. Antiangiogenic therapy may stabilize tumor vasculature and enhance delivery of drugs to developing neoplasms.
7. Biologic therapies may inadvertently alter tissue programming and therefore should be fully explored in preclinical animal models of human disease pathogenesis.

FUTURE DIRECTIONS/UNRESOLVED ISSUES

1. Stromal signaling pathways that operate at each distinct stage of carcinogenesis and in each cell type should be identified and targeted.
2. Critical epithelial–stromal signaling pathways as therapeutic targets during the earliest stages of premalignant development should be identified.
3. The mechanisms by which oncogenic signals from stroma facilitate generation of neoplastic epithelial cells should be elucidated.

ACKNOWLEDGMENTS

We acknowledge the UCSF Comprehensive Cancer Center Breast and Prostate tissue banks for providing tissues sections, Dr. Volkan Adsay for pancreatic micrographs, Dr. Karin de Visser for help with illustrations and critical discussion, and members of the Tlsty and Coussens laboratories for insightful comments. T.D.T. is supported by grants from the National Cancer Institute, AVON, the California Breast Cancer Research Program, and the Department of Defense. L.M.C. is supported by grants from the National Cancer Institute, National Institute of Diabetes & Digestive & Kidney Diseases, National Center for Research Resources, and the Department of Defense.

LITERATURE CITED

1. Bissell MJ, Radisky D. 2001. Putting tumors in context. *Nat. Rev. Cancer* 1:46–54
2. Tlsty TD. 2001. Stromal cells can contribute oncogenic signals. *Semin. Cancer Biol.* 11:97–104
3. Mueller MM, Fusenig NE. 2004. Friends or foes—bipolar effects of the tumour stroma in cancer. *Nat. Rev. Cancer* 4:839–49
4. Allinen M, Beroukhim R, Cai L, Brennan C, Lahti-Domenici J, et al. 2004. Molecular characterization of the tumor microenvironment in breast cancer. *Cancer Cell* 6:17–32

5. van den Hooff A. 1988. Stromal involvement in malignant growth. *Adv. Cancer Res.* 50:159–96
6. Ronnov-Jessen L, Petersen OW, Bissell MJ. 1996. Cellular changes involved in conversion of normal to malignant breast: importance of the stromal reaction. *Physiol. Rev.* 76:69–125
7. Mackie EJ, Chiquet-Ehrismann R, Pearson CA, Inaguma Y, Taya K, et al. 1987. Tenascin is a stromal marker for epithelial malignancy in the mammary gland. *Proc. Natl. Acad. Sci. USA* 84:4621–25
8. Sappino AP, Schurch W, Gabbiani G. 1990. Differentiation repertoire of fibroblastic cells: expression of cytoskeletal proteins as marker of phenotypic modulations. *Lab. Invest.* 63:144–61
9. Albertson DG, Collins C, McCormick F, Gray JW. 2003. Chromosome aberrations in solid tumors. *Nat. Genet.* 34:369–76
10. Weir B, Zhao X, Meyerson M. 2004. Somatic alterations in the human cancer genome. *Cancer Cell* 6:433–38
11. McCormick F. 2004. Cancer: survival pathways meet their end. *Nature* 428:267–69
12. Rous P, Kidd J. 1941. Conditional neoplasms and subthreshold neoplastic states: a study of the tar tumors of rabbits. *J. Exp. Med.* 73:365–89
13. Mackenzie IC, Rous P. 1941. The experimental disclosure of latent neoplastic changes in tarred skin. *J. Exp. Med.* 73:391–415
14. Knudson AG. 2001. Two genetic hits (more or less) to cancer. *Nat. Rev. Cancer* 1:157–62
15. Balmain A, Gray J, Ponder B. 2003. The genetics and genomics of cancer. *Nat. Genet.* 33:238–44
16. Fitzpatrick FA. 2001. Inflammation, carcinogenesis and cancer. *Int. Immuno.* 1:1651–67
17. Coussens LM, Werb Z. 2002. Inflammation and cancer. *Nature* 420:860–67
18. Dalgleish AG, O'Byrne KJ. 2002. Chronic immune activation and inflammation in the pathogenesis of AIDS and cancer. *Adv. Cancer Res.* 84:231–76
19. Farrow B, Evers BM. 2002. Inflammation and the development of pancreatic cancer. *Surg. Oncol.* 10:153–69
20. Shacter E, Weitzman SA. 2002. Chronic inflammation and cancer. *Oncology* 16:217–26
21. Pasche B, Serhan C. 2004. Is C-reactive protein an inflammation opsonin that signals colon cancer risk? *JAMA* 291:623–24
22. Thun MJ, Henley SJ, Gansler T. 2004. Inflammation and cancer: an epidemiological perspective. *Novartis Found. Symp.* 256:6–21
23. Balkwill F, Mantovani A. 2001. Inflammation and cancer: back to Virchow?*Lancet* 357:539–45
24. Clevers H. 2004. At the crossroads of inflammation and cancer. *Cell* 118:671–74
25. Duncan LM, Richards LA, Mihm MC. 1998. Increased mast cell density in invasive melanoma. *J. Cutan. Pathol.* 25:11–15
26. Imada A, Shijubo N, Kojima H, Abe S. 2000. Mast cells correlate with angiogenesis and poor outcome in stage I lung adenocarcinoma. *Eur. Respir. J.* 15:1087–93
27. Takanami I, Takeuchi K, Naruke M. 2000. Mast cell density is associated with angiogenesis and poor prognosis in pulmonary adenocarcinoma. *Cancer* 88:2686–92
28. Tomita M, Matsuzaki Y, Onitsuka T. 2000. Effect of mast cells on tumor angiogenesis in lung cancer. *Ann. Thorac. Surg.* 69:1686–90
29. Toth-Jakatics R, Jimi S, Takebayashi S, Kawamoto N. 2000. Cutaneous malignant melanoma: correlation between neovascularization and peritumor accumulation of mast cells overexpressing vascular endothelial growth factor. *Hum. Pathol.* 31:955–60

30. Shea CR, Prieto VG. 1994. Mast cells in angiolipomas and hemangiomas of human skin: are they important for angiogenesis? *J. Cutan. Pathol.* 21:247–51
31. Benitez-Bribiesca L, Wong A, Utrera D, Castellanos E. 2001. The role of mast cell tryptase in neoangiogenesis of premalignant and malignant lesions of the uterine cervix. *J. Histochem. Cytochem.* 49:1061–62
32. Esposito I, Menicagli M, Funel N, Bergmann F, Boggi U, et al. 2004. Inflammatory cells contribute to the generation of an angiogenic phenotype in pancreatic ductal adenocarcinoma. *J. Clin. Pathol.* 57:630–36
33. Teich N, Mossner J. 2004. Genetic aspects of chronic pancreatitis. *Med. Sci. Monit.* 10:RA325–28
34. Warzocha K, Ribeiro P, Bienvenu J, Roy P, Charlot C, et al. 1998. Genetic polymorphisms in the tumor necrosis factor locus influence non-Hodgkin's lymphoma outcome. *Blood* 91:3574–81
35. Kuper H, Adami HO, Trichopoulos D. 2000. Infections as a major preventable cause of human cancer. *J. Intern. Med.* 248:171–83
36. Ernst PB, Gold BD. 2000. The disease spectrum of *Helicobacter pylori*: the immunopathogenesis of gastroduodenal ulcer and gastric cancer. *Annu. Rev. Microbiol.* 54:615–40
37. Engle SJ, Ormsby I, Pawlowski S, Boivin GP, Croft J, et al. 2002. Elimination of colon cancer in germ-free transforming growth factor β1-deficient mice. *Cancer Res.* 62:6362–66
38. Garcia-Rodriguez LA, Huerta-Alvarez C. 2001. Reduced risk of colorectal cancer among long-term users of aspirin and nonaspirin nonsteroidal antiinflammatory drugs. *Epidemiology* 12:88–93
39. Gonzalez-Perez A, Rodriguez L, Lopez-Ridaura R. 2003. Effects of non-steroidal anti-inflammatory drugs on cancer sites other than the colon and rectum: a meta-analysis. *BMC Cancer* 3:1–12
40. Koki AT, Masferrer JL. 2002. Celecoxib: A specific COX-2 inhibitor with anticancer properties. *Cancer Control* 9:28–35
41. Turini ME, DuBois RN. 2002. Cyclooxygenase-2: a therapeutic target. *Annu. Rev. Med.* 53:35–37
42. Williams CS, Mann M, DuBois RN. 1999. The role of cyclooxygenases in inflammation, cancer, and development. *Oncogene* 18:7908–16
43. Meier CR, Schmitz S, Jick H. 2002. Association between acetaminophen or nonsteroidal antiinflammatory drugs and risk of developing ovarian, breast, or colon cancer. *Pharmacotherapy* 22:303–9
44. Sharpe CR, Collet JP, McNutt M, Belzile E, Boivin JF, Hanley JA. 2000. Nested case-control study of the effects of non-steroidal anti-inflammatory drugs on breast cancer risk and stage. *Br. J. Cancer* 83:112–20
45. Cotterchio M, Kreiger N, Sloan M, Steingart A. 2001. Nonsteroidal anti-inflammatory drug use and breast cancer risk. *Cancer Epidemiol. Biomarkers Prev.* 10:1213–17
46. Akre K, Ekstrom AM, Signorello LB, Hansson LE, Nyren O. 2001. Aspirin and risk for gastric cancer: a population-based case-control study in Sweden. *Br. J. Cancer* 84:965–68
47. Cerhan JR, Anderson KE, Janney CA, Vachon CM, Witzig TE, Habermann T. 2003. Association of aspirin and other non-steroidal anti-inflammatory drug use with incidence of non-Hodgkin lymphoma. *Int. J. Cancer* 106:784–88
48. Schernhammer ES, Kang JH, Chan AT, Michaud DS, Skinner HG, et al. 2004. A prospective study of aspirin use and the risk of pancreatic cancer in women. *J. Natl. Cancer Inst.* 96:22–28

49. Coussens LM, Tinkle CL, Hanahan D, Werb Z. 2000. MMP-9 supplied by bone marrow-derived cells contributes to skin carcinogenesis. *Cell* 103:481–90
50. Coussens LM, Raymond WW, Bergers G, Laig-Webster M, Behrendtsen O, et al. 1999. Inflammatory mast cells up-regulate angiogenesis during squamous epithelial carcinogenesis. *Genes Dev.* 13:1382–97
51. Greten FR, Eckmann L, Greten TF, Park JM, Li ZW, et al.2004. IKKβ links inflammation and tumorigenesis in a mouse model of colitis-associated cancer. *Cell* 118:285–96
52. Pikarsky E, Porat RM, Stein I, Abramovitch R, Amit S, et al. 2004. NF-κB functions as a tumour promoter in inflammation-associated cancer. *Nature* 431:461–66
53. Giraudo E, Inoue M, Hanahan D. 2004. An amino-bisphosphonate targets MMP-9-expressing macrophages and angiogenesis to impair cervical carcinogenesis. *J. Clin. Invest.* 114:623–33
54. Arbeit JM, Munger K, Howley PM, Hanahan D. 1994. Progressive squamous epithelial neoplasia in K14-human papillomavirus type 16 transgenic mice. *J. Virol.* 68:4358–68
55. Coussens LM, Hanahan D, Arbeit JM. 1996. Genetic predisposition and parameters of malignant progression in K14-HPV16 transgenic mice. *Am. J. Pathol.* 149:1899–917
56. de Visser KE, Coussens LM. (May 12, 2005) The interplay between innate and adaptive immunity regulates cancer development. *Cancer Immunol. Immunother*. 10.1007/s00262-005-0702-5
57. de Visser KE, Korets LV, Coussens LM. De novo carcinogenesis promoted by chronic inflammation is B lymphocyte dependent. *Cancer Cell* 7:411–23
58. Lin EY, Nguyen AV, Russell RG, Pollard JW. 2001. Colony-stimulating factor 1 promotes progression of mammary tumors to malignancy. *J. Exp. Med.* 193:727–40
59. Sparmann A, Bar-Sagi D. 2004. Ras-induced interleukin-8 expression plays a critical role in tumor growth and angiogenesis. *Cancer Cell* 6:447–58
60. Almand B, Clark JI, Nikitina E, van Beynen J, English NR, et al. 2001. Increased production of immature myeloid cells in cancer patients: a mechanism of immunosuppression in cancer. *J. Immunol.* 166:678–89
61. Serafini P, De Santo C, Marigo I, Cingarlini S, Dolcetti L, et al. 2004. Derangement of immune responses by myeloid suppressor cells. *Cancer Immunol. Immunother.* 53:64–72
62. Kusmartsev S, Gabrilovich DI. 2002. Immature myeloid cells and cancer-associated immune suppression. *Cancer Immunol. Immunother.* 51:293–98
63. Yang L, Debusk LM, Fukuda K, Fingleton B, Green-Jarvis B, et al. 2004. Expansion of myeloid immune suppressor Gr^+CD11b^+ cells in tumor-bearing host directly promotes tumor angiogenesis. *Cancer Cell* 6:409–21
64. Gabrilovich DI, Velders MP, Sotomayor EM, Kast WM. 2001. Mechanism of immune dysfunction in cancer mediated by immature $Gr\text{-}1^+$ myeloid cells. *J. Immunol.* 166:5398–406
65. Wilson CL, Heppner KJ, Labosky PA, Hogan BL, Matrisian LM. 1997. Intestinal tumorigenesis is suppressed in mice lacking the metalloproteinase matrilysin. *Proc. Natl. Acad. Sci. USA* 94:1402–7
66. Kobayashi A, Greenblatt RM, Anastos K, Minkoff H, Massad LS, et al. 2004. Functional attributes of mucosal immunity in cervical intraepithelial neoplasia and effects of HIV infection. *Cancer Res.* 64:6766–74
67. Lin EY, Gouon-Evans V, Nguyen AV, Pollard JW. 2002. The macrophage growth factor CSF-1 in mammary gland development and tumor progression. *J. Mammary Gland. Biol. Neopl.* 7:147–62

68. Skobe M, Hamberg LM, Hawighorst T, Schirner M, Wolf GL, et al. 2001. Concurrent induction of lymphangiogenesis, angiogenesis, and macrophage recruitment by vascular endothelial growth factor-C in melanoma. *Am. J. Pathol.* 159:893–903
69. Schoppmann S, Birner P, Stockl J, Kalt R, Ullrich R, et al. 2002. Tumor-associated macrophages express lymphatic endothelial growth factors and are related to peritumoral lymphangiogenesis. *Am. J. Pathol.* 161:947–56
70. Nesbit M, Schaider H, Miller TH, Herlyn M. 2001. Low-level monocyte chemoattractant protein-1 stimulation of monocytes leads to tumor formation in nontumorigenic melanoma cells. *J. Immunol.* 166:6483–90
71. Hiratsuka S, Nakamura K, Iwai S, Murakami M, Itoh T, et al. 2002. MMP9 induction by vascular endothelial growth factor receptor-1 is involved in lung-specific metastasis. *Cancer Cell* 2:289–300
72. Balkwill F. 2004. Cancer and the chemokine network. *Nat. Rev. Cancer* 4:540–50
73. Balkwill F. 2002. Tumor necrosis factor or tumor promoting factor?*Cytokine Growth Factor Rev.* 13:135–41
74. Maeda H, Akaike T. 1998. Nitric oxide and oxygen radicals in infection, inflammation, and cancer. *Biochemistry* 63:854–65
75. Balkwill F, Coussens LM. 2004. Cancer: an inflammatory link. *Nature* 431:405–6
76. Barbera-Guillem E, Nyhus JK, Wolford CC, Friece CR, Sampsel JW. 2002. Vascular endothelial growth factor secretion by tumor-infiltrating macrophages essentially supports tumor angiogenesis, and IgG immune complexes potentiate the process. *Cancer Res.* 62:7042–49
77. Bergers G, Brekken R, McMahon G, Vu TH, Itoh T, et al. 2000. Matrix metalloproteinase-9 triggers the angiogenic switch during carcinogenesis. *Nat. Cell Biol.* 2:737–44
78. de Visser KE, Coussens LM. 2004. Inflammation and matrix metalloproteinases: implications for cancer development. In *Cancer and Inflammation*, ed. DW Morgan, UJ Forssmann, MT Nakada, pp. 71–97. Basel, Switzerland: Birkhauser Verlag
79. Diaz RJ, Eichten AE, de Visser KE, Coussens LM. 2005. Matrix metalloproteinases: Mediators of tumour-host interactions. In *Fundamental Aspects of Cancer: Cancer Growth & Progression*, ed. G Meadows, pp. 781–126. Dordrecht, The Netherlands: Springer
80. Egeblad M, Werb Z. 2002. New functions for the matrix metalloproteinases in cancer progression. *Nat. Rev. Cancer* 2:161–74
81. de Visser KE, Korets LV, Coussens LM. 2004. Early neoplastic progression is complement independent. *Neoplasia* 6:768–76
82. van Kempen LCL, Rhee JS, Dehne K, Lee J, Edwards DR, Coussens LM. 2002. Epithelial carcinogenesis: dynamic interplay between neoplastic cells and their microenvironment. *Differentiation* 70:501–623
83. Dranoff G. 2003. Coordinated tumor immunity. *J. Clin. Invest.* 111:1116–18
84. Oshikiri T, Miyamoto M, Shichinohe T, Suzuoki M, Hiraoka K, et al. 2003. Prognostic value of intratumoral $CD8^+$ T lymphocyte in extrahepatic bile duct carcinoma as essential immune response. *J Surg. Oncol.* 84:224–28
85. Abe M, Kondo S, Hirano S, Ambo Y, Tanaka E, et al. 2003. Long-term survival after radical resection of advanced pancreatic cancer: a case report with special reference to $CD8^+$ T-cell infiltration. *Int. J. Gastrointest. Cancer* 33:107–10
86. Wakabayashi O, Yamazaki K, Oizumi S, Hommura F, Kinoshita I, et al. 2003. $CD4^+$ T cells in cancer stroma, not $CD8^+$ T cells in cancer cell nests, are associated with favorable prognosis in human non-small cell lung cancers. *Cancer Sci.* 94:1003–9

87. Nakakubo Y, Miyamoto M, Cho Y, Hida Y, Oshikiri T, et al. 2003. Clinical significance of immune cell infiltration within gallbladder cancer. *Br. J. Cancer* 89:1736–42
88. Funada Y, Noguchi T, Kikuchi R, Takeno S, Uchida Y, Gabbert HE. 2003. Prognostic significance of $CD8^+$ T cell and macrophage peritumoral infiltration in colorectal cancer. *Oncol. Rep.* 10:309–13
89. Dudley ME, Rosenberg SA. 2003. Adoptive-cell-transfer therapy for the treatment of patients with cancer. *Nat. Rev. Cancer* 3:666–75
90. Pardoll DM. 2002. Spinning molecular immunology into successful immunotherapy. *Nat. Rev. Immunol.* 2:227–38
91. Pardoll DM. 2002. T cells take aim at cancer. *Proc. Natl. Acad. Sci. USA* 99:15840–42
92. Pardoll DM. 2003. Does the immune system see tumors as foreign or self? *Annu. Rev. Immunol.* 21:807–39
93. Schaerli P, Ebert L, Willimann K, Blaser A, Roos RS, et al. 2004. A skin-selective homing mechanism for human immune surveillance T cells. *J. Exp. Med.* 199:1265–75
94. Kupper TS, Fuhlbrigge RC. 2004. Immune surveillance in the skin: mechanisms and clinical consequences. *Nat. Rev. Immunol.* 4:211–22
95. Fuchs E, Raghavan S. 2002. Getting under the skin of epidermal morphogenesis. *Nat. Rev. Genet.* 3:199–209
96. Seitz CS, Lin Q, Deng H, Khavari PA. 1998. Alterations in NF-κB function in transgenic epithelial tissue demonstrate a growth inhibitory role for NF-κB. *Proc. Natl. Acad. Sci. USA* 95:2307–12
97. Scott KA, Moore RJ, Arnott CH, East N, Thompson RG, et al. 2003. An anti-tumor necrosis factor-α antibody inhibits the development of experimental skin tumors. *Mol. Cancer Ther.* 2:445–51
98. Szlosarek PW, Balkwill FR. 2003. Tumour necrosis factor α: a potential target for the therapy of solid tumours. *Lancet Oncol.* 4:565–73
99. Coussens LM, B. Fingleton B, Matrisian LM. 2002. Matrix metalloproteinase inhibitors and cancer: trials and tribulations. *Science* 295:2387–92
100. Chang HY, Sneddon JB, Alizadeh AA, Sood R, West RB, et al. 2004. Gene expression signature of fibroblast serum response predicts human cancer progression: similarities between tumors and wounds. *PLoS Biol.* 2:E7
101. Bhowmick NA, Moses HL. 2005. Tumor-stroma interactions. *Curr. Opin. Genet. Dev.* 15:97–101
102. Bhowmick NA, Neilson EG, Moses HL. 2004. Stromal fibroblasts in cancer initiation and progression. *Nature* 432:332–37
103. Willis RA. 1967. The unusual in tumour pathology. *Can. Med. Assoc. J.* 97:1466–79
104. Bauer EA, Uitto J, Walters RC, Eisen AZ. 1979. Enhanced collagenase production by fibroblasts derived from human basal cell carcinomas. *Cancer Res.* 39:4594–99
105. Knudson W, Biswas C, Toole BP. 1984. Interactions between human tumor cells and fibroblasts stimulate hyaluronate synthesis. *Proc. Natl. Acad. Sci. USA* 81:6767–71
106. Rasmussen AA, Cullen KJ. 1998. Paracrine/autocrine regulation of breast cancer by the insulin-like growth factors. *Breast Cancer Res. Treat.* 47:219–33
107. Schor SL, Schor AM, Rushton G. 1988. Fibroblasts from cancer patients display a mixture of both foetal and adult-like phenotypic characteristics. *J. Cell Sci.* 90:401–7
108. Schor SL, Haggie JA, Durning P, Howell A, Smith L, et al. 1986. Occurrence of a fetal fibroblast phenotype in familial breast cancer. *Int. J. Cancer* 37:831–36
109. Olumi AF, Grossfeld GD, Hayward SW, Carroll PR, Tlsty TD, Cunha GR. 1999. Carcinoma-associated fibroblasts direct tumor progression of initiated human prostatic epithelium. *Cancer Res.* 59:5002–11

110. Camps JL, Chang SM, Hsu TC, Freeman MR, Hong SJ, et al. 1990. Fibroblast-mediated acceleration of human epithelial tumor growth in vivo. *Proc. Natl. Acad. Sci. USA* 87:75–79
111. Gleave M, Hsieh JT, Gao CA, von Eschenbach AC, Chung LW. 1991. Acceleration of human prostate cancer growth in vivo by factors produced by prostate and bone fibroblasts. *Cancer Res.* 51:3753–61
112. Atula S, Grenman R, Syrjanen S. 1997. Fibroblasts can modulate the phenotype of malignant epithelial cells in vitro. *Exp. Cell Res.* 235:180–87
113. Billingham RE, Orr JW, Woodhouse DL. 1951. Transplantation of skin components during chemical carcinogenesis with 20-methylcholanthrene. *Br. J. Cancer* 5:417–32
114. Hodges GM, Hicks RM, Spacey GD. 1977. Epithelial-stromal interactions in normal and chemical carcinogen-treated adult bladder. *Cancer Res.* 37:3720–30
115. Uchida K, Samma S, Momose H, Kashihara N, Rademaker A, Oyasu R. 1990. Stimulation of urinary bladder tumorigenesis by carcinogen-exposed stroma. *J. Urol.* 143:618–21
116. Barcellos-Hoff MH, Ravani SA. 2000. Irradiated mammary gland stroma promotes the expression of tumorigenic potential by unirradiated epithelial cells. *Cancer Res.* 60:1254–60
117. Ronnov-Jessen L, Petersen OW, Koteliansky VE, Bissell MJ. 1995. The origin of the myofibroblasts in breast cancer. Recapitulation of tumor environment in culture unravels diversity and implicates converted fibroblasts and recruited smooth muscle cells. *J. Clin. Invest.* 95:859–73
118. Roberts AB, Sporn MB, Assoian RK, Smith JM, Roche NS, et al. 1986. Transforming growth factor type β: rapid induction of fibrosis and angiogenesis in vivo and stimulation of collagen formation in vitro. *Proc. Natl. Acad. Sci. USA* 83:4167–71
119. Dvorak HF. 1986. Tumors: wounds that do not heal. Similarities between tumor stroma generation and wound healing. *N. Engl. J. Med.* 315:1650–59
120. Waite KA, Eng C. 2003. From developmental disorder to heritable cancer: it's all in the BMP/TGF-β family. *Nat. Rev. Genet.* 4:763–73
121. Sieweke MH, Thompson NL, Sporn MB, Bissell MJ. 1990. Mediation of wound-related Rous sarcoma virus tumorigenesis by TGF-β. *Science* 248:1656–60
122. Jacobs TW, Byrne C, Colditz G, Connolly JL, Schnitt SJ. 1999. Radial scars in benign breast-biopsy specimens and the risk of breast cancer. *N. Engl. J. Med.* 340:430–36
123. Linskens MH, Feng J, Andrews WH, Enlow BE, Saati SM, et al. 1995. Cataloging altered gene expression in young and senescent cells using enhanced differential display. *Nucleic Acids Res.* 23:3244–51
124. Serrano M, Lin AW, McCurrach ME, Beach D, Lowe SW. 1997. Oncogenic ras provokes premature cell senescence associated with accumulation of p53 and p16INK4a. *Cell* 88:593–602
125. Parrinello S, Coppe JP, Krtolica A, Campisi J. 2005. Stromal-epithelial interactions in aging and cancer: senescent fibroblasts alter epithelial cell differentiation. *J. Cell Sci.* 118:485–96
126. McCullough KD, Coleman WB, Smith GJ, Grishan JW. 1994. Age-dependent regulation of the tumorigenic potential of neoplastically transformed rat liver epithelial cells by the liver microenvironment. *Cancer Res.* 54:3668–71
127. Lukanova A, Kaaks R. 2005. Endogenous hormones and ovarian cancer: epidemiology and current hypotheses. *Cancer Epidemiol. Biomarkers Prev.* 14:98–107

128. Platz EA, Giovannucci E. 2004. The epidemiology of sex steroid hormones and their signaling and metabolic pathways in the etiology of prostate cancer. *J. Steroid Biochem. Mol. Biol.* 92:237–53
129. Muti P. 2005. The role of endogenous hormones in the etiology and prevention of breast cancer: the epidemiological evidence. *Recent Results Cancer Res.* 166:245–56
130. Hansen RK, Bissell MJ. 2000. Tissue architecture and breast cancer: the role of extracellular matrix and steroid hormones. *Endocr. Relat. Cancer* 7:95–113
131. Wang YZ, Wong YC. 1998. Sex hormone-induced prostatic carcinogenesis in the noble rat: the role of insulin-like growth factor-I (IGF-I) and vascular endothelial growth factor (VEGF) in the development of prostate cancer. *Prostate* 35:165–77
132. Xie B, Tsao SW, Wong YC. 1999. Sex hormone-induced mammary carcinogenesis in female Noble rats: expression of TGF-β1 and its receptors, TGF-α, and EGF-R in mammary carcinogenesis. *Breast Cancer Res. Treat.* 58:227–39
133. Jacoby RF, Schlack S, Cole CE, Skarbek M, Harris C, Meisner LF. 1997. A juvenile polyposis tumor suppressor locus at 10q22 is deleted from nonepithelial cells in the lamina propria. *Gastroenterology* 112:1398–403
134. Howe JR, Roth S, Ringold JC, Summers RW, Jarvinen HJ, et al. 1998. Mutations in the SMAD4/DPC4 gene in juvenile polyposis. *Science* 280:1086–88
135. Moinfar F, Man YG, Arnould L, Bratthauer GL, Ratschek M, Tavassoli FA. 2000. Concurrent and independent genetic alterations in the stromal and epithelial cells of mammary carcinoma: implications for tumorigenesis. *Cancer Res.* 60:2562–66
136. Whitfield ML, Finlay DR, Murray JI, Troyanskaya OG, Chi JT, et al. 2003. Systemic and cell type-specific gene expression patterns in scleroderma skin. *Proc. Natl. Acad. Sci. USA* 100:12319–24
137. Sternlicht MD, Lochter A, Sympson CJ, Huey B, Rougier JP, et al. 1999. The stromal proteinase MMP3/stromelysin-1 promotes mammary carcinogenesis. *Cell* 98:137–46
138. Folkman J. 2003. Fundamental concepts of the angiogenic process. *Curr. Mol. Med.* 3:643–51
139. Carmeliet P, Jain RK. 2000. Angiogenesis in cancer and other diseases. *Nature* 407:249–57
140. Carmeliet P. 2003. Angiogenesis in health and disease. *Nat. Med.* 9:653–60
141. Bergers G, Benjamin LE. 2003. Angiogenesis: tumorigenesis and the angiogenic switch. *Nat. Rev. Cancer* 3:401–10
142. Folkman J. 2002. Role of angiogenesis in tumor growth and metastasis. *Semin. Oncol.* 29:15–18
143. Hanahan D, Weinberg RA. 2000. The hallmarks of cancer. *Cell* 100:57–70
144. Giordano FJ, Johnson RS. 2001. Angiogenesis: the role of the microenvironment in flipping the switch. *Curr. Opin. Genet. Dev.* 11:35–40
145. Lafleur MA, Handsley MM, Edwards DR. 2003. Metalloproteinases and their inhibitors in angiogenesis. *Expert Rev. Mol. Med.* 5:1–39
146. McDonald DM, Baluk P. 2002. Significance of blood vessel leakiness in cancer. *Cancer Res.* 62:5381–85
147. Jain RK. 2005. Normalization of tumor vasculature: an emerging concept in antiangiogenic therapy. *Science* 307:58–62
148. Sternlicht MD, Werb Z. 2001. How matrix metalloproteinases regulate cell behavior. *Annu. Rev. Cell. Dev. Biol.* 17:463–516
149. Seandel M, Noack-Kunnmann K, Zhu D, Aimes RT, Quigley JP. 2001. Growth factor-induced angiogenesis in vivo requires specific cleavage of fibrillar type I collagen. *Blood* 97:2323–32

150. Bergers G, Coussens LM. 2000. Extrinsic regulators of epithelial tumor progression: metalloproteinases. *Curr. Opin. Genet. Dev.* 10:120–27
151. Yu WH, Woessner JF Jr, McNeish JD, Stamenkovic I. 2002. CD44 anchors the assembly of matrilysin/MMP-7 with heparin-binding epidermal growth factor precursor and ErbB4 and regulates female reproductive organ remodeling. *Genes Dev.* 16:307–23
152. Jain RK. 2003. Molecular regulation of vessel maturation. *Nat. Med.* 9:685–93
153. O'Reilly MS, Boehm T, Shing Y, Fukai N, Vasios G, et al. 1997. Endostatin: an endogenous inhibitor of angiogenesis and tumor growth. *Cell* 88:277–85
154. Hiraoka N, Allen E, Apel IJ, Gyetko MR, Weiss SJ. 1998. Matrix metalloproteinases regulate neovascularization by acting as pericellular fibrinolysins. *Cell* 95:365–77
155. Cornelius LA, Nehring LC, Harding E, Bolanowski M, Welgus HG, et al. 1998. Matrix metalloproteinases generate angiostatin: effects on neovascularization. *J. Immunol.* 161:6845–52
156. Hiller O, Lichte A, Oberpichler A, Kocourek A, Tschesche H. 2000. Matrix metalloproteinases collagenase-2, macrophage elastase, collagenase-3, and membrane type 1-matrix metalloproteinase impair clotting by degradation of fibrinogen and factor XII. *J. Biol. Chem.* 275:33008–13
157. McQuibban GA, Gong JH, Wong JP, Wallace JL, Clark-Lewis I, Overall CM. 2002. Matrix metalloproteinase processing of monocyte chemoattractant proteins generates CC chemokine receptor antagonists with anti-inflammatory properties in vivo. *Blood* 100:1160–67
158. Sottile J. 2004. Regulation of angiogenesis by extracellular matrix. *Biochim. Biophys. Acta* 1654:13–22
159. Kalluri R. 2003. Basement membranes: structure, assembly and role in tumour angiogenesis. *Nat. Rev. Cancer* 3:422–33
160. O'Reilly MS, Holmgren L, Shing Y, Chen C, Rosenthal RA, et al. 1994. Angiostatin: a novel angiogenesis inhibitor that mediates the suppression of metastases by a Lewis lung carcinoma. *Cell* 79:315–28
161. Bergers G, Javaherian K, Lo KM, Folkman J, Hanahan D. 1999. Effects of angiogenesis inhibitors on multistage carcinogenesis in mice. *Science* 284:808–12
162. Folkman J, Kalluri R. 2004. Cancer without disease. *Nature* 427:787
163. Ferreras M, Felbor U, Lenhard T, Olsen BR, Delaisse J. 2000. Generation and degradation of human endostatin proteins by various proteinases. *FEBS Lett.* 486:247–51
164. Ramchandran R, Dhanabal M, Volk R, Waterman MJ, Segal M. 1999. Antiangiogenic activity of restin, NC10 domain of human collagen XV: comparison to endostatin. *Biochem. Biophys. Res. Commun.* 255:735–39
165. Colorado PC, Torre A, Kamphaus G, Maeshima Y, Hopfer H, et al. 2000. Anti-angiogenic cues from vascular basement membrane collagen. *Cancer Res.* 60:2520–26
166. Kamphaus GD, Colorado PC, Panka DJ, Hopfer H, Ramchandran R, et al. 2000. Canstatin, a novel matrix-derived inhibitor of angiogenesis and tumor growth. *J. Biol. Chem.* 275:1209–15
167. Maeshima Y, Colorado PC, Torre A, Holthaus KA, Grunkemeyer JA, et al. 2000. Distinct antitumor properties of a type IV collagen domain derived from basement membrane. *J. Biol. Chem.* 275:21340–48
168. Maeshima Y, Colorado PC, Kalluri R. 2000. Two RGD-independent $\alpha v\beta 3$ integrin binding sites on tumstatin regulate distinct anti-tumor properties. *J. Biol. Chem.* 275:23745–50

169. Petitclerc E, Stromblad S, von Schalscha TL, Mitjans F, Piulats J, et al. 1999. Integrin $\alpha v\beta 3$ promotes M21 melanoma growth in human skin by regulating tumor cell survival. *Cancer Res.* 59:2724–30
170. Petitclerc E, Boutaud A, Prestayko A, Xu J, Sado Y, et al. 2000. New functions for non-collagenous domains of human collagen type IV. Novel integrin ligands inhibiting angiogenesis and tumor growth in vivo. *J. Biol. Chem.* 275:8051–61
171. Hamano Y, Zeisberg M, Sugimoto H, Lively JC, Maeshima Y, et al. 2003. Physiological levels of tumstatin, a fragment of collagen IV $\alpha 3$ chain, are generated by MMP-9 proteolysis and suppress angiogenesis via $\alpha V\beta 3$ integrin. *Cancer Cell* 3:589–601
172. Bissell MJ, Aggeler J. 1987. Dynamic reciprocity: How do extracellular matrix and hormones direct gene expression?*Prog. Clin. Biol. Res.* 249:251–62
173. Tlsty TD, Hein PW. 2001. Know thy neighbor: stromal cells can contribute oncogenic signals. *Curr. Opin. Genet. Dev.* 11:54–59
174. Aumailley M, Gayraud B. 1998. Structure and biological activity of the extracellular matrix. *J. Mol. Med.* 76:253–65
175. Howe A, Aplin AE, Alahari SK, Juliano RL. 1998. Integrin signaling and cell growth control. *Curr. Opin. Cell Biol.* 10:220–31
176. Weaver VM, Lelievre S, Lakins JN, Chrenek MA, Jones JC, et al. 2002. $\beta 4$ integrin-dependent formation of polarized three-dimensional architecture confers resistance to apoptosis in normal and malignant mammary epithelium. *Cancer Cell* 2:205–16
177. Bissell MJ, Radisky DC, Rizki A, Weaver VM, Petersen OW. 2002. The organizing principle: microenvironmental influences in the normal and malignant breast. *Differentiation* 70:537–46
178. Radisky D, Hagios C, Bissell MJ. 2001. Tumors are unique organs defined by abnormal signaling and context. *Semin. Cancer Biol.* 11:87–95
179. Hynes RO. 2002. Integrins: bidirectional, allosteric signaling machines. *Cell* 110:673–87
180. Bosman FT, Stamenkovic I. 2003. Functional structure and composition of the extracellular matrix. *J. Pathol.* 200:423–28
181. Ruiter D, Bogenrieder T, Elder D, Herlyn M. 2002. Melanoma-stroma interactions: structural and functional aspects. *Lancet Oncol.* 3:35–43
182. Hunzelman N, Risteli J, Risteli L. 1998. Circulating type I collagen degradation products in the urine of patients with scleroderma. *Br. J. Dermatol.* 139:1020–25
183. Zeisberg M, Maeshima Y, Mosterman B, Kalluri R. 2002. Renal fibrosis: extracellular matrix microenvironment regulates migratory behavior of activated tubular epithelial cells. *Am. J. Pathol.* 160:2001–8
184. Gheree-Kermani M, Phan M. 2001. Role of cytokines and cytokine therapy in wound healing and fibrotic disease. *Curr. Pharm. Des.* 7:1083–103
185. van Kempen LC, Ruiter DJ, van Muijen GN, Coussens LM. 2003. The tumor microenvironment: a critical determinant of neoplastic evolution. *Eur. J. Cell. Biol.* 82:539–48
186. Kinzler KW, Vogelstein B. 1998. Landscaping the cancer terrain. *Science* 280:1036–37
187. Fukino K, Shen L, Matsumoto S, Mutter GL, Eng C. 2004. Combined total genome loss of heterozygosity scan of breast cancer stroma and epithelium reveals multiplicity of stromal targets. *Cancer Res.* 64:7231–36
188. Kielty CM, Hopkindson I, Grant ME. 1993. Collagen: the collagen family: structure, assembly, and organization in the extracellular matrix. *Connect. Tissue Res.* 124:103–47
189. Vuorio E, de Crombrugghe B. 1990. The family of collagen genes. *Annu. Rev. Biochem.* 59:837–72

190. Zhu GG, Risteli L, Makinen M, Risteli J, Kauppila A, Stenback F. 1995. Immunohistochemical study of type I collagen and type I pN-collagen in benign and malignant ovarian neoplasms. *Cancer* 75:1010–17
191. Kauppila S, Stenback F, Risteli J, Jukkola A, Risteli L. 1998. Aberrant type I and type III collagen gene expression in human breast cancer in vivo. *J. Pathol.* 186:262–68
192. Santala M, Simojoki M, Risteli J, Risteli L, Kauppila A. 1999. Type I and III collagen metabolites as predictors of clinical outcome in epithelial ovarian cancer. *Clin. Cancer Res.* 5:4091–96
193. Burns-Cox N, Avery NC, Gingell JC, Bailey AJ. 2001. Changes in collagen metabolism in prostate cancer: a host response that may alter progression. *J. Urol.* 166:1698–701
194. Ylisirnio S, Hoyhtya M, Makitaro R, Paakko P, Risteli J, et al. 2001. Elevated serum levels of type I collagen degradation marker ICTP and tissue inhibitor of metalloproteinase (TIMP) 1 are associated with poor prognosis in lung cancer. *Clin. Cancer Res.* 7:1633–37
195. Guo YP, Martin LJ, Hanna W, Banerjee D, Miller N, et al. 2001. Growth factors and stromal matrix proteins associated with mammographic densities. *Cancer Epidemiol. Biomarkers Prev.* 10:243–48
196. Berking C, Takemoto R, Schaider H, Showe L, Satyamoorthy K, et al. 2001. Transforming growth factor-β1 increases survival of human melanoma through stroma remodeling. *Cancer Res.* 61:8306–16
197. Berndt A, Borsi L, Hyckel P, Kosmehl H. 2001. Fibrillary co-deposition of laminin-5 and large unspliced tenascin-C in the invasive front of oral squamous cell carcinoma in vivo and in vitro. *J. Cancer Res. Clin. Oncol.* 127:286–92
198. Clarijs R, Ruiter DJ, De Waal RM. 2003. Pathophysiological implications of stroma pattern formation in uveal melanoma. *J. Cell. Physiol.* 194:267–71
199. Clarijs R, Schalkwijk L, Ruiter DJ, de Waal RM. 2001. Lack of lymphangiogenesis despite coexpression of VEGF-C and its receptor Flt-4 in uveal melanoma. *Invest. Ophthalmol. Vis. Sci.* 42:1422–28
200. Clarijs R, Ruiter DJ, de Waal RM. 2001. Lymphangiogenesis in malignant tumours: Does it occur? *J. Pathol.* 193:143–46
201. Clarijs R, Otte-Holler I, Ruiter DJ, de Waal RM. 2002. Presence of a fluid-conducting meshwork in xenografted cutaneous and primary human uveal melanoma. *Invest. Ophthalmol. Vis. Sci.* 43:912–18
202. Hendrix MJ, Seftor EA, Hess AR, Seftor RE. 2003. Vasculogenic mimicry and tumour-cell plasticity: lessons from melanoma. *Nat. Rev. Cancer* 3:411–21
203. Hashizume H, Baluk P, Morikawa S, McLean JW, Thurston G, et al. 2000. Openings between defective endothelial cells explain tumor vessel leakiness. *Am. J. Pathol.* 156:1363–80
204. Ramanujan S, Pluen A, McKee TD, Brown EB, Boucher Y, Jain RK. 2002. Diffusion and convection in collagen gels: implications for transport in the tumor interstitium. *Biophys. J.* 83:1650–60
205. Saaristo A, Karpanen T, Alitalo K. 2000. Mechanisms of angiogenesis and their use in the inhibition of tumor growth and metastasis. *Oncogene* 19:6122–29
206. Herbst RS, Lee AT, Tran HT, Abbruzzese JL. 2001. Clinical studies of angiogenesis inhibitors: the University of Texas MD Anderson Center Trial of Human Endostatin. *Curr. Oncol. Rep.* 3:131–40
207. Willett CG, Boucher Y, Di Tomaso E, Duda DG, Munn LL, et al. 2004. Direct evidence that the VEGF-specific antibody bevacizumab has antivascular effects in human rectal cancer. *Nat. Med.* 10:145–47

208. Emmanouilides C, Pegram M, Robinson R, Hecht R, Kabbinavar F, Isacoff W. 2004. Anti-VEGF antibody bevacizumab (Avastin) with 5FU/LV as third line treatment for colorectal cancer. *Tech. Coloproctol.* 8:50–52

208a. U.S. Food and Drug Administration. 2004. *FDA approves first angiogenesis inhibitor to treat colorectal cancer*. **http://www.fda.gov/bbs/topics/NEWS/2004/NEW01027.html**

209. Autio P, Risteli J, Haukipuro K, Risteli L, Oikarinen A. 1994. Collagen synthesis in human skin in vivo: modulation by aging, ultraviolet B irradiation and localization. *Photodermatol. Photoimmunol. Photomed.* 10:212–16

210. Samet JM. 2000. Does idiopathic pulmonary fibrosis increase lung cancer risk?*Am. J. Respir. Crit. Care Med.* 161:1–2

211. Mossman BT, Churg A. 1998. Mechanisms in the pathogenesis of asbestosis and silicosis. *Am. J. Respir. Crit. Care Med.* 157:1666–80

212. Sassi M, Jukkola A, Riekki R, Hoyhtya M, Risteli L, et al. 2001. Type I collagen turnover and cross-linking are increased in irradiated skin of breast cancer patients. *Radiother. Oncol.* 58:317–23

213. McGaha T, Kodera T, Phelps R, Spiera H, Pines M, Bona C. 2002. Effect of halofuginone on the development of tight skin (TSK) syndrome. *Autoimmunity* 35:277–82

214. McGaha TL, Kodera T, Spiera H, Stan AC, Pines M, Bona CA. 2002. Halofuginone inhibition of COL1A2 promoter activity via a c-Jun-dependent mechanism. *Arthritis Rheum.* 46:2748–61

215. Spira G, Mawasi N, Paizi M, Anbinder N, Genina O, et al. 2002. Halofuginone, a collagen type I inhibitor improves liver regeneration in cirrhotic rats. *J. Hepatol.* 37:331–39

215a. Doctor's Guide. 2000. *Halofuginone receives FDA orphan drug status for scleroderma.* **http://www.pslgroup.com/dg/18dff6.htm**

215b. Clinical Trials. 2005. *Halofuginone Hydrobromide in treating patients with progressive advanced solid tumors*. **http://www.clinicaltrials.gov/ct/show/NCT00027677**

216. Jackson CJ, Jenkins KL. 1991. Type I collagen fibrils promote rapid vascular tube formation upon contact with the apical side of cultured endothelium. *Exp. Cell Res.* 192:319–23

217. Elkin M, Miao HQ, Nagler A, Aingorn E, Reich R, et al. 2000. Halofuginone: a potent inhibitor of critical steps in angiogenesis progression. *FASEB J.* 14:2477–85

218. Gavish Z, Pinthus JH, Barak V, Ramon J, Nagler A, et al. 2002. Growth inhibition of prostate cancer xenografts by halofuginone. *Prostate* 51:73–83

219. Di Lullo G, Sweeney S, Korkko J, Ala-Kokkor P, San Antonio J. 2002. Mapping the ligand-binding sites and disease-associated mutations on the most abundant protein in the human-type I collagen. *J. Biol. Chem.* 277:4223–31

220. Thurston G, Maas K, Labarbara A, McLean JW, McDonald DM. 2000. Microvascular remodeling in chronic airway inflammation in mice. *Clin. Exp. Pharmacol. Physiol.* 27:836–41

221. Eichten AE, Shen H-CJ, Coussens LM. 2005. Three-dimensional visualization of blood and lymphatic vasculature in tissue whole mounts using confocal microscopy. In *Current Protocols in Cytometry*, ed. JP Robinson, New Jersey: John Wiley & Sons, Inc. pp. 12.5.1–11

Neurodegenerative Diseases: New Concepts of Pathogenesis and Their Therapeutic Implications

Daniel M. Skovronsky,[1] Virginia M.-Y. Lee,[2] and John Q. Trojanowski[2]

[1]Avid Radiopharmaceuticals, Inc., Philadelphia, Pennsylvania 19104; email: skovronsky@avidrp.com

[2]Center for Neurodegenerative Disease Research, Institute on Aging, University of Pennsylvania, Philadelphia, Pennsylvania 19104; email: trojanow@mail.med.upenn.edu; vmylee@mail.med.upenn.edu

Annu. Rev. Pathol. Mech. Dis. 2006. 1:151–70

First published online as a Review in Advance on October 11, 2005

The *Annual Review of Pathology: Mechanisms of Disease* is online at pathmechdis.annualreviews.org

doi: 10.1146/annurev.pathol.1.110304.100113

1553-4006/06/0114-0151$20.00

Key Words

amyloid, Alzheimer's disease, Parkinson's disease, neurodegeneration, misfolding

Abstract

Neurodegenerative diseases as diverse as Alzheimer's, Parkinson's, and Creutzfeldt-Jakob disease share a common pathogenetic mechanism involving aggregation and deposition of misfolded proteins, which leads to progressive central nervous system disease. Although the type of aggregated protein and the regional and cellular distribution of deposition vary from disease to disease, these disorders may all be linked by similar pathways of protein aggregation with fibril formation and amyloid deposition. This perspective on pathogenesis suggests that a wide variety of neurodegenerative diseases can be grouped mechanistically as brain amyloidoses, an outlook that yields novel insights into potential therapeutic approaches that may be applicable across the broad spectrum of neurodegenerative disease.

Amyloid: protein aggregates that share specific traits, including cross β-sheet quaternary structure

AMYLOID AS A COMMON THEME IN NEURODEGENERATIVE DISEASE

Neurodegenerative disorders such as Alzheimer's and Parkinson's disease account for a significant and increasing proportion of morbidity and mortality in the developed world (1, 2). Largely as a result of increased life expectancy and changing population demographics (i.e., the aging of baby boomers), neurodegenerative dementias and neurodegenerative movement disorders are becoming more common (3, 4). As our population ages, an improved understanding of these diseases will be vital to developing more effective therapies and combating the staggering personal, social, and economic costs of these diseases (5). Unifying theories of pathogenesis in neurodegenerative disease provide an avenue for developing therapeutic strategies with broad applicability for disease prevention and an opportunity for decreasing morbidity and mortality from these disorders in the elderly population (6).

Converging lines of investigation have revealed a potential single common pathogenic mechanism underlying many diverse neurodegenerative disorders, i.e., the aggregation and deposition of misfolded proteins. As summarized in **Table 1**, nearly every major neurodegenerative disease is characterized pathologically by the insidious accumulation of insoluble filamentous aggregates of normally soluble proteins in the central nervous system (CNS). Because these filamentous aggregates display the ultrastructural and tinctorial properties of amyloid (i.e., ~10-nm-wide fibrils with crossed β-pleated sheet structures that stain with Congo red, thioflavin-S, or other related dyes), these diseases can be grouped together as brain amyloidoses.

What, then, accounts for the striking phenotypic diversity seen in these diseases? Each of the related brain amyloidoses is distinguished by (*a*) distinct temporal and regional patterns of deposition of aggregates, (*b*) varying cellular hosts or extracellular locales of the aggregates, and (*c*) different protein constituents of the aggregates (**Table 1**). Each of these characteristics, combined with the patient's own innate and variable response to the aggregates, may in turn alter the cascade of events leading to a particular temporal and regional pattern of neuronal dysfunction and death, which manifests as a specific clinical syndrome such as dementia in Alzheimer's disease or a movement disorder in Parkinson's disease. Thus, from a pathological standpoint, neurodegenerative entities are defined by the type and pattern of amyloid deposition in the brain. Unfortunately, the type and pattern of brain amyloidosis does not always correlate well with the observed clinical phenotype. This disconnect has led to a perplexing nosology that sometimes requires clinicians to describe phenotypes on the basis of the presumed presence of pathological lesions (e.g., dementia with Lewy bodies) and sometimes requires pathologists to describe lesions using clinical language regardless of the patient's actual clinical presentation (e.g., progressive supranuclear palsy, PSP). The best way to circumvent this morass may be the use some day of chemical analytes of biological fluids and neuroimaging biomarkers that allow clinicians to distinguish between

COMMON MOTIFS IN NEURODEGENERATIVE DISEASE

The major pathological lesions are accumulations of insoluble filamentous aggregates that take the form of amyloid. The aggregates are composed of a normal, soluble protein or peptide that has been misfolded. This amyloidogenic protein constituent differs among various neurodegenerative diseases. The amyloidogenic protein is typically expressed systemically, but accumulates only in the CNS. The aggregates accumulate early in the lifetime of the individual, but only manifest clinically in middle or late life. Most cases are sporadic, but genetic forms can be caused by mutations in the gene encoding the amyloidgenic protein that make it more prone to misfold and aggregate.

TABLE 1 Common neurodegenerative diseases characterized by deposition of aggregated proteins

Disease	Microscopic lesion	Location	Aggregated protein
Alzheimer's disease	Amyloid plaque	Extracellular	Amyloid-β (Aβ)
	Neurofibrillary tangle	Intracytoplasmic (neurons)	Tau
	Lewy bodies (seen in Lewy body variant)	Intracytoplasmic (neurons)	α-synuclein
Amyotrophic lateral sclerosis	Hyaline inclusions	Intracytoplasmic (neurons)	Superoxide dismutase-1 (SOD1)
Cortical basal degeneration/ progressive supranuclear palsy	Tau positive inclusions	Intracytoplasmic (neurons, oligodendroglia and astrocyes)	Tau
Dementia with Lewy bodies	Lewy bodies	Intracytoplasmic (neurons)	α-synuclein
Huntington disease	Neuronal inclusions	Intranuclear (neurons)	Huntington (containing polyglutamine repeat expansion)
Multiple system atrophy	Glial cytoplasmic inclusions	Intracytoplasmic (oligodendroglia)	α-synuclein
Parkinson's disease	Lewy bodies	Intracytoplasmic (neurons)	α-synuclein
Pick's disease	Pick bodies	Intracytoplasmic (neurons)	Tau
Prion diseases	Prion plaques	Extracellular	Protease-resistant prion protein (PrP)
Spinocerebellar ataxia	Neuronal inclusions	Intranuclear (neurons)	Ataxin (containing polyglutamine repeat expansion)

these related brain amyloidoses on the basis of the nature and extent of the brain pathology as well as the specific amyloidogenic protein(s) involved in disease pathogenesis.

Recognizing that all these related neurodegenerative diseases share common mechanisms involving CNS accumulation of misfolded proteins suggests that these disorders may have similar targets for the development of diagnostic and therapeutic agents. This review highlights these potential targets, focusing on three prototypical and common amyloidgenic proteins: Aβ, tau, and synuclein. Within this context, Alzheimer's disease, the tauopathies (Pick's disease, cortical basal degeneration, and PSP), and the synucleinopathies (dementia with Lewy bodies, Parkinson's disease, and multiple system atrophy) are discussed as exemplars or models of the brain amyloidoses that occur in many aging-related neurodegenerative disorders.

General Mechanisms of Brain Amyloid Formation

Brain amyloidosis begins with the production of a soluble native protein that is misfolded to yield the precursor for fibril formation (**Figure 1**). The misfolded protein can self-associate to form oligomers, protofibrils, or other intermediates en route to fibril formation (reviewed in Reference 7). Oligomers of Aβ can be detected in vitro (8), in cell culture and transgenic mouse models of Alzheimer's disease (9–11), and in postmortem Alzheimer's disease brain specimens (12). Although oligomers of Aβ have been the most well studied, it is apparent that other amyloidogenic proteins such as α-synuclein or polyglutamine-containing proteins can also form oligomers. Remarkably, oligomers composed of each of these amyloidogenic proteins (which share no primary sequence homology) show a similar

Amyloidogenic: property of being prone to aggregation and amyloid formation

Aβ (also amyloid-β or β-amyloid): 39–43 amino acid peptide generated by proteolytic cleavage of the amyloid precursor protein, which is prone to aggregating as amyloid

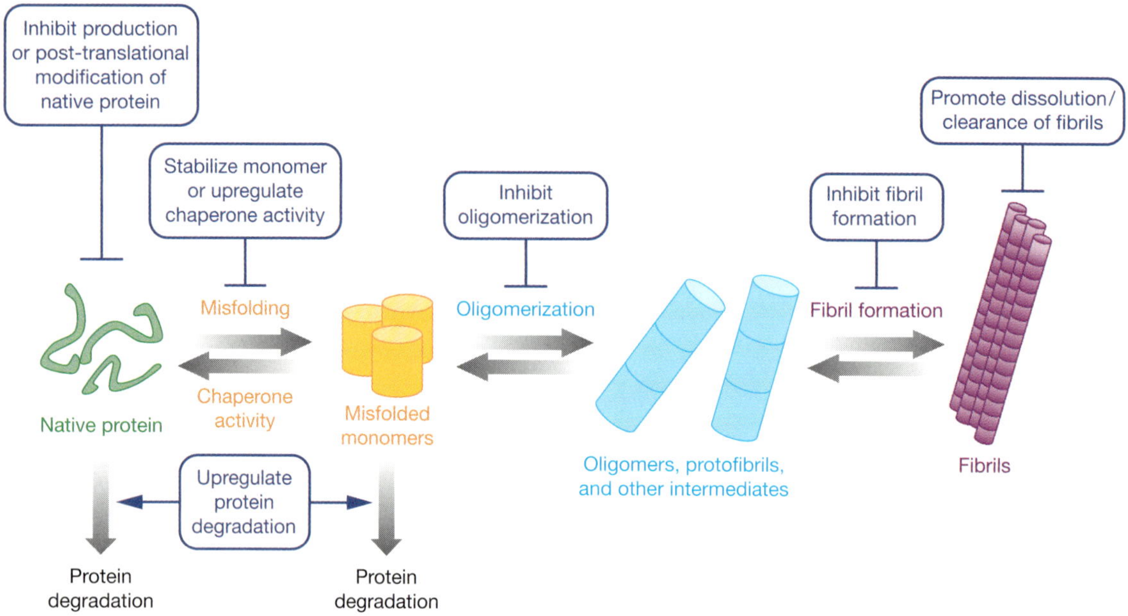

Figure 1

Model for protein misfolding and fibrillization. Soluble native protein is misfolded and associates in the form of oligomers and other intermediates that eventually give rise to fibrils. Potential opportunities for theapeutic intervention are shown in blue boxes.

conformation-dependent structure (12). These studies may suggest a common mechanism of amyloid formation that depends upon structural determinants within the oligomers. Further support for this hypothesis comes from the observation that different forms of amyloid interact with one another in vitro. For example, α-synuclein can initiate fibrillization of tau, and coincubation of tau and α-synuclein synergistically promotes fibrillization of both proteins (13).

In vivo, various factors may influence the balance between native protein, misfolded protein, oligomers, and fibrils. For example, in the disease state, overproduction of the amyloidogenic protein constituent, inappropriate covalent modification or cleavage, failed degradation, or insufficient molecular chaperone activity may all contribute in shifting the balance towards misfolded protein and oligomer formation. Each of these steps represents a potential target for therapeutic intervention, with therapies being developed currently for different forms of amyloid.

Consequences of Brain Amyloidosis

Although accumulation of brain amyloid is clearly a unifying characteristic of many neurodegenerative diseases, the mechanisms by which brain amyloid leads to neuronal death or dysfunction are ill defined, but likely to be numerous and diverse. For example, evidence suggests that brain amyloid is linked mechanistically to impairments in axonal transport (14–17), inhibition of proteasomal activity (18, 19), defects in DNA transcription (20), increased levels of oxidative stress (21, 22), and apoptosis (23, 24). Despite a wealth of experimental data, there is still no consensus on whether oligomers, protofibrils, or mature fibrils (or some combination of these) are the important toxic species that mediate neurodegeneration, nor do we understand the mechanisms by which they compromise the function and viability of selectively vulnerable CNS cells.

Aβ: THE EXTRACELLULAR AMYLOID OF ALZHEIMER'S DISEASE

Alzheimer's Disease: The Prototype Aβ Amyloidosis

The sina qua non of Alzheimer's disease, as defined originally by Alois Alzheimer, is the presence of extracellular amyloid plaques and intraneuronal neurofibrillary tangles (NFTs). In addition to these two cardinal lesions, >50% of sporadic and familial Alzheimer's patients have coexisting cortical Lewy bodies (25–28). Indeed, these three types of amyloid lesions define the Lewy body variant of Alzheimer's disease, the most common pathological subtype of this widespread dementia disorder. Because each of these three lesions is composed of filamentous aggregates of distinctly different misfolded proteins, the Lewy body variant of Alzheimer's disease is a triple amyloidosis. Specifically, amyloid plaques are comprised of fibrils formed by 39–42 amino acid long Aβ peptides, tangles are comprised of fibrils of hyperphosphorylated tau protein, and Lewy bodies are comprised of filamentous α-synuclein.

Other triple brain amyloidoses that can display Aβ, tau, and α-synuclein pathology include Down's syndrome (29) and Guam Parkinson's dementia complex (30). Examples of double amyloidoses (two forms of brain amyloid) include the majority of Alzheimer's disease patients (Aβ and tau), certain Parkinson's disease patients (e.g., patients of the Contursi kindred, who show both abundant tau and α-synuclein pathology) (31), and subsets of patients with Niemann-Pick type C disease (some have tau and Aβ pathology, whereas others have tau and α-synuclein pathology) (32, 33). Notably, Aβ pathology is accompanied by other forms of amyloidosis in all neurodegenerative dementias, but pure Aβ amyloidosis is seen in cerebral amyloid angiopathy, which manifests clinically as a stroke syndrome.

The Role of Aβ Pathology in Alzheimer's Disease

Amyloid plaques are not only a histopathological hallmark of Alzheimer's disease, but the aggregated Aβ of which they are composed likely plays a key role in the pathogenesis of Alzheimer's disease (summarized by the amyloid cascade hypothesis) (34). The most direct evidence supporting this hypothesis stems from studies of gene mutations that cause autosomal-dominant inherited forms of Alzheimer's disease. As illustrated in **Figure 2**, most but not all of these mutations lead to increased production and accumulation of specific Aβ species (Aβ42), either through effects on the amyloid precursor protein (APP) itself (35) or through effects on presenilin 1 or 2 (36), which form part of γ-secretase, one of the proteolytic complexes that cleaves APP to generate Aβ (37). Aggregated amyloid (in the form of oligomers, protofibrils, or fibrils) is toxic to neurons in most but not all culture conditions (38, 39), and in primary neuronal culture and mouse models, Aβ may act synergistically with neurofibrillary tangle pathology (40, 41). These observations have led to the hypothesis that increased production, aggregation, and accumulation of Aβ initiates a cascade of events leading to neurotoxicity and eventually to clinical symptoms of Alzheimer's disease (34), as summarized in **Figure 3**. Autopsy studies of patients with genetic forms of Alzheimer's disease, Down's syndrome, or mild cognitive impairment (which appears to be a prodromal phase of Alzheimer's disease) have shown that accumulation of Aβ may precede clinical development of Alzheimer's disease by as many as 10 years (42–45); importantly, the increased presence of Aβ correlates well with cognitive decline early in the course of the disease (46).

Thus, Aβ pathology (*a*) is required for the diagnosis of Alzheimer's disease, (*b*) plays a key role in the pathogenesis of Alzheimer's

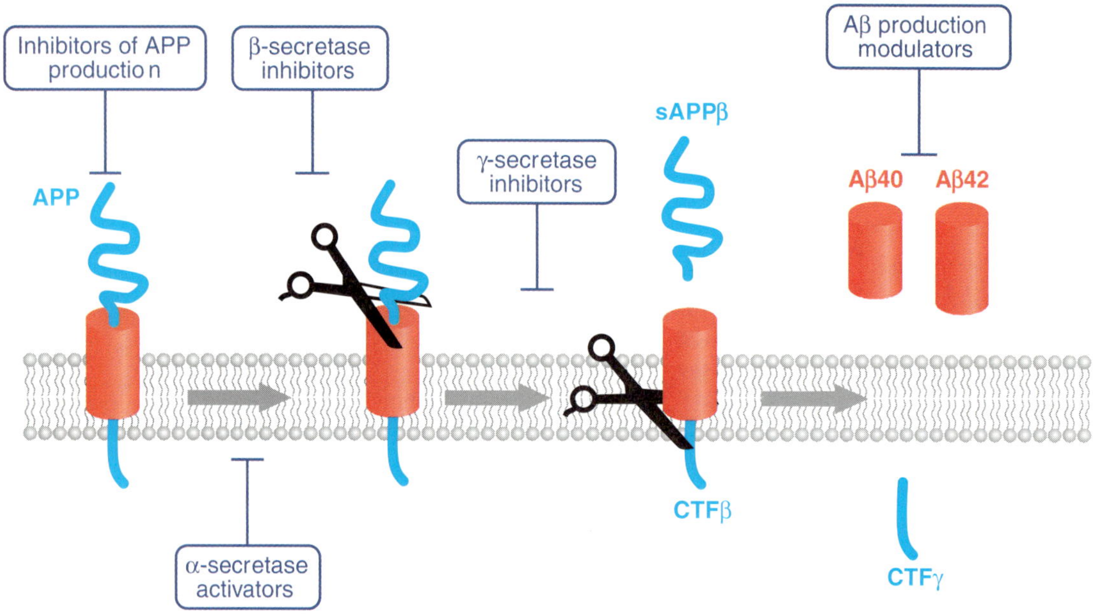

Figure 2

Aβ production. The integral membrane protein amyloid precursor protein (APP) is cleaved by the beta-site APP-cleaving enzyme (BACE, or β-secretase) to yield a secreted fragment of APP (sAPPβ) and a C-terminal fragment of APP (CTFβ). CTFβ is then cleaved by γ-secretase within the membrane to yield a smaller C-terminal fragment (CTFγ) and Aβ fragments of various lengths (*shown in red*). An alternate cleavage by α-secretase (not shown) cuts within the Aβ domain and thus precludes Aβ production. Potential opportunities for therapeutic intervention are shown in the blue boxes.

disease, and (*c*) develops prior to symptomatic manifestations of Alzheimer's disease. For these reasons, there has been great interest in developing therapies and diagnostic tools aimed at Aβ. Of the 66 drugs that are known currently to be in clinical trials for Alzheimer's disease, more than 40% target amyloid plaques or Aβ production.

Potential Therapeutic Interventions Suggested by Current Understanding of Aβ Amyloidosis

β-secretase inhibitors. The proteases that cleave APP to generate Aβ (**Figure 2**) provide some of the most alluring targets for drug development (47). The β-secretase protein referred to as beta-site APP-cleaving enzyme (BACE) may be a particularly good drug target because (*a*) knock-out of BACE in mice eliminates Aβ production without side effects (48), (*b*) BACE belongs to a well-studied class of proteases (aspartic proteases) for which inhibitors have been developed successfully for human use (i.e., renin and HIV protease inhibitors) (49), (*c*) the X-ray crystal structure of BACE has been published (50), and (*d*) peptidomimetic inhibitors of BACE with nanomolar activity have been generated (51). However, the development of small-molecule BACE inhibitors is complicated by the fact that the active-site cleft of the enzyme is larger and more open than other aspartic proteases (50).

γ-secretase inhibitors. The APP γ-secretase has been an active target for drug development, with multiple classes of potent inhibitors described (52–54). At the 2004 International Conference on Alzheimer's Disease and Related Disorders, investigators

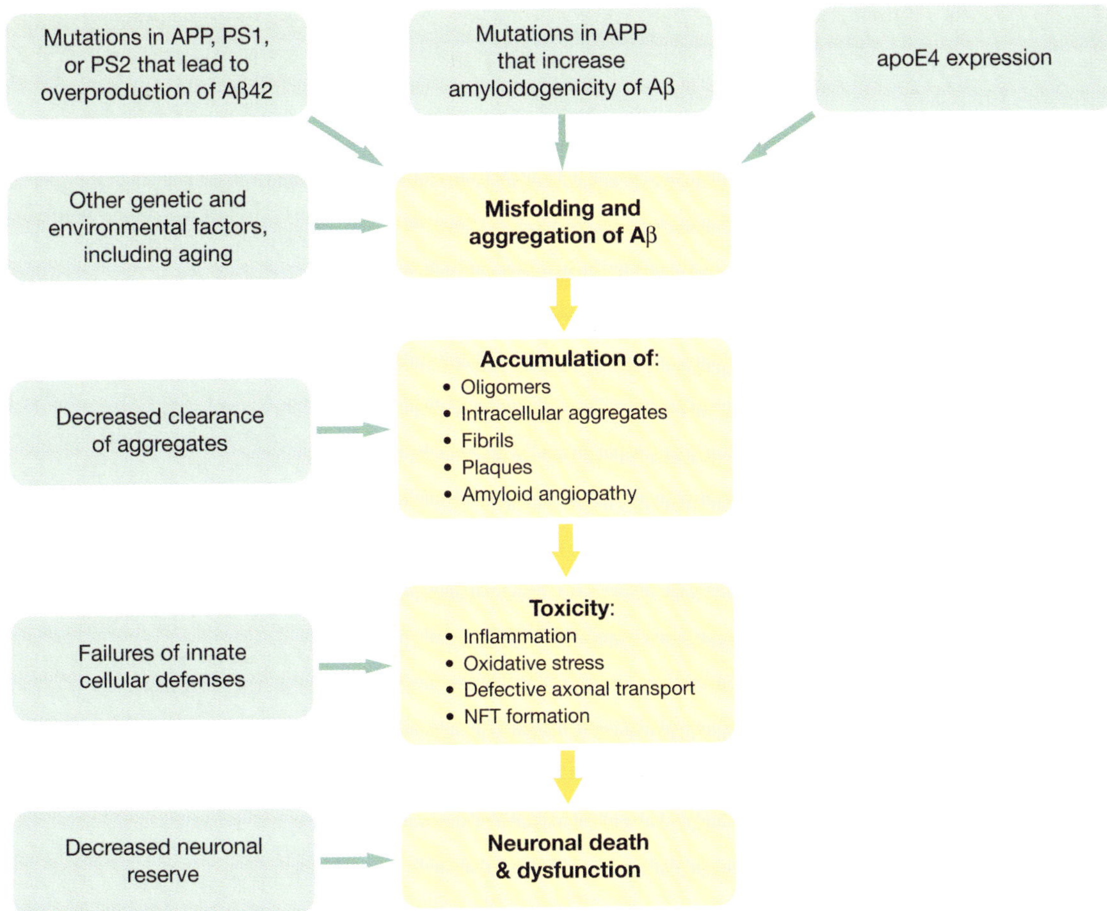

Figure 3

Amyloid cascade hypothesis. Increased aggregation of Aβ can occur as a result of (*a*) overproduction of Aβ42 [as in the case of most amyloid precursor protein (APP), presenilin 1 (PS1), and presenilin 2 (PS2) gene mutations], (*b*) expression of mutations in the Aβ domain of APP that increases its propensity for aggregation, (*c*) Apolipoprotein E4 (apoE4) expression, and (*d*) other genetic and environmental factors, including aging. Aggregated Aβ accumulates in various forms and locations, some or all of which may result in cellular toxicities mediated by a variety of mechanisms. Decreased clearance of aggregates and failures of cellular defenses to toxicity may exacerbate this process. The toxic effects of amyloid result eventually in neuronal death and dysfunction, manifesting as dementia. Patients with decreased neuronal reserve (perhaps as a result of existing comorbidities) may show increased sensitivity to neuronal loss. NFT, neurofibrillary tangles.

from Eli Lilly reported Phase I data with a γ-secretase inhibitor (LY450139), which reduced blood levels of Aβ, but did not alter levels of Aβ in cerebral spinal fluid (CSF). However, enthusiasm for the use of γ-secretase inhibitors is tempered by concerns regarding toxicity caused by interference with γ-secretase-mediated Notch signaling (55) or inhibition of signaling by other γ-secretase-cleaved substrates (56). Alternatively, indirect inhibition of γ-secretase may be one way to avoid this issue. For example, inhibitors of glycogen synthase kinase 3 (GSK3), such as lithium and kenpaullones as well as small interfering RNAs directed against GSK3α, reduce Aβ production in cells and transgenic mice by inhibiting γ-secretase cleavage, without altering Notch cleavage (57).

Aβ vaccination. Aβ vaccination has proven to be one of the most exciting and novel strategies for removing amyloid plaques from the brain (reviewed in Reference 58). Immunization of transgenic mice with Aβ peptides (active immunization) or with monoclonal antibodies directed against Aβ (passive immunization) results in dramatic clearance of plaques (59, 60). Immunization also results in improved cognitive performance in several different transgenic mouse models of Alzheimer's disease (61, 62). Various mechanisms for immunization have been hypothesized, including antibody-mediated microglial clearance of plaques, clearance of brain Aβ oligomers, and peripheral clearance of soluble Aβ. A combination of mechanisms may be required for maximal effect of immunization. Human studies of active Aβ immunization were halted because of cases of meningoencephalitis in treated patients (63, 64). However, active and passive immunization strategies that decrease the risk of this serious side effect are currently under preclinical and clinical development (58). Provocatively, preliminary analysis of the Phase II data from the first vaccination study suggested that patients who generated antiplaque antibodies showed a slower rate of cognitive decline (65).

NSAIDS. Several nonsteroidal anti-inflammatory drugs (NSAIDs) selectively lower Aβ42 through a mechanism independent of cyclooxygenase but likely involves the modulation of γ-secretase (66, 67). Indeed, preclinical studies on R-flurbiprofen, the pure R enantiomer of the NSAID flurbiprofen, show that it does not inhibit cyclooxygenase enzymes, but it does reduce Aβ42 levels in vitro and in vivo, and it also reduces Aβ amyloid pathology in the brain (68). Not surprisingly, this compound recently entered Phase III trials for Alzheimer's disease (Myriad genetics). The approach using NSAIDs and related compounds for treatment of Alzheimer's disease is bolstered by epidemiological evidence linking NSAID use to decreased risk of the disease (69).

Statins. Epidemiological studies suggest that high levels of cholesterol may contribute to the pathogenesis of Alzheimer's disease (70; reviewed in Reference 71). Retrospective studies indicate that the cholesterol-lowering drugs or statins can protect against Alzheimer's disease, in some cases reducing the relative risk of Alzheimer's by more than 70% (72, 73). These data prompted prospective studies of statins in Alzheimer's disease. Preliminary data from one such study has shown a reduction of Aβ40 in the CSF and slight improvement in cognitive function (74) with simvastatin treatment. However, results from a larger-scale trial of a different design (named Prospective Study of Pravastatin in the Elderly at Risk, PROSPER) have not shown similar improvements (75). The mechanisms by which statins affect brain Aβ deposition remains an area of active investigation (71). Nonetheless, there is growing evidence that high cholesterol levels increase Aβ generation and plaque deposition (76, 77), and these effects appear to be offset or reversed by statins (78–80).

Clioquinol. The metal-protein-attenuating compound (MPAC) clioquinol (iodochlorhydroxyquin) dissociates amyloid plaques in postmortem human brain samples by a mechanism that may involve chelating Cu^{2+} and Zn^{2+} (81). Strikingly, clioquinol decreases brain Aβ deposition in a transgenic mouse model of Alzheimer's disease (82), and preliminary data from a Phase II study of clioquinol in Alzheimer's patients has shown decreased plasma Aβ42 levels as well as slowed cognitive deterioration in clioquinol-treated patients (83).

Glycosaminoglycans mimetics. Another strategy to prevent the formation of Aβ fibrils in Alzheimer's disease capitalized on the role of glycosaminoglycans (GAGs) in amyloid formation (reviewed in Reference 84). Small-molecule GAG mimetics compete with binding of GAGs to amyloid fibrils and thus prevent fibril formation. Encouragingly, the biotechnology company Neurochem reports that one such GAG mimetic is currently in Phase III clinical trials for Alzheimer's disease (reviewed in Reference 85).

TAU: A PROTOYPICAL INTRACELLULAR AMYLOID

Tauopathies

Tau pathology is not only a prominent feature of Alzheimer's disease, but it is also seen in a variety of other related neurodegenerative diseases. Indeed, Pick's disease, corticobasal degeneration (CBD), PSP, and frontal temporal dementia with parkinsonism linked to chromosome 17 (FTDP-17) are all defined by specific regional and cellular distributions of abnormally aggregated tau filaments. There is now unequivocal evidence demonstrating that abnormalities in tau are sufficient to cause neurodegenerative disease. These abonormalities include (*a*) the presence of causative mutations in the gene for tau in patients with FTDP-17 (86, 87), (*b*) the linkage of specific tau haplotypes to PSP and CBD (88), (*c*) the absence of other disease-specific neuropathological abnormalities in many tauopathies, and (*d*) the generation of tau transgenic mice that recapitulate the key phenotypic hallmarks of authentic human neurodegenerative tauopathies (89).

Although tau dysfunction alone is sufficient to induce neurodegeneration in the absence of other brain amyloids, the frequency with which tau pathology occurs in a wide variety of other neurodegenerative diseases has led to the hypothesis that tau plays a role in a final, common pathway leading to neuronal death or dysfunction, which can be activated by other initiating events. In transgenic mice expressing tau, coexpression of APP or α-synuclein results in the acceleration of tau pathology, which suggests that neurodegeneration mediated by tau pathology may also be activated downstream of disease pathways resulting from accumulations of both Aβ and α-synuclein amyloidogenesis. This fits well with observations from human disease that patients with APP mutations show abundant Aβ and tau pathology, but patients with tau mutations show primarily tau pathology alone.

Mechanisms of Tau-Induced Pathogenesis

Tau is a microtubule-associated protein that binds to and stabilizes microtubules. There are now more than 30 distinct mutations or pathogenic nucleotide substitutions in the gene for tau that have been shown to cause FTDP-17 in more than 50 different kindreds (reviewed in Reference 90), representative examples of which are shown in **Figure 4**. These mutations may lead to neurodegenerative disease by one or more distinct mechanisms: (*a*) alterations in tau splicing, leading to abnormal patterns of tau-isoform expression (91), (*b*) compromise of tau's ability to bind to and stabilize microtubules (92, 93), and (*c*) enhanced fibrillization of tau (94). Thus, as illustrated in **Figure 5**, tau mutations, and by analogy tau dysfunction in sporadic disease, may be pathogenic through mechanisms involving both loss of function (decreased microtubule stabilization) and toxic gain of function (increased fibril formation). Reflecting this fundamental dichotomy, therapies targeted at both mechanisms are currently in development.

Potential Therapeutic Interventions Suggested by Current Understanding of Tau Amyloidosis

Microtubule-stabilizing drugs. Because tauopathies may be caused in part by the failure of tau to appropriately stabilize microtubules, microtubule-stabilizing drugs may be therapeutically beneficial for these diseases (95). Transgenic mice that overexpress tau

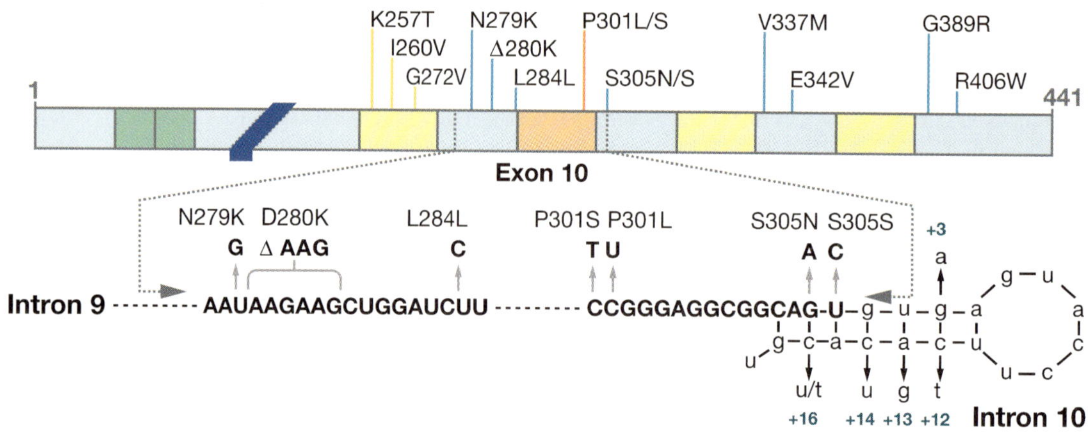

Mutations that impair tau protein function

G272V
Δ280K
P301S
G389R
R406W
P301L
V337M

Mutations that promote tau aggregation

G272V
P301S
P301L
V337M

Mutations that alter exon-10 splicing

N279K
Δ280K
S305N
L284L
S305S
Intron-10 mutations

Figure 4

Tau mutations cause frontal temporal dementia with parkinsonism linked to chromosome 17 (FTDP-17) by different mechanisms. Tau mutations may lead to neurodegenerative disease by impairing tau's ability to bind to and stabilize microtubules, promoting tau aggregation, and altering exon-10 splicing.

accumulate filamentous tau inclusions and show reductions in microtubules and impaired fast axonal transport, in addition to neurodegeneration and motor weakness (96). When these mice are treated with the microtubule-stabilizing drug paclitaxel they show improvements in microtubule numbers and fast axonal transport, accompanied by improved motor abilities, thus providing in vivo evidence that microtubule-stabilizing drugs may have a therapeutic benefit for human tauopathies (97).

Inhibitors of tau filament and tau phosphorylation. There has been a growing emphasis on designing inhibitors of tau filament formation in an attempt to generate drugs that ameliorate tau pathology in neurodegenerative diseases. Rational-design approaches and screening of small-molecule libraries have revealed a number of different classes of inhibitors (98–101), although in vivo data are not yet available. Similarly, inhibition of tau phosphorylation has presented a tempting target for drug design, with most efforts focused on inhibiting GSK3β (reviewed in Reference 102). However difficulties generating inhibitors with appropriate specificity for GSK3β as well as issues with target-mediated toxicity complicate this approach.

α-SYNUCLEIN: THE INTRACELLULAR AMYLOID OF PARKINSON'S DISEASE

Parkinson's Disease and Other α-Synucleinopathies

Although the molecular identities of the amyloidogenic proteins that define Alzheimer's disease and tauopathies were discovered by biochemical methods, the molecular identity

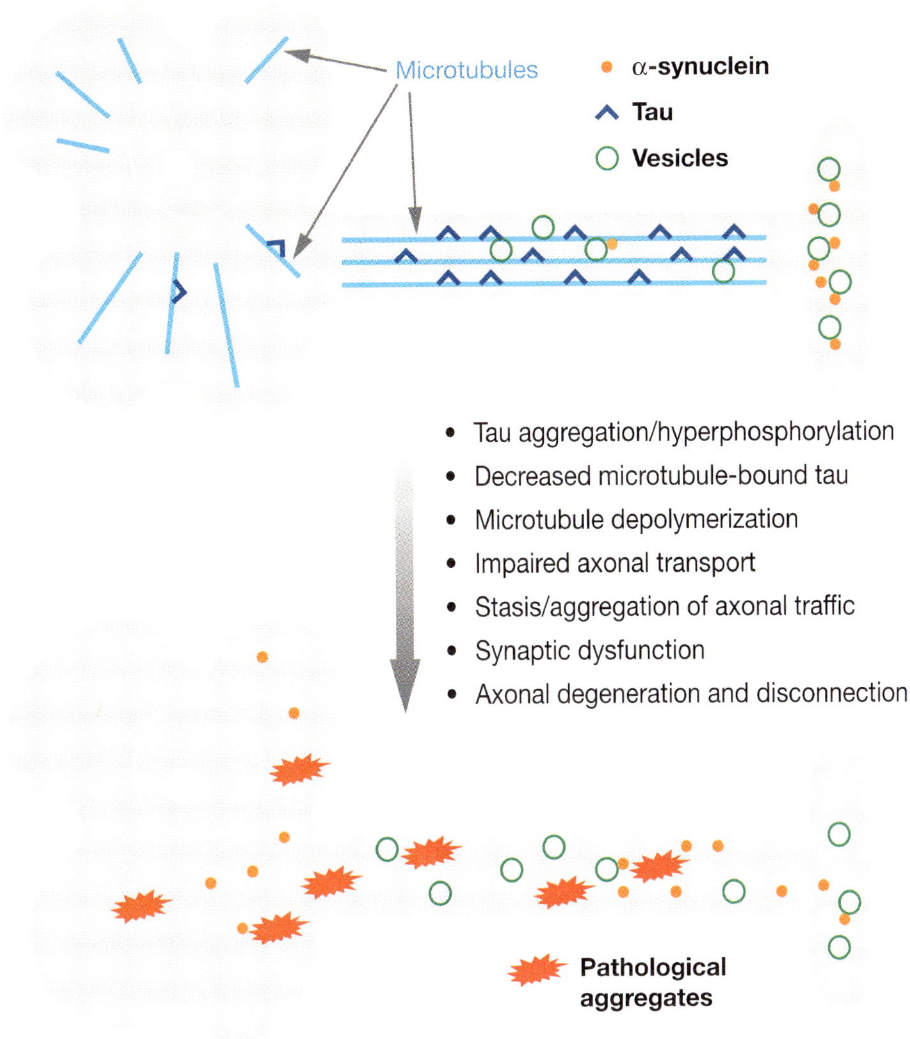

Figure 5

Deleterious effects of tau amyloidosis. Tau hyperphosphorylation and aggregation may lead to neuronal dysfunction through a variety of mechanisms, including microtubule depolymerization. This in turn may lead to impaired axonal transport, causing synaptic dysfunction and eventually axonal degeneration.

of the amyloidogenic protein in Parkinson's disease was first suggested by genetic studies. The discovery that familial forms of Parkinson's disease may be caused by mutations in the gene for α-synuclein (103) provided the rationale for studies demonstrating that the Lewy bodies that define Parkinson's disease are composed of filamentous aggregates of α-synuclein (104). Similar studies have demonstrated extensive α-synuclein pathology in dementia with Lewy bodies, multiple system atrophy, and other seemingly distinct disorders that, because they are characterized by inclusions formed by the same protein, are now classified together as α-synculeinopathies (105–107).

Mechanisms of α-Synuclein-Induced Pathogenesis

Because mutations or duplications in the gene for α-synuclein lead to genetic forms of autosomal-dominantly inherited Parkinson's disease and dementia with Lewy bodies (103, 108), it has been hypothesized that increased expression, aggregation, and accumulation of α-synuclein in the brain plays a key role in the pathogenesis of neurodegeneration (reviewed in Reference 109). Further support for the role of α-synuclein in disease has come from transgenic mice engineered to overexpress mutant forms of α-synuclein, which show both α-synuclein pathology and neurodegeneration (110–112). Importantly, in human disease, deposition of brain α-synuclein may precede disease symptoms by more than a decade, providing a window for therapeutic intervention (113, 114).

Environmental factors may also play a crucial role in the pathogenesis of synucleinopathies, and epidemiological studies suggest an association between Parkinson's disease and environmental toxins such as pesticides (115). Chronic systemic treatment of rats with rotenone, a pesticide known to inhibit mitochondria, causes selective nigrostriatal dopaminergic degeneration with associated inclusions containing fibrillar α-synuclein (116). Rotenone treatment may induce an increase in oxidative stress in the dopaminergic neurons, which in turn may facilitate fibrillization of α-synuclein, providing a link between oxidative stress and pathogenesis of synucleionopathies (117–119).

Potential Therapeutic Interventions Suggested by Current Understanding of α-Synuclein Amyloidosis

Inhibition of aggregation. Inhibition of α-synuclein aggregation is an attractive target for drug development, and several groups have identified small-molecule and peptide-based inhibitors of aggregation (120–124). A number of catecholamines, including dopamine, have been found to inhibit synuclein fibril formation (124). The inhibitory activity of dopamine depends on its oxidation and leads to accumulation of α-synuclein protofibrils (124). The link between dopamine and α-synuclein may provide insights into the potential mechanisms underlying the selective vulnerability of dopaminergic neurons in Parkinson's disease, although many other types of neurons as well as glial cells are selectively affected by accumulations of α-synuclein inclusions.

Induction of chaperones. A complementary approach to inhibiting α-synuclein-induced toxicity has been suggested by *Drosophila* studies, which show that expression of the molecular chaperone Hsp70 prevents the dopaminergic neuron loss associated with α-synuclein expression and that interference with endogenous chaperone activity accelerates α-synuclein toxicity (125). Treatment of *Drosophila* flies with the drug geldanamycin protects neurons against α-synuclein toxicity, likely through enhanced chaperone activation (125–127).

SUMMARY

Neurodegenerative diseases have long been defined by the properties of the neuropathological lesions observed in the brain. We now know that these lesions are not just markers for neurodegenerative diseases, but are tied intrinsically to their pathogenesis. Moreover, the striking similarities between many neurodegenerative diseases suggest common mechanisms in the etiology of these disorders. The repeated theme of protein misfolding leading to amyloid formation and neurotoxicity is reinforced by a striking message from genetic studies: In each case of dominantly inherited neurodegeneration, the disease-causing mutations can be linked directly to amyloid formation. These clues have now come into sharp focus and neurodegenerative properties are better understood, and they have provided a strong rationale for the in vitro experiments, mouse models, and epidemiological studies that have gone a long way towards verifying this hypothesis. These experiments have laid a solid groundwork for a number of potential therapeutics that are now in preclinical and clinical development. Over the next five years the efficacy of a large number of these drugs will be tested, and there is a growing optimism that the results of these trials will confirm current notions of the etiology of neurodegenerative diseases.

SUMMARY POINTS

1. Most neurodegenerative diseases are characterized by pathological lesions composed of accumulations of amyloid.
2. Mutations that cause familial forms of these diseases are linked to accumulation of the amyloid, and mouse models that recapitulate features of these diseases can be generated by engineering amyloid accumulation in the brain.
3. In different diseases the amyloid is composed of different protein constituents, but in each case there are likely to be quite similar pathways of misfolding, oligomerization, and fibril formation.
4. Each step in these pathways may provide targets for therapeutic drug development.

FUTURE DIRECTIONS/UNRESOLVED ISSUES

1. What causes amyloid deposition in sporadic (nonfamilial) cases of neurodegenerative disease?
2. Why does amyloid take decades to accumulate and become symptomatic?
3. Which intermediates along the pathway from misfolded protein to amyloid fibrils are the toxic species?
4. What are the mechanisms underlying the toxicity of these species?
5. What accounts for the striking selective vulnerability of different brain regions to amyloid and its effects?
6. Why is the brain so prone to amyloidosis?

ACKNOWLEDGMENTS

During the writing of this review, the authors were supported by grants from the National Institute on Aging and the National Institute of Neurological Disorders and Stroke of the National Institutes of Health (grant numbers AG-09215; AG-10124; AG-14382; AG-17586; AG-17628; and NS-44233), the Marian S. Ware Alzheimer Drug Discovery Program, and the Picower Foundation. V.M.Y.L. is the John H. Ware 3rd Professor for Alzheimer's Disease Research and J.Q.T. is the William Maul Measey-Truman G. Schnabel Jr. M.D. Professor of Geriatric Medicine and Gerontology.

LITERATURE CITED

1. Hebert LE, Beckett LA, Scherr PA, Evans DA. 2001. Annual incidence of Alzheimer disease in the United States projected to the years 2000 through 2050. *Alzheimer Dis. Assoc. Disord.* 15:169–73
2. Hebert LE, Scherr PA, Bienias JL, Bennett DA, Evans DA. 2003. Alzheimer disease in the US population: prevalence estimates using the 2000 census. *Arch. Neurol.* 60:1119–22

3. Brookmeyer R, Gray S, Kawas C. 1998. Projections of Alzheimer's disease in the United States and the public health impact of delaying disease onset. *Am. J. Public Health* 88:1337–42
4. Samii A, Nutt JG, Ransom BR. 2004. Parkinson's disease. *Lancet* 363:1783–93
5. Ernst RL, Hay JW, Fenn C, Tinklenberg J, Yesavage JA. 1997. Cognitive function and the costs of Alzheimer disease. An exploratory study. *Arch. Neurol.* 54:687–93
6. Forman MS, Trojanowski JQ, Lee VM. 2004. Neurodegenerative diseases: a decade of discoveries paves the way for therapeutic breakthroughs. *Nat. Med.* 10:1055–63
7. Caughey B, Lansbury PT. 2003. Protofibrils, pores, fibrils, and neurodegeneration: separating the responsible protein aggregates from the innocent bystanders. *Annu. Rev. Neurosci.* 26:267–98
8. Huang TH, Yang DS, Plaskos NP, Go S, Yip CM, et al. 2000. Structural studies of soluble oligomers of the Alzheimer beta-amyloid peptide. *J. Mol. Biol.* 297:73–87
9. Walsh DM, Tseng BP, Rydel RE, Podlisny MB, Selkoe DJ. 2000. The oligomerization of amyloid beta-protein begins intracellularly in cells derived from human brain. *Biochemistry* 39:10831–39
10. Podlisny MB, Walsh DM, Amarante P, Ostaszewski BL, Stimson ER, et al. 1998. Oligomerization of endogenous and synthetic amyloid beta-protein at nanomolar levels in cell culture and stabilization of monomer by Congo red. *Biochemistry* 37:3602–11
11. Takahashi RH, Almeida CG, Kearney PF, Yu F, Lin MT, et al. 2004. Oligomerization of Alzheimer's beta-amyloid within processes and synapses of cultured neurons and brain. *J. Neurosci.* 24:3592–99
12. Kayed R, Head E, Thompson JL, McIntire TM, Milton SC, et al. 2003. Common structure of soluble amyloid oligomers implies common mechanism of pathogenesis. *Science* 300:486–89
13. Giasson BI, Forman MS, Higuchi M, Golbe LI, Graves CL, et al. 2003. Initiation and synergistic fibrillization of tau and alpha-synuclein. *Science* 300:636–40
14. Stokin GB, Lillo C, Falzone TL, Brusch RG, Rockenstein E, et al. 2005. Axonopathy and transport deficits early in the pathogenesis of Alzheimer's disease. *Science* 307:1282–88
15. Hiruma H, Katakura T, Takahashi S, Ichikawa T, Kawakami T. 2003. Glutamate and amyloid beta-protein rapidly inhibit fast axonal transport in cultured rat hippocampal neurons by different mechanisms. *J. Neurosci.* 23:8967–77
16. Roy S, Zhang B, Lee VM, Trojanowski JQ. 2005. Axonal transport defects: a common theme in neurodegenerative diseases. *Acta Neuropathol.* 109:5–13
17. Morfini G, Pigino G, Brady ST. 2005. Polyglutamine expansion diseases: failing to deliver. *Trends Mol. Med.* 11:64–70
18. Stefanis L, Larsen KE, Rideout HJ, Sulzer D, Greene LA. 2001. Expression of A53T mutant but not wild-type alpha-synuclein in PC12 cells induces alterations of the ubiquitin-dependent degradation system, loss of dopamine release, and autophagic cell death. *J. Neurosci.* 21:9549–60
19. Tanaka Y, Engelender S, Igarashi S, Rao RK, Wanner T, et al. 2001. Inducible expression of mutant alpha-synuclein decreases proteasome activity and increases sensitivity to mitochondria-dependent apoptosis. *Hum. Mol. Genet.* 10:919–26
20. Steffan JS, Bodai L, Pallos J, Poelman M, McCampbell A, et al. 2001. Histone deacetylase inhibitors arrest polyglutamine-dependent neurodegeneration in Drosophila. *Nature* 413:739–43
21. Behl C, Davis JB, Lesley R, Schubert D. 1994. Hydrogen peroxide mediates amyloid beta protein toxicity. *Cell* 77:817–27

22. Stefanova N, Reindl M, Neumann M, Haass C, Poewe W, et al. 2005. Oxidative stress in transgenic mice with oligodendroglial {alpha}-synuclein overexpression replicates the characteristic neuropathology of multiple system atrophy. *Am. J. Pathol.* 166:869–76
23. Nakagawa T, Zhu H, Morishima N, Li E, Xu J, et al. 2000. Caspase-12 mediates endoplasmic-reticulum-specific apoptosis and cytotoxicity by amyloid-beta. *Nature* 403:98–103
24. Xu J, Kao SY, Lee FJ, Song W, Jin LW, Yankner BA. 2002. Dopamine-dependent neurotoxicity of alpha-synuclein: a mechanism for selective neurodegeneration in Parkinson disease. *Nat. Med.* 8:600–6
25. Brown DF, Risser RC, Bigio EH, Tripp P, Stiegler A, et al. 1998. Neocortical synapse density and Braak stage in the Lewy body variant of Alzheimer disease: a comparison with classic Alzheimer disease and normal aging. *J. Neuropathol. Exp. Neurol.* 57:955–60
26. Brown DF, Dababo MA, Bigio EH, Risser RC, Eagan KP, et al. 1998. Neuropathologic evidence that the Lewy body variant of Alzheimer disease represents coexistence of Alzheimer disease and idiopathic Parkinson disease. *J. Neuropathol. Exp. Neurol.* 57:39–46
27. Lippa CF, Fujiwara H, Mann DM, Giasson B, Baba M, et al. 1998. Lewy bodies contain altered alpha-synuclein in brains of many familial Alzheimer's disease patients with mutations in presenilin and amyloid precursor protein genes. *Am. J. Pathol.* 153:1365–70
28. Hamilton RL. 2000. Lewy bodies in Alzheimer's disease: a neuropathological review of 145 cases using alpha-synuclein immunohistochemistry. *Brain Pathol.* 10:378–84
29. Lippa CF, Schmidt ML, Lee VM, Trojanowski JQ. 1999. Antibodies to alpha-synuclein detect Lewy bodies in many Down's syndrome brains with Alzheimer's disease. *Ann. Neurol.* 45:353–57
30. Sebeo J, Hof PR, Perl DP. 2004. Occurrence of alpha-synuclein pathology in the cerebellum of Guamanian patients with parkinsonism-dementia complex. *Acta Neuropathol.* 107:497–503
31. Duda JE, Giasson BI, Mabon ME, Miller DC, Golbe LI, et al. 2002. Concurrence of alpha-synuclein and tau brain pathology in the Contursi kindred. *Acta Neuropathol.* 104:7–11
32. Saito Y, Suzuki K, Hulette CM, Murayama S. 2004. Aberrant phosphorylation of alpha-synuclein in human Niemann-Pick type C1 disease. *J. Neuropathol. Exp. Neurol.* 63:323–28
33. Saito Y, Suzuki K, Nanba E, Yamamoto T, Ohno K, Murayama S. 2002. Niemann-Pick type C disease: accelerated neurofibrillary tangle formation and amyloid beta deposition associated with apolipoprotein E epsilon 4 homozygosity. *Ann. Neurol.* 52:351–55
34. Hardy J, Selkoe DJ. 2002. The amyloid hypothesis of Alzheimer's disease: progress and problems on the road to therapeutics. *Science* 297:353–56
35. Goate A, Chartier-Harlin MC, Mullan M, Brown J, Crawford F, et al. 1991. Segregation of a missense mutation in the amyloid precursor protein gene with familial Alzheimer's disease. *Nature* 349:704–6
36. Scheuner D, Eckman C, Jensen M, Song X, Citron M, et al. 1996. Secreted amyloid beta-protein similar to that in the senile plaques of Alzheimer's disease is increased in vivo by the presenilin 1 and 2 and APP mutations linked to familial Alzheimer's disease. *Nat. Med.* 2:864–70
37. Wolfe MS, Xia W, Moore CL, Leatherwood DD, Ostaszewski B, et al. 1999. Peptidomimetic probes and molecular modeling suggest that Alzheimer's gamma-secretase is an intramembrane-cleaving aspartyl protease. *Biochemistry* 38:4720–27
38. Yankner BA. 1996. Mechanisms of neuronal degeneration in Alzheimer's disease. *Neuron* 16:921–32

39. Kayed R, Head E, Thompson JL, McIntire TM, Milton SC, et al. 2003. Common structure of soluble amyloid oligomers implies common mechanism of pathogenesis. *Science* 300:486–89
40. Rapoport M, Dawson HN, Binder LI, Vitek MP, Ferreira A. 2002. Tau is essential to beta-amyloid-induced neurotoxicity. *Proc. Natl. Acad. Sci. USA* 99:6364–69
41. Lewis J, Dickson DW, Lin WL, Chisholm L, Corral A, et al. 2001. Enhanced neurofibrillary degeneration in transgenic mice expressing mutant tau and APP. *Science* 293:1487–91
42. Mann DM, Brown A, Prinja D, Davies CA, Landon M, et al. 1989. An analysis of the morphology of senile plaques in Down's syndrome patients of different ages using immunocytochemical and lectin histochemical techniques. *Neuropathol. Appl. Neurobiol.* 15: 317–29
43. Lemere CA, Lopera F, Kosik KS, Lendon CL, Ossa J, et al. 1996. The E280A presenilin 1 Alzheimer mutation produces increased A beta 42 deposition and severe cerebellar pathology. *Nat. Med.* 2:1146–50
44. Smith MJ, Kwok JB, McLean CA, Kril JJ, Broe GA, et al. 2001. Variable phenotype of Alzheimer's disease with spastic paraparesis. *Ann. Neurol.* 49:125–29
45. Morris JC, Storandt M, McKeel DW Jr, Rubin EH, Price JL, et al. 1996. Cerebral amyloid deposition and diffuse plaques in "normal" aging: Evidence for presymptomatic and very mild Alzheimer's disease. *Neurology* 46:707–19
46. Naslund J, Haroutunian V, Mohs R, Davis KL, Davies P, et al. 2000. Correlation between elevated levels of amyloid beta-peptide in the brain and cognitive decline. *JAMA* 283:1571–77
47. Golde TE. 2003. Alzheimer disease therapy: can the amyloid cascade be halted? *J. Clin. Invest.* 111:11–18
48. Roberds SL, Anderson J, Basi G, Bienkowski MJ, Branstetter DG, et al. 2001. BACE knockout mice are healthy despite lacking the primary beta-secretase activity in brain: implications for Alzheimer's disease therapeutics. *Hum. Mol. Genet.* 10:1317–24
49. Gruninger-Leitch F, Schlatter D, Kung E, Nelbock P, Dobeli H. 2002. Substrate and inhibitor profile of BACE (beta-secretase) and comparison with other mammalian aspartic proteases. *J. Biol. Chem.* 277:4687–93
50. Hong L, Koelsch G, Lin X, Wu S, Terzyan S, et al. 2000. Structure of the protease domain of memapsin 2 (beta-secretase) complexed with inhibitor. *Science* 290:150–53
51. Sinha S, Anderson JP, Barbour R, Basi GS, Caccavello R, et al. 1999. Purification and cloning of amyloid precursor protein beta-secretase from human brain. *Nature* 402:537–40
52. Li Y-M, Xu M, Lai M-T, Huang Q, Castro JL, et al. 2000. Photoactivated gamma-secretase inhibitors directed to the active site covalently label presenilin 1. *Nature* 405:689–94
53. Wolfe MS, Esler WP, Das C. 2002. Continuing strategies for inhibiting Alzheimer's gamma-secretase. *J. Mol. Neurosci.* 19:83–87
54. Esler WP, Kimberly WT, Ostaszewski BL, Diehl TS, Moore CL, et al. 2000. Transition-state analogue inhibitors of gamma-secretase bind directly to presenilin-1. *Nat. Cell Biol.* 2:428–34
55. De Strooper B, Annaert W, Cupers P, Saftig P, Craessaerts K, et al. 1999. A presenilin-1-dependent gamma-secretase-like protease mediates release of Notch intracellular domain. *Nature* 398:518–22
56. Ni C-Y, Murphy MP, Golde TE, Carpenter G. 2001. gamma-Secretase cleavage and nuclear localization of ErbB-4 receptor tyrosine kinase. *Science* 294:2179–81

57. Phiel CJ, Wilson CA, Lee VMY, Klein PS. 2003. GSK-3alpha regulates production of Alzheimer's disease amyloid-beta peptides. *Nature* 423:435–39
58. Schenk D. 2004. Hopes remain for an Alzheimer's vaccine. *Nature* 431:398
59. Schenk D, Barbour R, Dunn W, Gordon G, Grajeda H, et al. 1999. Immunization with amyloid-beta attenuates Alzheimer-disease-like pathology in the PDAPP mouse. *Nature* 400:173–77
60. Bard F, Cannon C, Barbour R, Burke RL, Games D, et al. 2000. Peripherally administered antibodies against amyloid beta-peptide enter the central nervous system and reduce pathology in a mouse model of Alzheimer disease. *Nat. Med.* 6:916–19
61. Janus C, Pearson J, McLaurin J, Mathews PM, Jiang Y, et al. 2000. A beta peptide immunization reduces behavioural impairment and plaques in a model of Alzheimer's disease. *Nature* 408:979–82
62. Morgan D, Diamond DM, Gottschall PE, Ugen KE, Dickey C, et al. 2000. A beta peptide vaccination prevents memory loss in an animal model of Alzheimer's disease. *Nature* 408:982–85
63. Nicoll JA, Wilkinson D, Holmes C, Steart P, Markham H, Weller RO. 2003. Neuropathology of human Alzheimer disease after immunization with amyloid-beta peptide: a case report. *Nat. Med.* 9:448–52
64. Orgogozo JM, Gilman S, Dartigues JF, Laurent B, Puel M, et al. 2003. Subacute meningoencephalitis in a subset of patients with AD after Abeta42 immunization. *Neurology* 61:46–54
65. Hock C, Konietzko U, Streffer JR, Tracy J, Signorell A, et al. 2003. Antibodies against beta-amyloid slow cognitive decline in Alzheimer's disease. *Neuron* 38:547–54
66. Weggen S, Eriksen JL, Das P, Sagi SA, Wang R, et al. 2001. A subset of NSAIDs lower amyloidogenic A[beta]42 independently of cyclooxygenase activity. *Nature* 414:212–16
67. Lim GP, Yang F, Chu T, Chen P, Beech W, et al. 2000. Ibuprofen suppresses plaque pathology and inflammation in a mouse model for Alzheimer's disease. *J. Neurosci.* 20:5709–14
68. Eriksen JL, Sagi SA, Smith TE, Weggen S, Das P, et al. 2003. NSAIDs and enantiomers of flurbiprofen target gamma-secretase and lower Abeta42 in vivo. *J. Clin. Invest.* 112:440–49
69. Stewart WF, Kawas C, Corrada M, Metter EJ. 1997. Risk of Alzheimer's disease and duration of NSAID use. *Neurology* 48:626–32
70. Jarvik GP, Wijsman EM, Kukull WA, Schellenberg GD, Yu C, Larson EB. 1995. Interactions of apolipoprotein E genotype, total cholesterol level, age, and sex in prediction of Alzheimer's disease: a case-control study. *Neurology* 45:1092–96
71. Puglielli L, Tanzi RE, Kovacs DM. 2003. Alzheimer's disease: the cholesterol connection. *Nat. Neurosci.* 6:345–51
72. Wolozin B, Kellman W, Ruosseau P, Celesia GG, Siegel G. 2000. Decreased prevalence of Alzheimer disease associated with 3-hydroxy-3-methyglutaryl coenzyme A reductase inhibitors. *Arch. Neurol.* 57:1439–43
73. Jick H, Zornberg GL, Jick SS, Seshadri S, Drachman DA. 2000. Statins and the risk of dementia. *Lancet* 356:1627–31
74. Simons M, Schwarzler F, Lutjohann D, von Bergmann K, Beyreuther K, et al. 2002. Treatment with simvastatin in normocholesterolemic patients with Alzheimer's disease: A 26-week randomized, placebo-controlled, double-blind trial. *Ann. Neurol.* 52:346–50
75. Shepherd J, Blauw GJ, Murphy MB, Bollen EL, Buckley BM, et al. 2002. Pravastatin in elderly individuals at risk of vascular disease (PROSPER): a randomised controlled trial. *Lancet* 360:1623–30

76. Refolo LM, Malester B, LaFrancois J, Bryant-Thomas T, Wang R, et al. 2000. Hypercholesterolemia accelerates the Alzheimer's amyloid pathology in a transgenic mouse model. *Neurobiol. Dis.* 7:321–31
77. Frears ER, Stephens DJ, Walters CE, Davies H, Austen BM. 1999. The role of cholesterol in the biosynthesis of beta-amyloid. *NeuroReport* 10:1699–705
78. Refolo LM, Pappolla MA, LaFrancois J, Malester B, Schmidt SD, et al. 2001. A cholesterol-lowering drug reduces beta-amyloid pathology in a transgenic mouse model of Alzheimer's disease. *Neurobiol. Dis.* 8:890–99
79. Simons M, Keller P, De Strooper B, Beyreuther K, Dotti CG, Simons K. 1998. Cholesterol depletion inhibits the generation of beta-amyloid in hippocampal neurons. *Proc. Natl. Acad. Sci. USA* 95:6460–64
80. Fassbender K, Simons M, Bergmann C, Stroick M, Lutjohann D, et al. 2001. Simvastatin strongly reduces levels of Alzheimer's disease beta-amyloid peptides Abeta 42 and Abeta 40 in vitro and in vivo. *Proc. Natl. Acad. Sci. USA* 98:5856–61
81. Cherny RA, Legg JT, McLean CA, Fairlie DP, Huang X, et al. 1999. Aqueous dissolution of Alzheimer's disease Abeta amyloid deposits by biometal depletion. *J. Biol. Chem.* 274:23223–28
82. Cherny RA, Atwood CS, Xilinas ME, Gray DN, Jones WD, et al. 2001. Treatment with a copper-zinc chelator markedly and rapidly inhibits beta-amyloid accumulation in Alzheimer's disease transgenic mice. *Neuron* 30:665–76
83. Ritchie CW, Bush AI, Mackinnon A, Macfarlane S, Mastwyk M, et al. 2003. Metal-protein attenuation with iodochlorhydroxyquin (clioquinol) targeting Abeta amyloid deposition and toxicity in Alzheimer disease: a pilot phase 2 clinical trial. *Arch. Neurol.* 60:1685–91
84. Gervais F, Chalifour R, Garceau D, Kong X, Laurin J, et al. 2001. Glycosaminoglycan mimetics: a therapeutic approach to cerebral amyloid angiopathy. *Amyloid* 1(Suppl. 8):28–35
85. Geerts H. 2004. NC-531 (Neurochem). *Curr. Opin. Investig. Drugs* 5:95–100
86. Goedert M, Crowther RA, Spillantini MG. 1998. Tau mutations cause frontotemporal dementias. *Neuron* 21:955–58
87. Clark LN, Poorkaj P, Wszolek Z, Geschwind DH, Nasreddine ZS, et al. 1998. Pathogenic implications of mutations in the tau gene in pallido-ponto-nigral degeneration and related neurodegenerative disorders linked to chromosome 17. *Proc. Natl. Acad. Sci. USA* 95:13103–7
88. Houlden H, Baker M, Morris HR, MacDonald N, Pickering-Brown S, et al. 2001. Corticobasal degeneration and progressive supranuclear palsy share a common tau haplotype. *Neurology* 56:1702–6
89. Lee VM, Kenyon TK, Trojanowski JQ. 2005. Transgenic animal models of tauopathies. *Biochim. Biophys. Acta* 1739:251–59
90. Goedert M, Jakes R. 2005. Mutations causing neurodegenerative tauopathies. *Biochim. Biophys. Acta* 1739:240–50
91. D'Souza I, Poorkaj P, Hong M, Nochlin D, Lee VM, et al. 1999. Missense and silent tau gene mutations cause frontotemporal dementia with parkinsonism-chromosome 17 type, by affecting multiple alternative RNA splicing regulatory elements. *Proc. Natl. Acad. Sci. USA* 96:5598–603
92. Hasegawa M, Smith MJ, Goedert M. 1998. Tau proteins with FTDP-17 mutations have a reduced ability to promote microtubule assembly. *FEBS Lett.* 437:207–10

93. Hong M, Zhukareva V, Vogelsberg-Ragaglia V, Wszolek Z, Reed L, et al. 1998. Mutation-specific functional impairments in distinct tau isoforms of hereditary FTDP-17. *Science* 282:1914–17
94. Goedert M, Jakes R, Crowther RA. 1999. Effects of frontotemporal dementia FTDP-17 mutations on heparin-induced assembly of tau filaments. *FEBS Lett.* 450:306–11
95. Lee VM, Daughenbaugh R, Trojanowski JQ. 1994. Microtubule stabilizing drugs for the treatment of Alzheimer's disease. *Neurobiol. Aging* 15(Suppl. 2):S87–89
96. Ishihara T, Hong M, Zhang B, Nakagawa Y, Lee MK, et al. 1999. Age-dependent emergence and progression of a tauopathy in transgenic mice overexpressing the shortest human tau isoform. *Neuron* 24:751–62
97. Zhang B, Maiti A, Shively S, Lakhani F, McDonald-Jones G, et al. 2005. Microtubule-binding drugs offset tau sequestration by stabilizing microtubules and reversing fast axonal transport deficits in a tauopathy model. *Proc. Natl. Acad. Sci. USA* 102:227–31
98. Wischik CM, Edwards PC, Lai RYK, Roth M, Harrington CR. 1996. Selective inhibition of Alzheimer disease-like tau aggregation by phenothiazines. *Proc. Natl. Acad. Sci. USA* 93:11213–18
99. Taniguchi S, Suzuki N, Masuda M, Hisanaga S-I, Iwatsubo T, et al. 2005. Inhibition of heparin-induced Tau filament formation by phenothiazines, polyphenols, and porphyrins. *J. Biol. Chem.* 280:7614–23
100. Chirita C, Necula M, Kuret J. 2004. Ligand-dependent inhibition and reversal of tau filament formation. *Biochemistry* 43:2879–87
101. Pickhardt M, Gazova Z, von Bergen M, Khlistunova I, Wang Y, et al. 2005. Anthraquinones inhibit tau aggregation and dissolve Alzheimer's paired helical filaments in vitro and in cells. *J. Biol. Chem.* 280:3628–35
102. Bhat RV, Budd Haeberlein SL, Avila J. 2004. Glycogen synthase kinase 3: a drug target for CNS therapies. *J. Neurochem.* 89:1313–17
103. Polymeropoulos MH, Lavedan C, Leroy E, Ide SE, Dehejia A, et al. 1997. Mutation in the alpha-synuclein gene identified in families with Parkinson's disease. *Science* 276:2045–47
104. Spillantini MG, Schmidt ML, Lee VM, Trojanowski JQ, Jakes R, Goedert M. 1997. Alpha-synuclein in Lewy bodies. *Nature* 388:839–40
105. Spillantini MG, Crowther RA, Jakes R, Hasegawa M, Goedert M. 1998. alpha-Synuclein in filamentous inclusions of Lewy bodies from Parkinson's disease and dementia with lewy bodies. *Proc. Natl. Acad. Sci. USA* 95:6469–73
106. Baba M, Nakajo S, Tu PH, Tomita T, Nakaya K, et al. 1998. Aggregation of alpha-synuclein in Lewy bodies of sporadic Parkinson's disease and dementia with Lewy bodies. *Am. J. Pathol.* 152:879–84
107. Tu PH, Galvin JE, Baba M, Giasson B, Tomita T, et al. 1998. Glial cytoplasmic inclusions in white matter oligodendrocytes of multiple system atrophy brains contain insoluble alpha-synuclein. *Ann. Neurol.* 44:415–22
108. Singleton AB, Farrer M, Johnson J, Singleton A, Hague S, et al. 2003. alpha-synuclein locus triplication causes Parkinson's disease. *Science* 302:841
109. Eriksen JL, Dawson TM, Dickson DW, Petrucelli L. 2003. Caught in the act: alpha-synuclein is the culprit in Parkinson's disease. *Neuron* 40:453–56
110. Giasson BI, Duda JE, Quinn SM, Zhang B, Trojanowski JQ, Lee VM. 2002. Neuronal alpha-synucleinopathy with severe movement disorder in mice expressing A53T human alpha-synuclein. *Neuron* 34:521–33
111. Maries E, Dass B, Collier TJ, Kordower JH, Steece-Collier K. 2003. The role of alpha-synuclein in Parkinson's disease: insights from animal models. *Nat. Rev. Neurosci.* 4:727–38

112. Masliah E, Rockenstein E, Veinbergs I, Mallory M, Hashimoto M, et al. 2000. Dopaminergic loss and inclusion body formation in alpha-synuclein mice: implications for neurodegenerative disorders. *Science* 287:1265–69
113. Braak H, Del Tredici K, Bratzke H, Hamm-Clement J, Sandmann-Keil D, Rub U. 2002. Staging of the intracerebral inclusion body pathology associated with idiopathic Parkinson's disease (preclinical and clinical stages). *J. Neurol.* 249(Suppl. 3):III/1–5
114. Gibb WR, Lees AJ. 1988. The relevance of the Lewy body to the pathogenesis of idiopathic Parkinson's disease. *J. Neurol. Neurosurg. Psychiatry* 51:745–52
115. Gorell JM, Johnson CC, Rybicki BA, Peterson EL, Richardson RJ. 1998. The risk of Parkinson's disease with exposure to pesticides, farming, well water, and rural living. *Neurology* 50:1346–50
116. Betarbet R, Sherer TB, MacKenzie G, Garcia-Osuna M, Panov AV, Greenamyre JT. 2000. Chronic systemic pesticide exposure reproduces features of Parkinson's disease. *Nat. Neurosci.* 3:1301–6
117. Giasson BI, Lee VM. 2000. A new link between pesticides and Parkinson's disease. *Nat. Neurosci.* 3:1227–28
118. Giasson BI, Duda JE, Murray IV, Chen Q, Souza JM, et al. 2000. Oxidative damage linked to neurodegeneration by selective alpha-synuclein nitration in synucleinopathy lesions. *Science* 290:985–89
119. Ischiropoulos H, Beckman JS. 2003. Oxidative stress and nitration in neurodegeneration: cause, effect, or association? *J. Clin. Invest.* 111:163–69
120. Bodles AM, El-Agnaf OM, Greer B, Guthrie DJ, Irvine GB. 2004. Inhibition of fibril formation and toxicity of a fragment of alpha-synuclein by an N-methylated peptide analogue. *Neurosci. Lett.* 359:89–93
121. El-Agnaf OM, Paleologou KE, Greer B, Abogrein AM, King JE, et al. 2004. A strategy for designing inhibitors of alpha-synuclein aggregation and toxicity as a novel treatment for Parkinson's disease and related disorders. *FASEB J.* 18:1315–17
122. Lee EN, Cho HJ, Lee CH, Lee D, Chung KC, Paik SR. 2004. Phthalocyanine tetrasulfonates affect the amyloid formation and cytotoxicity of alpha-synuclein. *Biochemistry* 43:3704–15
123. Fornai F, Lenzi P, Gesi M, Ferrucci M, Lazzeri G, et al. 2003. Recent knowledge on molecular components of Lewy bodies discloses future therapeutic strategies in Parkinson's disease. *Curr. Drug Targets CNS Neurol. Disord.* 2:149–52
124. Conway KA, Rochet JC, Bieganski RM, Lansbury PT Jr. 2001. Kinetic stabilization of the alpha-synuclein protofibril by a dopamine-alpha-synuclein adduct. *Science* 294:1346–49
125. Auluck PK, Chan HY, Trojanowski JQ, Lee VM, Bonini NM. 2002. Chaperone suppression of alpha-synuclein toxicity in a Drosophila model for Parkinson's disease. *Science* 295:865–68
126. Auluck PK, Meulener MC, Bonini NM. 2005. Mechanisms of suppression of {alpha}-synuclein neurotoxicity by geldanamycin in Drosophila. *J. Biol. Chem.* 280:2873–78
127. Rekas A, Adda CG, Aquilina JA, Barnham KJ, Sunde M, et al. 2004. Interaction of the molecular chaperone alphaB-crystallin with alpha-synuclein: effects on amyloid fibril formation and chaperone activity. *J. Mol. Biol.* 340:1167–83

The Endothelium as a Target for Infections

Gustavo Valbuena[1] and David H. Walker[2]

[1]School of Medicine, Universidad de Los Andes, Bogota, Colombia; email: gvalbuen@utmb.edu

[2]Department of Pathology, University of Texas Medical Branch, Galveston, Texas 77555; email: dwalker@utmb.edu

Annu. Rev. Pathol. Mech. Dis. 2006. 1:171–98

First published online as a Review in Advance on October 20, 2005

The *Annual Review of Pathology: Mechanisms of Disease* is online at pathmechdis.annualreviews.org

doi: 10.1146/annurev.pathol.1.110304.100031

1553-4006/06/0114-0171$20.00

Key Words

rickettsia, bartonella, hantavirus, herpesvirus 8, inflammation

Abstract

The endothelial cells lining vascular and lymphatic vessels are targets of several infectious agents, including viruses and bacteria, that lead to dramatic changes in their functions. Understanding the pathophysiological mechanisms that cause the clinical manifestations of those infections has been advanced through the use of animal models and in vitro systems; however, there are also abundant studies that explore the consequences of endothelial infection in vitro without supporting evidence that endothelial cells are actual in vivo targets of infection in human diseases. This article defines criteria for considering an infection as truly endothelium-targeted and reviews the literature that offers insights into the pathogenesis of human endothelial-target infections.

INTRODUCTION

Chemokines: family of chemotactic cytokines that differentially attract specific subtypes of leucocytes via G protein–coupled receptors

The endothelium consists of a single layer of flat cells (endothelial cells) that line the vasculature. Its critical location allows endothelial cells to serve regulatory functions in angiogenesis, hemostasis, permeability, solute exchange, vascular tone, and inflammation (1, 2). This last function is particularly important because endothelial cells constitute the interface between circulating leukocytes and possible sites of inflammation (owing to infection, tumor growth, or autoimmunity). Leukocyte recruitment is one function of the endothelium that has been investigated extensively; much is known about the mechanisms that lead to the migration of leukocytes from the vessel lumen into the tissue parenchyma (3–5). Moreover, there is now evidence that a common embryonic precursor to both hematopoietic and endothelial lineages exists (6). Its existence was identified from human embryonic stem cells that do not express CD45 and are positive for PECAM-1 (CD-31), Flk-1 (receptor for VEGF), and VE-Cadherin (CD-144); clonal analysis of these cells in culture demonstrated that their progeny is hematopoietic or endothelial and, in very few cases, both. Such a common origin is in agreement with a view of the endothelium as an immunological organ; the capacity of endothelial cells to secrete cytokines and chemokines, express adhesion molecules, and present antigens reinforces this view. From this perspective, most infectious pathogens have some relationship with the endothelium and its functions, ranging from surface colonization leading to endothelial activation (i.e., expression of an inflammatory phenotype) to intracellular infection leading to a variety of effects including activation of endothelial pathogen killing mechanisms. However, a broad discussion covering this topic is beyond the scope of the present review, which instead will focus on microorganisms that specifically and consistently target the endothelium.

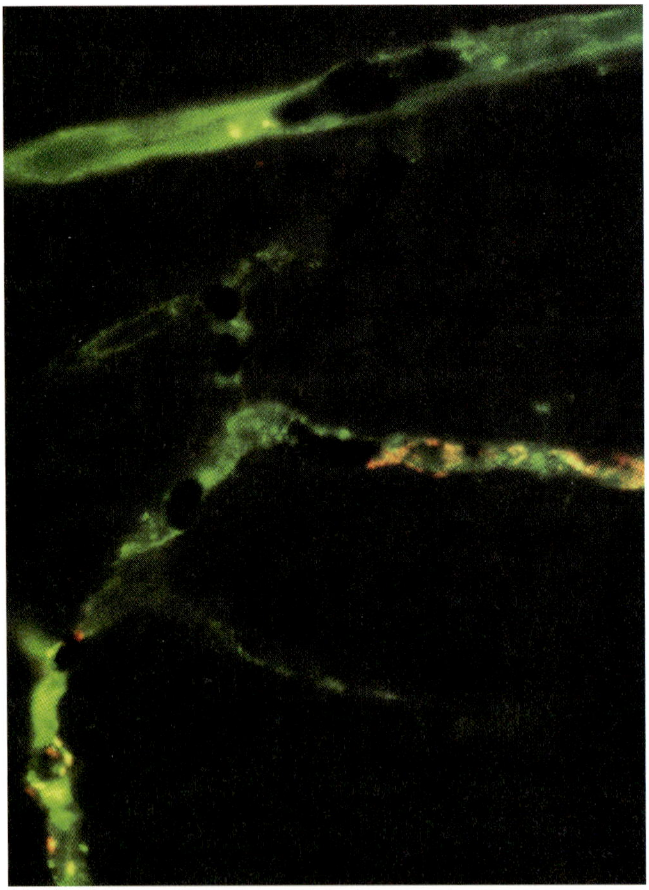

Figure 1

Mouse retinal whole mount preparation five days after inoculation with a lethal dose of *Rickettsia conorii*. Immunofluorescent detection of *R. conorii* (*orange*) and ICAM-1 (CD54) (*green*). Colocalized antigens appear yellow-orange. The multifocal infection is limited to the vasculature.

CRITERA FOR THE OCCURRENCE OF ENDOTHELIAL INFECTION

There are at least four criteria that should be considered when deciding whether an infection is truly endothelial or not: (*a*) The infectious agent's intracellular location must be demonstrated in endothelial cells of human cases or animal models that closely mimic the pathological characteristics of the human infection (**Figure 1**); (*b*) the infectious agents must be able to replicate inside endothelial cells; (*c*) the endothelium must be a consistent target of the infection throughout the course of the disease, and (*d*) evidence of in vitro infection of endothelial cells is not sufficient by itself.

The techniques, samples, and timing of the studies or experimental procedures are also relevant. Immunological detection of a microorganism's antigens by immunohistochemistry or immunofluorescence should be interpreted cautiously because many endothelial cells are capable of phagocytosis (such as those of the liver sinusoids) or pinocytosis, and the intracellular detection of antigens could reflect staining of immune complexes or dead organisms; this is particularly relevant if the pathogen establishes high levels of viremia or bacteremia. Electron microscopy is thus a very powerful technique because it allows the assessment of the agent's integrity, intracellular compartment localization, and replication of the infectious agents inside endothelial cells. Alternatively, in situ hybridization of the microorganism's RNA permits cellular localization and constitutes supportive evidence for active microbial metabolism. Furthermore, in RNA viruses, detection of sense RNA opposite to that present in the virion supports the possibility of active virus replication. The timing of sampling is also important. One of the problems with the interpretation of postmortem studies is that endothelial cells can become late targets of infection when the immune system has been overwhelmed. Better sources are biopsies from living individuals at various times during the course of infection or appropriate animal models sampled at multiple time points. The strains of bacteria or viruses used for experimental studies introduce yet another variable: After multiple passages in the laboratory, some strains may change their tissue tropism and/or lose their pathogenicity, or may even gain new properties; therefore, researchers prefer recently isolated strains, especially if they originate from infected human cases, for experimental studies. Nonetheless, there are strains of differing virulence both for humans and in the animal models. Lastly, the immune status of affected individuals is important because different types of immune deficiencies can allow shifts in tissue tropism. For example, in cat-scratch disease, immunocompetent patients develop immune-mediated lesions of the lymph nodes. In contrast, immunocompromised patients infected with *Bartonella henselae* develop vasoproliferative lesions in the skin and viscera.

HUVECs: human umbilical vein endothelial cells

CONSIDERATIONS REGARDING IN VITRO STUDIES OF ENDOTHELIAL INFECTION

Once the criteria for endothelial infection have been met, the results from in vitro studies with endothelial cells become more relevant. However, there are several important considerations concerning these types of studies. Endothelial cells are functionally and phenotypically very heterogeneous, with marked differences in receptor expression, permeability, adhesion molecule expression, and activation response in different organs and different regions of each organ's vascular bed (i.e., arteries, arterioles, capillaries, venules, and veins) (1, 7, 8). This point must be considered when confronted with generalizations derived from the in vitro analysis of endothelial cells of restricted origin. Such is the case for human umbilical vein endothelial cells (HUVECs), the most frequently used cellular model owing to wide availability and ease of isolation. These cells originate in a large vessel of the placenta, an organ not found in the vast majority of patients. Ideally, in vitro results with these cells should be confirmed in other types of primary endothelial cells, particularly in microvascular endothelial cells because they represent the great majority of infected cells in vivo. Additionally, it is now known that endothelial cells in culture acquire a phenotype different from that of endothelial cells in situ (9); furthermore, high-passage cells differ from low-passage cells. Moreover, culture conditions and methods of purification of primary endothelial cells, including purity of the preparations, introduce variables that may affect the results. For all these reasons, it is important

BSL-3/4: biosafety level necessary for work with infectious agents; BSL-3 agents may cause severe or potentially lethal diseases; BSL-4 agents are novel and/or dangerous microorganisms that have a high fatality rate

to correlate the results of cell culture models with in vivo results through the use of appropriate animal models or the study of archival material from human cases (i.e., biopsy or autopsy).

DEFINING *BONA-FIDE* ENDOTHELIUM-TARGETING INFECTIOUS AGENTS

Microbial pathogens that have been claimed to have human endothelial cells as one of their targets include the following: cytomegalovirus, rickettsiae, *Orientia tsutsugamushi*, Kaposi's sarcoma–associated herpes virus (human herpesvirus 8, HHV8), *Chlamydia (Chlamydophila) pneumoniae*, bartonellae, Nipah virus, *Francisella tularensis*, *Listeria monocytogenes*, and hemorrhagic fever viruses, which include bunyaviruses (such as hantavirus, nairovirus, and the phlebovirus that causes Rift Valley fever), flaviviruses such as dengue, filoviruses such as Ebola and Marburg, and some arenaviruses that cause Lassa fever and South American hemorrhagic fevers. The main reason for suggesting that some of these agents infect the endothelium is because hemorrhage is an important component of the clinical presentation of some of these infections. In addition, some claims about the relevance of endothelial cells as targets of these infections originated from in vitro studies showing permissiveness to intracellular replication and hypotheses that the pathophysiology of those diseases would place endothelial cells as logical targets. This is the case for many hemorrhagic fevers (10, 11) in which immunopathogenic mechanisms (i.e., excessive production of cytokines such as tumor necrosis factor-α (TNF-α) and others) may play a predominant role in the hemorrhagic manifestations (12). Moreover, proof from clinical and experimental in vivo studies is insufficient or lacking because many of these diseases are endemic to underdeveloped areas without adequate experimental laboratory infrastructure or because the studies are dangerous and require high-grade containment laboratories (BSL-3 or BSL-4).

To illustrate these points, despite the evidence of in vitro replication of the filovirus Ebola (a BSL-4 agent that causes a hemorrhagic fever) inside endothelial cells and the demonstration of endothelial cytotoxicity mediated by the virion glycoprotein (13, 14), recent studies in a primate model showed that, in vivo, endothelial cells are late targets of infection and are in fact minimally disrupted (15). It is likely, therefore, that the human endothelial infection documented in a postmortem study (16) occurs late and is not fundamental in the pathogenesis of the disease. This is consistent with the hypothesis that vascular hemorrhage is not a consequence of endothelial destruction, but most likely secondary to functional changes of the endothelium through direct and indirect (i.e., mediated by secreted factors) interactions with infected leukocytes. Similarly, there is no evidence that Rift Valley fever virus causes significant in vivo endothelial infection despite the production of prominent in vitro endothelial infection (17); neither is there evidence of dengue viral replication in the endothelium from fatal cases of dengue infection as assessed by a combination of immunohistochemistry and in situ hybridization (18). Interestingly, in this study dengue antigens were immunolocalized to the cytoplasm of endothelial cells in the lungs and liver; however, no viral RNA was detectable. This raises an important issue: What is the appropriate interpretation of immunohistochemical signals in phagocytic cells, including liver endothelial cells, which are scavenger cells (19), and lung endothelial cells, which may serve a similar function through pinocytosis? Such an antigen could consist of dead phagocytosed viruses or immune complexes. Therefore, localization of viral nucleic acids is often necessary to establish the presence of true infection and viral replication. This analysis was not performed in a reported fatal case in which dengue virus antigen was immunolocalized to brain endothelial cells among other cells (20). Because of the lack of convincing and consistent evidence of in vivo endothelial infection by dengue virus, we will not discuss the abundant literature regarding the effects of this viral infection on cultured endothelial cells.

Another interesting case is *C. pneumoniae*, publicized because of its possible role in atherogenesis (21, 22). Although there are abundant descriptions of the effects of these bacteria on endothelial cells in vitro (23), there is no firm evidence that they infect endothelial cells in vivo. Although the data from human samples show the presence of *C. pneumoniae* in atherosclerotic plaques (24), in general a description of its specific location is lacking (25–27) and, when described, the antigen has been localized to macrophages and smooth muscle cells (28–32) or attached to debris within the atherosclerotic plaque (33). In one report, the antigen was predominantly localized to smooth muscle cells and macrophages and only occasionally to endothelial cells; however, no photographic documentation was presented (34). Recent evidence indicates that antichlamydial antibodies used in immunohistochemistry may cross-react with ceroid deposits within atherosclerotic plaques (35). Nevertheless, detection of chlamydial DNA and protein in atherosclerotic plaques suggests that *C. pneumoniae* possibly plays a role in the development of atherosclerosis and its complications (36); the possible role of the endothelium may be related to the interaction with infected macrophages and smooth muscle cells within the plaque. Because there is no definitive proof that *C. pneumoniae* infects the vascular endothelium in vivo, it will not be considered further in this review.

Other infectious agents have been described as infecting endothelial cells in vivo, but not consistently. That is the case, for instance, of a polyomavirus closely related to BK virus, which caused a disseminated endothelial infection in a patient with type-1 diabetes who received a transplanted kidney (37). Endothelial cells do not represent, however, an important part of the spectrum of tissue tropism of these viruses. Interestingly, hamsters inoculated with the human polyomavirus JC showed brain endothelial cell infection, which was even more prominent when the animals were immunosuppressed with cyclophosphamide (38). Another example is *F. tularensis*. Antigens from these bacteria have been described in endothelial cells of an infected human lymph node from a patient who exhibited the ulceroglandular variety of tularemia (39); however, no other in vivo evidence has been published and the relevance of this finding has not been investigated. In fact, in vitro, very few *F. tularensis* survive inside HUVECs as indicated by a 24-hour gentamicin protection assay (40). In a 48-hour assay, the recovery of bacteria is extremely low, suggesting that endothelial cells are an unlikely site of *F. tularensis* replication and survival. Macrophages most likely are the principal target of these bacteria in vivo (41). A final example is *L. monocytogenes*, facultative intracellular gram-positive bacteria that produce food-borne infections that lead to chorioamnionitis (with consequent abortion or stillbirth), neonatal meningitis, and meningoencephalitis in adults (elderly and immunocompromised persons). All these syndromes probably occur only when the immune system does not clear the subclinical pyogranulomatous hepatitis that is established after listeriae cross the intestinal barrier. The involvement of the brain parenchyma may reflect a tropism for the microvascular endothelium (42). The evidence of endothelial infection in vivo is, however, scant: There is one report of intraendothelial listeriae in an autopsy case of meningoencephalitis (43).

Researchers have postulated that interaction with endothelial cells is a prerequisite for meningeal and brain invasion of all pathogens that cause meningitis or meningoencephalitis. For the best-investigated agent-causing meningitis, *Escherichia coli*, evidence shows that endothelial cells of the blood-brain barrier must be invaded in order for the microorganisms to gain access to the meninges

Transcytosis: transfer of macromolecules or microorganisms from one extracellular space to another through an endocytic vesicle that traverses the cell cytoplasm

NFκB: nuclear factor kappa B

EBV: Epstein-Barr virus

RANTES: regulated on activation, normal T cell expressed and secreted (also known as CCL5)

HHV8: human herpesvirus 8

CMV: cytomegalovirus

Apoptosis: regulated process of cell death produced by the activation of a protease cascade that leads to collapse of the cytoplasm and nucleus and DNA break-up

and brain through a process of transcytosis (44, 45). Similar processes have not been investigated in relevant animal models to understand the hematogenous dissemination of infectious organisms to other organs. Nonetheless, the response of the endothelium to such invasion [which is known to include the activation of proinflammatory transcription factors such as nuclear factor kappa B (NFκB)] should be important in the pathogenesis of these infections. We will not review the literature (consisting almost exclusively of in vitro studies) in this regard because we are limiting our discussion to infectious agents that consistently target the endothelium.

Post-transplant lymphoproliferative disease (PTLD), an entity associated with Epstein-Barr virus (EBV), is one disease in which no formal proof of in vivo endothelial infection exists, yet there is indirect evidence that it may occur. Serum interleukin (IL)-6 (a growth factor for EBV-immortalized cells) is elevated in patients with PTLD, and a culture of disaggregated PTLD tissue showed that adherent cells, possibly endothelial cells, were the source of IL-6 (46). Later, it was demonstrated that EBV infects cultured primary human endothelial cells, leading to secretion of high levels of IL-6 (47). This effect is probably mediated by prolonged NFκB activation induced by EBV infection as was demonstrated in another in vitro study that also showed expression of other genes induced by NFκB, namely IL-1, IL-8 (or CXCL8), RANTES (regulated on activation, normal T cell expressed and secreted; or CCL5), MCP-1 (or CCL2), E-selectin, ICAM-1, and VCAM-1 (48). Recently, there has been indirect evidence that in vivo EBV endothelial infection may occur: Endothelial expression of Bcl-2 (an antiapoptotic protein that can be induced by EBV) in liver allografts was associated with EBV infection. Patients with those conditions did not show rejection despite lowering or cessation of immunosuppressive therapy (49). It is now important to establish that EBV infects endothelial cells in vivo.

TRUE ENDOTHELIUM-TARGETING INFECTIOUS AGENTS

There is convincing clinical or experimental in vivo evidence of endothelial infection for the Nipah virus (50), cytomegalovirus (51–53), Crimean-Congo hemorrhagic fever virus (54), hantavirus (55, 56), HHV8 (57, 58), *Bartonella bacilliformis* (59), *O. tsutsugamushi* (60), and rickettsiae (61–69) (**Table 1**). In addition, arenaviruses causing Lassa fever and South American hemorrhagic fevers have been reported to infect endothelial cells, although the evidence has been published only as part of a review article (11), an abstract (S.R. Zaki, personal communication), and in two studies of experimental animal infections. In one of them, an animal model with Pichinde virus, the virus was identified in cells that correspond morphologically to endothelial cells but that were not clearly labeled as such at the time (70). In another study, infection of a New World primate with Junin virus resulted in the infection of small vessels of the brain; however, other cell types, including macrophages, hepatocytes, and neurons, were more prominently infected (71).

All but three of the agents that infect endothelial cells in vivo, namely hantaviruses, HHV8, and rickettsiae, also infect other cell types as prominently as, or frequently more prominently than, endothelial cells.

Cytomegaloviral Infection of the Endothelium

Cytomegalovirus (CMV), for instance, can infect almost any cell type, although mainly in immunocompromised patients (72, 73). In fact, endothelial infection by CMV may occur only when apoptosis is inhibited by a viral product, which was recently identified in murine CMV through random transposon mutagenesis and demonstrated by the loss of ability to grow in endothelial cells when compared with growth in fibroblasts that were infected in parallel (74). The gene encoding

Table 1 Endothelial-target pathogens and their characteristics

Pathogens	Diseases	Mechanism of transmission or vectors	Pathophysiology related to endothelial cells	Endothelial cells as main targets	Adequate animal model
Rickettsiae, spotted fever group	Rocky Mountain spotted fever, Mediterranean spotted fever, and other spotted fevers	Ticks and mites	Oxidative damage Endothelial cell activation[1] Inhibition of apoptosis	Yes. Monocytes and hepatocytes are secondary targets	Yes. C3H/HeN mice infected with *Rickettsia conorii*
Rickettsiae, typhus group	Epidemic and murine typhus	Human body louse and fleas	Burst lysis Endothelial cell activation[1] Inhibition of apoptosis	Yes. Monocytes and hepatocytes are secondary targets	Yes. C3H/HeN mice infected with *Rickettsia typhi*
Orientia tsutsugamushi	Scrub typhus	Chiggers	Possibly similar to rickettsiae (more research needed)	Yes	No
Human herpesvirus 8 (HHV8)	Kaposi's sarcoma, primary effusion lymphoma, variant of Castleman's disease	Not clearly established	Activation of angiogenic program Activation of endothelial cells[1]	Yes. Also infects leukocytes	No
Hantaviruses	Hemorrhagic fever with renal syndrome Hantavirus pulmonary syndrome	Inhalation of aerosols from excreta of infected rodents	Immunopathology Direct viral effects leading to activation of endothelial cells[1]	Yes. Principally in certain vascular beds	Yes. Syrian golden hamster
Bartonella bacilliformis	Oroya fever and verruga peruana	Sandfly	Inhibition of apoptosis Production of angiogenic factors Activation of endothelial cells[1]	No. Erythrocytes are major target cells. Intimate extracellular bacterial contact with endothelial cells but few are intracellular	No
Other bartonellae	Bacillary angiomatosis, bacillary peliosis, cat-scratch disease, trench fever, endocarditis, bacteremia	Several arthropods	Inhibition of apoptosis Production of angiogenic factors Activation of endothelial cells[1]	No. Intra-erythrocytic infection in natural host. Intimate contact with endothelial cells but few are intracellular	No
Nipah virus	Encephalitis	Possibly airborne and contact with infected pigs	Not investigated	No. Also infects neurons	No

(*Continued*)

Table 1 (*Continued*)

Pathogens	Diseases	Mechanism of transmission or vectors	Pathophysiology related to endothelial cells	Endothelial cells as main targets	Adequate animal model
Cytomegalovirus	Systemic infection in immuno-compromised patients Accelerated atherosclerosis in transplanted grafts Congenital and others	Oral, trans-placental, venereal, transfusions, transplants	Inhibition of apoptosis Endothelial cells as vehicle of systemic dissemination Activated phenotype in endothelial cells[1]	No. Also infects leukocytes and many other cell types	Yes. Infection of mice with mouse cytomegalovirus
Crimean-Congo hemorrhagic fever virus	Hemorrhagic fever	Ticks Aerosols from infected animals and humans	Disseminated intravascular coagulation hypothesized but not proven	No. Also infects monocytes and hepatocytes	No

[1]Activated endothelial cells secrete cytokines (such as IL-1 and IL-6) and chemokines (such as IL-8, RANTES, and MCP-1) and express adhesion molecules including ICAM-1, VCAM-1, and E-selectin. The specific expressed or secreted proteins vary depending on the activation stimulus.

this antiapoptotic protein (M45) has a homologue in human CMV (UL45). In any case, CMV-infected endothelial cells circulate in patients with active disease, so they can be a vehicle of systemic dissemination (52, 53). On the other hand, endothelial cells may not be a site of latency because CMV DNA is not detected in endothelial cells of immunocompetent seropositive individuals, whereas it is detectable in monocytes of the same individuals (75).

In vitro, CMV infection of primary human endothelial cells results in expression of the cytokine IL-6, the chemokines CXCL8 and CCL2, and the adhesion molecules ICAM-1, VCAM-1, and E-selectin (76). The products of the viral-immediate early genes lead directly to increased activity of an E-selectin promoter-reporter vector in endothelial cells (77). There are two possible consequences of these changes: (*a*) The attraction and adhesion of leukocytes could increase the likelihood of CMV dissemination by cell-to-cell contact, or (*b*) the combination of chemoattraction and adhesion of leukocytes could result in inflammation within the vascular wall. Evidence suggests that CMV infection is associated with the development of atherosclerosis and, particularly, transplant-associated accelerated atherosclerosis (78).

Other Viral Infections of the Endothelium

Nipah virus infection of endothelial cells in the brain is associated with vasculitis, thrombosis, and tissue necrosis; however, Nipah virus also infects neurons. This tropism contributes to the pathogenesis of the human disease, which is characterized by a severe acute encephalitic syndrome in the majority of patients (50). Crimean-Congo hemorrhagic fever virus infects monocytes and hepatocytes as well, and arenaviruses infect mesothelial cells and mononuclear blood cells (12, 70).

Bartonella Infection and the Endothelium

B. bacilliformis (the agent of Oroya fever and verruga peruana) and other bartonellae constitute a special case among endothelial-target infectious agents because they maintain a close relationship with endothelial cells, mainly as extracellular agents in direct contact with the endothelium, and trigger an angioproliferative response. In fact, there has been evidence of in vivo intracellular endothelial infection only for *B. bacilliformis* (59). The organisms are found within vacuoles, particularly in cells with (Rocha-Lima) inclusions that stain red with Giemsa; these organisms are, however, few compared with the great majority, which are extracellular. The formation of those inclusions may be related to a novel mechanism of cellular invasion that has been described only in bartonellae. It consists of an actin-dependent active process that takes 18 to 24 hours during which bacteria accumulate and aggregate on a focal area of endothelial cells before they are engulfed to form a structure christened the invasome (79).

There are seven other species of bartonellae that cause human infections in which the pathogenesis involves endothelial cells, but there is no in vivo evidence of intracellular endothelial infection (80). In fact, in patients with endocarditis caused by *Bartonella quintana*, an electron microscopy study showed evidence of intracellular infection in cells of the valvular vegetations (81); unfortunately, the phenotype of the infected cells was not identified and, again, the majority of the bacteria were extracellular. Most bartonella infections are transmitted by arthropod vectors resulting, in immunocompromised patients, in angioproliferative lesions termed bacillary angiomatosis and bacillary peliosis (caused by *B. henselae* and *B. quintana*), the latter consisting of lesions in the liver and spleen (82). In immunocompetent patients, bartonella infections result in cat-scratch disease, trench fever, endocarditis, and bacteremia.

B. bacilliformis is the one member of the *Bartonella* genus that causes angioproliferative lesions (verruga peruana) in apparently immunocompetent individuals, but its distribution is restricted to the Andes of Peru, Ecuador, Colombia, and Bolivia where its vectors, the nocturnal sandflies (e.g., *Lutzomyia verrucarum*) exist. The disease begins classically with a febrile anemia that results from invasion of erythrocytes (Oroya fever) and is followed by angioproliferative lesions of the skin that can persist for years. Intracellular endothelial infection is, however, not required for the development of these lesions. This was determined by an in vivo angiogenesis assay in rats, in which sponges containing *B. bacilliformis* homogenates were implanted subcutaneously (83); there was a 2.5-fold increase in the number of vessels as compared with controls. In fact, culture supernatants of *B. henselae* were sufficient to induce proliferation of HUVECs in vitro (84).

VEGF: vascular endothelial growth factor

The mechanisms involved in triggering the angiogenic response during bartonella infections include the inhibition of endothelial apoptosis and induction of angiogenic cytokine secretion. The antiapoptotic mechanism, which is active only for bartonella-infected endothelial cells, appears to involve the inhibition of the caspase proteolytic cascade that underlies apoptosis. Specifically, caspases 3 and 8 are inhibited (85). The bacterial factor causing this effect can be secreted because the medium in which *Bartonella* has been cultivated has an antiapoptotic effect, albeit not all the antiapoptotic activity can be explained in this manner, suggesting that other factors requiring direct contact may be necessary. In regards to the secretion of angiogenic factors, *Bartonella* nonfimbrial adhesin A (BadA) mediated the adherence of *B. henselae* to endothelial cells through β1 integrins and triggered the activation of a luciferase reporter construct under the control of the vascular endothelial growth factor (VEGF) promoter (86). This promoter is activated by the angiogenic transcription factor HIF-1; therefore BadA activates the proangiogenic program through HIF-1. Moreover, VEGF is secreted both in vitro and in vivo during bartonella infection (87). In addition, mRNA of angiopoietin-2 and the receptors VEGFR1 and VEGFR2 (an angiogenic system) can be detected in endothelial cells in verruga peruana lesions by in situ hybridization (88). This study also revealed that the major expression of VEGF mRNA was in the suprabasal keratinocytes of these lesions. Another source of VEGF may be infected

Operon: cluster of prokaryotic genes transcribed as a single unit; encodes proteins that participate in various steps of the same process or function

Trans-complementation: capacity of a nonchromosomal DNA element to restore the normal phenotype in cells whose corresponding chromosomal DNA element had been mutated

monocytes because these cells infiltrate bartonella lesions, and in vitro infection of the macrophage cell line THP-1 with *B. henselae* induces the expression of VEGF (89). Thus, in addition to an autocrine loop, a paracrine angiogenic loop may be established between infiltrating monocytes/macrophages and endothelial cells. Of note, *B. bacilliformis* (but not *B. henselae*) secretes a proteinaceous factor that is directly mitogenic to endothelial cells in vitro; this factor could be GroEL as evidenced by the neutralization of this effect with specific antibodies (90). The mechanism of GroEL action is unknown, and it could involve the production of angiogenic cytokines, including CXCL8.

Unfortunately, an adequate animal model of bartonella pathogenesis has not been established. There are, however, in vitro models of angiogenesis that can be used to study this pathogen's virulence factors. For instance, *B. henselae* infection of endothelial cells in an in vitro cord formation assay, in which endothelial cells overlaid with a type-I collagen gel form a network of interconnected cells, increases the viability of endothelial cells forming the cords for a longer time than VEGF (91). Also, bartonella infection of endothelial cells in a three-dimensional collagen tube formation assay (trypsinized endothelial cells resuspended in a collagen gel migrate to form capillary-like tubular structures) allows cells to invade the matrix, survive in it, and form tubes; neither uninfected control cells nor VEGF-treated cells were capable of any of these activites (91).

Endothelial cells respond to in vitro bartonella infections with the activation of the transcription factor NFκB and the consequent development of an inflammatory phenotype that includes the expression of adhesion molecules, specifically E-selectin and ICAM-1 (92, 93). Such a response can be mimicked by purified bartonella outer membrane proteins. Also, a recent study revealed one possible trigger of the inflammatory response of endothelial cells exposed to bartonellae: *B. henselae* has a VirB type-IV secretion system, which is induced upon infection of endothelial cells in vitro (94). The study of a mutant strain for the VirB operon and comparison with a trans-complemented strain demonstrated that this system mediates invasome-mediated entry as well as the proinflammatory and antiapoptotic responses of endothelial cells interacting with bartonellae (95). The future description of the function of proteins translocated by VirB into the cytoplasm of endothelial cells will be extremely important for the study of endothelial biology. A recent exhaustive review provides further information on the pathogenesis of bartonella infections (96).

INFECTIOUS AGENTS THAT USE ENDOTHELIAL CELLS AS THEIR MAJOR TARGET

In contrast to all the pathogens above, *O. tsutsugamushi*, rickettsiae, HHV8, and hantaviruses are the only human infectious pathogens that use endothelial cells as their main targets of intracellular infection.

Hantaviruses and Endothelial Cells

Hantaviruses that infect the endothelium are transmitted by direct contact or inhalation of viral aerosols from excreta of persistently infected rodents. They produce hemorrhagic fever with renal syndrome (Hantaan, Seoul, Puumala and Belgrade) and hantavirus pulmonary syndrome (Sin Nombre, Andes, and other viruses). In both cases, increased vascular permeability is the hallmark of infection; however, hantaviruses do not produce cytopathic effects in endothelial cells in vitro (97) or in vivo (55), and neither do they cause increased endothelial permeability in vitro (98). In fact, evidence suggests that the characteristic microvascular leakage observed clinically results from the action of inflammatory mediators and immune cells that target endothelial cells (i.e., the immune response against the virus) (99, 100). However, it appears that pathogenic hantaviruses bind and enter endothelial cells through endothelial β3 integrins (101–103), which are important in the regulation of vascular permeability through ligand-binding interactions (104, 105), and thus these events may explain some of the pathophysiological phenomena observed in infected patients.

In addition, pathogenic hantaviruses produce distinctive endothelial transcriptional patterns when compared with nonpathogenic hantaviruses, including the induction of stronger proinflammatory responses, which could directly explain some of the features of the clinical syndromes associated with hantavirus infection (106, 107). For instance, the pathogenic Sin Nombre virus induces expression of many more genes in infected HUVECs than the nonpathogenic Prospect Hill virus (175 genes versus 36 genes), including increased expression of CC-chemokines such as CCL5 (RANTES), which can attract leukocytes capable of secreting cytokines (such as TNF-α) that can increase vascular permeability (98, 108). Nonpathogenic hantaviruses trigger an early response of interferon-responsive genes, whereas pathogenic hantaviruses do so later. In particular, the antiviral MxA protein is expressed earlier in HUVECs infected with nonpathogenic viruses. Similarly, in HUVECs, a nonpathogenic hantavirus triggers a rapid upregulation of major histocompatibility complex (MHC) class-I molecules, whereas the response to a pathogenic hantavirus is more gradual (peak levels at 2–3 days postinfection versus 4–5 days postinfection, respectively) (107). Such upregulation is mediated by interferon-beta (IFN-β) as demonstrated by antibody-mediated neutralization of nearly 80% of the response. These data contrasting the kinetics of antiviral mechanisms in endothelial cells infected with pathogenic and nonpathogenic hantaviruses could explain, at least partially, the limited replication of nonpathogenic hantaviruses after infection and the efficient replication of pathogenic hantaviruses (106, 107). The transcriptional response of endothelial cells infected with hantaviruses associated with the renal syndrome and pulmonary syndrome groups is different; it is possible that analysis of the differentially expressed genes may provide clues about the pathogenesis and vascular bed preferences of hantaviruses that infect different vascular beds.

MHC: major histocompatibility complex

Another recent interesting finding is that the pathogenic Hantaan virus does not increase the permeability of HUVECs as determined by an unchanged transmonolayer electrical resistance (TER) and unchanged passive diffusion of bovine serum albumin (109). These observations are in agreement with a previous report (98). Unexpectedly, hantavirus-infected HUVECs respond with prolonged increased permeability to physiological concentrations of TNF-α that could be produced by adherent monocytes (109). In uninfected monolayers of HUVECs, the decreased TER triggered by TNF-α begins to return to control levels at 48 hours and is similar to control levels at 72 hours, whereas infected HUVECs still have a low TER at 96 hours that could be inhibited by neutralizing anti-TNF-α antibodies and that was neither associated with disruption of the monolayer nor decreased cell viability. It was also not associated with nitric oxide, IL-6, or prostaglandin synthesis. These data help reconcile the two hypotheses about the pathogenesis of hantavirus-associated diseases: immunopathogenesis and direct effects of the virus on endothelial cells.

HHV8 and Endothelial Cells

HHV8 causes Kaposi's sarcoma (110, 111), a spindle-cell neoplasm of endothelial origin that is the most frequent neoplasm in patients with AIDS (it is an AIDS-defining illness) and is also a frequent endemic tumor in equatorial Africa. It was originally described as a rare tumor in elderly men of Eastern European origin. In addition, HHV8 is associated with body cavity–based B cell lymphoma (also known as primary effusion lymphoma) (112) and the plasmablastic variant of multicentric Castleman's disease (113). The virus infects peripheral blood mononuclear cells in addition to endothelial cells (114); however, HHV8 attaches to endothelial cells in vitro better than to monocytes and B lymphocytes; this attachment results in infection and transcription of lytic and latent viral genes (115).

vGPCR: viral G protein–coupled receptor

vCyc: viral cyclin

EGFP: enhanced green fluorescent protein

At least two HHV8 products are important in the pathogenesis of Kaposi's sarcoma. One is encoded by open reading frame 74 and consists of a constitutively active viral G protein–coupled receptor (vGPCR) homologous to the CXCL8 receptors CXCR1 and CXCR2 (116, 117). The expression of this vGPCR (which should be transient because it is a lytic gene) may be dysregulated in Kaposi's sarcoma by factors such as other viral infections (e.g., HIV, CMV) or inflammatory stimuli (118). The other viral product is open reading frame 72, which encodes a viral cyclin (vCyc) that inactivates retinoblastoma protein (pRB), a physiological inhibitor of entry into S phase (119, 120). The importance of vGPCR in the pathogenesis of Kaposi's sarcoma was well demonstrated through retroviral gene transfer targeted specifically to the endothelium (121). Transgenic mice that express the avian leukosis virus (ALV) receptor (TVA) under the control of the endothelial-specific *TIE2* promoter were transduced with an ALV vector encoding vGPCR; those animals developed Kaposi's sarcoma-like tumors. Several other candidate genes (including latent genes, such as vCyc, expressed in Kaposi's sarcoma in vivo) were tested, but none of them produced the tumoral phenotype. vGPCR was, however, not expressed in all tumor cells. Moreover, when nude mice were injected with a mixture of endothelial cell lines expressing either vGPCR or the nononcogenic fluorescent protein EGFP (enhanced green fluorescent protein), vascular tumors composed of a mixture of cells expressing either one of these proteins were formed. Furthermore, when the injected mixture consisted of endothelial cells expressing either vGPCR or the latent genes vFLIP and vCyc, mixed cell tumors grew in which most cells were derived from cells expressing the latent genes, thus showing that vGPCR can unmask the tumorigenic potential of other genes that are not oncogenic by themselves. The mechanism triggered by vGPCR is probably paracrine, involving the secretion of VEGF, other cytokines (e.g., IL-6), and angiogenic chemokines (e.g., CCCL5 and CXCL8) (122) through the activation of signaling pathways, particularly Akt (123), that lead to activation of transcription factors NFκB and AP-1 (124). Paracrine recruitment of noninfected endothelial cells is probably important in Kaposi's sarcoma pathogenesis; the lack of HHV8 detection in many tumor cells in human Kaposi's sarcoma is in agreement with this view. Even when vGPCR is expressed only by hematopoietic cells in a transgenic model, the animals develop vascular tumors (125). There are many other viral genes that are hypothesized to participate in the oncogenic process triggered by HHV8; they have been reviewed recently (118) and will not be discussed further here.

Other factors that may play a role in the pathogenesis of Kaposi's sarcoma include stimulation of tumor growth, neoangiogenesis and antiapoptotic mechanisms through CD40 expressed by Kaposi's sarcoma cells (126) (the ligand of CD40, CD154, is expressed by infiltrating leukocytes), downregulation of MHC class-I molecules (127), induction of the c-*kit* gene (encoding the stem cell factor receptor) (128), and promotion of an angiogenic phenotype by IFN-γ secreted from tumor-infiltrating CD8+ T cells (129).

A final interesting aspect of HHV8 infection of endothelial cells is that it induces a phenotype closely related (but not identical) to that of lymphatic endothelial cells. This has been confirmed by oligonucleotide microarray analysis of biopsy samples after the removal of the signal contributed by nontumoral cells (130), and by microarray analysis of human dermal microvascular endothelial cells infected with HHV8 in vitro (131, 132). The gene expression profile of Kaposi's sarcoma samples was more closely related to the profile of lymphatic endothelial cells than vascular endothelial cells. More importantly, in vitro infection of vascular endothelial cells with HHV8 changed the expression profile of these cells to one more closely related to that of lymphatic endothelial cells. Also, infection of lymphatic endothelial cells altered the expression profile of these cells moving it away from that of uninfected lymphatic endothelial cells. In addition, the expression analysis revealed several autocrine growth loops including VEGF-D and its receptor VEGFR3.

Rickettsiae and Endothelial Cells

Rickettsiae are strictly intracellular bacteria that reside free in the cytoplasm of mammalian endothelial cells and many arthropod cells including salivary gland epithelium and ova. They are transmitted by arthropods and cause severe febrile illnesses with systemic multiorgan involvement; cases are frequently fatal even in young immunocompetent individuals if appropriate antibiotics are not administered early (133–135). That is particularly true for tick-transmitted Rocky Mountain spotted fever (caused by *Rickettsia rickettsii*) and louse-borne epidemic typhus (caused by *Rickettsia prowazekii*) (136, 137), whose causative agents are now considered select agents with restricted possession and transfer by the Centers for Disease Control because they can potentially be used as bioweapons (138).

Rickettsiae are divided into two main groups: (*a*) spotted fever group rickettsiae, which include *R. rickettsii* and the agent of boutonneuse fever, *Rickettsia conorii*, among others; and (*b*) typhus group rickettsiae, which include *R. prowazekii* and the agent of murine or endemic typhus, *Rickettsia typhi* (137). The spotted fever group rickettsiae differ from the typhus group rickettsiae in their capacity to stimulate host cell actin polymerization for cell-to-cell movement (139–141), a lipopolysaccharide that is specific for each group (142), and the presence of the rickettsial outer membrane protein A (OmpA) (143). The capacity of the spotted fever group rickettsiae to stimulate polymerization of host cell actin to move directionally within and between cells is mediated by the protein RickA through activation of the host cell complex Arp2/3, which leads to the formation of actin filaments that resemble those of filopodia (144, 145). Surprisingly, that activity does not seem to disrupt the stability of the cytoskeleton and the interendothelial adherens junctions (145a).

Adherens junctions: specialized cellular attachment that links the actin cytoskeleton of two neighboring cells through transmembrane adhesion proteins

A closely related microorganism, *O. tsutsugamushi*, another intracellular bacterium that infects endothelial cells (60), is transmitted by larval trombiculid mites (chiggers) and causes a disease similar to typhus (with the addition of an inoculation eschar and regional lymphadenitis) named scrub typhus, chigger-borne rickettsiosis, or tsutsugamushi disease. This disease occurs in Asia, northern Australia, and adjacent islands of the Pacific and Indian Oceans.

Research in rickettsiology has been advanced by the development of animal models that faithfully replicate most of the clinical, pathological, and immunological characteristics of rickettsioses in humans. They consist of intravenous *R. typhi* infection of C3H/HeN mice for the typhus group rickettsioses (69) and intravenous *R. conorii* infection of C3H/HeN mice for the spotted fever group rickettsioses (68). Two important characteristics of both models are endothelial-target infection (**Figure 2**) and a range of lethal to sublethal infectious doses, the latter stimulating strong protective immunity. In addition, investigations on *Ehrlichia* (formerly *Cowdria*) *ruminantium*, a tick-borne rickettsial pathogen of ruminants that infects endothelial cells and causes heartwater, has the potential to provide clues about the pathogenesis of human rickettsioses because increased capillary permeability is a central feature of this disease, as it is for the human rickettsioses (**Figure 3**). Also, some aspects of the pathogenesis may be common, including endothelial nitric oxide production as an antimicrobial mechanism (146) and the importance of T cell responses in antirickettsial immunity (147).

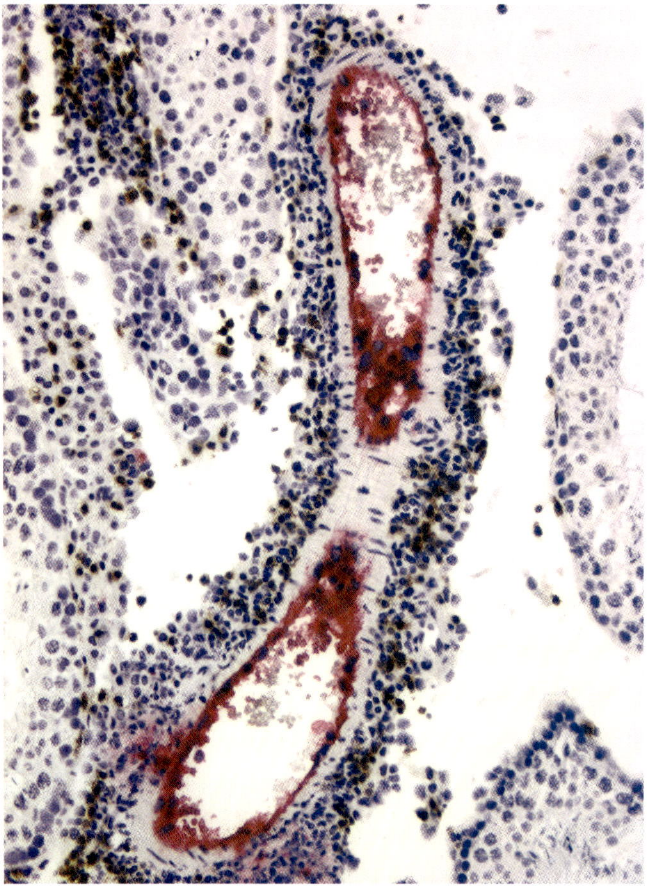

Figure 2

Immunohistochemical detection of *Rickettsia conorii* (*red*) in the endothelium of testes vessels from C3H/HeN mice inoculated with a lethal dose five days earlier. Infiltrating CD8+ T cells are stained brown.

Focal adhesions: specialized cellular attachment that links the actin cytoskeleton to the extracellular matrix through transmembrane adhesion proteins

One of the strategies that rickettsiae use to survive inside infected cells involves the inhibition of endothelial apoptosis (148, 149). This antiapoptotic effect appears to be mediated by rickettsia-triggered NFκB activation (148). In contrast, *O. tsutsugamushi* does not seem to have this effect (150). Moreover, it has been suggested that *O. tsutsugamushi*-triggered apoptosis is a consequence of diminished focal adhesions associated with the infection, although this change is evident only in heavily infected cells, and the mechanistic link has not been established (151).

Endothelial cells become activated upon in vitro rickettsial infection resulting in the secretion of cytokines such as IL-1, IL-6, and CXCL8 (152, 153) and the expression of adhesion molecules such as E-selectin, VCAM-1, and ICAM-1 (154, 155). Such a response may be initiated by direct rickettsia-triggered activation of the transcription factor NFκB (156–158). This is likely the same stimulus of chemokine expression in rickettsial diseases. We have demonstrated, in *R. conorii*–infected C3H/HeN mice, the endothelial expression of the chemokines CCL2, CCL3, CCL4, CCL12, CX3CL1, CXCL9, and CXCL10 in vivo (159, 160). Furthermore, the expression of the T cell chemoattractants CXCL9 and CXCL10 occurs in brain endothelial cells of fatal cases of Rocky Mountain spotted fever (159). Also, *O. tsutsugamushi* infection of an endothelial-like cell line as well as infection of a human dermal microvascular endothelial cell line induce or upregulate the expression of CXCL8, CCL5, and CCL2 (150, 161). These effects can be reproduced by heat-inactivated *O. tsutsugamushi* and are not mediated by NFκB activation in this experimental model; instead, the transcription factor AP-1 is the likely mediator because its binding activity increases upon *Orientia* infection. This finding has been confirmed with HUVECs infected with *O. tsutsugamushi* (162); however, *Orientia* infection of HUVECs also triggers activation of NFκB (although inhibition of this pathway did not affect the chemokine expression). These contrasting outcomes show that results from in vitro models are variable and depend upon multiple factors including origin of the cells (i.e., macrovascular, microvascular, venular, arterial, different organs, etc.), whether such cells are cell lines or primary cultures, and culture conditions.

Intraendothelial rickettsial infection also modulates the endothelial regulatory function on coagulation. In vitro, rickettsial infection of HUVECs results in endothelial synthesis of platelet-activating factor (163), increased secretion of arachidonic acid derivatives such as prostacyclin and PGE2 (164), increased expression of tissue factor (165, 166) and von Willebrand factor (167), increased secretion of plasminogen activator inhibitor-1 (168), and decreased expression of thrombomodulin (167). All these changes fit the laboratory findings in patients with rickettsioses (i.e., consumption of procoagulants and thrombocytopenia) as well as the nonocclusive thrombi (a manifestation of physiological hemostasis) found in autopsy cases. There is a good correlation of these in vitro findings with clinical studies that have been previously evaluated in depth (169).

One aspect that has seldom been investigated in endothelial-target infectious diseases is the mechanism(s) of pathogen clearance from the infected endothelium. The rickettsial model offers interesting answers: Mouse endothelial cell lines can kill rickettsiae after IFN-γ- and TNF-α-induced activation through a mechanism involving nitric oxide synthesis (by inducible nitric oxide synthase, iNOS). This effect was demonstrated by the abrogation of iNOS activity with N^G-monomethyl-L-arginine (N^GMMLA), a nitric oxide synthesis inhibitor (170). The in vivo relevance of this finding is indicated by the overwhelming infection resulting from IFN-γ and/or TNF-α neutralization, which is associated with decreased nitric oxide production and a similar increased growth of rickettsiae in mice treated with N^GMMLA (171). In the mouse endothelial cell line SVEC4–10, hydroxyl radicals, hydrogen peroxide, and limitation of tryptophan availability also contribute to the rickettsicidal effect (172). In HUVECs, part of the antirickettsial effect is due to hydrogen peroxide; moreover, iNOS activity could not be detected in all lots of HUVECs studied (173).

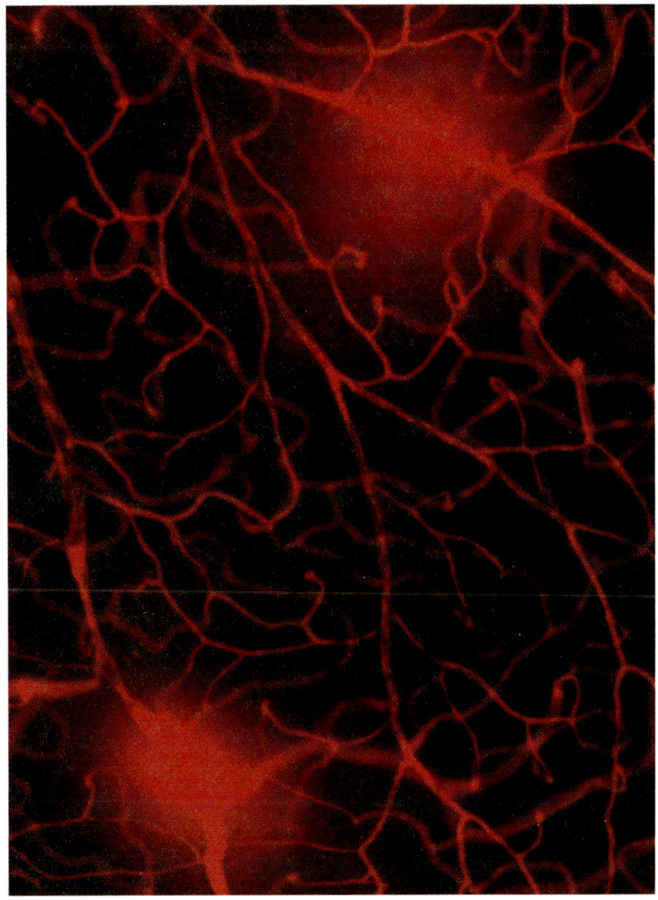

Figure 3

Mouse retinal whole mount preparation five days after inoculation with a lethal dose of *Rickettsia conorii*. Fluorescent detection of Evans blue-bound serum proteins (*red*). Rickettsiae-infected animals show leakage, whereas control animals have an intact blood-retinal barrier (not shown).

PATHOPHYSIOLOGICAL CONSEQUENCES OF ENDOTHELIAL INFECTION

There are common patterns of endothelial response to intracellular infection as assessed mainly by in vitro studies. They include acquisition of a spindled shape with expression of prominent actin stress fibers, increased permeability, activation of the inflammatory response through transcription factors including NFκB, and consequent expression of cytokines, chemokines, and adhesion molecules. Unfortunately, some protein expression data from in vitro studies have motivated in vitro functional studies that may not be relevant to the infection in vivo. For instance, most of the true endothelial infections lead to the in vitro expression of E-selectin, which is an

Antigenic cross-presentation: uptake and processing of antigens from outside the antigen-presenting cell (APC) for presentation in the context of the APC's major histocompatibility complex (MHC) class-I molecules

adhesion molecule important in the recruitment of neutrophils; however, neutrophil infiltration is not a prominent feature of any of these infections in vivo. This again emphasizes the need to confirm the relevance of in vitro findings through the study of human tissue or valid animal models.

The bulk of the infected endothelial cells, particularly those in the microvasculature (arterioles, capillaries, and venules), have frequent close contacts with circulating T cells. This physiological characteristic together with normal human constitutive endothelial expression of MHC class I and class II molecules (only class I for mice) makes endothelial cells uniquely positioned for the function of antigen presentation (174, 175). This aspect has been investigated almost exclusively from the perspective of organ transplants (174, 176) and has not been explored in the more physiological situation of an endothelial-target infection. Such research is important because there is evidence that T cell activation and proliferation is triggered by endothelial antigen presentation (177, 178). In addition, the antigen-presenting function of the endothelium mediates antigen-specific translocation of T cells into the interstitium (179, 180), a mechanism that implies antigenic cross-presentation, and that was demonstrated in other models as well (181).

Although the capacity of endothelial cells to activate secondary (memory) T cell responses has been demonstrated (albeit not in infectious disease models) and is well accepted (174, 175, 182), the debate regarding their ability to stimulate primary immune responses, particularly those of CD8+ T cells (the most important cells in the elimination of intracellular pathogens) is still open. Endothelial cells express various costimulatory molecules through which they can activate primary immune T cell responses (174). In vitro studies reveal that mouse endothelial cells, which use CD80 for costimulation, can activate alloreactive naïve CD8+ T cells, which leads to a phenotype that includes expression of perforin, FAS ligand, and IFN-γ, and IL-2 secretion (183). More importantly, evidence suggests that endothelial cells can activate naïve CD8+ T cells in vivo (183, 184). CD8+ T cells from CBA (H-2K^k) mice that recognize H-2K^b were adoptively transferred into B6 mice (H-2K^b) whose hematopoietic antigen-presenting cells (APCs) had been replaced by APCs expressing H-2K^k MHC class-I molecules (B6-CBA mice). The transferred CD8+ T cells were activated in vivo in a fashion similar to their direct in vitro activation by purified endothelial cells of B6 origin. Furthermore, hearts from B6-CBA mice transplanted into CD4+ T cell–depleted CBA mice were acutely rejected. Interestingly, in SCID/bg mice transplanted with human vessels, purified human T cells are activated and destroy the human endothelial cells but not mouse endothelial cells (185). Unfortunately, the transferred human T cells were not selected to contain only naïve cells, so the relative contribution of memory T cells to that response remains unknown.

CONCLUSIONS

Endothelial-target infections offer a pathophysiologically relevant model to study two important aspects of the immunological mechanisms of the endothelium, namely antigen presentation and antigen-specific interactions with T lymphocytes. These topics have not been investigated adequately from the perspective of microbial pathogens that directly infect the endothelium. Such research will surely offer new insights into the physiology of endothelial immunological functions in general and specifically into the physiology of endothelial antigen presentation and the interaction between endothelial cells and T cells, which have not been revealed by the transplantation model.

SUMMARY POINTS

1. Because endothelial cells line the vasculature, their position allows them to interact with any pathogen that can access the circulating blood and its cells; however, the microorganisms that consistently target endothelial cells are relatively few, namely, Nipah virus, cytomegalovirus, Crimean-Congo hemorrhagic fever virus, hantavirus, HHV8, bartonellae, *O. tsutsugamushi*, and rickettsiae.
2. The infectious agents whose main target is the endothelium are hantaviruses, rickettsiae, *O. tsutsugamushi*, and HHV8.
3. The majority of pathogens causing hemorrhagic diseases do not infect endothelial cells as their main target. Immunopathological mechanisms explain the phenotype of many of these diseases in which endothelial pathophysiology is potentially critical.
4. Phenotypic changes in infected endothelial cells should be correlated with in vivo findings before proceeding with in vitro mechanistic studies. Unfortunately, animal models of endothelial infection exist only for some of these (**Table 1**).
5. Pathophysiological studies on agents such as Nipah virus or Crimean-Congo hemorrhagic fever virus have not been performed, at least in part owing to the scarcity of BSL-4 facilities that are required for these studies.
6. Endothelial infection results in the expression of an inflammatory phenotype that is mediated, at least in part, by the transcription factor NFκB.
7. The role of the infected endothelium in antigen presentation and activation of pathogen-specific primary and secondary T cell specific responses needs to be explored.

FUTURE DIRECTIONS/UNRESOLVED ISSUES

1. Future research should determine the various elements of cellular tropism of endothelium-targeting infectious agents, including the identification of the cellular receptors used by the microbes.
2. It is necessary to develop valid animal models that faithfully replicate the human disease, including target cells and organs, clinical course, biochemical markers, and development of immunity. The use of mice with a reconstituted human immune system as well as human microvessels is particularly promising.
3. Implementation of in vitro experimental systems that include low-passage primary endothelial cells from relevant organs and shear flow would better simulate the physiological characteristics of in vivo infections.
4. The study of endothelial-target infectious agents offers the possibility of developing endothelium-specific vectors that could be used for delivering genes in a cell-specific fashion for therapeutic purposes.

LITERATURE CITED

1. Cines DB, Pollak ES, Buck CA, Loscalzo J, Zimmerman GA, et al. 1998. Endothelial cells in physiology and in the pathophysiology of vascular disorders. *Blood* 91:3527–61
2. Michiels C. 2003. Endothelial cell functions. *J. Cell. Physiol.* 196:430–43
3. Biedermann BC. 2001. Vascular endothelium: checkpoint for inflammation and immunity. *News Physiol. Sci.* 16:84–88
4. Luscinskas FW, Ma S, Nusrat A, Parkos CA, Shaw SK. 2002. The role of endothelial cell lateral junctions during leukocyte trafficking. *Immunol. Rev.* 186:578–67
5. Luscinskas FW, Ma S, Nusrat A, Parkos CA, Shaw SK. 2002. Leukocyte transendothelial migration: a junctional affair. *Semin. Immunol.* 14:105–13
6. **Wang L, Li L, Shojaei F, Levac K, Cerdan C, et al. 2004. Endothelial and hematopoietic cell fate of human embryonic stem cells originates from primitive endothelium with hemangioblastic properties. *Immunity* 21:31–41**

Suggests a common origin for endothelial and hematopoietic cells.

7. Lim YC, Garcia-Cardena G, Allport JR, Zervoglos M, Connolly AJ, et al. 2003. Heterogeneity of endothelial cells from different organ sites in T-cell subset recruitment. *Am. J. Pathol.* 162:1591–601
8. Garlanda C, Dejana E. 1997. Heterogeneity of endothelial cells. Specific markers. *Arterioscler. Thromb. Vasc. Biol.* 17:1193–202
9. **Durr E, Yu J, Krasinska KM, Carver LA, Yates JR, et al. 2004. Direct proteomic mapping of the lung microvascular endothelial cell surface in vivo and in cell culture. *Nat. Biotechnol.* 22:985–92**

Highlights the remarkable phenotypic differences between endothelial cells in culture and in vivo.

10. Chen JP, Cosgriff TM. 2000. Hemorrhagic fever virus-induced changes in hemostasis and vascular biology. *Blood Coagul. Fibrinolysis* 11:461–83
11. Peters CJ, Zaki SR. 2002. Role of the endothelium in viral hemorrhagic fevers. *Crit. Care Med.* 30:S268–73
12. Peters CJ. 2002. Human infection with arenaviruses in the Americas. *Curr. Top. Microbiol. Immunol.* 262:65–74
13. Yang ZY, Duckers HJ, Sullivan NJ, Sanchez A, Nabel EG, Nabel GJ. 2000. Identification of the Ebola virus glycoprotein as the main viral determinant of vascular cell cytotoxicity and injury. *Nat. Med.* 6:886–89
14. Yang ZY, Delgado R, Xu L, Todd RF, Nabel EG, et al. 1998. Distinct cellular interactions of secreted and transmembrane Ebola virus glycoproteins. *Science* 279:1034–37
15. **Geisbert TW, Young HA, Jahrling PB, Davis KJ, Larsen T, et al. 2003. Pathogenesis of Ebola hemorrhagic fever in primate models: evidence that hemorrhage is not a direct effect of virus-induced cytolysis of endothelial cells. *Am. J. Pathol.* 163:2371–82**

Exemplifies how the pathological study of an appropriate animal model at various time points may reveal important issues not shown by postmortem human studies.

16. Zaki SR, Goldsmith CS. 1999. Pathologic features of filovirus infections in humans. *Curr. Top. Microbiol. Immunol.* 235:97–116
17. Cosgriff TM, Morrill JC, Jennings GB, Hodgson LA, Slayter MV, et al. 1989. Hemostatic derangement produced by Rift Valley fever virus in rhesus monkeys. *Rev. Infect. Dis.* 11(Suppl. 4):S807–14
18. **Jessie K, Fong MY, Devi S, Lam SK, Wong KT. 2004. Localization of dengue virus in naturally infected human tissues, by immunohistochemistry and in situ hybridization. *J. Infect. Dis.* 189:1411–18**

Detection of antigen by immunohistochemistry may be explained by other processes besides microorganismal replication.

19. Seternes T, Sorensen K, Smedsrod B. 2002. Scavenger endothelial cells of vertebrates: a nonperipheral leukocyte system for high-capacity elimination of waste macromolecules. *Proc. Natl. Acad. Sci. USA* 99:7594–97

20. Ramos C, Sanchez G, Pando RH, Baquera J, Hernandez D, et al. 1998. Dengue virus in the brain of a fatal case of hemorrhagic dengue fever. *J. Neurovirol.* 4:465–68
21. Saikku P. 2000. Epidemiologic association of *Chlamydia pneumoniae* and atherosclerosis: the initial serologic observation and more. *J. Infect. Dis.* 181(Suppl. 3):S411–13
22. Saikku P, Leinonen M, Mattila K, Ekman MR, Nieminen MS, et al. 1988. Serological evidence of an association of a novel *Chlamydia*, TWAR, with chronic coronary heart disease and acute myocardial infarction. *Lancet* 2:983–86
23. Summersgill JT, Molestina RE, Miller RD, Ramirez JA. 2000. Interactions of *Chlamydia pneumoniae* with human endothelial cells. *J. Infect. Dis.* 181(Suppl. 3):S479–82
24. Kuo C, Campbell LA. 2000. Detection of *Chlamydia pneumoniae* in arterial tissues. *J. Infect. Dis.* 181(Suppl. 3):S432–36
25. Kuo CC, Grayston JT, Campbell LA, Goo YA, Wissler RW, Benditt EP. 1995. *Chlamydia pneumoniae* (TWAR) in coronary arteries of young adults (15–34 years old). *Proc. Natl. Acad. Sci. USA* 92:6911–14
26. Kuo CC, Shor A, Campbell LA, Fukushi H, Patton DL, Grayston JT. 1993. Demonstration of *Chlamydia pneumoniae* in atherosclerotic lesions of coronary arteries. *J. Infect. Dis.* 167:841–49
27. Ong G, Thomas BJ, Mansfield AO, Davidson BR, Taylor-Robinson D. 1996. Detection and widespread distribution of *Chlamydia pneumoniae* in the vascular system and its possible implications. *J. Clin. Pathol.* 49:102–6
28. Shor A, Kuo CC, Patton DL. 1992. Detection of *Chlamydia pneumoniae* in coronary arterial fatty streaks and atheromatous plaques. *S. Afr. Med. J.* 82:158–61
29. Kuo CC, Gown AM, Benditt EP, Grayston JT. 1993. Detection of *Chlamydia pneumoniae* in aortic lesions of atherosclerosis by immunocytochemical stain. *Arterioscler. Thromb.* 13:1501–4
30. Campbell LA, O'Brien ER, Cappuccio AL, Kuo CC, Wang SP, et al. 1995. Detection of *Chlamydia pneumoniae* TWAR in human coronary atherectomy tissues. *J. Infect. Dis.* 172:585–88
31. Shor A, Phillips JI, Ong G, Thomas BJ, Taylor-Robinson D. 1998. *Chlamydia pneumoniae* in atheroma: consideration of criteria for causality. *J. Clin. Pathol.* 51:812–17
32. Juvonen J, Juvonen T, Laurila A, Alakarppa H, Lounatmaa K, et al. 1997. Demonstration of *Chlamydia pneumoniae* in the walls of abdominal aortic aneurysms. *J. Vasc. Surg.* 25:499–505
33. Muhlestein JB, Hammond EH, Carlquist JF, Radicke E, Thomson MJ, et al. 1996. Increased incidence of *Chlamydia* species within the coronary arteries of patients with symptomatic atherosclerotic versus other forms of cardiovascular disease. *J. Am. Coll. Cardiol.* 27:1555–61
34. Ouchi K, Fujii B, Kudo S, Shirai M, Yamashita K, et al. 2000. *Chlamydia pneumoniae* in atherosclerotic and nonatherosclerotic tissue. *J. Infect. Dis.* 181(Suppl. 3):S441–43
35. Hoymans VY, Bosmans JM, Ursi D, Martinet W, Wuyts FL, et al. 2004. Immunohistostaining assays for detection of *Chlamydia pneumoniae* in atherosclerotic arteries indicate cross-reactions with nonchlamydial plaque constituents. *J. Clin. Microbiol.* 42:3219–24
36. Blasi F, Fagetti L, Allegra L. 2000. *Chlamydia pneumoniae* detection in atherosclerotic plaques in Italy. *J. Infect. Dis.* 181(Suppl. 3):S444–46
37. Petrogiannis-Haliotis T, Sakoulas G, Kirby J, Koralnik IJ, Dvorak AM, et al. 2001. BK-related polyomavirus vasculopathy in a renal-transplant recipient. *N. Engl. J. Med.* 345:1250–55

38. Ressetar HG, Webster HD, Stoner GL. 1992. Brain vascular endothelial cells express JC virus large tumor antigen in immunocompetent and cyclophosphamide-treated hamsters. *Proc. Natl. Acad. Sci. USA* 89:8170–74
39. Guarner J, Greer PW, Bartlett J, Chu MC, Shieh WJ, Zaki SR. 1999. Immunohistochemical detection of *Francisella tularensis* in formalin-fixed paraffin-embedded tissue. *Appl. Immunohistochem. Mol. Morphol.* 7:122–26
40. Forestal CA, Benach JL, Carbonara C, Italo JK, Lisinski TJ, Furie MB. 2003. *Francisella tularensis* selectively induces proinflammatory changes in endothelial cells. *J. Immunol.* 171:2563–70
41. Fortier AH, Green SJ, Polsinelli T, Jones TR, Crawford RM, et al. 1994. Life and death of an intracellular pathogen: *Francisella tularensis* and the macrophage. *Immunol. Ser.* 60:349–61
42. Vazquez-Boland JA, Kuhn M, Berche P, Chakraborty T, Dominguez-Bernal G, et al. 2001. Listeria pathogenesis and molecular virulence determinants. *Clin. Microbiol. Rev.* 14:584–640
43. Kirk J. 1993. Diagnostic ultrastructure of *Listeria monocytogenes* in human central nervous tissue. *Ultrastruct. Pathol.* 17:583–92
44. Kim KS. 2001. *Escherichia coli* translocation at the blood-brain barrier. *Infect. Immun.* 69:5217–22
45. Kim KS. 2003. Pathogenesis of bacterial meningitis: from bacteraemia to neuronal injury. *Nat. Rev. Neurosci.* 4:376–85
46. Tosato G, Jones K, Breinig MK, McWilliams HP, McKnight JL. 1993. Interleukin-6 production in posttransplant lymphoproliferative disease. *J. Clin. Invest.* 91:2806–14
47. Jones K, Rivera C, Sgadari C, Franklin J, Max EE, et al. 1995. Infection of human endothelial cells with Epstein-Barr virus. *J. Exp. Med.* 182:1213–21
48. Xiong A, Clarke-Katzenberg RH, Valenzuela G, Izumi KM, Millan MT. 2004. Epstein-Barr virus latent membrane protein 1 activates nuclear factor-kappa B in human endothelial cells and inhibits apoptosis. *Transplantation* 78:41–49
49. Millan MT, Natkunam Y, Clarke-Katzenberg R, Desai D, Prapong W, et al. 2002. Epstein-Barr virus infection is associated with endothelial Bcl-2 expression in transplant liver allografts. *Transplantation* 73:465–69
50. **Wong KT, Shieh WJ, Kumar S, Norain K, Abdullah W, et al. 2002. Nipah virus infection: pathology and pathogenesis of an emerging paramyxoviral zoonosis. *Am. J. Pathol.* 161:2153–67**

Highlights the importance of pathology techniques for the study of emerging infectious diseases.

51. Percivalle E, Revello MG, Vago L, Morini F, Gerna G. 1993. Circulating endothelial giant cells permissive for human cytomegalovirus (HCMV) are detected in disseminated HCMV infections with organ involvement. *J. Clin. Invest.* 92:663–70
52. Grefte A, Blom N, van der Giessen M, van Son W, The TH. 1993. Ultrastructural analysis of circulating cytomegalic cells in patients with active cytomegalovirus infection: evidence for virus production and endothelial origin. *J. Infect. Dis.* 168:1110–18
53. Grefte A, van der Giessen M, van Son W, The TH. 1993. Circulating cytomegalovirus (CMV)-infected endothelial cells in patients with an active CMV infection. *J. Infect. Dis.* 167:270–77
54. Burt FJ, Swanepoel R, Shieh WJ, Smith JF, Leman PA, et al. 1997. Immunohistochemical and in situ localization of Crimean-Congo hemorrhagic fever (CCHF) virus in human tissues and implications for CCHF pathogenesis. *Arch. Pathol. Lab. Med.* 121:839–46

55. Zaki SR, Greer PW, Coffield LM, Goldsmith CS, Nolte KB, et al. 1995. Hantavirus pulmonary syndrome. Pathogenesis of an emerging infectious disease. *Am. J. Pathol.* 146:552–79
56. Milazzo ML, Eyzaguirre EJ, Molina CP, Fulhorst CF. 2002. Maporal viral infection in the Syrian golden hamster: a model of hantavirus pulmonary syndrome. *J. Infect. Dis.* 186:1390–95
57. Boshoff C, Schulz TF, Kennedy MM, Graham AK, Fisher C, et al. 1995. Kaposi's sarcoma-associated herpesvirus infects endothelial and spindle cells. *Nat. Med.* 1:1274–78
58. Li JJ, Huang YQ, Cockerell CJ, Friedman-Kien AE. 1996. Localization of human herpes-like virus type 8 in vascular endothelial cells and perivascular spindle-shaped cells of Kaposi's sarcoma lesions by in situ hybridization. *Am. J. Pathol.* 148:1741–48
59. Arias-Stella J, Lieberman PH, Erlandson RA, Arias-Stella J Jr. 1986. Histology, immunohistochemistry, and ultrastructure of the verruga in Carrion's disease. *Am. J. Surg. Pathol.* 10:595–610
60. Moron CG, Popov VL, Feng HM, Wear D, Walker DH. 2001. Identification of the target cells of *Orientia tsutsugamushi* in human cases of scrub typhus. *Mod. Pathol.* 14:752–59
61. Walker DH, Harrison A, Henderson F, Murphy FA. 1977. Identification of *Rickettsia rickettsii* in a guinea pig model by immunofluorescent and electron microscopic techniques. *Am. J. Pathol.* 86:343–58
62. Kim J, Smith KJ, Naefie R, Skelton H. 2004. Histopathologic features of and lymphoid populations in the skin of patients with the spotted fever group of rickettsiae: southern Africa. *Int. J. Dermatol.* 43:188–94
63. Walker DH, Crawford CG, Cain BG. 1980. Rickettsial infection of the pulmonary microcirculation: the basis for interstitial pneumonitis in Rocky Mountain spotted fever. *Hum. Pathol.* 11:263–72
64. Moe JB, Ruch GL, Kenyon RH, Burek JD, Stookey JL. 1976. Pathology of experimental Rocky Mountain spotted fever in rhesus monkeys. *Vet. Pathol.* 13:69–77
65. Moe JB, Mosher DF, Kenyon RH, White JD, Stookey JL, et al. 1976. Functional and morphologic changes during experimental Rocky Mountain spotted fever in guinea pigs. *Lab. Invest.* 35:235–45
66. Bradford WD, Croker BP, Tisher CC. 1979. Kidney lesions in Rocky Mountain spotted fever: a light-, immunofluorescence-, and electron-microscopic study. *Am. J. Pathol.* 97:381–92
67. Walker DH, Parks FM, Betz TG, Taylor JP, Muehlberger JW. 1989. Histopathology and immunohistologic demonstration of the distribution of *Rickettsia typhi* in fatal murine typhus. *Am. J. Clin. Pathol.* 91:720–24
68. **Walker DH, Popov VL, Wen J, Feng HM. 1994. *Rickettsia conorii* infection of C3H/HeN mice. A model of endothelial-target rickettsiosis. *Lab. Invest.* 70:358–68**

Description of one of the best animal models of an endothelial-target infection to date.

69. Walker DH, Popov VL, Feng HM. 2000. Establishment of a novel endothelial target mouse model of a typhus group rickettsiosis: evidence for critical roles for gamma interferon and CD8 T lymphocytes. *Lab. Invest.* 80:1361–72
70. Murphy FA, Buchmeier MJ, Rawls WE. 1977. The reticuloendothelium as the target in a virus infection. Pichinde virus pathogenesis in two strains of hamsters. *Lab. Invest.* 37:502–15

71. Gonzalez PH, Laguens RP, Frigerio MJ, Calello MA, Weissenbacher MC. 1983. Junin virus infection of *Callithrix jacchus*: pathologic features. *Am. J. Trop. Med. Hyg.* 32:417–23
72. Myerson D, Hackman RC, Nelson JA, Ward DC, McDougall JK. 1984. Widespread presence of histologically occult cytomegalovirus. *Hum. Pathol.* 15:430–39
73. Sinzger C, Grefte A, Plachter B, Gouw AS, The TH, Jahn G. 1995. Fibroblasts, epithelial cells, endothelial cells and smooth muscle cells are major targets of human cytomegalovirus infection in lung and gastrointestinal tissues. *J. Gen. Virol.* 76:741–50
74. Brune W, Menard C, Heesemann J, Koszinowski UH. 2001. A ribonucleotide reductase homolog of cytomegalovirus and endothelial cell tropism. *Science* 291:303–5
75. Reeves MB, Coleman H, Chadderton J, Goddard M, Sissons JG, Sinclair JH. 2004. Vascular endothelial and smooth muscle cells are unlikely to be major sites of latency of human cytomegalovirus in vivo. *J. Gen. Virol.* 85:3337–41
76. Ricotta D, Alessandri G, Pollara C, Fiorentini S, Favilli F, et al. 2001. Adult human heart microvascular endothelial cells are permissive for non-lytic infection by human cytomegalovirus. *Cardiovasc. Res.* 49:440–48
77. Guetta E, Scarpati EM, DiCorleto PE. 2001. Effect of cytomegalovirus immediate early gene products on endothelial cell gene activity. *Cardiovasc. Res.* 50:538–46
78. Epstein SE, Speir E, Zhou YF, Guetta E, Leon M, Finkel T. 1996. The role of infection in restenosis and atherosclerosis: focus on cytomegalovirus. *Lancet* 348(Suppl. 1):S13–17
79. Dehio C, Meyer M, Berger J, Schwarz H, Lanz C. 1997. Interaction of *Bartonella henselae* with endothelial cells results in bacterial aggregation on the cell surface and the subsequent engulfment and internalisation of the bacterial aggregate by a unique structure, the invasome. *J. Cell Sci.* 110:2141–54
80. Reed JA, Brigati DJ, Flynn SD, McNutt NS, Min KW, et al. 1992. Immunocytochemical identification of *Rochalimaea henselae* in bacillary (epithelioid) angiomatosis, parenchymal bacillary peliosis, and persistent fever with bacteremia. *Am. J. Surg. Pathol.* 16:650–57
81. Brouqui P, Raoult D. 1996. *Bartonella quintana* invades and multiplies within endothelial cells in vitro and in vivo and forms intracellular blebs. *Res. Microbiol.* 147:719–31
82. Manders SM. 1996. Bacillary angiomatosis. *Clin. Dermatol.* 14:295–99
83. Garcia FU, Wojta J, Broadley KN, Davidson JM, Hoover RL. 1990. *Bartonella bacilliformis* stimulates endothelial cells in vitro and is angiogenic in vivo. *Am. J. Pathol.* 136:1125–35
84. Maeno N, Oda H, Yoshiie K, Wahid MR, Fujimura T, Matayoshi S. 1999. Live *Bartonella henselae* enhances endothelial cell proliferation without direct contact. *Microb. Pathog.* 27:419–27
85. Kirby JE, Nekorchuk DM. 2002. Bartonella-associated endothelial proliferation depends on inhibition of apoptosis. *Proc. Natl. Acad. Sci. USA* 99:4656–61
86. Riess T, Andersson SG, Lupas A, Schaller M, Schafer A, et al. 2004. Bartonella adhesin A mediates a proangiogenic host cell response. *J. Exp. Med.* 200:1267–78
87. Kempf VA, Volkmann B, Schaller M, Sander CA, Alitalo K, et al. 2001. Evidence of a leading role for VEGF in *Bartonella henselae*-induced endothelial cell proliferations. *Cell. Microbiol.* 3:623–32
88. Cerimele F, Brown LF, Bravo F, Ihler GM, Kouadio P, Arbiser JL. 2003. Infectious angiogenesis: *Bartonella bacilliformis* infection results in endothelial production of angiopoietin-2 and epidermal production of vascular endothelial growth factor. *Am. J. Pathol.* 163:1321–27
89. Resto-Ruiz SI, Schmiederer M, Sweger D, Newton C, Klein TW, et al. 2002. Induction of a potential paracrine angiogenic loop between human THP-1 macrophages and

human microvascular endothelial cells during *Bartonella henselae* infection. *Infect. Immun.* 70:4564–70
90. Minnick MF, Smitherman LS, Samuels DS. 2003. Mitogenic effect of *Bartonella bacilliformis* on human vascular endothelial cells and involvement of GroEL. *Infect. Immun.* 71:6933–42
91. Kirby JE. 2004. In vitro model of *Bartonella henselae*-induced angiogenesis. *Infect. Immun.* 72:7315–17
92. Fuhrmann O, Arvand M, Gohler A, Schmid M, Krull M, et al. 2001. *Bartonella henselae* induces NF-kappaB-dependent upregulation of adhesion molecules in cultured human endothelial cells: possible role of outer membrane proteins as pathogenic factors. *Infect. Immun.* 69:5088–97
93. Maeno N, Yoshiie K, Matayoshi S, Fujimura T, Mao S, et al. 2002. A heat-stable component of *Bartonella henselae* upregulates intercellular adhesion molecule-1 expression on vascular endothelial cells. *Scand. J. Immunol.* 55:366–72
94. Schmiederer M, Arcenas R, Widen R, Valkov N, Anderson B. 2001. Intracellular induction of the *Bartonella henselae* virB operon by human endothelial cells. *Infect. Immun.* 69:6495–502
95. Schmid MC, Schulein R, Dehio M, Denecker G, Carena I, Dehio C. 2004. The VirB type IV secretion system of *Bartonella henselae* mediates invasion, proinflammatory activation and antiapoptotic protection of endothelial cells. *Mol. Microbiol.* 52:81–92
96. Dehio C. 2004. Molecular and cellular basis of bartonella pathogenesis. *Annu. Rev. Microbiol.* 58:365–90
97. Yanagihara R, Silverman DJ. 1990. Experimental infection of human vascular endothelial cells by pathogenic and nonpathogenic hantaviruses. *Arch. Virol.* 111:281–86
98. Sundstrom JB, McMullan LK, Spiropoulou CF, Hooper WC, Ansari AA, et al. 2001. Hantavirus infection induces the expression of RANTES and IP-10 without causing increased permeability in human lung microvascular endothelial cells. *J. Virol.* 75:6070–85
99. Khaiboullina SF, St Jeor SC. 2002. Hantavirus immunology. *Viral Immunol.* 15:609–25
100. Peters CJ, Simpson GL, Levy H. 1999. Spectrum of hantavirus infection: hemorrhagic fever with renal syndrome and hantavirus pulmonary syndrome. *Annu. Rev. Med.* 50:531–45
101. Gavrilovskaya IN, Peresleni T, Geimonen E, Mackow ER. 2002. Pathogenic hantaviruses selectively inhibit beta3 integrin directed endothelial cell migration. *Arch. Virol.* 147:1913–31
102. Gavrilovskaya IN, Brown EJ, Ginsberg MH, Mackow ER. 1999. Cellular entry of hantaviruses which cause hemorrhagic fever with renal syndrome is mediated by beta3 integrins. *J. Virol.* 73:3951–59
103. Gavrilovskaya IN, Shepley M, Shaw R, Ginsberg MH, Mackow ER. 1998. beta3 Integrins mediate the cellular entry of hantaviruses that cause respiratory failure. *Proc. Natl. Acad. Sci. USA* 95:7074–79
104. Tsukada H, Ying X, Fu C, Ishikawa S, McKeown-Longo P, et al. 1995. Ligation of endothelial alpha v beta 3 integrin increases capillary hydraulic conductivity of rat lung. *Circ. Res.* 77:651–59
105. Hodivala-Dilke KM, McHugh KP, Tsakiris DA, Rayburn H, Crowley D, et al. 1999. Beta3-integrin-deficient mice are a model for Glanzmann thrombasthenia showing placental defects and reduced survival. *J. Clin. Invest.* 103:229–38

Reveals the power of genome-age techniques such as oligonucleotide microarrays for the study of infectious diseases.

Exemplifies and illustrates the power of modern in vivo techniques that use genetically modified animals.

106. Geimonen E, Neff S, Raymond T, Kocer SS, Gavrilovskaya IN, Mackow ER. 2002. Pathogenic and nonpathogenic hantaviruses differentially regulate endothelial cell responses. *Proc. Natl. Acad. Sci. USA* 99:13837–42

107. Kraus AA, Raftery MJ, Giese T, Ulrich R, Zawatzky R, et al. 2004. Differential antiviral response of endothelial cells after infection with pathogenic and nonpathogenic hantaviruses. *J. Virol.* 78:6143–50

108. Khaiboullina SF, Rizvanov AA, Otteson E, Miyazato A, Maciejewski J, St Jeor S. 2004. Regulation of cellular gene expression in endothelial cells by Sin Nombre and Prospect Hill viruses. *Viral Immunol.* 17:234–51

109. Niikura M, Maeda A, Ikegami T, Saijo M, Kurane I, Morikawa S. 2004. Modification of endothelial cell functions by Hantaan virus infection: prolonged hyper-permeability induced by TNF-alpha of Hantaan virus-infected endothelial cell monolayers. *Arch. Virol.* 149:1279–92

110. Chang Y, Cesarman E, Pessin MS, Lee F, Culpepper J, et al. 1994. Identification of herpesvirus-like DNA sequences in AIDS-associated Kaposi's sarcoma. *Science* 266:1865–69

111. Dictor M, Rambech E, Way D, Witte M, Bendsoe N. 1996. Human herpesvirus 8 (Kaposi's sarcoma-associated herpesvirus) DNA in Kaposi's sarcoma lesions, AIDS Kaposi's sarcoma cell lines, endothelial Kaposi's sarcoma simulators, and the skin of immunosuppressed patients. *Am. J. Pathol.* 148:2009–16

112. Cesarman E, Chang Y, Moore PS, Said JW, Knowles DM. 1995. Kaposi's sarcoma-associated herpesvirus-like DNA sequences in AIDS-related body-cavity-based lymphomas. *N. Engl. J. Med.* 332:1186–91

113. Soulier J, Grollet L, Oksenhendler E, Cacoub P, Cazals-Hatem D, et al. 1995. Kaposi's sarcoma-associated herpesvirus-like DNA sequences in multicentric Castleman's disease. *Blood* 86:1276–80

114. Whitby D, Howard MR, Tenant-Flowers M, Brink NS, Copas A, et al. 1995. Detection of Kaposi sarcoma associated herpesvirus in peripheral blood of HIV-infected individuals and progression to Kaposi's sarcoma. *Lancet* 346:799–802

115. Dezube BJ, Zambela M, Sage DR, Wang JF, Fingeroth JD. 2002. Characterization of Kaposi sarcoma-associated herpesvirus/human herpesvirus-8 infection of human vascular endothelial cells: early events. *Blood* 100:888–96

116. Bais C, Santomasso B, Coso O, Arvanitakis L, Raaka EG, et al. 1998. G-protein-coupled receptor of Kaposi's sarcoma-associated herpesvirus is a viral oncogene and angiogenesis activator. *Nature* 391:86–89

117. Arvanitakis L, Geras-Raaka E, Varma A, Gershengorn MC, Cesarman E. 1997. Human herpesvirus KSHV encodes a constitutively active G-protein-coupled receptor linked to cell proliferation. *Nature* 385:347–50

118. Sodhi A, Montaner S, Gutkind JS. 2004. Does dysregulated expression of a deregulated viral GPCR trigger Kaposi's sarcomagenesis? *FASEB J.* 18:422–27

119. Chang Y, Moore PS, Talbot SJ, Boshoff CH, Zarkowska T, et al. 1996. Cyclin encoded by KS herpesvirus. *Nature* 382:410

120. Godden-Kent D, Talbot SJ, Boshoff C, Chang Y, Moore P, et al. 1997. The cyclin encoded by Kaposi's sarcoma-associated herpesvirus stimulates cdk6 to phosphorylate the retinoblastoma protein and histone H1. *J. Virol.* 71:4193–98

121. Montaner S, Sodhi A, Molinolo A, Bugge TH, Sawai ET, et al. 2003. Endothelial infection with KSHV genes in vivo reveals that vGPCR initiates Kaposi's

sarcomagenesis and can promote the tumorigenic potential of viral latent genes. *Cancer Cell* 3:23–36

122. Pati S, Cavrois M, Guo HG, Foulke JS Jr, Kim J, et al. 2001. Activation of NF-kappaB by the human herpesvirus 8 chemokine receptor ORF74: evidence for a paracrine model of Kaposi's sarcoma pathogenesis. *J. Virol.* 75:8660–73
123. Sodhi A, Montaner S, Patel V, Gomez-Roman JJ, Li Y, et al. 2004. Akt plays a central role in sarcomagenesis induced by Kaposi's sarcoma herpesvirus-encoded G protein–coupled receptor. *Proc. Natl. Acad. Sci. USA* 101:4821–26
124. Schwarz M, Murphy PM. 2001. Kaposi's sarcoma-associated herpesvirus G protein-coupled receptor constitutively activates NF-kappa B and induces proinflammatory cytokine and chemokine production via a C-terminal signaling determinant. *J. Immunol.* 167:505–13
125. Yang TY, Chen SC, Leach MW, Manfra D, Homey B, et al. 2000. Transgenic expression of the chemokine receptor encoded by human herpesvirus 8 induces an angioproliferative disease resembling Kaposi's sarcoma. *J. Exp. Med.* 191:445–54
126. Biancone L, Cantaluppi V, Boccellino M, Del Sorbo L, Russo S, et al. 1999. Activation of CD40 favors the growth and vascularization of Kaposi's sarcoma. *J. Immunol.* 163:6201–8
127. Tomescu C, Law WK, Kedes DH. 2003. Surface downregulation of major histocompatibility complex class I, PE-CAM, and ICAM-1 following de novo infection of endothelial cells with Kaposi's sarcoma-associated herpesvirus. *J. Virol.* 77:9669–84
128. Moses AV, Jarvis MA, Raggo C, Bell YC, Ruhl R, et al. 2002. Kaposi's sarcoma-associated herpesvirus-induced upregulation of the c-kit proto-oncogene, as identified by gene expression profiling, is essential for the transformation of endothelial cells. *J. Virol.* 76:8383–99
129. Fiorelli V, Gendelman R, Sirianni MC, Chang HK, Colombini S, et al. 1998. Gamma-interferon produced by CD8+ T cells infiltrating Kaposi's sarcoma induces spindle cells with angiogenic phenotype and synergy with human immunodeficiency virus-1 Tat protein: an immune response to human herpesvirus-8 infection? *Blood* 91:956–67
130. Wang HW, Trotter MW, Lagos D, Bourboulia D, Henderson S, et al. 2004. Kaposi sarcoma herpesvirus-induced cellular reprogramming contributes to the lymphatic endothelial gene expression in Kaposi sarcoma. *Nat. Genet.* 36:687–93
131. Hong YK, Foreman K, Shin JW, Hirakawa S, Curry CL, et al. 2004. Lymphatic reprogramming of blood vascular endothelium by Kaposi sarcoma-associated herpesvirus. *Nat. Genet.* 36:683–85
132. Carroll PA, Brazeau E, Lagunoff M. 2004. Kaposi's sarcoma-associated herpesvirus infection of blood endothelial cells induces lymphatic differentiation. *Virology* 328:7–18
133. Centers for Disease Control and Prevention. 2004. Fatal cases of Rocky Mountain spotted fever in family clusters—three states, 2003. *MMWR* 53:407–10
134. Paddock CD, Greer PW, Ferebee TL, Singleton J Jr, McKechnie DB, et al. 1999. Hidden mortality attributable to Rocky Mountain spotted fever: immunohistochemical detection of fatal, serologically unconfirmed disease. *J. Infect. Dis.* 179:1469–76
135. Paddock CD, Holman RC, Krebs JW, Childs JE. 2002. Assessing the magnitude of fatal Rocky Mountain spotted fever in the United States: comparison of two national data sources. *Am. J. Trop. Med. Hyg.* 67:349–54
136. Walker DH. 2001. Typhus group rickettsioses. In *Essentials of Tropical Infectious Diseases*, ed. RL Guerrant, DH Walker, PF Weller, pp. 274–78. New York: Churchill Livingstone

137. Walker DH, Bouyer DH. 2003. Rickettsia. In *Manual of Clinical Microbiology*, ed. PL Murray, EJ Baron, JH Jorgensen, MA Pfaller, RH Yolken, pp. 1005–14. Washington, DC: ASM

138. Walker DH. 2003. Principles of the malicious use of infectious agents to create terror: reasons for concern for organisms of the genus *Rickettsia*. *Ann. NY Acad. Sci.* 990:739–42

139. Heinzen RA, Hayes SF, Peacock MG, Hackstadt T. 1993. Directional actin polymerization associated with spotted fever group rickettsia infection of Vero cells. *Infect. Immun.* 61:1926–35

140. Heinzen RA, Grieshaber SS, Van Kirk LS, Devin CJ. 1999. Dynamics of actin-based movement by *Rickettsia rickettsii* in Vero cells. *Infect. Immun.* 67:4201–7

141. Van Kirk LS, Hayes SF, Heinzen RA. 2000. Ultrastructure of *Rickettsia rickettsii* actin tails and localization of cytoskeletal proteins. *Infect. Immun.* 68:4706–13

142. Vishwanath S. 1991. Antigenic relationships among the rickettsiae of the spotted fever and typhus groups. *FEMS Microbiol. Lett.* 65:341–44

143. Hackstadt T. 1996. The biology of rickettsiae. *Infect. Agents Dis.* 5:127–43

144. Gouin E, Egile C, Dehoux P, Villiers V, Adams J, et al. 2004. The RickA protein of *Rickettsia conorii* activates the Arp2/3 complex. *Nature* 427:457–61

Explains the mechanisms of intracellular movement of spotted fever group rickettsiae while providing new tools for the study of cytoskeletal physiological processes.

145. Jeng RL, Goley ED, D'Alessio JA, Chaga OY, Svitkina TM, et al. 2004. A *Rickettsia* WASP-like protein activates the Arp2/3 complex and mediates actin-based motility. *Cell. Microbiol.* 6:761–69

145a. Valbuena G, Walker DH. 2005. Changes in the adherens junctions of human endothelial cells infected with spotted fever group rickettsiae. *Virchows Archiv.* 446:379–82

146. Mutunga M, Preston PM, Sumption KJ. 1998. Nitric oxide is produced by *Cowdria ruminantium*-infected bovine pulmonary endothelial cells in vitro and is stimulated by gamma interferon. *Infect. Immun.* 66:2115–21

147. Mwangi DM, Mahan SM, Nyanjui JK, Taracha EL, McKeever DJ. 1998. Immunization of cattle by infection with *Cowdria ruminantium* elicits T lymphocytes that recognize autologous, infected endothelial cells and monocytes. *Infect. Immun.* 66:1855–60

148. Clifton DR, Goss RA, Sahni SK, van Antwerp D, Baggs RB, et al. 1998. NF-kappa B-dependent inhibition of apoptosis is essential for host cell survival during *Rickettsia rickettsii* infection. *Proc. Natl. Acad. Sci. USA* 95:4646–51

149. Joshi SG, Francis CW, Silverman DJ, Sahni SK. 2003. Nuclear factor kappa B protects against host cell apoptosis during *Rickettsia rickettsii* infection by inhibiting activation of apical and effector caspases and maintaining mitochondrial integrity. *Infect. Immun.* 71:4127–36

150. Kim MK, Kee SH, Cho KA, Chung MH, Lim BU, et al. 1999. Apoptosis of endothelial cell line ECV304 persistently infected with *Orientia tsutsugamushi*. *Microbiol. Immunol.* 43:751–57

151. Kee SH, Cho KA, Kim MK, Lim BU, Chang WH, Kang JS. 1999. Disassembly of focal adhesions during apoptosis of endothelial cell line ECV304 infected with *Orientia tsutsugamushi*. *Microb. Pathog.* 27:265–71

152. Sporn LA, Marder VJ. 1996. Interleukin-1 alpha production during *Rickettsia rickettsii* infection of cultured endothelial cells: potential role in autocrine cell stimulation. *Infect. Immun.* 64:1609–13

153. Kaplanski G, Teysseire N, Farnarier C, Kaplanski S, Lissitzky JC, et al. 1995. IL-6 and IL-8 production from cultured human endothelial cells stimulated by infection with *Rickettsia conorii* via a cell-associated IL-1 alpha-dependent pathway. *J. Clin. Invest.* 96:2839–44

154. Sporn LA, Lawrence SO, Silverman DJ, Marder VJ. 1993. E-selectin-dependent neutrophil adhesion to *Rickettsia rickettsii*-infected endothelial cells. *Blood* 81:2406–12
155. Dignat-George F, Teysseire N, Mutin M, Bardin N, Lesaule G, et al. 1997. *Rickettsia conorii* infection enhances vascular cell adhesion molecule-1- and intercellular adhesion molecule-1-dependent mononuclear cell adherence to endothelial cells. *J. Infect. Dis.* 175:1142–52
156. Sahni SK, Van Antwerp DJ, Eremeeva ME, Silverman DJ, Marder VJ, Sporn LA. 1998. Proteasome-independent activation of nuclear factor kappaB in cytoplasmic extracts from human endothelial cells by *Rickettsia rickettsii*. *Infect. Immun.* 66:1827–33
157. Sahni SK, Rydkina E, Joshi SG, Sporn LA, Silverman DJ. 2003. Interactions of *Rickettsia rickettsii* with endothelial nuclear factor-kappaB in a "cell-free" system. *Ann. NY Acad. Sci.* 990:635–41
158. Sporn LA, Sahni SK, Lerner NB, Marder VJ, Silverman DJ, et al. 1997. *Rickettsia rickettsii* infection of cultured human endothelial cells induces NF-kappaB activation. *Infect. Immun.* 65:2786–91
159. Valbuena G, Bradford W, Walker DH. 2003. Expression analysis of the T-cell-targeting chemokines CXCL9 and CXCL10 in mice and humans with endothelial infections caused by rickettsiae of the spotted fever group. *Am. J. Pathol.* 163:1357–69
160. Valbuena G, Walker DH. 2004. Expression of CX3CL1 (fractalkine) in mice with endothelial-target rickettsial infection of the spotted-fever group. *Virchows Arch.* 446:21–27
161. Cho NH, Seong SY, Choi MS, Kim IS. 2001. Expression of chemokine genes in human dermal microvascular endothelial cell lines infected with *Orientia tsutsugamushi*. *Infect. Immun.* 69:1265–72
162. Cho NH, Seong SY, Huh MS, Kim NH, Choi MS, Kim IS. 2002. Induction of the gene encoding macrophage chemoattractant protein 1 by *Orientia tsutsugamushi* in human endothelial cells involves activation of transcription factor activator protein 1. *Infect. Immun.* 70:4841–50
163. Walker TS, Mellott GE. 1993. Rickettsial stimulation of endothelial platelet-activating factor synthesis. *Infect. Immun.* 61:2024–29
164. Walker TS, Brown JS, Hoover CS, Morgan DA. 1990. Endothelial prostaglandin secretion: effects of typhus rickettsiae. *J. Infect. Dis.* 162:1136–44
165. Sporn LA, Haidaris PJ, Shi RJ, Nemerson Y, Silverman DJ, Marder VJ. 1994. *Rickettsia rickettsii* infection of cultured human endothelial cells induces tissue factor expression. *Blood* 83:1527–34
166. Sporn LA, Shi RJ, Lawrence SO, Silverman DJ, Marder VJ. 1991. *Rickettsia rickettsii* infection of cultured endothelial cells induces release of large von Willebrand factor multimers from Weibel-Palade bodies. *Blood* 78:2595–602
167. Teysseire N, Arnoux D, George F, Sampol J, Raoult D. 1992. von Willebrand factor release and thrombomodulin and tissue factor expression in *Rickettsia conorii*-infected endothelial cells. *Infect. Immun.* 60:4388–93
168. Shi RJ, Simpson-Haidaris PJ, Marder VJ, Silverman DJ, Sporn LA. 1996. Increased expression of plasminogen activator inhibitor-1 in *R. rickettsii*-infected endothelial cells. *Thromb. Haemost.* 75:600–6
169. Elghetany MT, Walker DH. 1999. Hemostatic changes in Rocky Mountain spotted fever and Mediterranean spotted fever. *Am. J. Clin. Pathol.* 112:159–68

Uniquely explains the antimicrobial effector mechanisms of endothelial cells.

170. Walker DH, Popov VL, Crocquet-Valdes PA, Welsh CJ, Feng HM. 1997. Cytokine-induced, nitric oxide-dependent, intracellular antirickettsial activity of mouse endothelial cells. *Lab. Invest.* 76:129–38

171. Feng HM, Popov VL, Walker DH. 1994. Depletion of gamma interferon and tumor necrosis factor alpha in mice with *Rickettsia conorii*-infected endothelium: impairment of rickettsicidal nitric oxide production resulting in fatal, overwhelming rickettsial disease. *Infect. Immun.* 62:1952–60

172. Feng HM, Whitworth T, Popov V, Walker DH. 2004. Effect of antibody on the rickettsia-host cell interaction. *Infect. Immun.* 72:3524–30

173. Feng HM, Walker DH. 2000. Mechanisms of intracellular killing of *Rickettsia conorii* in infected human endothelial cells, hepatocytes, and macrophages. *Infect. Immun.* 68:6729–36

174. Choi J, Enis DR, Koh KP, Shiao SL, Pober JS. 2004. T lymphocyte-endothelial cell interactions. *Annu. Rev. Immunol.* 22:683–709

175. Pober JS. 1999. Immunobiology of human vascular endothelium. *Immunol. Res.* 19:225–32

176. Valujskikh A, Heeger PS. 2003. Emerging roles of endothelial cells in transplant rejection. *Curr. Opin. Immunol.* 15:493–98

177. Epperson DE, Pober JS. 1994. Antigen-presenting function of human endothelial cells. Direct activation of resting CD8 T cells. *J. Immunol.* 153:5402–12

178. Savage CO, Brooks CJ, Harcourt GC, Picard JK, King W, et al. 1995. Human vascular endothelial cells process and present autoantigen to human T cell lines. *Int. Immunol.* 7:471–79

179. Savinov AY, Wong FS, Stonebraker AC, Chervonsky AV. 2003. Presentation of antigen by endothelial cells and chemoattraction are required for homing of insulin-specific CD8+ T cells. *J. Exp. Med.* 197:643–56

180. Marelli-Berg FM, James MJ, Dangerfield J, Dyson J, Millrain M, et al. 2004. Cognate recognition of the endothelium induces HY-specific CD8+ T-lymphocyte transendothelial migration (diapedesis) in vivo. *Blood* 103:3111–16

181. Valujskikh A, Lantz O, Celli S, Matzinger P, Heeger PS. 2002. Cross-primed CD8(+) T cells mediate graft rejection via a distinct effector pathway. *Nat. Immun.* 3:844–51

182. Rothermel AL, Wang Y, Schechner J, Mook-Kanamori B, Aird WC, et al. 2004. Endothelial cells present antigens in vivo. *BMC Immunol.* 5:5

183. Kreisel D, Krupnick AS, Balsara KR, Riha M, Gelman AE, et al. 2002. Mouse vascular endothelium activates CD8+ T lymphocytes in a B7-dependent fashion. *J. Immunol.* 169:6154–61

Suggests that endothelial cells can prime naïve CD8+ T lymphocytes in vivo.

184. Kreisel D, Krupnick AS, Gelman AE, Engels FH, Popma SH, et al. 2002. Nonhematopoietic allograft cells directly activate CD8+ T cells and trigger acute rejection: an alternative mechanism of allorecognition. *Nat. Med.* 8:233–39

185. Zheng L, Gibson TF, Schechner JS, Pober JS, Bothwell AL. 2004. Bcl-2 transduction protects human endothelial cell synthetic microvessel grafts from allogeneic T cells in vivo. *J. Immunol.* 173:3020–26

Genetic Regulation of Cardiogenesis and Congenital Heart Disease

Deepak Srivastava

Gladstone Institute of Cardiovascular Disease and Department of Pediatrics, University of California, San Francisco, San Francisco, California 94158; email: dsrivastava@gladstone.ucsf.edu

Annu. Rev. Pathol. Mech. Dis. 2006. 1:199–213

First published online as a Review in Advance on October 24, 2005

The *Annual Review of Pathology: Mechanisms of Disease* is online at pathmechdis.annualreviews.org

doi: 10.1146/annurev.pathol.1.110304.100039

1553-4006/06/0114-0199$20.00

Key Words

cardiac development, molecular biology, signaling, transcription factors, stem cells

Abstract

Developmental heart disorders are the most common of all human birth defects and occur in nearly one percent of the population. Survivors of congenital heart malformations are an increasing population, and it is becoming clear that genetic mutations that cause developmental anomalies may result in cardiac dysfunction later in life. This review highlights the progress in understanding the underlying molecular basis for cardiac formation and how disruption of the intricate steps of cardiogenesis can lead to congenital heart defects. The lessons learned from examining the early steps of heart formation are essential for informing the prevention of malformations and their long-term consequences, as well as for approaches to guide stem cells into cardiac lineages.

INTRODUCTION

The heart has for centuries been the subject of fascination for anatomists, embryologists, biologists, and physicians. As the organ most essential for life, the heart is the first to form in an embryo and also must support the rapidly growing embryo before it has the opportunity to shape itself into a four-chambered organ. The combination of complex morphogenetic events necessary for cardiogenesis and its superimposed hemodynamic influences may contribute to the exquisite sensitivity of the heart to perturbations. This phenomenon is reflected in the estimated 10% incidence of severe cardiac malformations observed in early miscarriages. The fraction of congenital heart malformations hemodynamically compatible with intra-uterine circulation comprise the spectrum of congenital heart defects (CHDs) that are observed clinically.

Although genetic approaches have been important in understanding human CHD, detailed molecular analysis of cardiac development in humans has been difficult. Genetic pathways that dictate cardiac development are highly conserved across vastly diverse species from flies to humans, and this has resulted in a rapid expansion of information from studies in more tractable biological models (1, 2). Despite the diversity of body structures adopted by different species, a common genetic program for the early formation of a circulatory system seems to exist. Cardiovascular systems have developed increasing complexity in order to adapt to specific environments. For example, in a simplified view, higher organisms appear to have retained the morphologic steps utilized by lower organisms and built complexity into the heart as needed. In particular, the specification of chamber structures and the advent of a parallel circulation through chamber duplication and outflow-tract division by neural crest derivatives have facilitated the development of larger, air-breathing organisms that utilize complex circulatory systems.

Clinical lessons combined with experimental studies have led to a model suggesting that unique regions and segments of the heart have been added in a modular fashion during evolution. In such a scheme, defects in particular regions of the heart may arise from specific genetic and environmental effects during discrete developmental windows. To simplify the complex events of cardiogenesis and CHD, this review considers different regions of the developing heart individually in the context described above, weaving knowledge from model systems and human genetics when available.

CARDIOMYOCYTE AND HEART TUBE FORMATION

The heart is the first organ to form in vertebrates, and it arises through a complex series of morphogenetic interactions involving cells from several embryonic origins (**Figure 1**). Progenitor cells within the anterior lateral plate mesoderm become committed to a cardiogenic fate soon after gastrulation [at approximately embryonic day (E) 15 in humans] in response to an inducing signal thought to emanate from the adjacent endoderm (3). The specific signaling molecule(s) responsible for cardiogenic commitment remains to be identified, although bone morphogenetic proteins, fibroblast growth factors (Fgfs), and Wnts appear to be critical for this step (4–6). Cardiac precursors form a bilaterally symmetric cardiogenic field that develops further into parallel cardiac primordia, which fuse at the midline to form the primitive cardiac tube (7). This straight heart tube contains an outer myocardium and an inner endocardium separated by an extracellular matrix (ECM) known as the cardiac jelly. The tubular heart initiates rhythmic contractions at approximately E23.0 in humans.

Fruitflies have a primitive heart-like structure known as the dorsal vessel, which is analogous to the straight heart tube of the vertebrate embryo. It contracts rhythmically and pumps hemolymph through an open

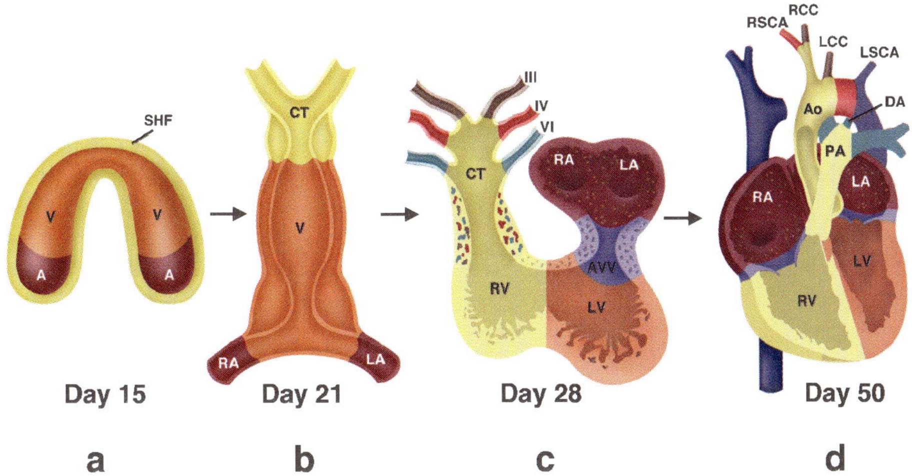

Figure 1

Schema of cardiac morphogenesis. Illustrations depict cardiac development, with morphologically related regions color-coded, seen from a ventral view. (*a*) Two distinct cardiogenic precursor fields form a crescent that is specified to form specific regions of the heart tube (A, artery; V, ventricle), which is patterned to form the various regions and chambers of the looped and mature heart. (*b*) The secondary heart field (SHF) contributes to much of the right ventricle and outflow tract as the heart loops. (*c*) Each cardiac chamber balloons from the outer curvature of the looped heart tube in a segmental fashion. Neural crest cells populate the bilaterally symmetric aortic arch arteries (III, IV, and VI) and aortic sac that together contribute to specific segments of the mature aortic arch, also color-coded. (*c*, *d*) Mesenchymal cells form the cardiac valves from the conotruncal (CT) and atrioventricular valve (AVV) segments, which divide into separate left- and right-sided valves. Corresponding days of human embryonic development are indicated. RV, right ventricle; LV, left ventricle; RA, right atrium; LA, left atrium; PA, pulmonary artery; Ao, aorta; DA, ductus arteriosus; RSCA, right subclavian artery; RCC, right common carotid; LCC, left common carotid; LSCA, left subclavian artery.

circulatory system. Formation of the dorsal vessel in flies is dependent upon a protein, tinman, whose name is based on the Wizard of Oz character that lacks a heart (8). Tinman belongs to the homeodomain family of proteins and was described initially to play a role in establishing regional identity of cells and organs during embryogenesis.

In contrast to the requirement of *tinman* gene for heart formation in flies, its mammalian orthologue, *Nkx2.5*, is not essential for specification of the cardiac lineage in mice, which suggests that either other genes may share functions with *Nkx2.5* or cardiogenesis in flies and vertebrates differs with respect to its dependence on this family of homeobox genes (9, 10). The possibility of functional redundancy between *Nkx2.5* and other cardiac-expressed homeobox genes in vertebrates is supported by the ability of dominant negative versions of Nkx2.5 transcription factor to block cardiogenesis in frog and zebrafish embryos (11, 12). Similarly, the transcriptional coactivator, myocardin, is necessary and sufficient in frogs for cardiac gene expression, likely through activation of serum response factor–dependent genes (13, 14).

The cardiac outflow tract (conotruncus) and parts of the right ventricle, which arise from a distinct population of cardiac precursors, are the last segments to form and appear to be added to the most anterior portion of the heart tube. A group of cells that lie dorsal and anterior to the cardiac precursors described above ultimately become part of the pharyngeal mesoderm (15–17). These cells appear to migrate to the conotruncus between E8.0 and E9.5, prior to neural crest invasion, and give rise to the outflow-tract myocardium and much of the right ventricle (**Figure 1**). Secreted signals from the conotruncus apparently induce the migration of cells from the pharyngeal region, although neither the nature of the signals nor the transcriptional regulation of these cells has been established. Fgf10 is expressed in this population of cells, but its role in their development remains unknown (17).

The pharyngeal mesoderm cells described above represent a second cardiac progenitor pool that differentiates into cardiomyocytes in the arterial pole of the heart tube and is therefore often referred to as a secondary heart field. The transcription factor Tbx1, which appears to be a cause of cardiac and craniofacial disorders in humans (18–21), is a major transcriptional regulator of the secondary heart field and is necessary for proper development of conotruncal myocardium and fibroblast growth factor secretion (22–24). Islet1, a basic helix-loop-helix (bHLH) transcription factor involved in pancreatic development, also marks this population and is necessary for its development (25). Interestingly, these cells mark niches of cardiac progenitor cells in the postnatal heart (26), which suggests that understanding the regulation of secondary heart field–derived progenitor pools may be useful in developing approaches for cardiac repair.

In addition to anterior-posterior (AP) patterning, a discrete dorsal-ventral polarity is also present in the primitive heart tube. As the heart tube loops to the right, the ventral surface of the tube rotates, becoming the outer curvature of the looped heart with the dorsal surface forming the inner curvature. The outer curvature becomes the site of active growth, and remodeling of the inner curvature is essential for ultimate alignment of the inflow and outflow tracts of the heart. Researchers have proposed a model in which individual chambers balloon from the outer curvature in a segmental fashion (27). Consistent with this model, numerous genes, including the transcription factor Hand1, are expressed on specific sites of the ventral and outer curvature of the heart (28, 29). Remodeling of the inner curvature occurs, allowing migration of the inflow tract to the right and outflow tract to the left. This process facilitates proper alignment and separation of right- and left-sided circulations (**Figure 2**). Defects of inner curvature remodeling may underly a host of human congenital heart malformations that involve improper alignment of the atria, ventricles, and outflow tract and are often observed in the setting of left-right (LR) asymmetry abnormalities, whereas other cardiac defects are a result of the disruption of discrete developmental events (**Table 1**).

CARDIAC LOOPING AND LEFT-RIGHT ASYMMETRY

The pathways that control the direction of cardiac looping along the LR axis are now well-established (30). The heart is the first organ to break the bilateral symmetry that characterizes the early embryo, and the rightward direction of its looping reflects a more global establishment of LR asymmetry, which affects the lungs, liver, spleen, and gut. Defects in establishment of LR asymmetry in humans are associated with a wide range of cardiac alignment defects.

A cascade of signaling molecules that regulate the establishment of embryonic LR asymmetry was revealed initially from studies of chick embryonic development (31). Before the formation of organs in the developing embryo, asymmetric expression of the morphogen Sonic hedgehog (Shh) on the left side of Hensen's node leads to the expression of nodal and lefty, members of the transforming growth factor-β (TGF-β) family, in the left lateral mesoderm. Left-sided expression of nodal induces the rightward looping of the midline heart tube. Fibroblast growth factor and activin receptor–mediated pathways suppress right-sided nodal expression. The above signaling pathways are active in the lateral plate mesoderm, but not in the heart or other organs that actually display LR asymmetry. Ultimately, the nodal-dependent pathways

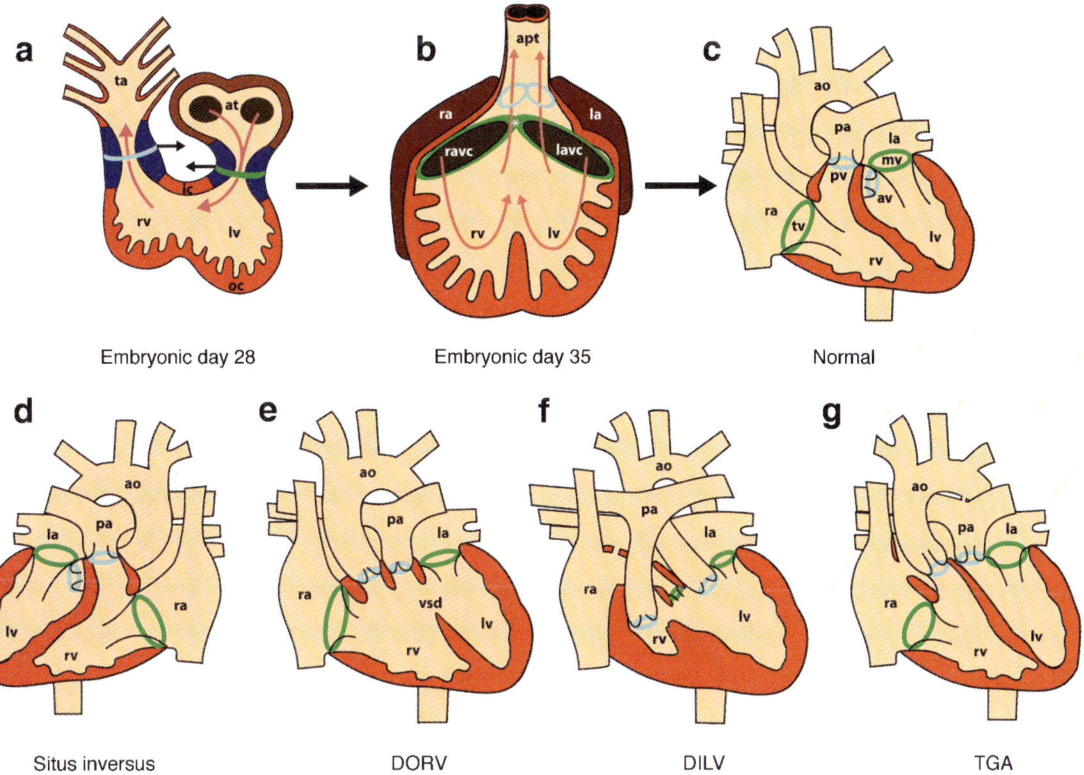

Figure 2

Normal and abnormal cardiac morphogenesis associated with left-right (LR) signaling. (*a*) As the linear heart tube loops rightward with inner curvature (ic) remodeling and outer curvature (oc) proliferation, the endocardial cushions (*dark blue*) of the inflow (*green*) and outflow (*light blue*) tracts become adjacent to one another. Subsequently, the atrioventricular septum (AVS) shifts to the right, while the aortopulmonary trunk (apt) shifts to the left. (*b*) The inflow tract is divided into the right (ravc) and left atrioventricular canal (lavc) by the AVS. The outflow tract, known as the truncus arteriosus (ta), becomes the apt upon septation. (*c*) Ultimately, the left (la) and right atrium (ra) are aligned with the left (lv) and right ventricle (rv), respectively. The lv and rv become aligned with the aorta (ao) and pulmonary artery (pa), respectively, after 180° rotation of the great vessels. (*d*) If the determinants of the LR axis are coordinately reversed, then a condition known as situs inversus results. (*e*) If the apt fails to shift to the left, then a condition known as double-outlet right ventricle (DORV) results, in which the right ventricle is aligned with both the aorta and pulmonary artery. (*f*) Likewise, if the AVS fails to shift to the right, both atria communicate with the left ventricle in a condition known as double-inlet left ventricle (DILV). (*g*) Transposition of the great arteries (TGA) results if the apt fails to twist, resulting in communication of the rv with ao and lv with pa. at, atrium; pv, pulmonary valve; av, aortic valve; mv, mitral valve; tv, tricuspid valve; vsd, ventricular septal defect. (Reproduced with permission from Reference 82).

result in expression of a homeodomain protein, Pitx2, on the left side of visceral organs and repression of Pitx2 on the right (32). Asymmetric expression of Pitx2 is sufficient for establishing the LR asymmetry of the heart, lungs, and gut, and this may occur via differential regulation of Wnt-dependent cell cycle pathways downstream of Pitx2 (33).

Genetic analysis of mouse mutants with abnormalities in LR asymmetry have illuminated some of the mechanisms controlling directionality of cardiac looping. Mice homozygous for mutation in the *LR dynein* gene

Table 1 Developmental pathway disruptions that may contribute to congenital heart defects in humans

Disruption of neural crest and SHF[1] contribution to the aortic arch	
	Right aortic arch
	Interrupted aortic arch
	Aberrant left subclavian artery origins
	Vascular "rings" and "slings"
Disruption of neural crest and SHF contribution to the outflow tract	
	Tetralogy of Fallot
	Persistent truncus arteriosus
	Membranous ventricular septal defects
	Double-outlet right ventricle
Disruption of aortic valve development	
	Aortic valve stenosis
	Aortic valve atresia
	Hypoplastic left heart syndrome
	Calcific aortic stenosis
Disruption of pulmonary valve development	
	Pulmonary valve stenosis
	Pulmonary valve atresia
	Hypoplastic right ventricle with PA and an intact ventricular septum
Disruption of atrioventricular valve development	
	Complete or partial atrioventricular septal defects
	Primum atrial septal defects
	Cleft mitral valves
	Tricuspid atresia
	Mitral stenosis/insufficiency
	Tricuspid stenosis/insufficiency
	Ebstein's anomaly
Disruption of right ventricular development	
	Tricuspid atresia with ventricular septal defect
	Ebstein's anomaly
Disruption of left ventricular development	
	Mitral atresia with ventricular septal defect
	Left ventricular noncompaction
Disruption of left-right asymmetry pathways affecting alignment	
	Double-outlet right ventricle
	Double-inlet left ventricle
	Tetralogy of Fallot
	Atrioventricular septal defects, particularly unbalanced
	Anomalous pulmonary venous return

[1]SHF, secondary heart field.

(*iv/iv*) display random LR orientation of the heart and viscera (34, 35). In the situs inversus (*inv*) mouse model, there is nearly a 100% reversal of LR asymmetry, although the function of the *inv* gene remains unknown. *Inv* mutant mice express nodal and Pitx2 along the right lateral mesoderm rather than the left, displaying complete reversal of the LR signals (32, 36, 37). In contrast, *iv/iv* mutant mice display bilaterally symmetric, absent, or random nodal and Pitx2 expression. *Pitx2* mutant mice have abnormal LR asymmetry of the lungs and a low penetrance of reversed cardiac looping, similar to *Shh* and *Fgf8* mutant mice (38). Oddly, the initial LR asymmetry and roles of Fgf and Shh are reversed in mice and chicks; however the LR sidedness of later events involving nodal and Pitx2 are conserved (39). Additional understanding of the early events will likely lead to convergence of LR mechanisms across species.

Although the necessity of LR asymmetric gene expression is obvious, how the initial asymmetry of gene expression is established remains in question. Initial clues came from studies of immotile cilia syndrome, also known as Kartagener's syndrome, in which individuals expressed situs inversus totalis, a condition causing mirror-image reversal of all organs (40). It has been described that, prior to organ formation, Hensen's node contains ciliary processes that beat in a counter-clockwise vortical fashion (41). Whether ciliary beating moves morphogens to the left side of the embryo or if bending of cilia induced by directional flow causes subsequent asymmetric gene expression remains controversial (42). In either case, mice lacking ciliary movement in the node display abnormal LR patterning, which is consistent with that notion that nodal cilia plays a critical role in LR asymmetry (35, 43–45).

PATTERNING OF THE DEVELOPING HEART TUBE

Studies using model organisms have begun to reveal the genetic basis of a segmental, ballooning model of cardiogenesis. Numerous transcription factors in mice are expressed in a region-specific fashion, which provides a possible explanation for how distinct segments of the heart assume their respective fates. Two related bHLH transcription factors, Hand2 and Hand1, are expressed predominantly in the primitive right- and left-ventricle segments, respectively, during mouse heart development (46, 47). Deletion of Hand2 in mice results in hypoplasia of the right ventricular segment and a thin left ventricular myocardium (47), suggesting a role for Hand2 in regulating derivatives of the secondary heart field. Hand1 is downregulated in Nkx2.5-deficient mice, who fail to segment the heart tube precisely and die around the stage of cardiac looping (29). Disruption of both Hand2 and Nkx2.5 results in the absence of the right and left ventricle, suggesting that the combined function of Hand2 and Nkx2.5, possibly through its regulation of Hand1, is necessary for ventricular formation (48). Indeed, compound loss of Hand1 and Hand2 in mice results in progressive ventricular defects with failure of ventricular expansion in mice lacking both genes (49). Consistent with the idea of an evolutionarily conserved role of Hand in ventricular expansion, zebrafish lacking the single fish Hand orthologue, Hand2, fail to expand the pool of ventricular precursors and do not develop a ventricular chamber (50).

Epigenetic factors may also contribute to ventricular morphogenesis as disruption of the chromatin remodeling protein Smyd1 (also known as mBop) results in a phenotype reminiscent of *Hand2* mutants, including a small right ventricular segment and poor development of the left ventricular myocardium (51). Smyd1 contains a SET domain that harbors histone methyltransferase activity and a MYND domain that recruits histone deacetylase activity that together are responsible for the transcriptional repression of target genes (51). Smyd1 activity is necessary for Hand2 expression in cardiac precursors of the primary heart field, likely through an intermediate that is unknown, consistent with the similar phenotype observed in targeted deletion of Hand2 or Smyd1 in mice. Interestingly, Smyd1 is a direct target of Mef2c (51a), a MADS box–containing transcription factor that is also required for right- and left-ventricle development. This suggests that a transcriptional cascade involving *Mef2c*, *Bop*, and *Hand* genes regulate ventricular cardiomyocyte development.

CONOTRUNCAL AND AORTIC ARCH DEVELOPMENT

Congenital cardiac defects involving the cardiac outflow tract, aortic arch, ductus arteriosus, and proximal pulmonary arteries account for 20%–30% of all CHDs. This region of the heart undergoes extensive and rather complex morphogenetic changes with contributions from the secondary heart field (discussed above) and neural crest–derived mesenchyme. Mutations in many signaling cascades affect neural crest migration or development, which includes the endothelin and semaphorin pathways, resulting in outflow-tract defects (52). Similarly, disruption of secondary heart field development by mutation of genes such as *Tbx1*, *Fgf8*, and *Islet1* results in persistent truncus arteriosus and malalignment of the outflow tract of the heart with the ventricular chambers (21, 25, 53, 54).

Neural crest cells are a unique population of cells along the crest of the neural folds that migrate away from the neural folds and retain the ability to differentiate into multiple cell types and are therefore pluripotent. Their migratory path and ultimate cell fates are dependent upon their relative position of origin along the anterior-posterior axis. Such neural crest cells differentiate and contribute to diverse embryonic structures, including the cranial ganglia, peripheral nervous system, adrenal glands, and melanocytes. Neural crest cells that arise from the otic placode to the third somite migrate through the developing pharyngeal arches and populate the mesenchyme of each of the pharyngeal and aortic arch arteries, the conotruncus and conotruncal septum (55). Because of their migratory path, this segment of the neural crest is often referred to as the cardiac neural crest.

Ablation of the cardiac neural crest prior to its migration away from the neural folds in chick embryos demonstrates a critical role for neural crest cells during cardiogenesis. Embryos deficient in cardiac neural crest cells display a variety of cardiac outflow-tract and aortic-arch defects similar to those seen in humans. These include tetralogy of Fallot (TOF), persistent truncus arteriosus, double-outlet right ventricle, and conotruncal ventricular septal defects. Within the aortic arch, a broad spectrum of aortic arch anomalies were observed, including interruption of the aortic arch, aberrant origins of the right subclavian artery, and persistence of the right aortic arch rather than the left aortic arch. Thus, defects in neural crest migration or differentiation likely underlie the many conotruncal and aortic arch defects seen in humans. Indeed, human mutations of the neural crest–enriched transcription factor TFAP2b results in persistent patency of the ductus arteriosus, a specialized aortic-arch vessel essential for fetal cardiac physiology (56), and it is likely that other genetic mutations affect specific regions of the aortic arch.

CARDIAC VALVE FORMATION

Appropriate placement and function of cardiac valves is essential for chamber septation and unidirectional blood flow through the heart. During early heart tube formation, cushions of ECM between the endocardium and myocardium precede valve formation at each end of the heart tube. Reciprocal signaling, mediated in part by TGF-β family members, between the myocardium and endocardium in the cushion region induces a transformation of endocardial cells into mesenchymal cells that migrate into the cushion of ECM. These mesenchymal cells differentiate into the fibrous tissue of the valves and are involved in septation of the common atrioventricular canal into right- and left-sided orifices. The transcription factor NFATc is expressed specifically during the formation of embryonic valves, and targeted deletion of NFATc in mice results in the absence of cardiac valve formation (57, 58).

Although lack of cardiac valve leaflets is a rare cardiac anomaly, thickened valve leaflets resulting in stenotic valves are a common form of CHD. In mouse models, the absence of the *Ptpn11* gene, which encodes the protein tyrosine phosphatase Shp-2, results in dysplastic semilunar valves via its involvement in a signaling pathway mediated by epidermal growth factor receptor (59). The importance of *PTPN11* in congenital heart disease was shown by the identification of point mutations in *PTPN11* in patients with Noonan syndrome, whose phenotype commonly includes pulmonic valve stenosis (60).

The Smad proteins are intracellular transcriptional mediators of signaling initiated by TGF-β ligands. Smad6 is expressed specifically in the atrioventricular cushions and outflow tract during cardiogenesis and is a negative regulator of TGF-β signaling. Targeted disruption of *Smad6* in mice results in thickened and gelatinous atrioventricular and semilunar valves, similar to those observed in human aortic and pulmonary valve disease (61). As with loss of Smad6 in mice, lack of Ephrin B2 also results in thickened valves, although the mechanism for this remains unclear (62).

The Notch signaling pathway is required for cell fate and differentiation decisions in the embryo (63), but has only recently been implicated in cardiovascular development. In fish and frogs, Notch appears to be involved in the development of the endocardial cushions that contribute to valve tissue (64). Consistent with this observation, the authors recently discovered that nonsyndromic, autosomal-dominant pedigrees with aortic valve disease segregate with missense mutations in *NOTCH1* (65). The *NOTCH1* mutations cause a developmental anomaly in the aortic valve in which two of the three valve leaflets fail to separate, resulting in a bicuspid rather than tricuspid aortic valve. *NOTCH1* mutations cause a wide spectrum of aortic valve diseases, ranging from severe newborn-onset cardiac disease to milder valve disease, which is initially asymptomatic but manifests in the fourth or fifth decade of life as severe and premature valve calcification.

The finding that *NOTCH1* mutations segregate with severe aortic valve calcification led to the recognition that Notch1 negatively regulates a central regulator of osteoblast-specific gene expression, Runx2, and may do so in the valve through the physical interaction of the hairy-related transcriptional repressor Hrt with Runx2 (65–67). It is possible that *NOTCH1* variants may be predictors of individuals at higher risk for developing valve calcification, providing an opportunity to identify genetically those who may benefit from more aggressive management of other known risk factors such as hypercholesterolemia and diabetes. This is another example of how identification of genetic causes of cardiac malformations may lead to prevention of related adult-onset cardiac disease.

Genetic studies of Alagille syndrome also support an important role for Notch signaling in human disease. Alagille syndrome is an autosomal-dominant disorder characterized by biliary atresia and cardiac defects, typically in the form of pulmonary artery stenosis and TOF, which is caused by mutations in *JAGGED-1*, a ligand for the Notch receptor (68, 69). Isolated pulmonary stenosis, or TOF, has also been associated with *JAGGED-1* mutations, consistent with the notion that it plays a role in valve development (70).

GENETICS OF HUMAN VALVULOSEPTAL DEFECTS

The study of chromosomal disorders and autosomal-dominant syndromes in the setting of CHD, and genetic linkage analysis of rare pedigrees with milder forms of CHD, have been informative, particularly in conjunction with functional studies in model organisms. Recent genetic studies of cardiac transcription factors NKX2.5, TBX5, and GATA4 exemplify the parallels in etiology between model organisms and human genetic studies of CHD. Numerous point mutations have been identified in *NKX2.5* in families with atrial septal defects and cardiac conduction abnormalities (71). Sporadic mutations of *NKX2.5* have also been found in patients with TOF and tricuspid valve anomalies (72). How these mutations result in cardiac defects is unknown, but the linkage of specific types of loss-of-function mutations with distinct abnormalities suggests that different structural determinants of NKX2.5 have unique functions in developmental decisions in the heart. Mutations in *NKX2.5* cause not only a developmental defect, but may also cause cardiac disease later in life, which highlights the notion that genetic causes of CHD may also underlie adult disease. This realization may provide an avenue to study preventive approaches for the later sequelae of congenital heart malformations and adult-onset heart disease (73, 74).

Humans with Holt-Oram syndrome, caused by mutations in *TBX5*, are characterized by cardiac anomalies similar to those with *NKX2.5* mutations (atrial and ventricular septal defects) and also limb abnormalities (75, 76). Intriguingly, mutations responsible for defects in the heart and limbs are clustered in different regions of the protein, which suggests that TBX5 engages different downstream genes or cofactors in these tissues that depend upon unique structural motifs in the protein.

Like individuals with *NKX2.5* and *TBX5* mutations, nonsyndromic, autosomal-dominant pedigrees that harbored mutations in the zinc finger–containing protein GATA4 were recently described (77). GATA4 or its relatives are essential for cardiogenesis in flies, fish, and mice (78–81). Interestingly, *GATA4* mutations cause atrial and ventricular septal defects that are very similar to those observed in the setting of *NKX2.5* and *TBX5* mutations. Correspondingly, GATA4 and TBX5 interact and cooperate physically to activate transcription (76). A familial *GATA4* point mutation disrupts GATA4's ability to interact with TBX5, and several human TBX5 mutations disrupt its interaction with GATA4, which suggests that the two cooperate in cardiac septation events (77). A genetic interaction between the two proteins has been confirmed as mice heterozygous for *Gata4* and *Tbx5* die during embryogenesis from severe hypoplasia of the endocardial cushion tissue necessary for valuloseptal development (V. Garg & D. Srivastava, unpublished observations). The endocardial cushion defect is similar to that observed in the setting of Trisomy 21 (Down Syndrome) in humans, and it will be interesting to determine if *GATA4*, *TBX5*, or other related genes are modifier genes for the cardiac phenotype of Trisomy 21.

CONCLUSIONS

Over the past decade investigators have witnessed remarkable advances in our understanding of cardiogenesis, and the heart has become one of the most well-understood organs in biology. This knowledge is now being used to discover the underlying genetics of CHD and the basis for many adult-onset diseases that have their origin in mutations of developmental genes. What is lacking is a coherent picture of the hierarchical pathways that govern most developmental processes and the mechanisms through which such pathways regulate the cell biology of morphogenesis. Such knowledge will require a better understanding of the target genes of critical transcriptional and signaling pathways that control cardiogenesis. Research in this area will be an essential step, as the targets will be the most amenable sites of intervention, both in a therapeutic sense and for the purpose of prevention. For example, identification of dietary substances that modulate key developmental pathways such as folic acid, which prevents neural tube defects, will be necessary for preventive efforts. In addition, early genetic identification of those at risk for adult-onset disease originating from a cardiac developmental defect, such as the age-related calcification that occurs in bicuspid aortic valve, will provide ample time for intervention to slow the progression of disease. The convergence of additional developmental knowledge and improved genetic tools should make this vision a reality in the coming years.

ACKNOWLEDGMENTS

D.S. was supported by grants from the National Heart, Lung, and Blood Institute/National Institutes of Health, March of Dimes Birth Defects Foundation, and American Heart Association's Established Investigator Award.

LITERATURE CITED

1. Srivastava D, Olson EN. 2000. A genetic blueprint for cardiac development. *Nature* 407:221–26
2. Chien KR, Olson EN. 2002. Converging pathways and principles in heart development and disease: CV@CSH. *Cell* 110:153–62
3. Schultheiss TM, Xydas S, Lassar AB. 1995. Induction of avian cardiac myogenesis by anterior endoderm. *Development* 121:4203–4
4. Schultheiss TM, Burch JB, Lassar AB. 1997. A role for bone morphogenetic proteins in the induction of cardiac myogenesis. *Genes Dev.* 11:451–62
5. Schneider VA, Mercola M. 2001. Wnt antagonism initiates cardiogenesis in *Xenopus laevis*. *Genes Dev.* 15:304–15
6. Marvin MJ, Di Rocco G, Gardiner A, Bush SM, Lassar AB. 2001. Inhibition of Wnt activity induces heart formation from posterior mesoderm. *Genes Dev.* 15:316–27
7. DeHaan RL. 1965. Development of pacemaker tissue in the embryonic heart. *Ann. NY Acad. Sci.* 127:7–18

8. Bodmer R. 1993. The gene tinman is required for specification of the heart and visceral muscles in *Drosophila*. *Development* 118:719–29
9. Lyons I, Parsons LM, Hartley L, Li R, Andrews JE, et al. 1995. Myogenic and morphogenetic defects in the heart tubes of murine embryos lacking the homeo box gene Nkx2-5. *Genes Dev.* 9:1654–66
10. Tanaka M, Wechsler SB, Lee IW, Yamasaki N, Lawitts JA, et al. 1999. Complex modular cis-acting elements regulate expression of the cardiac specifying homeobox gene Csx/Nkx2.5. *Development* 126:1439–50
11. Fu Y, Yan W, Mohun TJ, Evans SM. 1998. Vertebrate tinman homologues XNkx2–3 and XNkx2–5 are required for heart formation in a functionally redundant manner. *Development* 125:4439–49
12. Grow MW, Krieg PA. 1998. Tinman function is essential for vertebrate heart development: Elimination of cardiac differentiation by dominant inhibitory mutants of the tinman-related genes, XNkx2–3 and XNkx2–5. *Dev. Biol.* 204:187–96
13. Wang D, Chang PS, Wang Z, Sutherland L, Richardson JA, et al. 2001. Activation of cardiac gene expression by myocardin, a transcriptional cofactor for serum response factor. *Cell* 105:851–62
14. Small EM, Warkman AS, Wang DZ, Sutherland LB, Olson EN, et al. 2005. Myocardin is sufficient and necessary for cardiac gene expression in Xenopus. *Development* 132:987–97
15. Mjaatvedt CH, Nakaoka T, Moreno-Rodriguez R, Norris RA, Kern MJ, et al. 2001. The outflow tract of the heart is recruited from a novel heart-forming field. *Dev. Biol.* 238:97–109
16. Waldo KL, Kumiski DH, Wallis KT, Stadt HA, Hutson MR, et al. 2001. Conotruncal myocardium arises from a secondary heart field. *Development* 128:3179–88
17. Kelly RG, Brown NA, Buckingham ME. 2001. The arterial pole of the mouse heart forms from Fgf10-expressing cells in pharyngeal mesoderm. *Dev. Cell* 1:435–40
18. Lindsay EA, Botta A, Jurecic V, Carattini-Rivera S, Cheah YC, et al. 1999. Congenital heart disease in mice deficient for the DiGeorge syndrome region. *Nature* 401:379–83
19. Lindsay EA, Vitelli F, Su H, Morishima M, Huynh T, et al. 2001. Tbx1 haploinsufficieny in the DiGeorge syndrome region causes aortic arch defects in mice. *Nature* 410:97–101
20. Merscher S, Funke B, Epstein JA, Heyer J, Puech A, et al. 2001. TBX1 is responsible for cardiovascular defects in velo-cardio-facial/DiGeorge syndrome. *Cell* 104:619–29
21. Jerome LA, Papaioannou VE. 2001. DiGeorge syndrome phenotype in mice mutant for the T-box gene, Tbx1. *Nat. Genet.* 27:286–91
22. Yamagishi H, Maeda J, Hu T, McAnally J, Conway SJ, et al. 2003. Tbx1 is regulated by tissue-specific forkhead proteins through a common Sonic hedgehog-responsive enhancer. *Genes Dev.* 17:269–81
23. Hu T, Yamagishi H, Maeda J, McAnally J, Yamagishi C, et al. 2004. Tbx1 regulates fibroblast growth factors in the anterior heart field through a reinforcing autoregulatory loop involving forkhead transcription factors. *Development* 131:5491–502
24. Xu H, Morishima M, Wylie JN, Schwartz RJ, Bruneau BG, et al. 2004. Tbx1 has a dual role in the morphogenesis of the cardiac outflow tract. *Development* 131:3217–27
25. Cai CL, Liang X, Shi Y, Chu PH, Pfaff SL, et al. 2003. Isl1 identifies a cardiac progenitor population that proliferates prior to differentiation and contributes a majority of cells to the heart. *Dev. Cell* 5:877–89

26. Laugwitz KL, Moretti A, Lam J, Gruber P, Chen Y, et al. 2005. Postnatal isl1+ cardioblasts enter fully differentiated cardiomyocyte lineages. *Nature* 433:647–53
27. Moorman AF, Christoffels VM. 2003. Cardiac chamber formation: Development, genes, and evolution. *Physiol. Rev.* 83:1223–67
28. Thomas T, Kurihara H, Yamagishi H, Kurihara Y, Yazaki Y, et al. 1998. A signaling cascade involving endothelin-1, dHAND and msx1 regulates development of neural-crest-derived branchial arch mesenchyme. *Development* 125:3005–14
29. Biben C, Harvey RP. 1997. Homeodomain factor Nkx2–5 controls left/right asymmetric expression of bHLH gene eHand during murine heart development. *Genes Dev.* 11:1357–69
30. Palmer AR. 2004. Symmetry breaking and the evolution of development. *Science* 306:828–33
31. Levin M, Johnson RL, Stern CD, Kuehn M, Tabin C. 1995. A molecular pathway determining left-right asymmetry in chick embryogenesis. *Cell* 82:803–14
32. Piedra ME, Icardo JM, Albajar M, Rodriguez-Rey JC, Ros MA. 1998. Pitx2 participates in the late phase of the pathway controlling left-right asymmetry. *Cell* 94:319–24
33. Kioussi C, Briata P, Baek SH, Rose DW, Hamblet NS, et al. 2002. Identification of a Wnt/Dvl/beta-Catenin → Pitx2 pathway mediating cell-type-specific proliferation during development. *Cell* 111:673–85
34. Supp DM, Witte DP, Potter SS, Brueckner M. 1997. Mutation of an axonemal dynein affects left-right asymmetry in inversus viscerum mice. *Nature* 389:963–66
35. Supp DM, Brueckner M, Kuehn MR, Witte DP, Lowe LA, et al. 1999. Targeted deletion of the ATP binding domain of left-right dynein confirms its role in specifying development of left-right asymmetries. *Development* 126:5495–504
36. Ryan AK, Blumberg B, Rodriguez-Esteban C, Yonei-Tamura S, Tamura K, et al. 1998. Pitx2 determines left-right asymmetry of internal organs in vertebrates. *Nature* 394:545–51
37. Campione M, Steinbeisser H, Schweickert A, Deissler K, van Bebber F, et al. 1999. The homeobox gene Pitx2: Mediator of asymmetric left-right signaling in vertebrate heart and gut looping. *Development* 126:1225–34
38. Meyers EN, Martin GR. 1999. Differences in left-right axis pathways in mouse and chick: functions of FGF8 and SHH. *Science* 285:403–6
39. Rodriguez Esteban C, Capdevila J, Economides AN, Pascual J, Ortiz A, et al. 1999. The novel Cer-like protein Caronte mediates the establishment of embryonic left-right asymmetry. *Nature* 401:243–51
40. Afzelius BA. 1976. A human syndrome caused by immotile cilia. *Science* 193:317–19
41. Nonaka S, Tanaka Y, Okada Y, Takeda S, Harada A, et al. 1998. Randomization of left-right asymmetry due to loss of nodal cilia generating leftward flow of extraembryonic fluid in mice lacking KIF3B motor protein. *Cell* 95:829–37
42. McGrath J, Somlo S, Makova S, Tian X, Brueckner M. 2003. Two populations of node monocilia initiate left-right asymmetry in the mouse. *Cell* 114:61–73
43. Okada Y, Nonaka S, Tanaka Y, Saijoh Y, Hamada H, et al. 1999. Abnormal nodal flow precedes situs inversus in iv and inv mice. *Mol. Cell* 4:459–68
44. Marszalek JR, Ruiz-Lozano P, Roberts E, Chien KR, Goldstein LS. 1999. Situs inversus and embryonic ciliary morphogenesis defects in mouse mutants lacking the KIF3A subunit of kinesin-II. *Proc. Natl. Acad. Sci. USA* 96:5043–48

45. Takeda S, Yonekawa Y, Tanaka Y, Okada Y, Nonaka S, et al. 1999. Left-right asymmetry and kinesin superfamily protein KIF3A: New insights in determination of laterality and mesoderm induction by kif3A$^{-/-}$ mice analysis. *J. Cell Biol.* 145:825–36
46. Srivastava D, Cserjesi P, Olson EN. 1995. A subclass of bHLH proteins required for cardiac morphogenesis. *Science* 270:1995–99
47. Srivastava D, Thomas T, Lin Q, Kirby ML, Brown D, Olson EN. 1997. Regulation of cardiac mesodermal and neural crest development by the bHLH transcription factor, dHAND. *Nat. Genet.* 16:154–60
48. Yamagishi H, Yamagishi C, Nakagawa O, Harvey RP, Olson EN, et al. 2001. The combinatorial activities of Nkx2.5 and dHAND are essential for cardiac ventricle formation. *Dev. Biol.* 239:190–203
49. McFadden DG, Barbosa AC, Richardson JA, Schneider MD, Srivastava D, et al. 2005. The Hand1 and Hand2 transcription factors regulate expansion of the embryonic cardiac ventricles in a gene dosage-dependent manner. *Development* 132:189–201
50. Yelon D, Ticho B, Halpern ME, Ruvinsky I, Ho RK, et al. 2000. The bHLH transcription factor hand2 plays parallel roles in zebrafish heart and pectoral fin development. *Development* 127:2573–82
51. Gottlieb PD, Pierce SA, Sims RJ, Yamagishi H, Weihe EK, et al. 2002. Bop encodes a muscle-restricted protein containing MYND and SET domains and is essential for cardiac differentiation and morphogenesis. *Nat. Genet.* 31:25–32
51a. Phan D, Rasmussen TL, Nakagawa O, McAnally J, Gottlieb PD, et al. 2005. Bop, a regulator of right ventricular heart development, is a direct transcriptional activator of Mef2c in the developing heart. *Development* 132:2669–78
52. Hutson MR, Kirby ML. 2003. Neural crest and cardiovascular development: A 20-year perspective. *Birth Defects Res. C Embryo Today* 69:2–13
53. Abu-Issa R, Smyth G, Smoak I, Yamamura K, Meyers EN. 2002. Fgf8 is required for pharyngeal arch and cardiovascular development in the mouse. *Development* 129:4613–25
54. Frank DU, Fotheringham LK, Brewer JA, Muglia LJ, Tristani-Firouzi M, et al. 2002. An Fgf8 mouse mutant phenocopies human 22q11 deletion syndrome. *Development* 129:4591–603
55. Kirby ML, Waldo KL. 1995. Neural crest and cardiovascular patterning. *Circ. Res.* 77:211–15
56. Satoda M, Zhao F, Diaz GA, Burn J, Goodship J, et al. 2000. Mutations in TFAP2B cause Char syndrome, a familial form of patent ductus arteriosus. *Nat. Genet.* 25:42–46
57. Ranger AM, Grusby MJ, Hodge MR, Gravallese EM, de la Brousse FC, et al. 1998. The transcription factor NF-ATc is essential for cardiac valve formation. *Nature* 392:186–90
58. de la Pompa JL, Timmerman LA, Takimoto H, Yoshida H, Elia AJ, et al. 1998. Role of the NF-ATc transcription factor in morphogenesis of cardiac valves and septum. *Nature* 392:182–86
59. Chen B, Bronson RT, Klaman LD, Hampton TG, Wang JF, et al. 2000. Mice mutant for Egfr and Shp2 have defective cardiac semilunar valvulogenesis. *Nat. Genet.* 24:296–99
60. Tartaglia M, Mehler EL, Goldberg R, Zampino G, Brunner HG, et al. 2001. Mutations in PTPN11, encoding the protein tyrosine phosphatase SHP-2, cause Noonan syndrome. *Nat. Genet.* 29:465–68
61. Galvin KM, Donovan MJ, Lynch CA, Meyer RI, Paul RJ, et al. 2000. A role for Smad6 in development and homeostasis of the cardiovascular system. *Nat. Genet.* 24:171–74

62. Cowan CA, Yokoyama N, Saxena A, Chumley MJ, Silvany RE, et al. 2004. Ephrin-B2 reverse signaling is required for axon pathfinding and cardiac valve formation but not early vascular development. *Dev. Biol.* 271:263–71
63. Artavanis-Tsakonas S, Rand MD, Lake RJ. 1999. Notch signaling: Cell fate control and signal integration in development. *Science* 284:770–76
64. Timmerman LA, Grego-Bessa J, Raya A, Bertran E, Perez-Pomares JM, et al. 2004. Notch promotes epithelial-mesenchymal transition during cardiac development and oncogenic transformation. *Genes Dev.* 18:99–115
65. Garg V, Heistein LC, Eapen RS, Muth AN, Schluterman MK, et al. 2005. Mutations in *NOTCH1* cause aortic valve disease. *Nature.* 437:270–74
66. Ducy P, Zhang R, Geoffroy V, Ridall AL, Karsenty G. 1997. Osf2/Cbfa1: A transcriptional activator of osteoblast differentiation. *Cell* 89:747–54
67. Nakagawa O, Nakagawa M, Richardson JA, Olson EN, Srivastava D. 1999. HRT1, HRT2, and HRT3: A new subclass of bHLH transcription factors marking specific cardiac, somitic, and pharyngeal arch segments. *Dev. Biol.* 216:72–84
68. Li L, Krantz ID, Deng Y, Genin A, Banta AB, et al. 1997. Alagille syndrome is caused by mutations in human Jagged1, which encodes a ligand for Notch1. *Nat. Genet.* 16:243–51
69. Oda T, Elkahloun AG, Pike BL, Okajima K, Krantz ID, et al. 1997. Mutations in the human Jagged1 gene are responsible for Alagille syndrome. *Nat. Genet.* 16:235–42
70. Krantz ID, Smith R, Colliton RP, Tinkel H, Zackai EH, et al. 1999. Jagged1 mutations in patients ascertained with isolated congenital heart defects. *Am. J. Med. Genet.* 84:56–60
71. Schott JJ, Benson DW, Basson CT, Pease W, Silberbach GM, et al. 1998. Congenital heart disease caused by mutations in the transcription factor NKX2–5. *Science* 281:108–11
72. Benson DW, Silberbach GM, Kavanaugh-McHugh A, Cottrill C, Zhang Y, et al. 1999. Mutations in the cardiac transcription factor NKX2.5 affect diverse cardiac developmental pathways. *J. Clin. Invest.* 104:1567–73
73. Pashmforoush M, Lu JT, Chen H, Amand TS, Kondo R, et al. 2004. Nkx2–5 pathways and congenital heart disease; loss of ventricular myocyte lineage specification leads to progressive cardiomyopathy and complete heart block. *Cell* 117:373–86
74. Srivastava D. 2004. Heart disease: An ongoing genetic battle?*Nature* 429:819–22
75. Basson CT, Bachinsky DR, Lin RC, Levi T, Elkins JA, et al. 1997. Mutations in human TBX5 cause limb and cardiac malformation in Holt-Oram syndrome. *Nat. Genet.* 15:30–35
76. Mori AD, Bruneau BG. 2004. TBX5 mutations and congenital heart disease: Holt-Oram syndrome revealed. *Curr. Opin. Cardiol.* 19:211–15
77. Garg V, Kathiriya IS, Barnes R, Schluterman MK, King IN, et al. 2003. GATA4 mutations cause human congenital heart defects and reveal an interaction with TBX5. *Nature* 424:443–47
78. Molkentin JD, Lin Q, Duncan SA, Olson EN. 1997. Requirement of the transcription factor GATA4 for heart tube formation and ventral morphogenesis. *Genes Dev.* 11:1061–72
79. Kuo CT, Morrisey EE, Anandappa R, Sigrist K, Lu MM, et al. 1997. GATA4 transcription factor is required for ventral morphogenesis and heart tube formation. *Genes Dev.* 11:1048–60

80. Reiter JF, Kikuchi Y, Stainier DY. 2001. Multiple roles for Gata5 in zebrafish endoderm formation. *Development* 128:125–35
81. Gajewski K, Zhang Q, Choi CY, Fossett N, Dang A, et al. 2001. Pannier is a transcriptional target and partner of Tinman during *Drosophila* cardiogenesis. *Dev. Biol.* 233:425–36
82. Kathiriya IS, Srivastava D. 2000. Left-right asymmetry and cardiac looping: Implications for cardiac development and congenital heart disease. *Am. J. Med. Genet.* 97:271–79

Regulation of Lung Inflammation in the Model of IgG Immune-Complex Injury

Hongwei Gao,[1] Thomas Neff,[2] and Peter A. Ward[1]

[1]Department of Pathology, University of Michigan Medical School, Ann Arbor, Michigan 48109; email: hgao@umich.edu, pward@umich.edu

[2]Department of Anesthesiology, University of Zurich Medical School, CH-8091 Zurich, Switzerland; email: thomas.neff@usz.ch

Annu. Rev. Pathol. Mech. Dis. 2006. 1:215–42

First published online as a Review in Advance on October 20, 2005

The *Annual Review of Pathology: Mechanisms of Disease* is online at pathmechdis.annualreviews.org

doi: 10.1146/annurev.pathol.1.110304.100155

1553-4006/06/0114-0215$20.00

Key Words

complement, acute lung injury, cytokine, chemokine, neutrophils

Abstract

Modern techniques of cell and molecular biology have rapidly uncovered the mechanisms underlying inflammatory injury of the lung. This expanding knowledge (which includes an understanding of complement, cell surface receptors, cytokines and chemokines, transcription factors, oxidants, proteinases, and endogenous inhibitors, as well as the role of leukocyte adhesion-promoting molecules) has provided new insights into the inflammatory system in general, as well as in the context of lung injury. In this review, we summarize recent progress in understanding the regulation of lung inflammation by using immunoglobulin G (IgG) immune complex–induced lung injury as a model. These studies have provided information on the role of various inflammatory mediators and their sequence of engagement. Insights into potential interventional approaches for the suppression of inflammatory processes in humans have emerged from those studies.

INTRODUCTION

Inflammatory response: tissue response initiated by a variety of conditions, including tissue injury, presence of infectious agents, and events related to ischemia reperfusion

IC: immune complex

BAL: bronchoalveolar lavage

Vascular permeability: an active process leading to a transient opening of the tight junctions between endothelial cells; also the rapid endocytic transport of plasma, water, and salt across the cytoplasmic confines of endothelial cells

ALI: acute lung injury

ROS: reactive oxygen species

Inflammation is usually a local, protective response to injury or invasive microbes. This host-defense response depends upon the engagement of the innate and adaptive immune systems to thwart pathogenic threats. On the basis of the relative rarity of sustained and severe infections, these immune systems are remarkably effective. However, these defenses are imperfect in that serious infections or evidence of inflammatory injury sometimes do occur. Nevertheless, the remarkable vigor with which leukocytes destroy pathogens and pathogen-infected cells, and dispose of dead cells and their products, has come at a price: Evolution has been incompletely successful in elaborating an immune system capable of discriminating perfectly between circumstances where potent destructive powers must be applied and where restraint must be exercised. The immune responses, for example, sometimes injure the host in both acute and chronic reactions. Tissue injury and destruction may result from either direct effects of the pathological agent or, more often, as a consequence of an inflammatory cell response. Thus, inflammation must be fine-tuned and carefully and precisely regulated.

Due to the instructive role of lung models of acute injury in the complicated cascade of events leading to injury, and because lung preservation is maintained by intricate immune mechanisms that promote a balance between host defense against injury and reactive inflammatory responses, the lung has been a focus of investigation for innate and adaptive immune responses. The lung inflammatory response triggered by deposition of immunoglobulin G (IgG) immune complexes (ICs) is probably not unique to the lung, but can be used to quantify and assess the inflammatory response. In many respects, the lung has advantages that are unavailable in virtually any other organ (**Table 1**). For instance, analysis of airway resistance to air flow, changes in gas exchange between the alveolar and vascular compartments, and alterations in pulmonary artery pressure can be evaluated in the lung. Airway challenges with antigens or other substances can also be performed. The resulting inflammatory responses can be evaluated using whole-lung homogenates or the content of bronchoalveolar lavage (BAL) fluids in which cellular and soluble components can be measured. Blood flowing into the lung (pulmonary artery) or exiting the lung (left arterial blood) can also be analyzed. As in other organs, the immune response in the lung is fundamentally protective, but it is now well-established that this response can, under certain conditions, be harmful. Injury to the lung may have long-term physiological effects, including decreased efficacy of gas exchange, increased vascular permeability, and irreversible lung fibrosis. Many pulmonary diseases may engage similar mechanisms that lead to injury of the lung. When lung injury occurs, it is typically the result of multiple mediators and several different signaling cascades.

In this review, we use IgG IC-induced acute lung injury (ALI) as a model to describe the mechanisms and regulation of acute immunological pulmonary alveolitis. The current understanding of the roles of adhesion molecules, chemokines, regulatory cytokines, reactive oxygen species (ROS), and

Table 1 Special features of the lung as a model for inflammation

Analysis of airway resistance to the flow of air
Evaluation of change in gas exchange between the alveolar and vascular compartments
Evaluation of alterations in pulmonary artery pressure
Challenge of airway with antigens or with other substances
Evaluation of inflammatory responses by using whole lung homogenates or content of bronchoalveolar lavage (BAL) fluids
Analysis of blood flowing into the lung (pulmonary artery) or exiting the lung (left arterial blood)

proteinases in IgG IC-induced lung injury are reviewed. We also describe the transcriptional regulation and divergent roles for complement/complement receptors and Fcγ receptors (FcγR) in acute immunological pulmonary alveolitis. Also discussed is the relationship of acute lung inflammatory injury to apoptosis and death signaling. Finally, we provide a brief discussion of what we think are promising areas of future research for mechanisms of IC-induced ALI.

Acute Immunological Pulmonary Alveolitis: IgG Immune Complex–Induced Acute Lung Injury as a Model

The use of animal models of lung inflammation has allowed researchers to investigate possible inflammation pathways responsible for injury. Although such animal models do not necessarily extrapolate to lung inflammatory diseases in humans, they have, nevertheless, permitted a detailed dissection of events that lead ultimately to damage of interstitial capillary endothelial cells and alveolar epithelial cells. The information obtained through animal models of the lung also has broad application to an understanding of inflammatory injury in other organs. In this respect, the IgG IC model in the rodent lung has been employed extensively to determine how tissue injury occurs, although in the clinical setting the role of IgG IC in ALI in humans may be limited largely to autoimmune diseases. Intra-alveolar deposition of IgG IC is achieved by the instillation of IgG antibody to bovine serum albumin (BSA) into the airway, followed by the intravenous injection of BSA (**Figure 1**). This results in an acutely damaging process that affects capillary endothelial cells and alveolar epithelial cells via pathophysiological events, as shown in **Figure 2**.

FcγR: Fcγ receptor

Complement activation: a group of proteins that generate mediators of chemotaxis, anaphylaxis, bacterial cell lysis, and opsonization

The formation of IC results in in situ generation of the complement activation product, C5a. Stimulation of lung macrophages occurs with the formation of IgG IC and generation of C5a. Activation of lung macrophages results in robust formation of the early response cytokines interleukin-1 (IL-1) and tumor necrosis factor α (TNFα). These cytokines cause upregulation of adhesion molecules on the pulmonary vascular endothelium, including intercellular adhesion molecule-1 (ICAM-1) and E-selectin, which enhance adhesiveness of neutrophils and facilitate their subsequent transmigration into the interstitial and distal airways of lung (1). The expression of alveolar, epithelial ICAM-1 enhances adhesiveness of alveolar macrophages to the epithelial cells, which intensifies the production of cytokines and chemokines, including both cysteine-containing amino acids separated by a non-cysteine amino acid (CXC) and side-by-side cysteines (CC) chemokines. CXC chemokines such as macrophage inflammatory protein (MIP)-2 and cytokine-induced neutrophil chemoattractant (CINC)

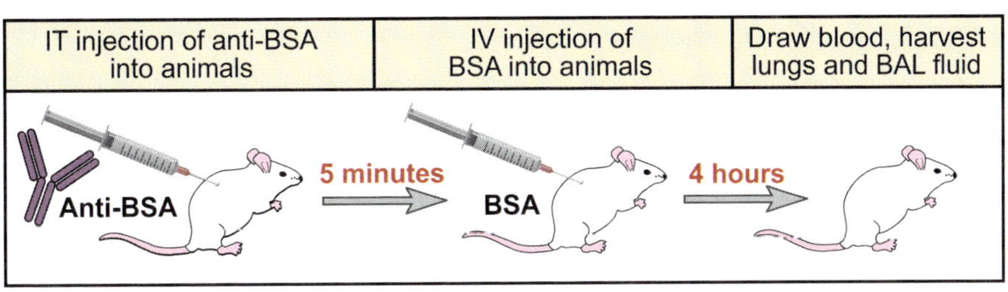

Figure 1

Flow diagram for IgG immune complex–induced lung injury model. IgG antibody to bovine serum albumin (BSA) is instilled into the airway. Five minutes later, BSA is injected intravenously. Four hours later, mice or rats are killed, blood is drawn, and lungs and bronchoalveolar lavage (BAL) fluid are harvested for analysis of lung injury. IT, intratracheal; IV, intravenous.

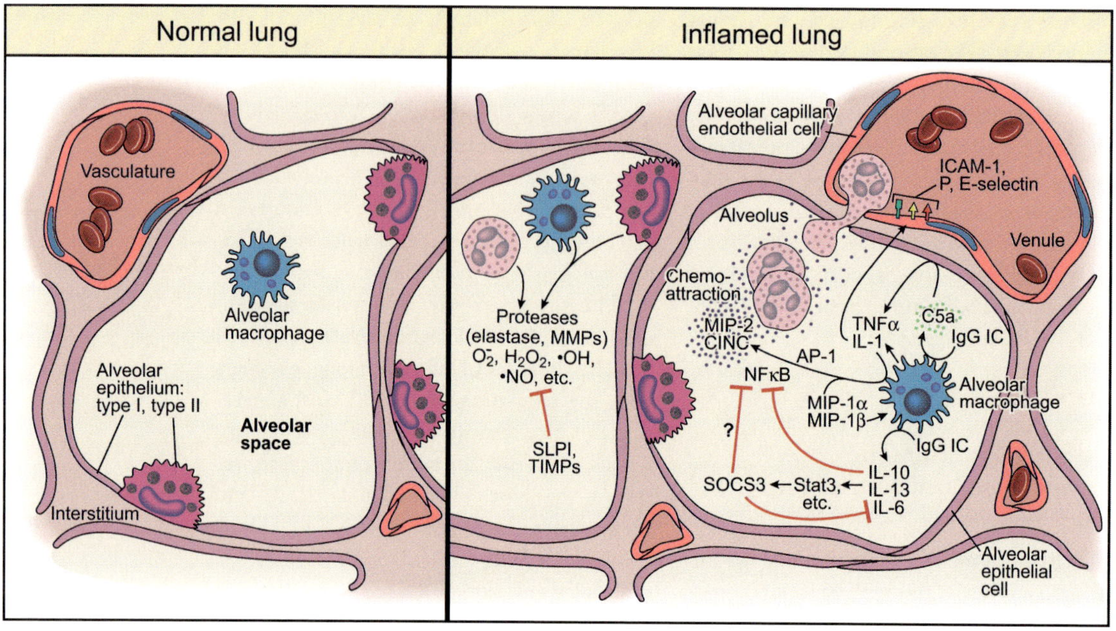

Figure 2

Schematic depiction of the pathogenesis and regulation of acute lung injury in response to IgG immune complex (IC) as compared with normal (noninflamed) lung. After onset of injury, the complement activation product, C5a, together with a number of other mediators [tumor necrosis factor α (TNFα) and interleukin-1 (IL-1)] generated and secreted by lung macrophages, initiates a pro-inflammatory cascade resulting in (*a*) activation of transcription factors such as NFκB, activator protein-1 (AP-1), and signal transducer and activators of transcription 3 (Stat3), (*b*) upregulation of vascular adhesion molecules [intercellular adhesion molecule-1 (ICAM-1) and P- and E-selectins], and (*c*) production of chemokines [macrophage inflammatory protein-2 (MIP-2) and cytokine-induced neutrophil chemoattractant (CINC)]. These events are followed by a recruitment of neutrophils into the interstitial and alveolar compartments. Activation of neutrophils, alveolar macrophages, and epithelial cells leads to the generation of reactive oxygen species and the release of proteinases, which cause lung injury. This inflammatory response is endogenously regulated by IL-6, IL-10, IL-13, as well as by secreted leukocyte proteinase inhibitor (SLPI) and tissue inhibitors of matrix metalloproteinases (TIMPs). MMPs, matrix metalloproteinase; SOCS3, suppressor of cytokine signaling 3.

IL: interleukin

SLPI: leukocyte proteinase inhibitor

produced in the lung form a chemoattractant gradient that recruits neutrophils into the lung. In humans, the IL-8 family of chemokines is induced.

CC chemokines such as MIP-1α and MIP-1β appear to operate as autocrine activators of alveolar macrophages, facilitating the acute inflammatory process (2, 3). Recruitment of neutrophils and their subsequent activation, as well as stimulation of lung macrophages by IgG IC and C5a, lead to the generation of oxidants and release of proteinases from both cell types, eventually causing lung injury characterized by increased vascular permeability and alveolar hemorrhage (4). Not surprisingly, many transcription factors such as NFκB, activator protein-1 (AP-1), and Stat3 (signal transducers and activators of transcription 3) are activated in the acute inflammatory reaction in the lung (5–7). This acute inflammatory response is regulated by IL-6, IL-10, and IL-13, with the last two cytokines found to inhibit NFκB activation (8). Other regulatory proteins during lung injury are the secreted leukocyte proteinase inhibitor (SLPI) and tissue inhibitors of matrix metalloproteinases (TIMPs), with SLPI shown to suppress activation of NFκB (9) (**Figure 2**).

Roles of Fcγ Receptors and Complement/Complement Receptors in Immune Complex Alveolitis

Although studies from mice deficient in FcγRs or complement have indicated distinct functions for these two systems in host immunity, recent results demonstrate that complement signaling, such as that induced by C5a, can be linked to FcγR-mediated responses in lung injury.

Role of Fcγ Receptors in IgG Immune Complex–Induced Lung Injury

IC initiation of lung inflammatory diseases is mediated, to a large extent, by FcγRs. Two general classes of FcγRs are currently recognized: the activation receptors, which are characterized by the presence of a cytoplasmic immunoreceptor tyrosine-based activation motif (ITAM) associated with the receptor, and the inhibitory receptor associated with an immunoreceptor tyrosine-based inhibition motif (ITIM) (10). Although the mechanisms by which IC initiates inflammation are not fully resolved, the specific contribution of each of the FcγR classes to in vivo immune reactions are reasonably established. Both the FcγRI and FcγRIII α chains utilize a disulfide-linked homodimer of the γ chain to transmit signals to the nucleus following ligation (11). The γ chain contains ITAM. Clustering of the FcγRI and FcγRIII by IgG IC induces phosphorylation of tyrosines within the ITAM motifs and initiates a cascade of downstream signaling events that leads eventually to a functional response such as phagocytosis. Whereas FcγRI is constitutively present on only monocytes and macrophages, FcγRIII is expressed in many tissues, including monocytes, macrophages, natural killer cells, mast cells, eosinophils, neutrophils, and platelets, but is absent in lymphocytes. FcγRII is present on almost all hematopoietic cells. In contrast to FcγRI and FcγRIII, FcγRII contains ITIMs, which can act as negative regulators of signals initiated by receptors containing ITAM (**Figure 3**).

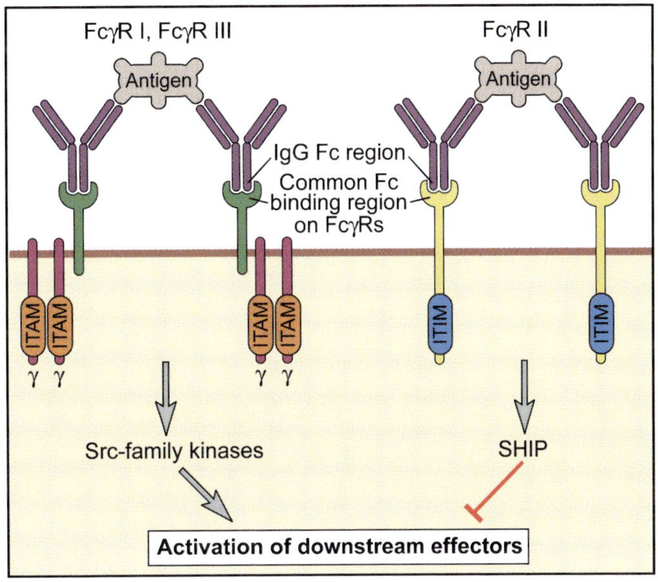

Figure 3

Activating and inhibitory Fc receptors. IgG immune complex causes aggregation of Fcγ receptors (FcγRs). The α chains of both FcγRI and FcγRIII have short cytoplasmic domains that lack activation motifs. Consequently, the γ chain is required to transduce the signals that induce activation of Src-family kinases. Co-engagement of FcγRII to FcγRI and FcγRIII leads to tyrosine phosphorylation of the immunoreceptor tyrosine-based inhibition motif (ITIM). Recruitment of inhibitory signaling molecule SH2 domain-containing inositol-5-phosphatase (SHIP) leads to the abrogation of activation signaling mediated by immunoreceptor tyrosine-based activation motif (ITAM).

TIMP: tissue inhibitors of matrix metalloproteinase

Recent studies using mice genetically deficient in the various FcγRs have provided invaluable insights into the ability of individual FcγRs to mediate IC-induced inflammatory response (**Table 2**). In the lung, the alveolar macrophage promotes IC injury through the production of cytokines, chemokines, and vasoactive substances (12). Alveolar macrophages express FcγRI, FcγRII, and FcγRIII. Mice lacking FcγR, FcγRI, or FcγRIII show impaired lung injury caused by

Table 2 Arthus reaction in various Fcγ receptor–deficient mice

Target	Lung	Other organs	References
$FcR\gamma^{-/-}$	Abolished immune complex–induced alveolitis	Impaired passive Arthus reaction (skin); abolished peritonitis	(16, 40, 148)
$Fc\gamma\ RI^{-/-}$	Not determined	Decreased immune complex–induced passive Arthus reaction (foot pad)	(17, 18)
$Fc\gamma\ RII^{-/-}$	Enhanced immune complex–induced alveolitis	Enhanced immune complex–induced peritonitis	(16, 149)
$Fc\gamma\ RIII^{-/-}$	Not determined	Impaired passive Arthus reaction (skin)	(75)

Edema: increased movement of fluid from the plasma into the extravascular space

TNFα: tumor necrosis factor α

MAC: membrane attack complex

IgG IC deposition, whereas FcγRII-deficient mice develop augmented inflammatory response in IC alveolitis, with increased hemorrhage, edema, and neutrophil infiltration (13–18). Moreover, the stronger phenotype of FcγRIII-deficient mice as compared with FcγRI-deficient mice, as well as the similarity of FcγRIII-deficient mice and FcγR-deficient mice, indicate that the critical role of FcγRs is mediated largely through FcγRIII (15). Relatively little is known about the phlogistic activity of ICs containing other types of immunoglobulins. FcγRs are also present on neutrophils and have been linked to neutrophil responses such as the respiratory burst and cell accumulation in immune-mediated inflammation (14, 19). Thus, the generation of mice selectively deficient for different FcγRs in macrophages and neutrophils is necessary for a more detailed understanding of FcγR function in lung inflammation (**Table 2**).

Complement/Complement Receptor Requirements in IgG Immune Complex–Induced Lung Injury

The role of complement activation products such as C5a, and the membrane attack complex (MAC) C5b-9, in the inflammatory response has been confirmed by a number of experimental studies (20, 21). C5a and MAC assume prominent roles in activating phagocytic cells, as well as endothelial cells. For example, intravenous treatment with anti-C5a IgG in cobra venom factor (CVF)-induced models of ALI results in complete abrogation of upregulation of lung vascular P-selectin, which indicates that upregulation of P-selectin is C5a-dependent (22). Furthermore, C5a induces increased expression of CD11b/CD18 on neutrophils, which contributes to increased adhesion of neutrophils to human umbilical vein endothelial cells (HUVECs) (23). Microarray assay demonstrates that there is an increased gene expression for adhesion molecules, cytokines, and chemokines in HUVECs following exposure to C5a (e.g., E-selectin, ICAM-1, and IL-6) (24). Additionally, both C3a and C5a induce the release of IL-1, TNFα, and prostaglandins from phagocytes (25). Moreover, C5a stimulates the production of plasminogen activator inhibitor-1 in human mast cells and basophils (26). Pre-exposure of mouse dermal microvascular endothelial cells to IL-6, lipopolysaccharide (LPS), or IFNγ followed by addition of C5a resulted in synergistic production of MIP-2 and monocyte chemoattractant protein-1 (MCP-1), which suggests that C5a in the presence of additional agonists may mediate pro-inflammatory effects in endothelial cells (27). Furthermore, MAC in sublytic concentrations enhances endothelial cell production of ICAM-1 and E-selectin in the presence of TNFα and directly induces endothelial cell production of IL-8, MCP-1, and activation of NFκB (28, 29). Because MAC inserts into the cell membrane in the absence of receptor engagement, the signaling pathways involved are unknown. These findings underscore the diverse roles of complement activation products in the inflammatory cascade that leads to tissue injury.

In the context of IgG IC-induced lung injury, compelling evidence indicates that complement activation products are required for the lung inflammatory response in this model (30). Both C5-deficient mice and in vivo blockade of C5a showed a significant decrease in vascular permeability and sharply diminished neutrophil accumulation, which suggests a dominant pro-inflammatory role for C5a (31, 32). The protective effects of anti-C5a IgG are related to its ability to suppress lung macrophage production of TNFα, a critical mediator for ICAM-1 upregulation. Moreover, complement activation in this model of lung inflammatory injury is compartmentalized: Only airway instillation of antibody, not intravenous infusion of anti-C5a IgG, is protective, which suggests that C5a activation is occurring chiefly in the distal airway compartment. Recent data indicate that C5a can be generated directly by activated lung macrophages, extending the potential sources of C5-cleaving enzymes beyond proteins present in the plasma (33). The dominant role of C5a in IgG IC-induced lung injury was demonstrated further by both in vitro and in vivo studies showing that, in the presence of IgG IC, C5a and MAC cause synergistic intrapulmonary generation of rat CXC (MIP-2 and CINC) and CC (MIP-1α, MIP-1β, and MCP-1) chemokines and increased neutrophil accumulation, as well as lung injury (34, 35). By using C5-deficient mice and specific antisera for C5a, it was demonstrated further that the upper airway hyper-reactivity induced by IgG IC was C5a-dependent (36). All these data suggest that activation of complement, especially generation of C5a, is an upstream event in the inflammatory cascade following IgG IC deposition in the lung (**Figure 4**).

Although the precise mechanism of C5a activation in lung injury is still unclear, the interaction of C5a with complement C5a receptor (C5aR) may be essential for the majority of complement-mediated inflammatory reactions. In addition to the well-known expression of C5aR on myeloid cells, it is also present on bronchial and alveolar epithelial cells (37, 38). Exposure of alveolar epithelial cells to LPS, IL-6, or TNFα causes increased binding of C5a, evidenced by its association with increased cellular levels of mRNA for C5aR (38). In vivo, mice deficient in C5aR were protected from IC-induced alveolitis (39, 40). A similar attenuation of lung injury after blocking C5a-C5aR interaction with specific C5aR antagonists indicates that the complement effect in IgG IC inflammation is mediated predominantly by C5aR (41). Both C5aR and FcγRs are expressed on alveolar macrophages. Although the strict requirement of FcγRs for the majority of IgG IC-induced inflammatory diseases may support the view that the participation of complement is independent of or secondary to FcγRs, complement and FcγRs play codominant roles in pulmonary IgG IC-induced reaction. This implies that FcγR-mediated responses can be integrated through C5aR activation (42–44). In the study that recently tested this hypothesis, C5a caused induction of FcγRIII and suppression of FcγRII on alveolar macrophages (40). Genetic ablation of C5aR expression completely abolished regulation of FcγRs and resulted in decreased TNFα and MIP-2 production and neutrophil infiltration in the lung. Formation of soluble IC also results in suppression of FcγRII and upregulation of FcγR III. However, in C5aR mutant mice, regulation of FcγR was absent. Therefore, C5a plays a critical role in regulating the inhibitory/activating FcγR II/III receptor pair to connect complement and FcγR effector pathways during inflammation (40). Acting upstream of C5, C3- and C4-deficient mice demonstrate similar reverse passive Arthus reaction in the skin as wild-type mice (43).

C5aR: complement C5a receptor

Transcriptional Mechanisms of IgG Immune Complex–Induced Alveolitis

One of the major cellular responses initiated by FcγR cross-linking in the lung is the activation of genes encoding important chemokines

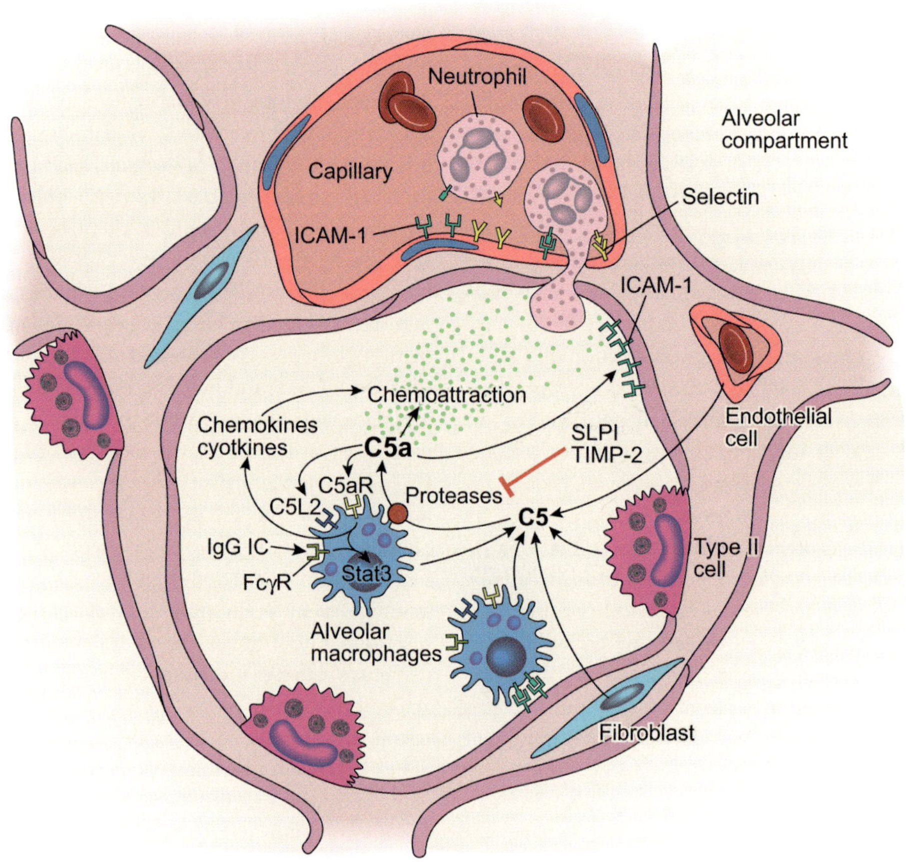

Figure 4

Generation and function of C5a in the alveolar compartment during IgG immune complex (IC)-induced lung injury. C5, produced locally from various types of lung cells, including alveolar macrophages, type II epithelial cells, and fibroblasts, is cleaved into C5a by enzymes released from macrophages. The enzymes appear to be inducible and can be blocked by naturally occurring secreted leukocyte proteinase inhibitors (SLPI) and tissue inhibitors of matrix metalloproteinases-2 (TIMP-2) (33, 119). C5a not only functions as a neutrophil chemoattractant, but it also regulates expression of adhesion molecules, cytokines, and chemokines. C5a also stimulates activation (phosphorylation) of transcription factors such as signal transducer and activators of transcription 3 (Stat3) for its maximal activity in the lung. ICAM-1, intercellular adhesion molecule-1; FcγR, Fcγ receptor.

and cytokines of inflammation. The resulting levels of these pro-inflammatory mediators, anti-inflammatory mediators, and their balance correlate with the magnitude of lung injury and its severity. Although the signaling pathway from FcγR to the nucleus is unclear, growing evidence indicates that the regulation of gene expression in the lung is mediated by a highly intricate network of transcription factors (45, 46). Recent studies in the IgG IC-induced lung injury model show that several transcription factors such as NFκB, AP-1, and Stat3 are activated in both alveolar macrophages and whole-lung extracts following IgG IC deposition (5–7). Thus, understanding the function of transcription factors involved in lung inflammation is of great interest.

Activation of NFκB During Lung Inflammatory Injury

NFκB proteins are a small group of closely related transcription factors, which in mammals consists of five members: c-Rel, p65 (RelA), RelB, p50, and p52. All five proteins have a Rel homology domain (RHD) that regulates their dimerization, DNA-binding, and principal regulatory domain (47). The nuclear-localization sequence at the C terminus of the RHD is rendered inactive in nonstimulated cells through binding of NFκB-specific inhibitors, IκB proteins (47). Activation of most NFκB depends upon phosphorylation-induced ubiquitination of IκB proteins, which is mediated by the IκB kinase complex and the $E3^{I\kappa B}$ ubiquitin ligase complex. Once poly-ubiquitinated, the IκBs undergo rapid degradation through the 26S proteasome; the liberated NFκB dimers translocate to the nucleus, where they participate in transcriptional activation of their target genes (48).

NFκB controls the expression of genes encoding a wide variety of pro-inflammatory mediators (including TNFα, IL-1β, many chemokines, and adhesion molecules) (47). All of these factors play an important role in lung inflammatory injury, suggesting that NFκB plays a critical role during the development of pulmonary inflammation and ALI. This was demonstrated further in vivo by showing that NFκB activation preceded transcriptional activation of the P-selectin, E-selectin, and ICAM-1 genes in the lung after administration of endotoxin (49). In the IgG IC model of lung injury, we found that activation of alveolar macrophages was characterized by increased nuclear translocation, DNA binding of NFκB, and subsequent production of TNFα and IL-1β (5, 8, 50, 51). TNFα and IL-1β further stimulate NFκB activation in neighboring lung cells such as alveolar epithelial and vascular endothelial cells. Depletion of alveolar macrophages or in vivo blockade of either TNFα or IL-1β substantially reduces lung NFκB activation and subsequent lung injury (5, 50–52). In addition, instillation of TNFα in the lungs of alveolar macrophage-depleted rats restored NFκB activation in whole-lung tissue (52). All these results suggest that activation of alveolar macrophages and NFκB is an initial event in the genesis of lung inflammatory reactions. NFκB activation, which is triggered by intrapulmonary deposition of IgG IC, is then propagated by products of alveolar macrophages into other lung cells.

It is well known that macrophage/neutrophil-derived ROS can activate NFκB (53). In the LPS-induced lung injury model, NFκB activation was impaired in NADPH (nicotinamide-adenine dinucleotide phosphate, reduced) oxidase-deficient mice, suggesting a role for ROS in in vivo lung NFκB activation (54). In the IgG IC model of lung injury, NFκB activation was suppressed by lung instillation of the antioxidant N-acetylcysteine (NAC), but not by catalase (5), which suggests that intracellular oxidant generation contributes to the activation of NFκB in lung tissue. However, how oxidants mediate well-coordinated NFκB signaling is still subject to intense debate. Furthermore, although the inhibitory action of NAC is widely believed to be due to its antioxidant activities, it seems difficult to envision any known protein in the signaling pathways associated with NFκB activation that would serve as a specific receptor for ROS. Recently, researchers demonstrated that NAC inhibits NFκB activity by selectively lowering the affinity of TNFα binding to its receptor, which is independent of its antioxidative function (55). Thus, NFκB activation does not seem to be a universal response to oxidative stress.

Activator Protein-1 Activation in Acute Lung Injury

The transcription factor complex, AP-1, is activated by a wide range of conditions and stresses, including oxidants, DNA damage, and pro-inflammatory cytokines (56). The AP-1 complex is a dimer composed of Jun/Jun, Fos/Jun, or ATF-2/Jun family proteins. Much of what is known about the biological function of AP-1 relates to its prominent roles in cell proliferation, differentiation, transformation, and apoptosis. Little is known regarding the function of AP-1 in lung inflammatory responses (56). The promoter regions of many inflammatory cytokines and chemokines contain AP-1 binding sites, which suggests that AP-1 activation may have a role in the induction of acute, cytokine-mediated inflammation (57, 58). Moreover, TNFα induces the activation of AP-1 in alveolar epithelial cells, which suggests that a positive-feedback mechanism exists (59). In vivo, AP-1 binding activity in the whole lung increases dramatically during both LPS-induced and IgG IC-induced lung injury (6, 60, 61). Like NFκB, the activation of AP-1 in the lung injury model of IgG IC is TNFα- and macrophage-, but not complement-, dependent (6). Considering that the transcription of many pro-inflammatory mediators requires cooperative transactivation of NFκB and AP-1 for optimal expression (62), it is likely that the role of AP-1 in the development of acute lung inflammatory injury is to cooperate with NFκB to regulate the expression of inflammatory mediators and the subsequent dissemination of the inflammatory response from alveolar macrophages to other cells within the lung (**Figure 5**).

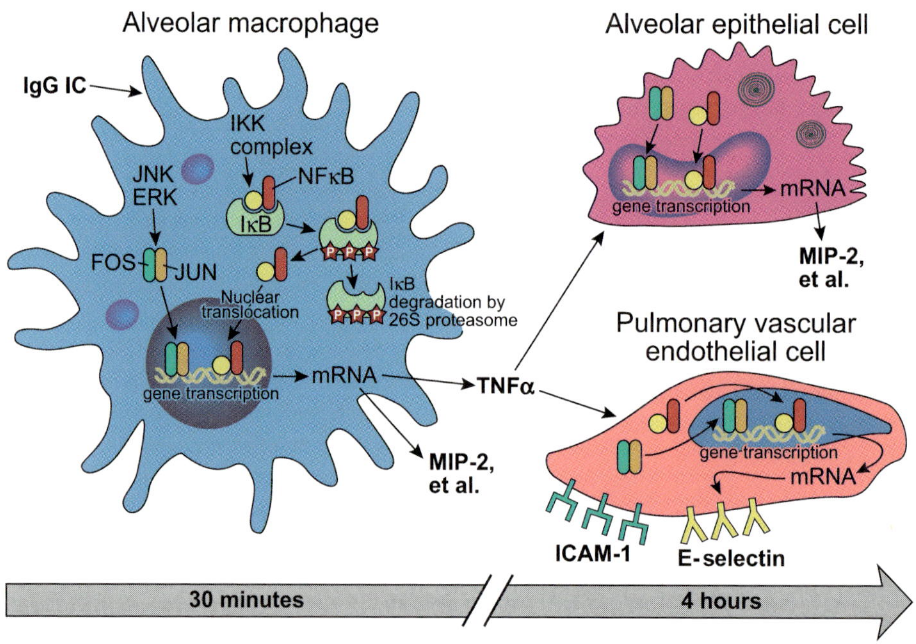

Figure 5

Possible roles for NFκB and activator protein-1 (AP-1) in the IgG immune complex (IC)-induced lung injury model. Intrapulmonary deposition of IgG ICs triggers intense activation of alveolar macrophages. Alveolar macrophage activation is characterized by increased nuclear translocation, DNA binding of NFκB and AP-1, and subsequent production of the pro-inflammatory mediators such as tumor necrosis factor α (TNFα) and macrophage inflammatory protein-2 (MIP-2). In this lung injury model, there are two waves of NFκB and AP-1 activation: an early wave (at 30 min) involving lung macrophages and a late wave (at 4 h) involving other lung cells, including alveolar epithelial and endothelial cells where NFκB dimers and AP-1 dimers can translocate into the nucleus and bind to relevant regions of DNA and initiate gene transcription such as intercellular adhesion molecule-1 (ICAM-1) and E-selectin. IKK, IKAPPAB kinase; JNK, c-JUN N-terminal kinase; ERK, extracellular signal-regulated protein kinase.

Stat3 Activation in Acute Lung Injury

Stats comprise a family of seven related polypeptides that participate in signaling pathways mediating a wide variety of cellular and organ responses to cytokines and growth factors. Although specific Stats generally mediate signals provided by relatively specific receptors, Stat3 participates in numerous pathways involving a large number of diverse growth factors and cytokines (63). Stat3 is activated by Janus kinase (JAKs)-induced phosphorylation. Phosphorylation mediates dimerization, nuclear translocation, and the subsequent activation of transcriptional targets. Although deletion of Stat3 causes early embryonic lethality, studies of tissue or cell-specific deletion of the Stat3 gene have suggested that Stat3 may play an important role during inflammation (63–65). Stat3 is expressed in various cell types in the lung, but its role in lung function and pathology is largely unknown. In vitro, Stat3 regulates the expression of surfactant protein B (66). Stimulation of alveolar macrophages through toll-like receptors 2, 4, or 9 is sufficient to inhibit phosphorylation and nuclear translocation of Stat3 (67). Moreover, altered IL-6-Stat3 signaling in lung fibroblasts from patients with idiopathic pulmonary fibrosis may contribute to the resistance of these cells to apoptosis (68). In vivo, Stat3 is activated rapidly in the lung after intranasal LPS administration in mice (69). Importantly, Stat3 activation requires ROS and occurs in other ALI models, such as hemorrhagic shock, gastric acid aspiration, and acute pancreatitis (69, 70). These observations suggest that Stat3 may be a common pathway for mediating ALI. In contrast, recent studies suggest that expression of Stat3 in respiratory epithelial cells plays a critical role in the maintenance of surfactant homeostasis and lung function during oxygen-induced injury (71, 72).

Stat3 activation was also demonstrated in lungs and alveolar macrophages after intrapulmonary deposition of IgG IC (7). Activation of Stat3 in lungs was macrophage- and neutrophil-dependent. Furthermore, both IL-6 and IL-10 contributed to Stat3 activation in inflamed lung (7). Thus, it is possible that IL-6 and IL-10 exert their regulatory function in vivo during ALI by activating Stat3, which then serves as a negative regulator of the acute inflammatory response. Supporting this hypothesis, overexpression of suppressor of cytokine signaling 3 (SOCS3), a feedback inhibitor of JAK-Stat signaling pathways, in the lung dramatically enhanced IgG IC-induced lung injury and inhibited Stat3 activation (Gao & Ward, unpublished data). Thus, the role of Stat3 in ALI is likely to be complex; more details of the Stat pathway are necessary for a better understanding of the mechanisms of ALI.

Roles of Cytokines in Acute Lung Injury

During the inflammatory response, production of early response cytokines such as TNFα and IL-1 defines not only the type of inflammation, but also the intensity of leukocyte accumulation. In the IgG IC model, both TNFα and IL-1 appear in BAL fluids obtained two to four hours after commencement of IgG IC deposition in lung (50, 51). Blocking of either cytokine [by antibodies, soluble TNFα receptor-1, or IL-1 receptor antagonist (IL-1Ra)] leads to a profound reduction in the neutrophil influx and eventual severity of lung injury (13, 50, 51), which suggests that these cytokines play a critical role in the development of IgG IC-induced lung injury. Recruitment of neutrophils into inflamed lung is initiated by TNFα and IL-1-induced expression of adhesion molecules on the lung vascular endothelium, which involve P-selectin, E-selectin, and ICAM-1 (73, 74). Moreover, TNFα and IL-1 directly or indirectly mediate neutrophil migration to the lung interstitium and alveoli by inducing a robust production of chemokines (CXC and CC) and cytokines in the lung via a NFκB-dependent mechanism (4, 5, 34). A recent study using mice either lacking the TNFα class I receptor or after treatment with neutralizing monoclonal antibody (mAb) to TNFα demonstrated that absence or in vivo blockade of TNFα, although effective in attenuating neutrophil influx, did not result in significantly reduced production of macrophage inflammatory protein 2 (MIP-2) and keratinocyte chemotactic factor (KC) chemokines. This result suggests that in IC-induced alveolitis, the activation of FcγRs may induce divergent downstream effector pathways to trigger the inflammatory response (13). Another member of the IL-1 family of ligands, IL-18, has also recently been shown to function as a pro-inflammatory cytokine during IgG IC-induced acute lung inflammation, and serves apparently as an autocrine activator of alveolar macrophages to bring about expression of other inflammatory mediators (75).

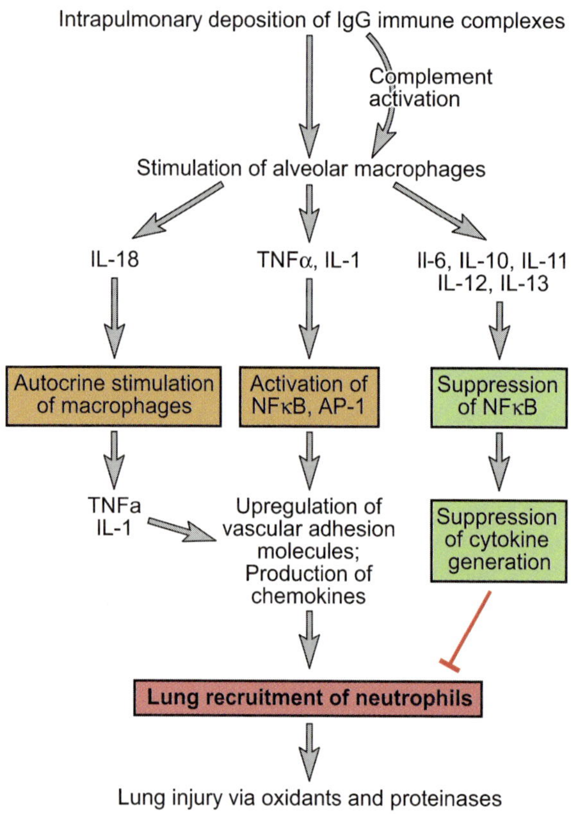

Figure 6

Role of cytokines in IgG immune complex (IC)-induced lung injury. Activation of alveolar macrophages and locally generated C5a by IgG IC results in the synthesis and release of tumor necrosis factor α (TNFα), interleukin-1 (IL-1), and IL-18, which represent a positive-feedback loop of lung inflammation. This inflammatory response is endogenously regulated by IL-6, IL-10, IL-11, IL-12, and IL-13, each of which interferes with either lung NFκB activation or some other undetermined signaling pathways. AP-1, activator protein-1.

The inflammatory response induced by intrapulmonary deposition of IgG IC is regulated by a number of endogenous anti-inflammatory cytokines. These include IL-4, IL-6, IL-10, IL-11, IL-12, and IL-13 (76). Although the molecular mechanisms by which these regulatory cytokines operate are incompletely defined, each is able to limit the extent of lung inflammation by reducing the production of TNFα and IL-1β (77–82). The anti-inflammatory effects of IL-10, IL-13, and IL-11 have been linked to their ability to suppress NFκB activation by either preventing IκBα degradation (IL-10 and IL-13) or inducing IκBα and IκBβ gene transcription (IL-11) (8, 79, 83). Although the precise mechanism by which IL-6 reduces lung injury is not defined, Kaplanski and colleagues recently suggested an attractive hypothesis in acute inflammation, namely that IL-6 exerts its protective role by favoring monocyte recruitment, which leads to inflammation resolution (84). Another important endogenous regulator capable of suppressing the IgG IC-induced neutrophil recruitment and ensuing lung injury is IL-1Ra (85). In the lung, alveolar macrophages and recruited neutrophils are the major sources of IL-1Ra, which competes with IL-1 to bind to the IL-1 receptor and inhibit IL-1 pro-inflammatory function (85). Taken together, a complex network of pro-inflammatory cytokines plays a major role in mediating, amplifying, and perpetuating the IgG IC-induced lung injury (**Figure 6**). Simultaneous production of anti-inflammatory cytokines counterbalances the effects of pro-inflammatory cytokines.

The Chemokine Network

Chemokines constitute a superfamily of small (8–10 kDa), inducible, and secreted polypeptides involved in a variety of immune mechanisms and inflammatory responses. The chemokines display highly conserved cysteine (C) amino acid residues. Four classes of chemokines (CXC, CC, C, and CX_3C-chemokines) have been defined on the basis of whether a nonconserved amino acid residue exists between the first two C amino acids of the primary structure (86).

Following intrapulmonary deposition of IgG IC in rodents, abundant neutrophil accumulation in the lungs is pivotal in the pathogenesis of acute lung inflammation (30). Early response cytokines (such as TNFα and IL-1β) together with C5a or sublytic forms of MAC initiate a pro-inflammatory cascade, including the generation of chemotactic chemokines (4). The rat CXC chemokines, MIP-2 and CINC (KC in mouse), are among the most potent chemoattractants for rodent neutrophils and play a key role by directly attracting neutrophils along a chemotactic gradient into the alveolar compartment and lung interstitium (77). Blocking studies with MIP-2 and CINC-specific antibodies showed significant decrease in myeloperoxidase (MPO) buildup and neutrophil content in BAL fluids, and attenuated lung injury after IC deposition in rats (77). In several human studies, IL-8, a member of the CXC-chemokine family, appears to be a main chemotactic factor for neutrophils and has been linked to the development and mortality caused by ALI/ARDS (acute lung injury/acute respiratory distress syndrome, respectively) (87). The possible role of IL-8 as a mediator in acute lung inflammatory reactions has also been investigated in various animal models. A rabbit model of lung ischemia-reperfusion injury has shown that IL-8 contributes significantly to maximal pulmonary neutrophil infiltration and lung injury (88). Passive immunization of animals with anti-IL-8 prior to ischemia-reperfusion attenuated lung injury. Similarly, in the IgG IC-induced lung injury model in rats, a neutralizing antibody to human recombinant IL-8 administered intratracheally at the onset of injury was highly protective against lung injury (89). The protective effects correlated with reduced accumulation of neutrophils in lung tissue, which suggest that in rats a homologue of IL-8 is functionally important for the development of ALI.

During the pathogenesis of lung injury in response to IgG IC deposition, the generation of the chemoattractant CXC chemokines (MIP-2 and CINC) appears to be amplified by CC chemokines (MIP-1α and MIP-1β). Both MIP-1α and MIP-1β seem to function as autocrine stimulators of pulmonary macrophages, priming them to respond to inflammatory stimuli with enhanced production of pro-inflammatory cytokines such as TNFα, which leads ultimately to exacerbated lung injury (2, 3). Researchers have also raised the question of whether two other CC chemokines, MCP-1 and RANTES (regulated on activation and normal T cells), are involved in this acute inflammatory response. Antibody-induced blockade of MCP-1 or RANTES did not affect lung neutrophil recruitment or the severity of lung injury (3). In contrast, the CC chemokine eotaxin, long known as a mediator of eosinophil recruitment into the lung during allergic airway inflammation, has been described recently as having a regulatory role in IgG IC-induced lung injury (90). In vivo blockade of eotaxin by antibody leads to increased MIP-2 and CINC production, enhanced neutrophil accumulation and, ultimately, intensified lung injury (90). The precise mechanism by which eotaxin-1 is able to affect the lung inflammatory response to IgG ICs remains to be defined. Thus, endogenous eotaxin seems to function as a regulatory chemokine by negatively regulating neutrophil migration through suppressed generation of MIP-2 and CINC.

Myeloperoxidase (MPO): cytoplasmic primary granules of neutrophils that contain several enzymes

Roles of Adhesion Molecules in Mediating Neutrophil Accumulation in Immune Complex–Mediated Lung Inflammation

Neutrophil accumulation is an early hallmark of IC-mediated inflammation. The earliest adhesive events involved in neutrophil recruitment in this lung injury model include the capture of blood neutrophils by activated endothelial cells, which is mediated by interactions between selectins and their glycoprotein/glycolipid counter-receptors [e.g., sialyl Lewis x-type (sLe^X) oligosaccharides]. By using either antiselectin antibodies or selectin-Ig chimeras, researchers demonstrated that L-, E-, and P-selectins are all required for the lung neutrophil accumulation and injury that ensues IgG IC deposition (73, 91–93). Studies of the effects of sLe^X oligosaccharides in IC-induced ALI have yielded conclusions consistent with those derived from the selectin-blocking experiments. In both rat IgG IC and CVF models of lung injury, for example, sLe^X preparations cause dose-dependent protective effects, as assessed by changes in lung vascular permeability, hemorrhage, and PMN buildup (94, 95). In contrast, in the model of IgA IC-induced lung injury, which does not involve participation of neutrophils, sLe^X preparations are not protective. Moreover, a truncated form of complement inhibitor soluble complement receptor type 1 (sCR1) possessing sLe^X moieties demonstrates greater protective effects than the non-sLe^X-decorated form of sCR1 in the IgG IC model (96). Enhanced protective effects correlate with greater lung vascular binding of sCR1-sLe^X as compared with sCR1 alone. These studies confirm that the interaction between selectins and their ligands and associated adhesive processes are essential for neutrophil recruitment in acute lung inflammation induced by IgG IC deposition, and provide support for efforts to diminish neutrophil recruitment and inflammation via blockade of selectin-dependent adhesion (**Figure 7**).

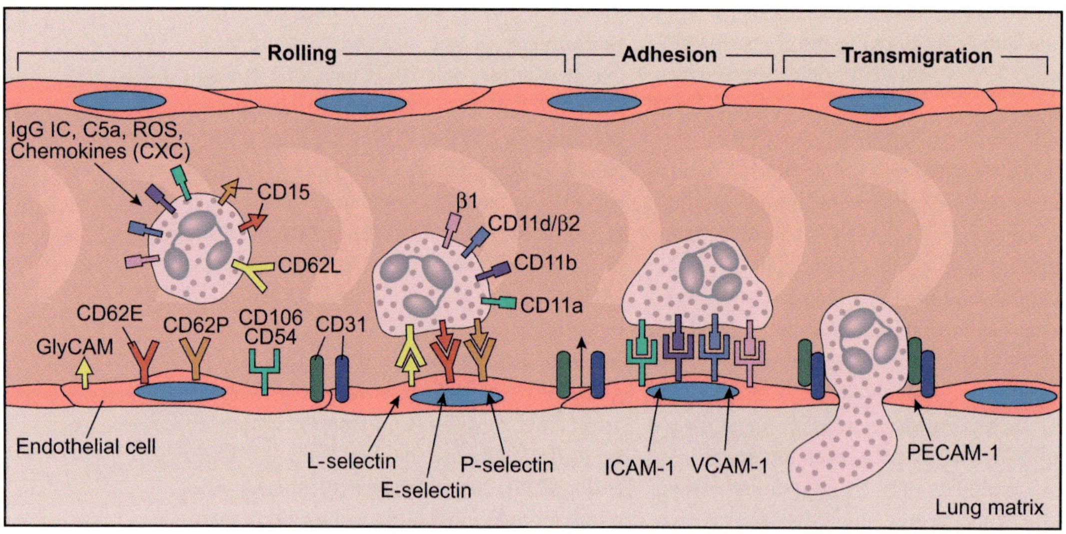

Figure 7

Adhesion molecule cascade during IgG immune complex (IC)-induced lung injury. The initial step involves activation of vascular endothelial cells, including upregulation of selectins (E-selectin and P-selectin). Neutrophil-rolling over the activated endothelium occurs by interacting with these selectins. As the neutrophils roll, the integrins, such as CD18 (CD11a/CD18 and CD11b/CD18), are engaged. The interactions between integrins on neutrophils and intercellular adhesion molecule-1 (ICAM-1) on endothelial cells mediate the firm adhesion of neutrophils. Platelet-endothelial cell adhesion molecule-1 (PECAM-1) contributes to the final neutrophil transmigration to lung interstitium. ROS, reactive oxygen species; CXC, cysteine containing amino acids separated by a noncysteine amino acid; GlyCAM, glycosylation-dependent cell adhesion molecule; VCAM-1, vascular cell adhesion molecule-1.

The firm adhesion of neutrophils to the lung vascular endothelium and their subsequent transmigration are modulated by certain types of integrins. The integrins are a family of transmembrane-spanning adhesion molecules expressed on the surface of leukocytes. Each functional unit consists of one α and one β chain. So far, at least 21 different α chains and eight different β chains that can associate to form heterodimers with different adhesive specificities have been identified (97). These molecules mediate adhesive interactions of leukocytes with ligands expressed on the endothelium such as ICAMs and vascular cell adhesion molecule-1 (VCAM-1). In the IgG IC model of ALI, the accumulation of neutrophils and ensuing injury require both β_2 integrins (CD11a, b, d/CD18) and β_1 integrins ($\alpha_4\beta_1$), as well as ICAM-1 (98–100). In addition, anti-CD11a only reduced lung MPO buildup and injury when given intravenously, whereas anti-CD11b was protective only when given intratracheally (99). These results suggest that CD11a/CD18 plays a key role in neutrophil adhesion to pulmonary vascular endothelium, whereas the role of CD11b/CD18 seems to be restricted to the distal airway compartment. Importantly, ICAM-1 plays roles in both the vascular and distal airway compartments (99). This is supported further by a study showing that soluble ICAM-1 can activate lung macrophages and enhance lung injury after intrapulmonary disposition of IC (101). The enhanced protective effects of combined adhesion molecule blockade in this lung injury model underscore further the concept that adhesion molecule participation in the inflammatory process may involve either the intravascular or extravascular compartment, or both (102).

Platelet-endothelial cell adhesion molecule-1 (PECAM-1) is a 130-kDa transmembrane glycoprotein expressed on the surface of platelets and most subsets of leukocytes, including macrophages and neutrophils. It is also found on endothelial cell intercellular junctions and is structurally related to ICAM-1 and VCAM-1. In the lung, PECAM-1 is expressed intensely in large- and small-vessel endothelium. By using both anti-PECAM-1 antibodies and PECAM-1 knock-out mice, researchers demonstrated that IgG IC-induced lung injury is PECAM-1-dependent (103, 104). Moreover, macrophages harvested from PECAM-1 knock-out mice showed decreased ability to secrete TNFα after exposure to IC-coated beads. In addition, the inhibition of IC-dependent lung inflammation was seen in bone marrow chimeric mice that had PECAM-null leukocytes, but not in mice with PECAM-null endothelial cells (104). Because PECAM-1-mediated transmigration requires homophilic neutrophil-endothelial cell interactions, these data suggest that the failure of neutrophil infiltration after PECAM-1 blockade was not caused by a block in transmigration, but rather by a specific deficit in the FcγR function of PECAM-null macrophages, although the exact mechanism is unclear (104).

Reactive Oxygen Species, Proteinases, Antiproteinases, and Lung Defense

During ALI, the activation and degranulation of migrated neutrophils and activation of resident macrophages result in the production of multiple toxic products of oxygen and L-arginine (such as $O_2^{\bullet}$, $HO^{\bullet}$, $^{\bullet}NO$, and $ONOO^{\bullet}$) and various proteinases, leading to structural damage of cells and connective tissue (**Figure 8**). ROS signaling in lung endothelium has an important role in in vivo pulmonary vascular permeability (105). In the IgG IC model, ROS are responsible for much of the cell and tissue damage that occurs in the injured lung because catalase and other antioxidant treatments greatly reduce lung injury (30, 106–109). Two pathways are suggested to be responsible for the production of ROS in the IgG IC inflamed lung (106, 109). The first pathway features stimulation of both alveolar macrophages and type II epithelial cells by the presence of the IC and is

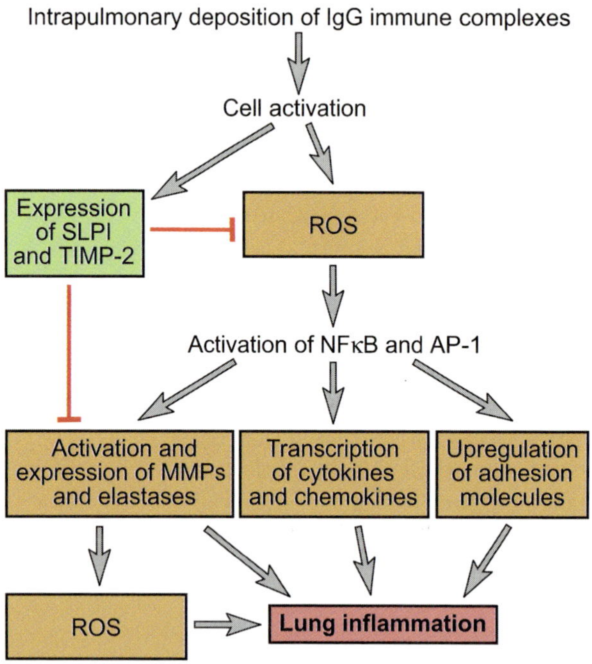

Figure 8

Roles of reactive oxygen species (ROS), proteinases, and proteinase inhibitors in the IgG immune complex (IC)-induced lung injury. IgG IC deposition in the lung triggers oxidative stress and stimulation of residential lung macrophages and recruited neutrophils via engagement of Fcγ receptors. ROS not only plays a destructive role in the lung, but also activates NFκB and activator protein-1 (AP-1), which lead to intense production of chemokines, cytokines, upregulation of adhesion molecules, activation, and expression of proteinases. These events further enhance influx of neutrophils into the lung, oxidative stress, and the subsequent lung injury. Proteinase inhibitor secreted by leukocyte proteinase inhibitor (SLPI) and tissue inhibitors of matrix metalloproteinases-2 (TIMP-2) are also induced rapidly after the pulmonary IgG IC deposition, which function as negative-feedback regulators of lung inflammation. MMPs, matrix metalloproteinases.

responsible for the production of •NO from L-arginine by inducible nitric oxide synthase (110). The second ROS-generating pathway features NADPH oxidase, an enzyme assembled on the surfaces of macrophages, monocytes, and neutrophils after cell activation by a variety of agonists, including IC. NADPH is responsible for the formation of $O_2^{\bullet}$ from oxygen (O_2), which can be reduced to H_2O_2. H_2O_2 can be reduced to $HO^{\bullet}$ or metabolized in the presence of MPO and chloride to produce hypochlorous acid, which is a potent oxidant and has the ability to convert latent collagenases and gelatinases to their active forms.

ROS may also mediate lung injury through regulating neutrophil accumulation directly, by modulating adhesion molecule expression, or indirectly, by mediating the activation of transcription factors, which lead to the enhanced expression of pro-inflammatory chemokine genes (4, 111). In addition, ROS can regulate FcγR signaling and function in both macrophages and neutrophils (112). ROS may also enhance the effects of proteinases in this lung injury model. It was shown recently that catalase suppresses matrix metalloproteinase-9 (MMP-9) elaboration concomitantly with its inhibition of IgG IC-induced lung injury (113), suggesting that oxidants and proteinases may interact to bring about inflammatory lung injury.

Besides ROS, proteinases are other leukocyte-derived toxic molecules that are considered important in the pathophysiology of ALI. Among the proteinases released during lung inflammation, elastase and MMPs have central roles in ALI (114). Elastase is a serine proteinase, is capable of degrading many components of extracellular matrix, and has cytotoxic effects on many cells such as neutrophils, endothelial cells, and airway epithelial cells (115–117). Three types of endogenous proteinase inhibitors suppress the activity of elastase, including α-1 proteinase inhibitor, α-2 macroglobulin, and SLPI. In the lung, SLPI is a central component of pulmonary defenses against proteinase-mediated lung injury (118). Endogenous SLPI has been detected and is upregulated during IgG IC-induced lung injury (119). Blockade of endogenous SLPI with neutralizing antibody causes enhanced pulmonary accumulation of neutrophils and increased lung vascular permeability, whereas intratracheal administration of recombinant human SLPI results in suppression of IgG IC-induced alveolitis (9, 119, 120). Thus, endogenous SLPI appears to be an important natural regulator of the inflammatory response.

However, recent studies demonstrate that SLPI functions as more than just a proteinase inhibitor. For example, SLPI augments glutathione production in the lung, which suggests that SLPI may be an important defense against oxidant-mediated lung injury (121). Moreover, SLPI modifies macrophage functions in mice, supported by the fact that ectopic expression of SLPI in macrophages increases their resistance to LPS (122). In contrast to wild-type macrophages, SLPI-deficient macrophages show activation of NFκB and higher production of IL-6 and high-mobility group-1 after cell exposure to LPS (123). These observations strongly suggest that SLPI is an important participant in innate immunity, acting as an anti-inflammatory molecule. Interestingly, SLPI may have a similar function in IgG IC-induced lung injury. In this model, the presence of SLPI results in a greatly reduced activation of NFκB and expression of ICAM-1 in whole lung (9). Because NFκB regulates the transcriptional activation of genes for ICAM-1, it is likely that SLPI reduces ICAM-1 expression through the suppression of endothelial NFκB activation. The mechanism by which SPLI impairs NFκB activation in the lung is distinct from the manner by which IL-10 and IL-13 inhibit NFκB activation. SLPI causes increased protein levels of lung IκBβ, but not IκBα (9). Thus, the inhibitory effects of SLPI on NFκB are related to the classical pathway for NFκB activation, but the exact mechanism of IκBβ buildup by SLPI is unclear.

Other important proteinases in the lung are MMPs. MMPs represent a pivotal family of zinc-dependent enzymes responsible for degradation of extracellular matrix components during normal remodeling and repair processes (124). In conditions such as pulmonary inflammation, high levels of MMPs are produced. These may facilitate tissue injury. Neutrophils and macrophages produce high levels of MMPs and seem to be the primary source of MMPs during inflammation (125, 126). Experimental models of lung injury suggest an important role for MMPs. Models of ALI induced by LPS, hyperoxia, or ozone have shown increased MMP activities in the lung (127–129). In the IgG IC-induced lung injury model, BAL fluid from injured lungs contained increased amounts of MMP-2, MMP-9, MMP-12, and MMP-13 as compared with control BAL fluid (120, 130). In mice genetically deficient in selected MMPs, Warner and colleagues showed that MMP-3, MMP-9, and MMP-12 were all involved in the pathogenesis of IgG IC-induced lung injury (131, 132). Moreover, in vitro production of MMP-3 and MMP-9 occurred in both rodent lung fibroblasts and type II epithelial cells (but not in endothelial cells) after either IgG IC or LPS stimulation (133). These observations provide insight into possible mechanisms by which tissue damage occurs in acute inflammation.

The potent proteolytic activities of MMPs are regulated mainly by specific TIMPs that inhibit MMP activities to a large degree. At least four TIMPs have been described so far (TIMP-1, -2, -3, and -4). Among them, TIMP-2 is released from a variety of lung cells and plays an important role in the regulation of tissue MMPs (134). In IgG IC-induced lung injury model, expression of TIMP-2 was upregulated in the inflamed lung (119). In addition, exogenously administered recombinant human TIMP-2 reduced the intensity of lung inflammatory injury after deposition of IgG IC, and blockade of endogenous TIMP-2 caused enhanced pulmonary accumulation of neutrophils and increased lung vascular permeability (119, 120). In contrast to SLPI, instillation of TIMP-2 into inflamed lung had no effect on the protein expression of either IκBα or IκBβ, suggesting that effects of SLPI on lung NFκB activation are specific to SLPI, not the general class of proteinase inhibitors. Interestingly, in this lung injury model, treatment with either anti-SLPI or anti-TIMP-2 resulted in a significant increase in C5a-related chemotactic activity, suggesting that enzymes regulated by these endogenous inhibitors facilitate the cleavage of C5 to generate C5a (119) (**Figure 4**). In summary, although the precise mechanisms of inflammatory-induced lung injury are still unknown, it can be concluded that the balance of endogenous proteinases and antiproteinases (SLPI and TIMPs) in the lung determines its outcome (**Figure 8**).

Role of Apoptosis and Death Signaling in Acute Lung Injury

An intact lung endothelial and epithelial barrier function are pivotal to preventing alveolar flooding with water, salt, and proteins from the vascular compartment. Besides the role of inflammatory cells in the pathogenesis of ALI, recent studies indicate that apoptosis of the alveolar epithelial and endothelial cells appear to be involved in the development of acute lung inflammatory changes (135). For example, alveolar epithelial cell apoptosis has been reported in humans who died in the course of ARDS, with increased Fas expression in the alveolar epithelium (136). Moreover, extensive alveolar endothelial and epithelial cell apoptosis has been found in murine models of endotoxin-induced lung injury (137–140) and in an acute IC alveolitis model using IgG antibodies against ovalbumin (141). More importantly, intranasal instillation of a Fas-activating antibody (Jo2) in mice causes alveolar epithelial cell apoptosis as assessed by TUNEL (terminal deoxynucleotidyltransferase-mediated dUTP nick end-labeling) assay and electron microscopy (142). In a recent study using the murine model of IgG IC-induced lung injury, an intact Fas/FasL system was required for the full development of lung injury (143). The activation of the Fas/FasL system was evidenced by upregulation of Fas protein and activated caspase-3, a key protein in the apoptotic signal transduction. In addition, mice lacking functional Fas or FasL were protected from acute lung inflammation and lung edema formation following intrapulmonary deposition of IgG IC. Intravenous injection of a pan-caspase inhibitor (Z-VAD-FMK) was also protective, as indicated by decreased lung permeability and wet lung weights (143). These results demonstrate clearly that apoptotic pathways are required in some manner for full expression of lung inflammatory response.

Extensive neutrophil trafficking into the alveolar air space is a hallmark of the acute lung inflammatory process. In response to pro-inflammatory stimuli, neutrophils develop respiratory burst activity and release toxic mediators and oxygen radicals. During this process, apoptosis is assumed to play an important role by eliminating activated neutrophils from the inflammatory site (by inducing their uptake by macrophages), thereby preventing release of damaging neutrophil products such as proteinases into the microenvironment (144, 145). Thus, apoptosis of neutrophils controls the duration and intensity of an inflammatory response and, therefore, the extent of neutrophil-mediated tissue damage. In the IgG IC-induced lung injury in rodents, CXC chemokines (mainly MIP-2 and KC) appear to play a pivotal role in neutrophil recruitment along a chemotactic gradient into the lung. Fas ligation stimulates production of various inflammatory mediators in different cell types, including bronchiolar epithelial cells (146) and murine peritoneal macrophages (147). Our own data showing significantly reduced levels of MIP-2 and KC in lungs of Fas-deficient mice after IgG IC deposition strongly suggest a direct role in neutrophil recruitment to the lungs through expression of CXC chemokines for the Fas/FasL system (143). In addition, in vivo administration into mouse lungs of Jo2 antibody leads to a significant stimulation of MIP-2 and KC release. In vitro incubation of alveolar mouse macrophages with Jo2 antibody shows increased MIP-2 production (143). These experiments confirm a key linkage between Fas-induced chemokine production, neutrophil recruitment, and lung inflammation at least in the IgG IC-induced pulmonary alveolitis.

CONCLUSIONS

Although the results discussed in this review are derived mostly from a lung injury model induced by IgG IC deposition, the data derived can be extrapolated to other acute inflammatory injury conditions. The balance between oxidants and antioxidants and between pro-inflammatory and anti-inflammatory cytokines, together with proteinases and antiproteinases in the inflamed lung, probably determines the outcome of an inflammatory insult. Besides chemokines, adhesion molecules, complement, the signalosomes (kinases, phosphatases, etc.), and downstream transcription factors induced by various mediators also contribute to the development of lung inflammatory process. Despite the advances in understanding how the signaling induced by these mediators is controlled in ALI, many challenges remain.

SUMMARY POINTS

1. IgG IC deposition triggers activation of complement and alveolar macrophages via engagement of FcγRs.
2. The pathogenesis of lung injury in response to IgG IC deposition is initiated by the production of early response cytokines (TNFα and IL-1) and the complement activation product c5a, all resulting in upregulation of vascular adhesion molecules followed by neutrophil migration into the interstitial and alveolar compartments.
3. CXC chemokines constitute a chemokine gradient to orchestrate neutrophil migration into the lung.
4. Transcription factors such as NFκB, AP-1, and Stat3 are activated in the IgG IC-injured lung.
5. ROS and proteases cause damage of alveolar epithelial cells and vascular endothelial cells; ROS can mediate activation of transcription factors such as NFκB, expression of inflammatory chemokines, and adhesion molecules.
6. IgG IC-induced lung inflammatory response is endogenously regulated by IL-6, IL-10, IL-13 signals, as well as by SLPI and TIMPs.
7. Apoptosis seems to be involved in IgG IC-induced lung injury.

FUTURE DIRECTIONS/UNRESOLVED ISSUES

1. Define the specific downstream signalling pathways (kinases and phosphatases) of FcγRs in a given stage and cell type of the immune response in the lung. Proteomics may assist in these studies.
2. Determine the exact mechanisms of C5a as a regulator of the inflammatory response. The contribution of the newly identified C5a binding receptor, C5L2 to C5a function, and how the C5a signalling through C5aR or C5L2 will affect inflammatory mediator production after IgG IC stimulation needs intensive investigation.
3. Understand the differential mechanisms of gene expression during injury, proliferation, and differentiation in lung endothelial cells and alveolar epithelial cells.

4. Establish a quantitative differential protein expression profile (proteome) of specific cell types isolated from normal lung and diseased lung tissue (and also BAL fluids) as needed. These will help to identify specific profiles and provide a better understanding of ALI processes.

ACKNOWLEDGMENTS

Work in the authors' laboratory is supported by grants GM-61656, GM-02957, and HL-31963 from the National Institute of Health. The authors thank Robin Kunkel for assistance in the preparation of the figures and Beverly Schumann for secretarial help.

LITERATURE CITED

1. Ward PA. 2003. Acute lung injury: how the lung inflammatory response works. *Eur. Respir. J. Suppl.* 44:S22–23
2. Shanley TP, Schmal H, Friedl HP, Jones ML, Ward PA. 1995. Role of macrophage inflammatory protein-1 alpha (MIP-1 alpha) in acute lung injury in rats. *J. Immunol.* 154:4793–802
3. Bless NM, Huber-Lang M, Guo RF, Warner RL, Schmal H, et al. 2000. Role of CC chemokines (macrophage inflammatory protein-1 beta, monocyte chemoattractant protein-1, RANTES) in acute lung injury in rats. *J. Immunol.* 164:2650–59
4. Guo RF, Ward PA. 2002. Mediators and regulation of neutrophil accumulation in inflammatory responses in lung: insights from the IgG immune complex model. *Free Radic. Biol. Med.* 33:303–10
5. Lentsch AB, Czermak BJ, Bless NM, Ward PA. 1998. NF-kappaB activation during IgG immune complex-induced lung injury: requirements for TNF-alpha and IL-1beta but not complement. *Am. J. Pathol.* 152:1327–36
6. Guo RF, Lentsch AB, Sarma JV, Sun L, Riedemann NC, et al. 2002. Activator protein-1 activation in acute lung injury. *Am. J. Pathol.* 161:275–82
7. Gao H, Guo RF, Speyer CL, Reuben J, Neff TA, et al. 2004. Stat3 activation in acute lung injury. *J. Immunol.* 172:7703–12
8. **Lentsch AB, Shanley TP, Sarma V, Ward PA. 1997. In vivo suppression of NF-kappa B and preservation of I kappa B alpha by interleukin-10 and interleukin-13. *J. Clin. Invest.* 100:2443–48**

First paper to link the in vivo protective effect of IL-10 and IL-13 to suppression of NFκB in acute lung injury.

9. Lentsch AB, Jordan JA, Czermak BJ, Diehl KM, Younkin EM, et al. 1999. Inhibition of NF-kappaB activation and augmentation of IkappaBbeta by secretory leukocyte proteinase inhibitor during lung inflammation. *Am. J. Pathol.* 154:239–47
10. Ravetch JV, Bolland S. 2001. IgG Fc receptors. *Annu. Rev. Immunol.* 19:275–90
11. Gerber JS, Mosser DM. 2001. Stimulatory and inhibitory signals originating from the macrophage Fc gamma receptors. *Microbes Infect.* 3:131–39
12. Ward PA. 1996. Role of complement, chemokines, and regulatory cytokines in acute lung injury. *Ann. NY Acad. Sci.* 796:104–12
13. Chouchakova N, Skokowa J, Baumann U, Tschernig T, Philippens KM, et al. 2001. Fc gamma RIII-mediated production of TNF-alpha induces immune complex alveolitis independently of CXC chemokine generation. *J. Immunol.* 166:5193–200

14. Coxon A, Cullere X, Knight S, Sethi S, Wakelin MW, et al. 2001. Fc gamma RIII mediates neutrophil recruitment to immune complexes: a mechanism for neutrophil accumulation in immune-mediated inflammation. *Immunity* 14:693–704
15. Takai T, Li M, Sylvestre D, Clynes R, Ravetch JV. 1994. FcR gamma chain deletion results in pleiotrophic effector cell defects. *Cell* 76:519–29
16. Clynes R, Maizes JS, Guinamard R, Ono M, Takai T, Ravetch JV. 1999. Modulation of immune complex-induced inflammation in vivo by the coordinate expression of activation and inhibitory Fc receptors. *J. Exp. Med.* 189:179–85
17. Barnes N, Gavin AL, Tan PS, Mottram P, Koentgen F, Hogarth PM. 2002. FcgammaRI-deficient mice show multiple alterations to inflammatory and immune responses. *Immunity* 16:379–89
18. Ioan-Facsinay A, de Kimpe SJ, Hellwig SM, van Lent PL, Hofhuis FM, et al. 2002. FcgammaRI (CD64) contributes substantially to severity of arthritis, hypersensitivity responses, and protection from bacterial infection. *Immunity* 16:391–402
19. Newbrough SA, Mocsai A, Clemens RA, Wu JN, Silverman MA, et al. 2003. SLP-76 regulates Fcgamma receptor and integrin signaling in neutrophils. *Immunity* 19:761–69
20. **Ward PA. 1996. Rous-Whipple Award Lecture. Role of complement in lung inflammatory injury. *Am. J. Pathol.* 149:1081–86**

A comprehensive review of complement role in acute lung injury.

21. Czermak BJ, Lentsch AB, Bless NM, Schmal H, Friedl HP, Ward PA. 1998. Role of complement in in vitro and in vivo lung inflammatory reactions. *J. Leukoc. Biol.* 64:40–48
22. Mulligan MS, Schmid E, Till GO, Hugli TE, Friedl HP, et al. 1997. C5a-dependent up-regulation in vivo of lung vascular P-selectin. *J. Immunol.* 158:1857–61
23. Jagels MA, Daffern PJ, Hugli TE. 2000. C3a and C5a enhance granulocyte adhesion to endothelial and epithelial cell monolayers: epithelial and endothelial priming is required for C3a-induced eosinophil adhesion. *Immunopharmacology* 46:209–22
24. Albrecht EA, Chinnaiyan AM, Varambally S, Kumar-Sinha C, Barrette TR, et al. 2004. C5a-induced gene expression in human umbilical vein endothelial cells. *Am. J. Pathol.* 164:849–59
25. Frank MM, Fries LF. 1991. The role of complement in inflammation and phagocytosis. *Immunol. Today* 12:322–26
26. Wojta J, Kaun C, Zorn G, Ghannadan M, Hauswirth AW, et al. 2002. C5a stimulates production of plasminogen activator inhibitor-1 in human mast cells and basophils. *Blood* 100:517–23
27. Laudes IJ, Chu JC, Huber-Lang M, Guo RF, Riedemann NC, et al. 2002. Expression and function of C5a receptor in mouse microvascular endothelial cells. *J. Immunol.* 169:5962–70
28. Kilgore KS, Shen JP, Miller BF, Ward PA, Warren JS. 1995. Enhancement by the complement membrane attack complex of tumor necrosis factor-alpha-induced endothelial cell expression of E-selectin and ICAM-1. *J. Immunol.* 155:1434–41
29. Kilgore KS, Schmid E, Shanley TP, Flory CM, Maheswari V, et al. 1997. Sublytic concentrations of the membrane attack complex of complement induce endothelial interleukin-8 and monocyte chemoattractant protein-1 through nuclear factor-kappa B activation. *Am. J. Pathol.* 150:2019–31
30. Johnson KJ, Ward PA. 1974. Acute immunologic pulmonary alveolitis. *J. Clin. Invest.* 54:349–57
31. **Larsen GL, Mitchell BC, Henson PM. 1981. The pulmonary response of C5 sufficient and deficient mice to immune complexes. *Am. Rev. Respir. Dis.* 123:434–39**

A key report describing requirement of C5a in acute lung injury.

32. Mulligan MS, Schmid E, Beck-Schimmer B, Till GO, Friedl HP, et al. 1996. Requirement and role of C5a in acute lung inflammatory injury in rats. *J. Clin. Invest.* 98:503–12
33. Huber-Lang M, Younkin EM, Sarma JV, Riedemann N, McGuire SR, et al. 2002. Generation of C5a by phagocytic cells. *Am. J. Pathol.* 161:1849–59
34. Czermak BJ, Sarma V, Bless NM, Schmal H, Friedl HP, Ward PA. 1999. In vitro and in vivo dependency of chemokine generation on C5a and TNF-alpha. *J. Immunol.* 162:2321–25
35. Czermak BJ, Lentsch AB, Bless NM, Schmal H, Friedl HP, Ward PA. 1999. Synergistic enhancement of chemokine generation and lung injury by C5a or the membrane attack complex of complement. *Am. J. Pathol.* 154:1513–24
36. Lukacs NW, Glovsky MM, Ward PA. 2001. Complement-dependent immune complex-induced bronchial inflammation and hyperreactivity. *Am. J. Physiol. Lung Cell Mol. Physiol.* 280:L512–18
37. Drouin SM, Kildsgaard J, Haviland J, Zabner J, Jia HP, et al. 2001. Expression of the complement anaphylatoxin C3a and C5a receptors on bronchial epithelial and smooth muscle cells in models of sepsis and asthma. *J. Immunol.* 166:2025–32
38. Riedemann NC, Guo RF, Sarma VJ, Laudes IJ, Huber-Lang M, et al. 2002. Expression and function of the C5a receptor in rat alveolar epithelial cells. *J. Immunol.* 168:1919–25
39. **Bozic CR, Lu B, Hopken UE, Gerard C, Gerard NP. 1996. Neurogenic amplification of immune complex inflammation. *Science* 273:1722–25**

The first paper to show the importance of the C5aR pathway in IC alveolitis.

40. **Shushakova N, Skokowa J, Schulman J, Baumann U, Zwirner J, et al. 2002. C5a anaphylatoxin is a major regulator of activating versus inhibitory FcgammaRs in immune complex-induced lung disease. *J. Clin. Invest.* 110:1823–30**

Describes how C5a plays a critical role in regulating the activating/inhibitory FcγRs in IC alveolitis.

41. Heller T, Hennecke M, Baumann U, Gessner JE, zu Vilsendorf AM, et al. 1999. Selection of a C5a receptor antagonist from phage libraries attenuating the inflammatory response in immune complex disease and ischemia/reperfusion injury. *J. Immunol.* 163:985–94
42. Baumann U, Kohl J, Tschernig T, Schwerter-Strumpf K, Verbeek JS, et al. 2000. A codominant role of Fc gamma RI/III and C5aR in the reverse Arthus reaction. *J. Immunol.* 164:1065–70
43. Ravetch JV, Clynes RA. 1998. Divergent roles for Fc receptors and complement in vivo. *Annu. Rev. Immunol.* 16:421–32
44. Trcka J, Moroi Y, Clynes RA, Goldberg SM, Bergtold A, et al. 2002. Redundant and alternative roles for activating Fc receptors and complement in an antibody-dependent model of autoimmune vitiligo. *Immunity* 16:861–68
45. Fan J, Ye RD, Malik AB. 2001. Transcriptional mechanisms of acute lung injury. *Am. J. Physiol. Lung Cell Mol. Physiol.* 281:L1037–50
46. Rahman I, MacNee W. 1998. Role of transcription factors in inflammatory lung diseases. *Thorax* 53:601–12
47. Hayden MS, Ghosh S. 2004. Signaling to NF-kappaB. *Genes Dev.* 18:2195–24
48. Karin M, Yamamoto Y, Wang QM. 2004. The IKK NF-kappa B system: a treasure trove for drug development. *Nat. Rev. Drug. Discov.* 3:17–26
49. Manning AM, Bell FP, Rosenbloom CL, Chosay JG, Simmons CA, et al. 1995. NF-kappa B is activated during acute inflammation in vivo in association with elevated endothelial cell adhesion molecule gene expression and leukocyte recruitment. *J. Inflamm.* 45:283–96
50. Warren JS, Yabroff KR, Remick DG, Kunkel SL, Chensue SW, et al. 1989. Tumor necrosis factor participates in the pathogenesis of acute immune complex alveolitis in the rat. *J. Clin. Invest.* 84:1873–82

51. Warren JS. 1991. Intrapulmonary interleukin 1 mediates acute immune complex alveolitis in the rat. *Biochem. Biophys. Res. Commun.* 175:604–10
52. Lentsch AB, Czermak BJ, Bless NM, Van Rooijen N, Ward PA. 1999. Essential role of alveolar macrophages in intrapulmonary activation of NF-kappaB. *Am. J. Respir. Cell Mol. Biol.* 20:692–98
53. Iles KE, Forman HJ. 2002. Macrophage signaling and respiratory burst. *Immunol. Res.* 26:95–105
54. Koay MA, Christman JW, Segal BH, Venkatakrishnan A, Blackwell TR, et al. 2001. Impaired pulmonary NF-kappaB activation in response to lipopolysaccharide in NADPH oxidase-deficient mice. *Infect. Immun.* 69:5991–96
55. Hayakawa M, Miyashita H, Sakamoto I, Kitagawa M, Tanaka H, et al. 2003. Evidence that reactive oxygen species do not mediate NF-kappaB activation. *EMBO J.* 22:3356–66
56. Karin M, Liu Z, Zandi E. 1997. AP-1 function and regulation. *Curr. Opin. Cell Biol.* 9:240–46
57. Roebuck KA, Carpenter LR, Lakshminarayanan V, Page SM, Moy JN, Thomas LL. 1999. Stimulus-specific regulation of chemokine expression involves differential activation of the redox-responsive transcription factors AP-1 and NF-kappaB. *J. Leukoc. Biol.* 65:291–98
58. Zagariya A, Mungre S, Lovis R, Birrer M, Ness S, et al. 1998. Tumor necrosis factor alpha gene regulation: enhancement of C/EBPbeta-induced activation by c-Jun. *Mol. Cell. Biol.* 18:2815–24
59. Rahman I. 2000. Regulation of nuclear factor-kappa B, activator protein-1, and glutathione levels by tumor necrosis factor-alpha and dexamethasone in alveolar epithelial cells. *Biochem. Pharmacol.* 60:1041–49
60. Rocksen D, Ekstrand-Hammarstrom B, Johansson L, Bucht A. 2003. Vitamin E reduces transendothelial migration of neutrophils and prevents lung injury in endotoxin-induced airway inflammation. *Am. J. Respir. Cell Mol. Biol.* 28:199–207
61. Bozinovski S, Jones JE, Vlahos R, Hamilton JA, Anderson GP. 2002. Granulocyte/macrophage-colony-stimulating factor (GM-CSF) regulates lung innate immunity to lipopolysaccharide through Akt/Erk activation of NFkappa B and AP-1 in vivo. *J. Biol. Chem.* 277:42808–14
62. Stein B, Baldwin AS Jr, Ballard DW, Greene WC, Angel P, Herrlich P. 1993. Cross-coupling of the NF-kappa B p65 and Fos/Jun transcription factors produces potentiated biological function. *EMBO J.* 12:3879–91
63. Levy DE, Lee CK. 2002. What does Stat3 do? *J. Clin. Invest.* 109:1143–48
64. Cheng F, Wang HW, Cuenca A, Huang M, Ghansah T, et al. 2003. A critical role for Stat3 signaling in immune tolerance. *Immunity* 19:425–36
65. Welte T, Zhang SS, Wang T, Zhang Z, Hesslein DG, et al. 2003. STAT3 deletion during hematopoiesis causes Crohn's disease-like pathogenesis and lethality: a critical role of STAT3 in innate immunity. *Proc. Natl. Acad. Sci. USA* 100:1879–84
66. Yan C, Naltner A, Martin M, Naltner M, Fangman JM, Gurel O. 2002. Transcriptional stimulation of the surfactant protein B gene by STAT3 in respiratory epithelial cells. *J. Biol. Chem.* 277:10967–72
67. Fernandez S, Jose P, Avdiushko MG, Kaplan AM, Cohen DA. 2004. Inhibition of IL-10 receptor function in alveolar macrophages by Toll-like receptor agonists. *J. Immunol.* 172:2613–20

68. Moodley YP, Misso NL, Scaffidi AK, Fogel-Petrovic M, McAnulty RJ, et al. 2003. Inverse effects of interleukin-6 on apoptosis of fibroblasts from pulmonary fibrosis and normal lungs. *Am. J. Respir. Cell Mol. Biol.* 29:490–98
69. Severgnini M, Takahashi S, Rozo LM, Homer RJ, Kuhn C, et al. 2004. Activation of the STAT pathway in acute lung injury. *Am. J. Physiol. Lung Cell Mol. Physiol.* 286:L1282–92
70. Meng ZH, Dyer K, Billiar TR, Tweardy DJ. 2001. Essential role for IL-6 in postresuscitation inflammation in hemorrhagic shock. *Am. J. Physiol. Cell Physiol.* 280:C343–51
71. Hokuto I, Ikegami M, Yoshida M, Takeda K, Akira S, et al. 2004. Stat-3 is required for pulmonary homeostasis during hyperoxia. *J. Clin. Invest.* 113:28–37
72. Yang L, Lian X, Cowen A, Xu H, Du H, Yan C. 2004. Synergy between signal transducer and activator of transcription 3 and retinoic acid receptor-alpha in regulation of the surfactant protein B gene in the lung. *Mol. Endocrinol.* 18:1520–32
73. Mulligan MS, Varani J, Dame MK, Lane CL, Smith CW, et al. 1991. Role of endothelial-leukocyte adhesion molecule 1 (ELAM-1) in neutrophil-mediated lung injury in rats. *J. Clin. Invest.* 88:1396–406
74. Mulligan MS, Vaporciyan AA, Miyasaka M, Tamatani T, Ward PA. 1993. Tumor necrosis factor alpha regulates in vivo intrapulmonary expression of ICAM-1. *Am. J. Pathol.* 142:1739–49
75. Jordan JA, Guo RF, Yun EC, Sarma V, Warner RL, et al. 2001. Role of IL-18 in acute lung inflammation. *J. Immunol.* 167:7060–68
76. Lentsch AB, Ward PA. 2001. Regulation of experimental lung inflammation. *Respir. Physiol.* 128:17–22
77. Shanley TP, Schmal H, Warner RL, Schmid E, Friedl HP, Ward PA. 1997. Requirement for C-X-C chemokines (macrophage inflammatory protein-2 and cytokine-induced neutrophil chemoattractant) in IgG immune complex-induced lung injury. *J. Immunol.* 158:3439–48
78. Shanley TP, Schmal H, Friedl HP, Jones ML, Ward PA. 1995. Regulatory effects of intrinsic IL-10 in IgG immune complex-induced lung injury. *J. Immunol.* 154:3454–60
79. Lentsch AB, Crouch LD, Jordan JA, Czermak BJ, Yun EC, et al. 1999. Regulatory effects of interleukin-11 during acute lung inflammatory injury. *J. Leukoc. Biol.* 66:151–57
80. Lentsch AB, Czermak BJ, Jordan JA, Ward PA. 1999. Regulation of acute lung inflammatory injury by endogenous IL-13. *J. Immunol.* 162:1071–76
81. Mulligan MS, Jones ML, Vaporciyan AA, Howard MC, Ward PA. 1993. Protective effects of IL-4 and IL-10 against immune complex-induced lung injury. *J. Immunol.* 151:5666–74
82. Mulligan MS, Warner RL, Foreback JL, Shanley TP, Ward PA. 1997. Protective effects of IL-4, IL-10, IL-12, and IL-13 in IgG immune complex-induced lung injury: role of endogenous IL-12. *J. Immunol.* 159:3483–89
83. Trepicchio WL, Wang L, Bozza M, Dorner AJ. 1997. IL-11 regulates macrophage effector function through the inhibition of nuclear factor-kappaB. *J. Immunol.* 159:5661–70
84. Kaplanski G, Marin V, Montero-Julian F, Mantovani A, Farnarier C. 2003. IL-6: a regulator of the transition from neutrophil to monocyte recruitment during inflammation. *Trends Immunol.* 24:25–29
85. Shanley TP, Peters JL, Jones ML, Chensue SW, Kunkel SL, Ward PA. 1996. Regulatory effects of endogenous interleukin-1 receptor antagonist protein in immunoglobulin G immune complex-induced lung injury. *J. Clin. Invest.* 97:963–70
86. Luster AD. 1998. Chemokines–chemotactic cytokines that mediate inflammation. *N. Engl. J. Med.* 338:436–45

87. Miller EJ, Cohen AB, Nagao S, Griffith D, Maunder RJ, et al. 1992. Elevated levels of NAP-1/interleukin-8 are present in the airspaces of patients with the adult respiratory distress syndrome and are associated with increased mortality. *Am. Rev. Respir. Dis.* 146:427–32
88. Sekido N, Mukaida N, Harada A, Nakanishi I, Watanabe Y, Matsushima K. 1993. Prevention of lung reperfusion injury in rabbits by a monoclonal antibody against interleukin-8. *Nature* 365:654–57
89. Mulligan MS, Jones ML, Bolanowski MA, Baganoff MP, Deppeler CL, et al. 1993. Inhibition of lung inflammatory reactions in rats by an anti-human IL-8 antibody. *J. Immunol.* 150:5585–95
90. Guo RF, Lentsch AB, Warner RL, Huber-Lang M, Sarma JV, et al. 2001. Regulatory effects of eotaxin on acute lung inflammatory injury. *J. Immunol.* 166:5208–18
91. Bless NM, Tojo SJ, Kawarai H, Natsume Y, Lentsch AB, et al. 1998. Differing patterns of P-selectin expression in lung injury. *Am. J. Pathol.* 153:1113–22
92. Mulligan MS, Miyasaka M, Tamatani T, Jones ML, Ward PA. 1994. Requirements for L-selectin in neutrophil-mediated lung injury in rats. *J. Immunol.* 152:832–40
93. Mulligan MS, Watson SR, Fennie C, Ward PA. 1993. Protective effects of selectin chimeras in neutrophil-mediated lung injury. *J. Immunol.* 151:6410–17
94. Mulligan MS, Lowe JB, Larsen RD, Paulson J, Zheng ZL, et al. 1993. Protective effects of sialylated oligosaccharides in immune complex-induced acute lung injury. *J. Exp. Med.* 178:623–31
95. Mulligan MS, Paulson JC, De Frees S, Zheng ZL, Lowe JB, Ward PA. 1993. Protective effects of oligosaccharides in P-selectin-dependent lung injury. *Nature* 364:149–51
96. Mulligan MS, Warner RL, Rittershaus CW, Thomas LJ, Ryan US, et al. 1999. Endothelial targeting and enhanced antiinflammatory effects of complement inhibitors possessing sialyl Lewisx moieties. *J. Immunol.* 162:4952–59
97. Johnston B, Kubes P. 1999. The alpha4-integrin: an alternative pathway for neutrophil recruitment? *Immunol. Today* 20:545–50
98. Mulligan MS, Wilson GP, Todd RF, Smith CW, Anderson DC, et al. 1993. Role of beta 1, beta 2 integrins and ICAM-1 in lung injury after deposition of IgG and IgA immune complexes. *J. Immunol.* 150:2407–17
99. Mulligan MS, Vaporciyan AA, Warner RL, Jones ML, Foreman KE, et al. 1995. Compartmentalized roles for leukocytic adhesion molecules in lung inflammatory injury. *J. Immunol.* 154:1350–63
100. Shanley TP, Warner RL, Crouch LD, Dietsch GN, Clark DL, et al. 1998. Requirements for alpha d in IgG immune complex-induced rat lung injury. *J. Immunol.* 160:1014–20
101. Schmal H, Czermak BJ, Lentsch AB, Bless NM, Beck-Schimmer B, et al. 1998. Soluble ICAM-1 activates lung macrophages and enhances lung injury. *J. Immunol.* 161:3685–93
102. Mulligan MS, Miyasaka M, Ward PA. 1996. Protective effects of combined adhesion molecule blockade in models of acute lung injury. *Proc. Assoc. Am. Physicians* 108:198–208
103. Vaporciyan AA, DeLisser HM, Yan HC, Mendiguren II, Thom SR, et al. 1993. Involvement of platelet-endothelial cell adhesion molecule-1 in neutrophil recruitment in vivo. *Science* 262:1580–82
104. Albelda SM, Lau KC, Chien P, Huang ZY, Arguiris E, et al. 2004. Role for platelet-endothelial cell adhesion molecule-1 in macrophage Fcgamma receptor function. *Am. J. Respir. Cell Mol. Biol.* 31:246–55
105. Frey RS, Malik AB. 2004. Oxidant signaling in lung cells. *Am. J. Physiol. Lung Cell Mol. Physiol.* 286:L1–3

106. Johnson KJ, Ward PA. 1981. Role of oxygen metabolites in immune complex injury of lung. *J. Immunol.* 126:2365–69
107. Johnson KJ, Fantone JC 3rd, Kaplan J, Ward PA. 1981. In vivo damage of rat lungs by oxygen metabolites. *J. Clin. Invest.* 67:983–93
108. Mulligan MS, Varani J, Warren JS, Till GO, Smith CW, et al. 1992. Roles of beta 2 integrins of rat neutrophils in complement- and oxygen radical-mediated acute inflammatory injury. *J. Immunol.* 148:1847–57
109. Mulligan MS, Hevel JM, Marletta MA, Ward PA. 1991. Tissue injury caused by deposition of immune complexes is L-arginine dependent. *Proc. Natl. Acad. Sci. USA* 88:6338–42
110. Warner RL, Paine R 3rd, Christensen PJ, Marletta MA, Richards MK, et al. 1995. Lung sources and cytokine requirements for in vivo expression of inducible nitric oxide synthase. *Am. J. Respir. Cell Mol. Biol.* 12:649–61
111. Chow CW, Herrera Abreu MT, Suzuki T, Downey GP. 2003. Oxidative stress and acute lung injury. *Am. J. Respir. Cell Mol. Biol.* 29:427–31
112. Pricop L, Salmon JE. 2002. Redox regulation of Fcgamma receptor-mediated phagocytosis: implications for host defense and tissue injury. *Antioxid. Redox Signal.* 4:85–95
113. Warner RL, Bless NM, Lewis CS, Younkin E, Beltran L, et al. 2000. Time-dependent inhibition of immune complex-induced lung injury by catalase: relationship to alterations in macrophage and neutrophil matrix metalloproteinase elaboration. *Free Radic. Biol. Med.* 29:8–16
114. Moraes TJ, Chow CW, Downey GP. 2003. Proteinases and lung injury. *Crit. Care Med.* 31:S189–94
115. Janoff A. 1985. Elastase in tissue injury. *Annu. Rev. Med.* 36:207–16
116. Trevani AS, Andonegui G, Giordano M, Nociari M, Fontan P, et al. 1996. Neutrophil apoptosis induced by proteolytic enzymes. *Lab. Invest.* 74:711–21
117. Nakamura H, Yoshimura K, McElvaney NG, Crystal RG. 1992. Neutrophil elastase in respiratory epithelial lining fluid of individuals with cystic fibrosis induces interleukin-8 gene expression in a human bronchial epithelial cell line. *J. Clin. Invest.* 89:1478–84
118. Sallenave JM, Si Tahar M, Cox G, Chignard M, Gauldie J. 1997. Secretory leukocyte proteinase inhibitor is a major leukocyte elastase inhibitor in human neutrophils. *J. Leukoc. Biol.* 61:695–702
119. Gipson TS, Bless NM, Shanley TP, Crouch LD, Bleavins MR, et al. 1999. Regulatory effects of endogenous proteinase inhibitors in acute lung inflammatory injury. *J. Immunol.* 162:3653–62
120. Mulligan MS, Desrochers PE, Chinnaiyan AM, Gibbs DF, Varani J, et al. 1993. In vivo suppression of immune complex-induced alveolitis by secretory leukoproteinase inhibitor and tissue inhibitor of metalloproteinases 2. *Proc. Natl. Acad. Sci. USA* 90:11523–27
121. Gillissen A, Birrer P, McElvaney NG, Buhl R, Vogelmeier C, et al. 1993. Recombinant secretory leukoproteinase inhibitor augments glutathione levels in lung epithelial lining fluid. *J. Appl. Physiol.* 75:825–32
122. Jin FY, Nathan C, Radzioch D, Ding A. 1997. Secretory leukocyte proteinase inhibitor: a macrophage product induced by and antagonistic to bacterial lipopolysaccharide. *Cell* 88:417–26
123. Nakamura A, Mori Y, Hagiwara K, Suzuki T, Sakakibara T, et al. 2003. Increased susceptibility to LPS-induced endotoxin shock in secretory leukoproteinase inhibitor (SLPI)-deficient mice. *J. Exp. Med.* 197:669–74
124. Ohbayashi H. 2002. Matrix metalloproteinases in lung diseases. *Curr. Protein. Pept. Sci.* 3:409–21

125. Shipley JM, Wesselschmidt RL, Kobayashi DK, Ley TJ, Shapiro SD. 1996. Metalloelastase is required for macrophage-mediated proteolysis and matrix invasion in mice. *Proc. Natl. Acad. Sci. USA* 93:3942–46
126. Palmgren MS, deShazo RD, Carter RM, Zimny ML, Shah SV. 1992. Mechanisms of neutrophil damage to human alveolar extracellular matrix: the role of serine and metalloproteinases. *J. Allergy Clin. Immunol.* 89:905–15
127. D'Ortho MP, Jarreau PH, Delacourt C, Macquin-Mavier I, Levame M, et al. 1994. Matrix metalloproteinase and elastase activities in LPS-induced acute lung injury in guinea pigs. *Am. J. Physiol. Lung Cell Physiol.* 266:L209–16
128. Pardo A, Selman M, Ridge K, Barrios R, Sznajder JI. 1996. Increased expression of gelatinases and collagenase in rat lungs exposed to 100% oxygen. *Am. J. Respir. Crit. Care Med.* 154:1067–75
129. Kleeberger SR, Bassett DJ, Jakab GJ, Levitt RC. 1990. A genetic model for evaluation of susceptibility to ozone-induced inflammation. *Am. J. Physiol. Lung Cell Physiol.* 258:L313–20
130. Gibbs DF, Warner RL, Weiss SJ, Johnson KJ, Varani J. 1999. Characterization of matrix metalloproteinases produced by rat alveolar macrophages. *Am. J. Respir. Cell Mol. Biol.* 20:1136–44
131. Warner RL, Beltran L, Younkin EM, Lewis CS, Weiss SJ, et al. 2001. Role of stromelysin 1 and gelatinase B in experimental acute lung injury. *Am. J. Respir. Cell Mol. Biol.* 24:537–44
132. Warner RL, Lewis CS, Beltran L, Younkin EM, Varani J, Johnson KJ. 2001. The role of metalloelastase in immune complex-induced acute lung injury. *Am. J. Pathol.* 158:2139–44

Describes the role of MMPs in acute lung inflammation.

133. Warner RL, Bhagavathula N, Nerusu KC, Lateef H, Younkin E, et al. 2004. Matrix metalloproteinases in acute inflammation: induction of MMP-3 and MMP-9 in fibroblasts and epithelial cells following exposure to pro-inflammatory mediators in vitro. *Exp. Mol. Pathol.* 76:189–95
134. Shapiro SD, Kobayashi DK, Welgus HG. 1992. Identification of TIMP-2 in human alveolar macrophages. Regulation of biosynthesis is opposite to that of metalloproteinases and TIMP-1. *J. Biol. Chem.* 267:13890–94
135. Martin TR, Nakamura M, Matute-Bello G. 2003. The role of apoptosis in acute lung injury. *Crit. Care Med.* 31:S184–88
136. Albertine KH, Soulier MF, Wang Z, Ishizaka A, Hashimoto S, et al. 2002. Fas and fas ligand are up-regulated in pulmonary edema fluid and lung tissue of patients with acute lung injury and the acute respiratory distress syndrome. *Am. J. Pathol.* 161:1783–96
137. Fujita M, Kuwano K, Kunitake R, Hagimoto N, Miyazaki H, et al. 1998. Endothelial cell apoptosis in lipopolysaccharide-induced lung injury in mice. *Int. Arch. Allergy Immunol.* 117:202–8
138. Kitamura Y, Hashimoto S, Mizuta N, Kobayashi A, Kooguchi K, et al. 2001. Fas/FasL-dependent apoptosis of alveolar cells after lipopolysaccharide-induced lung injury in mice. *Am. J. Respir. Crit. Care Med.* 163:762–69
139. Vernooy JH, Dentener MA, van Suylen RJ, Buurman WA, Wouters EF. 2001. Intratracheal instillation of lipopolysaccharide in mice induces apoptosis in bronchial epithelial cells: no role for tumor necrosis factor-alpha and infiltrating neutrophils. *Am. J. Respir. Cell. Mol. Biol.* 24:569–76
140. Kawasaki M, Kuwano K, Hagimoto N, Matsuba T, Kunitake R, et al. 2000. Protection from lethal apoptosis in lipopolysaccharide-induced acute lung injury in mice by a caspase inhibitor. *Am. J. Pathol.* 157:597–603

141. Nomoto Y, Kuwano K, Hagimoto N, Kunitake R, Kawasaki M, Hara N. 1997. Apoptosis and Fas/Fas ligand mRNA expression in acute immune complex alveolitis in mice. *Eur. Respir. J.* 10:2351–59
142. Matute-Bello G, Winn RK, Jonas M, Chi EY, Martin TR, Liles WC. 2001. Fas (CD95) induces alveolar epithelial cell apoptosis in vivo: implications for acute pulmonary inflammation. *Am. J. Pathol.* 158:153–61
143. Neff TA, Guo RF, Neff SB, Sarma JV, Speyer CL, et al. 2005. Relationship of acute lung inflammatory injury to Fas/FasL system. *Am. J. Pathol.* 166:685–94
144. Haslett C. 1999. Granulocyte apoptosis and its role in the resolution and control of lung inflammation. *Am. J. Respir. Crit. Care Med.* 160:S5–11
145. Cox G, Crossley J, Xing Z. 1995. Macrophage engulfment of apoptotic neutrophils contributes to the resolution of acute pulmonary inflammation in vivo. *Am. J. Respir. Cell Mol. Biol.* 12:232–37
146. Hagimoto N, Kuwano K, Kawasaki M, Yoshimi M, Kaneko Y, et al. 1999. Induction of interleukin-8 secretion and apoptosis in bronchiolar epithelial cells by Fas ligation. *Am. J. Respir. Cell Mol. Biol.* 21:436–45
147. Hohlbaum AM, Gregory MS, Ju ST, Marshak-Rothstein A. 2001. Fas ligand engagement of resident peritoneal macrophages in vivo induces apoptosis and the production of neutrophil chemotactic factors. *J. Immunol.* 167:6217–24

Integrative Biology of Prostate Cancer Progression

Scott A. Tomlins,[1] Mark A. Rubin,[3] and Arul M. Chinnaiyan[1,2]

[1]Departments of Pathology and Urology,[2] Comprehensive Cancer Center, University of Michigan Medical School, Ann Arbor, Michigan 48109; email: tomlinss@med.umich.edu; arul@umich.edu

[3]Department of Pathology, Brigham and Women's Hospital, Harvard Medical School, Boston, Massachusetts 02115; email: marubin@partners.org

Annu. Rev. Pathol. Mech. Dis. 2006. 1:243–71

First published online as a Review in Advance on October 24, 2005

The *Annual Review of Pathology: Mechanisms of Disease* is online at pathmechdis.annualreviews.org

doi: 10.1146/annurev.pathol.1.110304.100047

1553-4006/06/0114-0243$20.00

Key Words

candidate genes, microarrays, androgen receptor, hedgehog pathway

Abstract

Prostate cancer displays considerable clinical, morphological, and biological heterogeneity. Classical genetic techniques have provided only limited information about the pathogenesis of prostate cancer progression. Nevertheless, several candidate genes and pathways have been implicated in prostate cancer development. High-throughput techniques have exponentially expanded the number of candidate genes, including some whose role in prostate cancer pathogenesis has been studied. However, the techniques used to study the prostate cancer genome, transcriptome, and proteome generate massive amounts of data that have yet to be integrated and explored. To move beyond candidate gene identification and develop a comprehensive understanding of cancer pathogenesis, integrative approaches need to analyze this data on a global level. This review addresses candidate genes involved in prostate cancer pathogenesis in a biological and clinical context and demonstrates how integrated analysis of high-throughput data augments our understanding of prostate cancer.

INTRODUCTION

PCA: prostate cancer

PSA: prostate-specific antigen

PIN: prostatic intra-epithelial neoplasia

Gleason score: a system to assess the glandular architecture in prostate cancer on a scale of one to five

Although prostate cancer (PCA) has surpassed lung cancer as the most common noncutaneous cancer in American men, its etiology remains largely unknown. Retrospective studies suggest that by age 80, more than half of all American men have some cancer in their prostate (1), yet most men show no symptoms, and clinical treatment is not needed. However, some PCAs are aggressive and quickly spread locally and metastasize throughout the body. The advent of the prostate-specific antigen (PSA) screening test has led to increasing number of cancers being detected at an early stage. Together, these factors have complicated treatment decisions, and a more thorough understanding of PCA progression and pathogenesis is urgently needed.

Marked incidence differences between industrialized Western countries and East Asian countries suggest that lifestyle components contribute to PCA development. The higher incidence in Western countries is attributed commonly to dietary factors, such as increased meat and dairy intake, in addition to reduced fruit and vegetable consumption, although this is a matter of some controversy. Although there is evidence for a strong genetic component of PCA and several genetic loci have been implicated in hereditary PCA, the functional role of these genes in PCA pathogenesis is speculative (2). Traditionally, most human cancers are thought to develop through a series of sequentially accumulated genetic events, which culminates in carcinoma and metastatic disease, and these results are reflected at the histologic, genetic, and clinical level. Unfortunately, many aspects of PCA biology do not fit with this model, and it is unclear if this conceptual framework should be applied to understanding of PCA pathogenesis.

Histologically, PCA's progression to carcinoma is somewhat reminiscent of other epithelial cancers. In the normal prostate, the glandular epithelium consists of two cell layers: the basal layer and the differentiated luminal secretory layer, with rare neuroendocrine (NE) cells distributed mostly in the basal layer. Prostatic intra-epithelial neoplasia (PIN), characterized by nuclear and architectural changes in luminal epithelial cells with maintenance of the basal epithelium and basement membrane, is an accepted precursor lesion to frank adenocarcinoma. Proliferative inflammatory atrophy (PIA) is a lesion that has recently been proposed to be a candidate precursor lesion to PIN and/or PCA on the basis of the hypothesis that inflammation plays a role in the development of PCA (3–6). This hypothesis is consistent with epidemiological data, as the Western diet is presumed to be high in potential carcinogens and low in protective antioxidants. Furthermore, some candidate loci implicated in hereditary PCA encode viral and bacterial response genes, and some genetic events in sporadic cancer (see Glutathoine S-Transferase Pi below) are also consistent with this hypothesis (5).

PCA is also often multifocal, as several distinct foci of PIN and/or PCA can be found in a single prostate gland, each expressing different degrees of cellular dysplasia and tissue disorganization. PCA is most commonly graded by the method described by Gleason (7), which assigns a score on the basis of the glandular architecture (lower scores indicate a well-differentiated glandular pattern). The Gleason score is composed of the two most common patterns, as PCA is often multifocal with distinct patterns present in the same tumor. Even so, histologically identical tumors of the same stage can show remarkably different clinical courses, ranging from an indolent disease to one that is rapidly invasive and metastatic. Presently, it is unclear whether these histological and clinical differences are driven by corresponding molecular differences and what the implications are for the pathogenesis of PCA.

Candidate Genes Involved in Prostate Cancer Pathogenesis

The histological and clinical heterogeneity of PCA are also reflected at the molecular level. Little evidence exists for a clearly defined series of genetic events leading to PCA development. There are no obvious syndromes that predispose one to PCA, and although classical methods of identifying candidate genes have provided important candidates, few PCAs share all or even many of the same alterations. However, molecular studies have identified several candidate genes and pathways that are consistent with important aspects of the epidemiological and biological features of PCA and likely to be important in PCA pathogenesis and progression. The candidate genes and pathways described below are shown in the context of the histological progression of PCA in **Figure 1** and summarized in **Table 1**.

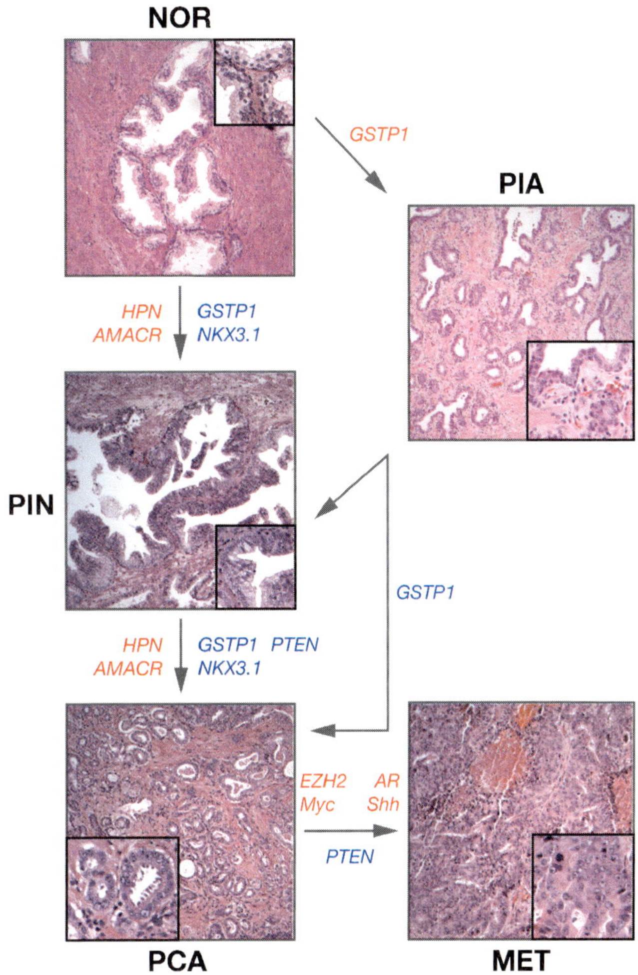

Figure 1

Genetic alterations during the histological progression of prostate cancer (PCA). Photomicrographs of hematoxylin and eosin–stained sections representative of the indicated tissue or lesion (10x original magnification, 40x inserts). Arrows indicate proposed routes of progression from normal (NOR) prostate glands to precursor lesions [prostatic intra-epithelial neoplasia (PIN) or proliferative inflammatory atrophy (PIA)] to localized PCA to metastatic disease (MET). Pathway and candidate gene names in blue or red represent genes and pathways underexpressed or overexpressed, respectively, during the indicated transition.

Glutathione S-Transferase Pi

Decreased expression of the pi-class glutathione S-transferase through somatic hypermethylation of the glutathoine S-transferase pi (*GSTP1*) locus is one of the most frequently reported events in PCA. Glutathione S-transferases are enzymes that protect against cancer development by catalyzing the conjugation of the chemical scavenger glutathione to reactive chemical species. Although *GSTP1* is normally expressed in basal cells but not in luminal secretory cells in benign prostate epithelium, *GSTP1* is transcriptionally silenced in almost all PCA cells (8). This silencing, mediated by hypermethylation of the CpG-island sequences in the *GSTP1* promoter, occurs in more than 90% of PCA cases (9). However, *GSTP1* does not appear to act as a classical tumor suppressor, as PCA lines forced to express *GSTP1* grow well in vitro and in vivo (10). Although the mechanism by which *GSTP1* is selectively targeted for methylation is unknown, this phenomenon provides important information about PCA pathogenesis.

GSTP1: glutathione S-transferase pi

Up to 60% of PIN, the accepted precursor lesion to PCA, also display loss of *GSTP1* expression through CpG-island hypermethylation (8). Furthermore, PIA lesions, the recently described candidate

Table 1 Candidate genes and pathways dysregulated during PCA progression

Gene or pathway	Function	Evidence	References
Hedgehog pathway	Development and regeneration	Marked activation of the hedgehog pathway has been reported in advanced PCA. Treatment with cyclopamide, a hedgehog inhibitor, inhibits growth and invasion of cell lines and xenografts.	(73–76)
α-methylacyl-CoA racemase (*AMACR*)	Fatty acid metabolism	This enzyme is involved in peroxisomal β-oxidation of branched-chain fatty acids. It is also one of the most overexpressed genes in PCA identified by microarray studies.	(85, 90, 105)
Fatty acid synthase (*FASN*)	Fatty acid metabolism	Highly expressed in aggressive localized and metastatic PCA. Expression in PCA is regulated by ubiquitin-specific protease-2a.	(100, 139, 140)
Myc	Growth control	One of the master regulators of cell proliferation. *Myc* is often amplified in localized and metastatic PCA. Myc expression in the mouse prostate results in PCA development.	(64–67)
PIM-1	Growth control	A serine-threonine kinase that interacts with Myc. Expression of PIM-1 characterizes a Myc-like signature in human PCA, and PIM-1 is highly expressed in murine PCA driven by Myc expression. High levels of PIM-1 predict recurrence in localized PCA.	(67, 68, 70)
Glutathione-S-transferase pi-class (*GSTP1*)	Protection from carcinogens	Glutathione S-transferases protect against reactive chemical species. Transcriptional silencing of *GSTP1* through promoter hypermethylation is one of the most frequent events in PCA (>90%). The precursor lesion PIN also shows *GSTP1* hypermethylation.	(8–10, 12)
Phosphatase and tensin homolog (*PTEN*)	PI3K signaling	PTEN antagonizes the PI3K/Akt signaling pathway and is frequently deleted in PCA. Loss of PTEN expression in mouse models results in PCA.	(13–15, 22–26, 28)
Cyclin-dependent kinase inhibitor 1B (*p27*)	PI3K signaling	Expression of this cyclin-dependent kinase inhibitor is often lost in PCA. The downregulation is mediated by PI3K and the ubiquitin ligase SKP2.	(27, 28, 141–144)
Neutral endopeptidase (*NEP*)	PI3K signaling	NEP is frequently lost in the development of PCA and stabilizes PTEN.	(36, 37, 145)
Hepsin (HPN)	Protease	This serine protease is one of the most consistently overexpressed genes reported in PCA profiling studies. Hepsin expression in the mouse prostate causes disruption of the basement membrane and weakening of epithelial-stroma adhesions.	(69, 70, 89)
Androgen receptor (*AR*)	Steroid receptor	Alterations to AR signaling mediate the transition to androgen-independent disease. A modest elevation in AR expression was necessary and sufficient for the transition to androgen independence in a xenograft model.	(50, 52–55, 57)
NKX3.1	Transcriptional regulation	The *NKX3.1* locus frequently demonstrates LOH in PIN and PCA. *NKX3.1* null mice develop PIN. *NKX3.1* acts as a haploinsuffcent tumor suppressor, and loss of one allele affects cellular proliferation and gene expression.	(38, 39, 41, 49)
Enhancer of Zeste homolog 2 (*EZH2*)	Transcriptional regulation	A polycomb group protein that acts as a transcriptional repressor, EZH2 is required for proliferation in different cell types. EZH2 protein is increased in metastatic PCA and high expression in localized PCA predicts recurrence.	(107, 108, 110–112)

precursor to PIN and PCA, typically display high levels of *GSTP1* expression (4), although approximately 6% show *GSTP1* hypermethylation (11). These observations support the hypothesis that inflammation is important to the pathogenesis of PCA, as described above. The consequence of *GSTP1* loss in PIN and PCA is likely to be increased vulnerability to electrophilic or oxidant carcinogens, such as 2-amino-1-methyl-6-phenylimidazo[4,5-*b*]pyridine (PhIP), which is found in well-done or charred meats. For example, PCA cell lines overexpressing *GSTP1* form significantly fewer PhIP-DNA adducts upon exposure to activated PhIP than do control cells (12). *GSTP1* expression in the androgen-dependent PCA cell line LNCaP also significantly inhibits the oxidation of DNA bases upon exposure to oxidant stresses (5). Although the mechanism of *GSTP1* silencing is unknown, its frequency in the context of known risk factors for PCA supports roles for *GSTP1* and inflammation in PCA development.

Phosphate and Tensin Homolog

In 1997, phosphatase and tensin homolog (*PTEN*) was cloned and mapped to chromosome 10q23, a region undergoing frequent deletion in a variety of tumors, including PCA (13–15). Germline *PTEN* mutations in families with the related hamartoma syndromes, Cowden syndrome and Bannayan-Riley-Ruvalcaba syndrome were shortly identified, confirming *PTEN* as a classic tumor suppressor gene (16, 17). The region containing *PTEN* is a frequent target for heterozygous deletion in primary and metastatic prostate tumors, where loss of heterozygosity (LOH) is found up to 60% of the time. Point mutations and deletions of the *PTEN* gene have also been reported in PCA cell lines and xenografts, as well as in primary and metastatic tumors (18). Although the occurrence of second mutational events is generally less frequent than LOH incidence, second *PTEN* mutations have been found in up to 50% of metastatic tumors (19). However, loss of PTEN protein expression also occurs in 20% of primary tumors, particularly in those with advanced-grade or stage tumors (20). Epigenetic inactivation of *PTEN* through promoter hypermethylation has been described in PCA xenografts, however the same phenomenon has not been identified in primary human tumors (18).

The protein encoded by *PTEN* antagonizes the phosphoinositide 3-kinase (PI3K)/Akt pathway. A summary of the PI3K/Akt pathway in PCA is depicted in **Figure 2**. PI3K phosphorylates phosphatidylinositol-4,5-biphosphate (PIP_2), generating phosphatidylinositol-3,4,5-triphosphate (PIP_3). PIP_3 acts as a second messenger that activates multiple downstream effectors, including Akt (protein kinase B), a serine threonine kinase that promotes cell growth, survival, invasiveness, and angiogenesis (18). Thus, PTEN serves to suppress the PI3K/Akt signaling pathway, and the loss of PTEN results in PI3K-signaling activation.

PTEN null mice are embryonic lethal (21), and $PTEN^{+/-}$ mice develop PIN with varying penetrance, although development of carcinoma is rare (one report of a 65-week-old mouse with invasive cancer showing LOH at the wild-type allele) (21–23). Consistent with its role in PCA development, the age of prostate tumorigenesis is accelerated in different PIN/PCA-prone backgrounds with *PTEN* haploinsufficiency, including $NKX3.1^{-/-}$ (24, 25), transgenic adenocarcinoma of mouse prostate [prostate-specific expression of simian virus (SV) 40 early genes] (26), and $p27^{-/-}$ (*CDKN1B*) (27, 28). Furthermore, prostate-specific deletion of both *PTEN* alleles in two mouse models resulted in completely penetrant high-grade PIN and carcinoma with varying rates of metastatic disease (29, 30). Recently, a hypomorphic *PTEN* mutant mouse series demonstrated that the extent of *PTEN* inactivation controls PCA incidence and progression in a dose-dependent manner (31). Consistent with the importance of downstream

PTEN: phosphatase and tensin homolog

Loss of heterozygosity (LOH): deletion of a portion of a chromosome; all polymorphic markers remaining within the region will appear to be homozygous

PI3K: phosphoinositide 3-kinase

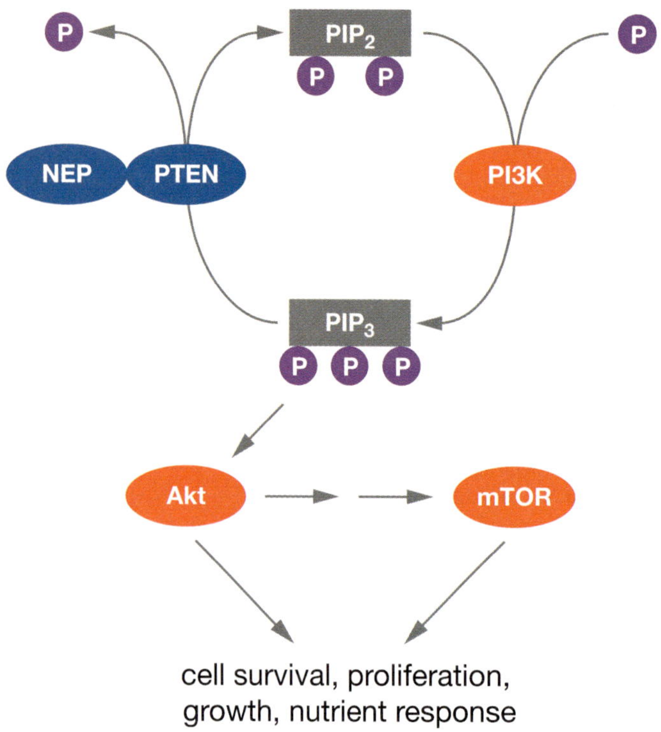

Figure 2

Components of the phosphoinositide 3-kinase (PI3K)/phosphatase and tensin homolog (PTEN) pathway involved in prostate cancer (PCA) development. Members of the PI3K pathway are indicated, with gene/protein products represented in ellipses, lipid signaling molecules in rectangles, and phosphate groups in purple circles. PI3K is recruited to the cell membrane by activated receptor tyrosine kinases, where it catalyzes the transfer of a phosphate group to phosphatidylinositol-4,5 bisphosphate (PIP_2), yielding phosphatidylinositol-3,4,5 trisphosphate (PIP_3). PIP_3 transmits signals through the kinase Akt and downstream members such as mammalian target of rapamycin (mTOR). The phosphatase PTEN inhibits the activity of the PI3K pathway through inactivation of PIP_3 to PIP_2, and neutral endopeptidase (NEP) binds directly and stabilizes PTEN. Proteins indicated in red demonstrate increased activity in PCA development or mouse models predisposed to PCA development, whereas proteins in blue show decreased activity in PCA through deletion or inactivation.

PI3K-signaling events in the development of PCA, expression of an activated allele of *Akt* in the mouse prostate results in a highly penetrant PIN phenotype (32). Treatment with the rapamycin derivative RAD001 eradicated the PIN, demonstrating that the mammalian target of rapamycin kinase, which is known to mediate Akt signaling pathways, controls PIN development in this model (33). Other lines of evidence from mouse and xenograft models implicate *PTEN* in controlling specifically the progression from localized PCA to metastasis (34, 35).

Researchers have investigated further mechanisms for the specific effects of *PTEN* on the prostate. Recently, neutral endopeptidase (NEP), also known as membrane metallo-endopeptidase, a protein frequently showing loss of expression in primary PCA (36), has been shown to directly bind PTEN (37). NEP recruits PTEN to the plasma membrane, which increases the stability and phosphatase activity of PTEN, resulting in Akt inactivation. In four PCA cell lines that were characterized, NEP and PTEN were never expressed simultaneously and the androgen insensitive PCA cell line PC-3, which expresses neither NEP nor PTEN, showed the strongest activation of Akt (37). Taken together, these results demonstrate the importance of *PTEN* loss to PCA pathogenesis and support dysregulation of PI3K signaling as a general feature of PCA.

NK3 Transcription Factor Related, Locus 1

A two-megabase region surrounding chromosome 8p21 is one of the most frequent sites of LOH in PCA (90% frequency) as well as PIN (60% frequency) (38, 39). Although it does not act as a classic tumor suppressor, the androgen-regulated NK3 transcription factor related, locus 1 (*NKX3.1*) homeobox gene is localized to this region (40) and plays roles in both prostate development and PCA pathogenesis. NKX3.1 is the earliest known marker of prostate formation during embryogenesis, and its expression in luminal epithelium continues through adulthood. Loss of *NKX3.1* causes defects in prostatic secretion and ductal morphogenesis in mice (41). Like other NKX homeobox proteins, NKX3.1 acts a transcriptional regulator, and cell-line experiments suggest that NKX3.1 can regulate PSA transcription (42).

Although expression of NKX3.1 in prostatic epithelium precedes androgen receptor (AR) expression, subsequent NKX3.1 expression is dependent upon androgen signaling (41). Depletion of androgen in cell culture medium downregulates *NKX3.1* expression in human PCA cells, and numerous studies have confirmed that *NKX3.1* is androgen regulated (40).

In addition to developmental defects, *NKX3.1* null mice also display increasing prostatic epithelial hyperplasia and dysplasia with age. By one to two years of age, the mice develop features similar to PIN, however they do not develop carcinoma (41). *NKX3.1*'s role in the promotion of PIN is independent of prostate development, as a prostate-specific deletion of a *NKX3.1* allele in adult mice results in PIN formation (43). Consistent with the idea that LOH at *NKX3.1* promotes PCA pathogenesis, *NKX3.1* cooperates with other tumor suppressors in mouse models of cancer. As described above, compound $PTEN^{+/-}$; *NKX3.1* $^{-/-}$ mutant mice show increased development of high-grade PIN with strong activation of Akt, and older mice show invasive carcinoma and develop metastases (24, 25, 44).

Although 8p21 is deleted at high frequency in PCA, as described above, the remaining *NKX3.1* allele does not undergo mutational inactivation, as would be expected for a classical tumor suppressor (45). $PTEN^{+/-}$; $NKX3.1^{+/-}$ compound heterozygotes are consistent with this idea, as the wild-type *PTEN* allele is lost, whereas the wild-type *NKX3.1* allele remains intact (24). However, NKX3.1 protein expression is downregulated in approximately 20% of PIN and localized PCA, in addition to 78% of metastases (46), although a recent study did not confirm the loss of expression (47). However, heterozygous $NKX3.1^{+/-}$ mice also demonstrate dysplasia and PIN formation and display loss of NKX3.1 protein expression after the development of PIN (43). Recent evidence also suggests that *NKX3.1* may be selectively methylated in PCA (48).

By utilizing *NKX3.1* $^{+/-}$ and *NKX3.1* $^{-/-}$ mice, Magee and colleagues clarified the mechanism of *NKX3.1* dosage-dependent tumor suppression (49). They demonstrated that *NKX3.1* controls the rate at which proliferating, luminal epithelial cells exit the cell cycle and that deletion of one or both alleles extends the proliferative phase during prostate regeneration. Through gene expression profiling, they identified discrete clusters of haploinsufficient and nonhaploinsufficient target genes. Interestingly, not all haploinsufficient genes exhibited the same response to loss of one *NKX3.1* allele, as some targets showed complete loss of expression, whereas others were less affected. Taken together, results from these experiments demonstrate a role for *NKX3.1* as a haploinsufficient tumor suppressor during the early pathogenesis of PCA.

AR: androgen receptor

Androgen Receptor

During the normal development of the prostate and the development of PCA, cell survival depends primarily upon the AR. Normally, the steroid receptor is bound to heat-shock proteins in the cytoplasm of prostate cells. Binding of the cognate ligand dihyrotestosterone causes dissociation of the AR, which translocates to the nucleus. After translocating to the nucleus, the AR dimerizes, binds to regulatory sequences of specific target genes, and activates their transcription. Most prostate tumors are initially responsive to androgen ablation, however almost all tumors eventually become androgen independent and proliferate despite androgen ablation. Determining how PCA cells become androgen independent is an area of intense investigation, and many of these studies have focused on the role of the AR.

Recent evidence suggests that the mechanisms of androgen independence can either involve or bypass the AR and that both types of mechanisms may co-exist in the same cancer. Pathways involving the AR include

DNA microarray: thousands of "probes" (cDNA clones or oligonucleotides) on a solid support that are hybridized with fluorescently tagged antisense RNA or complementary DNA

amplifications or mutations of the receptor, dysregulation of growth factors or cytokines, and alterations of coactivators. Several excellent reviews cover this subject in more detail than can be presented here and include a discussion of those pathways that do not involve the *AR* gene directly (50, 51). A summary of the role of the AR in the development of hormone-refractory PCA is presented in **Figure 3**.

Despite resistance to anti-androgen therapy, continued expression of the AR occurs frequently in metastatic PCA. Independent studies find increased *AR* mRNA in hormone-refractory cancers compared with hormone-dependent cancers, and 20%–30% of hormone-refractory cancers show an amplification of the *AR* gene (52–54). Androgen-refractory tumors also contain a variety of mutations in the *AR*, which increase the number of ligands that can activate the receptor, although there is some controversy as to how often this occurs in vivo (55). Interestingly, prostate-specific expression of a mutant *AR*, *AR*-E231G, in mice resulted in completely penetrant PCA and lung metastases, which demonstrates the oncogenic effects of *AR* mutations (56). Recently, evidence from a DNA microarray study by Chen and colleagues (57) elegantly demonstrated the importance of the *AR* to PCA progression, as summarized in **Figure 3*b***. By comparing

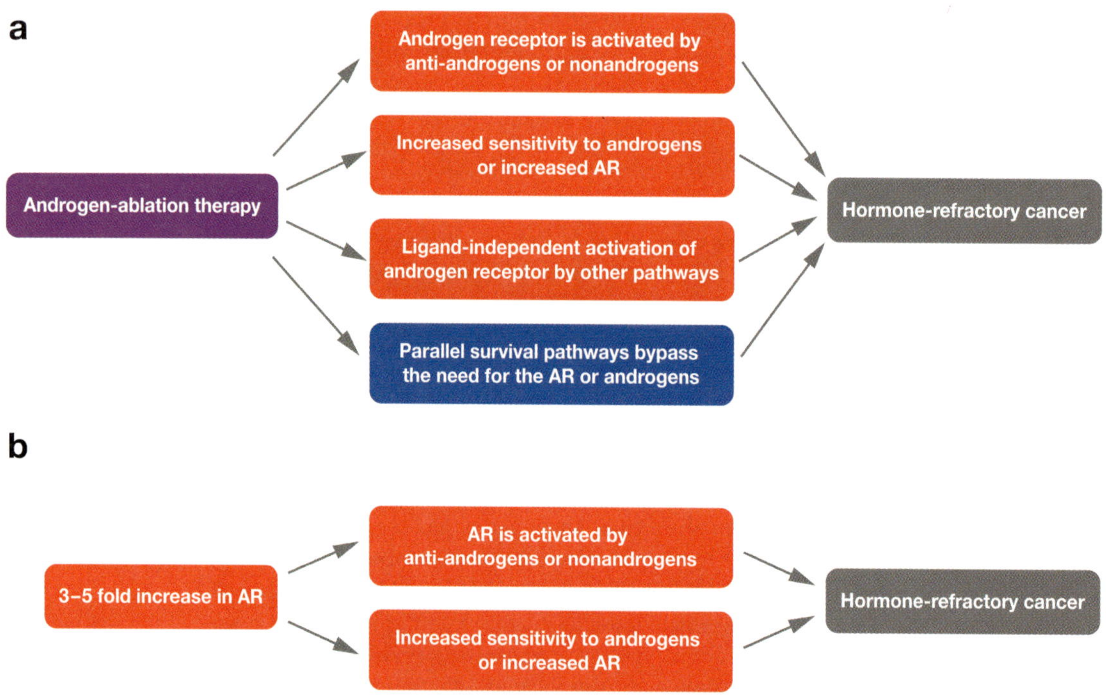

Figure 3

The role of the androgen receptor (AR) in the development of hormone-refractory prostate cancer (PCA). (*a*) Although PCA treated with hormone ablation initially responds clinically, hormone-refractory disease develops almost invariably. The AR is thought to play a crucial role in this progression and possible mechanisms, as described in the text (51), are shown in red, whereas mechanisms not involving the AR are shown in blue. (*b*) Chen and colleagues (57) identified a modest increase in the *AR* through gene expression profiling of seven isogenic pairs of hormone-dependent/refractory xenografts as the only consistent gene expression change. In animal models, the authors demonstrated that a modest increase in the level of *AR* expression resulted in hormone-refractory disease involving two of the mechanisms shown in part *a*.

microarray profiles of hormone-sensitive and hormone-refractory pairs of human prostate xenografts, the authors reported a two- to five-fold increase in the *AR* as the only gene expression change associated consistently with androgen independence (57). Furthermore, this modest increase was necessary and sufficient for hormone-independent progression in the animal models. Cells with modestly increased AR expression are also highly sensitive to androgens, and AR antagonists act as agonists. Taken together, the importance of the AR to the development of hormone-refractory disease suggests that strategies to downregulate the AR may also be important clinically. Studies of the role of the AR in PCA pathogenesis and progression will continue to be pursued with great interest.

Myc

Dysregulation of the *Myc* family of genes is one of the most common events in human cancer. In PCA, *c-Myc*, a strong positive regulator of cellular proliferation located at chromosome 8q24, appears to play a role in PCA pathogenesis. Gains in chromosome 8 are one of the most common amplifications in human prostate tumors, even at the early stage of PIN (58). However, entire copies of chromosome 8 are often gained, and many genes localized to 8q24 are also amplified in PCA, which suggests that other target genes in the region may be important (59–61). However, high-level amplification of *Myc* has been identified consistently during the progression to androgen-independent metastatic disease (62–64). Cell culture work has shown that androgen-dependent LNCaP cells overexpressing *Myc* form colonies in soft agar independently of androgens, and *Myc* appears to be an essential downstream target of the AR (65).

Two mouse models overexpressing *Myc* specifically in the prostate also indicate that *Myc* has an earlier role in PCA progression. These models demonstrate that *Myc* overexpression induces PIN (66) or overt carcinoma (67), depending upon the targeting promoter. In mice that overexpress *Myc* and develop carcinoma, microarray expression profiling studies defined a mouse Myc-PCA expression signature that shares features with human PCA, as shown in **Figure 4**. *NKX3.1* gene expression is lost during the transition from PIN to carcinoma, and this is confirmed at the protein level. Furthermore, one of the most consistently regulated genes in the mouse Myc-PCA signature that is also co-expressed in human cancers showing a Myc-like signature was *PIM-1*, which cooperates with Myc in other cancers (68). Increased PIM-1 protein expression has predicted PSA recurrence in patients with localized PCA (69, 70). These results suggest that *Myc* controls aspects of PCA progression, similar to its role in other human cancers.

Prostate-specific antigen (PSA) recurrence: multiple measurements of increasing PSA levels are used to indicate recurrence of the primary tumor

SHH: sonic hedgehog

PTCH: patched homolog

Hedgehog Pathway

Recent evidence also implicates the sonic hedgehog (SHH) pathway, known for its important role in prostate development, as crucial to the development of PCA metastasis (**Figure 5**). Secreted SHH molecules bind to the patched receptor (PTCH), relieving PTCH-mediated inhibition of smoothened, a seven-transmembrane G protein coupled receptor. Smoothened signaling leads to activation of downstream target genes through glioma-associated oncogene homolog (*GLI*)-dependent transcription. *PTCH* is also a target gene of *GLI*, which forms a negative-feedback mechanism (71). Hedgehog signaling is required for proper growth, patterning, and tissue polarity during prostate development, although hedgehog signaling has not been reported in normal adult prostate (72).

In 2004, four studies reported that the hedgehog pathway is activated in advanced PCA (73–76). Expression of *GLI-1*, *SHH*, and *PTCH* mRNA was reported with varying frequencies in benign prostate, localized PCA, or metastatic PCA. However increased expression during the progression to advanced or metastatic cancer was consistently reported

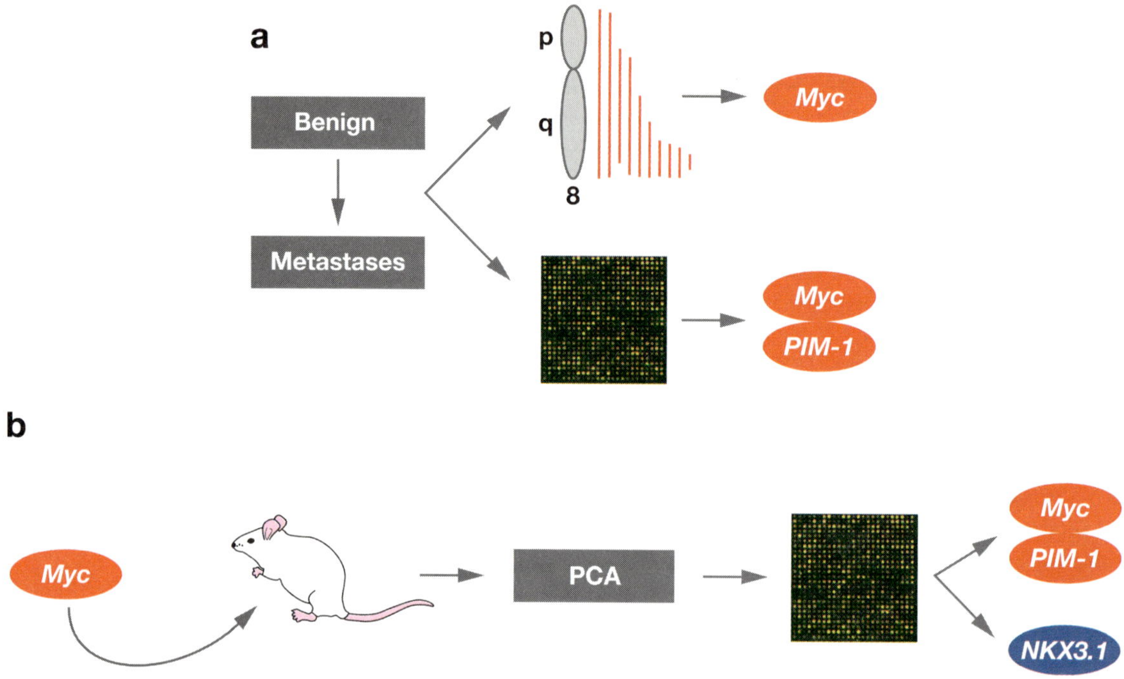

Figure 4

Integrative analyses reveal conserved *Myc* activation signatures in human prostate cancer (PCA) and mouse models. (*a*) During the transition from benign prostate to PCA and metastatic disease, multiple techniques, including comparative genomic hybridization, have demonstrated that one of the most frequently gained regions is chromosome 8q24, the locus of *Myc*. Gene expression profiling of localized and metastatic PCA also demonstrates increased expression of *Myc*, often in parallel with increased expression of *PIM-1*, a gene known to cooperate with *Myc* in other malignancies. (*b*) Prostate-specific expression of *Myc* in mouse models also results in PCA development, and gene expression profiling of these tumors reveal increased *PIM-1* expression, as seen in human tissue samples. These tumors also show decreased expression of *NKX3.1*, a prostate dosage-dependent tumor suppressor.

(73, 75, 76). Furthermore, treatment of PCA cell lines or xenografts with cyclopamide, a SHH pathway inhibitor, consistently inhibited growth, invasion, and metastasis both in vitro and in vivo (73, 75, 76). Sheng and colleagues also demonstrated that suppressor of fused (*SUFU*), an inhibitor of SHH pathway activity, showed decreased expression in high-grade tumors and identified two somatic mutations, suggesting a possible regulatory role for *SUFU* in PCA (76). Karhadkar and colleagues also demonstrated that constitutive activation of the SHH pathway can transform primitive prostate epithelial progenitor cells (75).

There are some discrepancies that will need to be resolved to understand completely the contribution of the SHH pathway to PCA pathogenesis. For example, Fan and colleagues demonstrated by in situ hybridization on benign and cancerous human tissue samples that *SHH* expression localizes to the epithelium, whereas *GLI-1* expression localizes to the surrounding stroma (74). This pattern was maintained in their xenograft models using LNCaP cells. However Sanchez and colleagues reported that GLI-1, PTCH, and SHH normally are co-expressed in epithelial cells and not in the surrounding stroma (73). Karhadkar and colleagues also demonstrated high levels of *SHH* and *PTCH* in the DU145 cell line, and treatment of these cells with cyclopamide inhibited cell growth significantly (75). In contrast, Sanchez and colleagues reported that DU145 cells did not express *SHH* or *PTCH*, and they found these cells to be insensitive to cyclopamide (73). It is interesting to note that although quantitative polymerase chain reaction revealed 10- to 100-fold changes between expression levels of SHH pathway members, no microarray studies have identified pathway members as being dysregulated between low- and high-grade tumors or localized and metastatic samples. The reasons for this discrepancy are unclear.

In addition to establishing a role for the SHH pathway in the development of metastatic PCA, Karhadkar and colleagues also demonstrated that the SHH pathway is required for epithelial cell regeneration after androgen ablation, followed by androgen re-treatment. Taken together with their other observations, the authors suggest that PCA may develop from the trapping of normal prostate stem cells in a SHH pathway–dependent state of continuous renewal (75). The involvement of prostate stem cells in PCA has been proposed previously (77), and the recent identification of cells with stem cell–like properties in other cancers has led to speculation that tissue-specific stem cells, through the SHH pathway, may drive many cancers, including PCA (78–80). The possibility of the SHH pathway mediating prostate stem cell behavior would be consistent with several aspects of PCA. The cycling between tissue damage and regeneration would promote the prolonged expansion of the stem cell pool, consistent with the idea that inflammation drives PCA. Subsequent genetic events could lock the stem cells into a state of continuous proliferation (78). A role for stem cells in PCA is also consistent with the clinical course of androgen-ablation therapy if the prostate tumor is thought to contain androgen-independent cancer stem cells and differentiated tumor cells that have become androgen dependent. The initial clinical response would result from selective killing of differentiated tumor cells that are androgen dependent, whereas the relapse would be a result of the expansion of androgen-independent stem cells (77). Although the hypothesis that stem cells are important to PCA is consistent with other observations, prospective markers to identify and isolate potential PCA stem cells are needed for experimental confirmation.

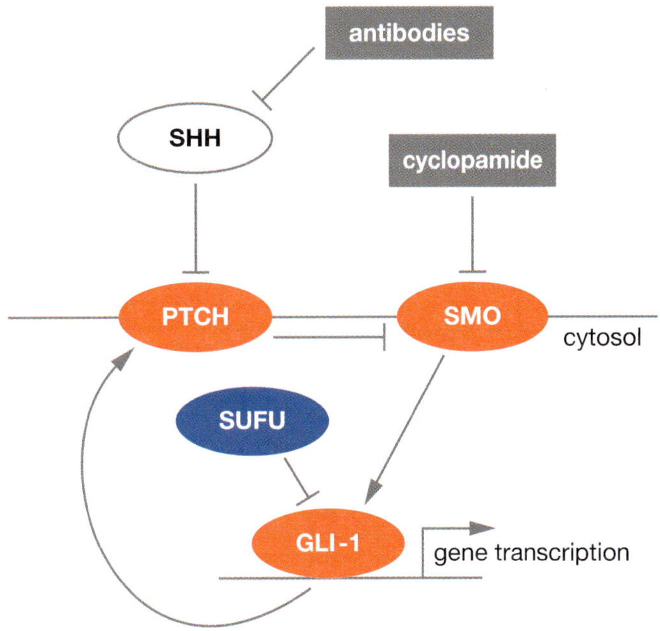

Figure 5

Activation and targeting of the hedgehog pathway in advanced prostate cancer (PCA). Components of the hedgehog pathway that have been implicated in advanced PCA are indicated. Protein components are indicated in ellipses, and specific pathway inhibitors are indicated in rectangles. The color of the ellipse indicates transcript abundance in advanced PCA, with red and blue representing increased and decreased activity, respectively. Positive (→) and negative (⊣) regulation between pathway members is indicated. SHH, sonic hedgehog; PTCH, patched receptor; SMO, smoothened; SUFU, suppressor of fused; GLI-1, glioma-associated oncogene homolog 1.

Prostate stem cell: undifferentiated cell in the prostate that can renew itself and differentiate to yield other prostate cells

Candidate Genes Identified Through DNA Microarrays

Although the candidate genes and pathways described above have provided profound insight into the pathogenesis of PCA,

HPN: hepsin

AMACR: α-methylacyl-CoA racemase

EZH2: enhancer of Zeste homolog 2

researchers are still far from understanding the key transitions in the progression and development of PCA. Due to the observed clinical and biological heterogeneity, many research groups have attempted to characterize PCA globally at the molecular level using DNA microarrays. DNA microarrays have become the standard research tool for high-throughput examination of genome-wide expression changes in PCA, with more than 25 published studies examining various aspects of PCA biology (catalogued at **http://www.oncomine.org**). Most of these studies have focused on distinguishing PCA from benign prostate tissue, and almost all studies report distinct expression profiles separating cancerous from benign tissues. Unfortunately, due to differences in technology, experimental design, and the output of hundreds to thousands of candidate genes, translating these profiles to candidate genes and pathways involved in the pathogenesis of PCA has been much more difficult. Nevertheless, several attractive candidates, including hepsin (*HPN*), α-methylacyl-CoA racemase (*AMACR*), and enhancer of Zeste homolog 2 (*EZH2*), have been identified, and functional studies have provided evidence for their involvement in the pathogenesis of PCA progression. Recently, Tomlins and colleagues (80a) have used novel methods of analyzing gene expression data to identify recurrent fusions of the androgen-regulated gene transmembrane protease, serine 2 (*TMPRSS2*) with *ETS* family members in a majority of PCAs. Furthermore, recent studies have shown the existence of distinct classes of tumors on the basis of their expression profiles (81–84), supporting the observed clinical heterogeneity of prostate tumors and suggesting that these profiles may represent underlying genetic changes during PCA pathogenesis and progression.

Hepsin

Marked overexpression of the type II serine protease *HPN* has been identified in nearly every DNA microarray study profiling PCA (85). *HPN* mRNA is upregulated in approximately 90% of prostate tumors, with expression confined to epithelial cells; however the role of *HPN* in PCA progression is still unclear. In humans, HPN protein expression is strongest at the PIN stage and decreases during the transition to metastatic cancer. Intensity of HPN protein expression in localized tumors is also inversely correlated with PSA recurrence after surgical treatment (70). However, other studies have found that *HPN* mRNA is highest in high-grade and stage tumors, although metastatic tissues were not examined (86, 87). Cell-line experiments support a role for *HPN* early in PCA pathogenesis, as forced expression of *HPN* in PC-3 cells, a metastasis-derived cell line that does not express endogenous *HPN*, decreases cell proliferation and invasion (88).

In an effort to understand the function of *HPN* in PCA, Klezovitch and colleagues created transgenic mice with forced expression of *HPN* specifically in the prostate (89). Although these mice show no obvious abnormalities in proliferation or apoptosis in the prostate, weakening of epithelial-stromal adhesion and disorganization and disruption of the basement membrane occurs. To determine the effect on cancer progression, these transgenic mice were crossed with the *LPB-Tag* mouse, which expresses the SV40 large T antigen specifically in the prostate through the probasin promoter. *LPB-Tag* mice develop high-grade PIN and limited adenocarcinoma by 20 weeks of age, with no metastases. However, in addition to developing focal carcinoma, up to 55% of *HPN*/*LPB-Tag* mice develop prominent metastases. Although these metastatic lesions show NE differentiation, it is unclear if this is owing to *HPN*, as other metastases from *LPB-Tag*-driven models also show NE differentiation. Crossing these transgenic *HPN* mice with other mouse models that do not develop NE differentiation ($NKX3.1^{-/-}$ or $PTEN^{+/-}$) should clarify the role of *HPN* in PCA progression. In addition to these experimental results, the magnitude and consistency of overexpression in PCA suggest that *HPN* plays a role in PCA pathogenesis.

Alpha-methylacyl-CoA Racemase

The enzyme AMACR, which is involved in peroxisomal β-oxidation of dietary branched-chain fatty acids, has also been identified as an important contributor to PCA. The functionally active protein is specifically overexpressed in PCA epithelium compared with benign epithelium, and DNA microarrays consistently reveal *AMACR* to be one of the most upregulated transcripts from normal to cancerous tissue (85, 90–92). *AMACR* is also overexpressed in PIN (90, 91, 93). In addition to studies demonstrating it as a possible biomarker (94–96), epidemiologic, genetic, and functional studies point to a role for *AMACR* and fatty acid metabolism in general in PCA pathogenesis.

The major dietary sources of branched-chain fatty acids, meat and dairy products, have been implicated in the increased incidence of PCA in Western countries, as described in the introduction. Compared with control patients, recent evidence also suggests that PCA patients have higher levels of phytanic acid, which is caused primarily by dietary intake of dairy and red meat and requires AMACR for its metabolism (97). Branched-chain fatty acids also induce AMACR protein expression, but not transcript expression, in PCA cells in vitro (98). In addition, other enzymes involved in fatty acid metabolism, including D-bifunctional protein (99), fatty acid synthase (FASN) (100), and sterol-CoA desaturase (101), are also dysregulated in PCA. These observations suggest general dysregulation of lipid metabolism, possibly though the generation of reactive oxygen species during β-oxidation, as a feature of PCA. Genome scans for linkage in families with hereditary PCA suggest that the locus of *AMACR* (at chromosome 5p13) contains a PCA susceptibility gene (102, 103), and *AMACR* single-nucleotide polymorphisms (SNP) cosegregate with PCA in hereditary PCA families (104). Finally, knockdown of *AMACR* expression in an androgen-dependent PCA cell line also inhibits cellular proliferation (105). Future experiments, including the generation of transgenic mice that express *AMACR* in the prostate, should provide more information about the role of *AMACR* in PCA pathogenesis.

Enhancer of Zeste Homolog 2

Although most microarray studies profiling PCA are designed to identify genes differentially expressed between normal and cancerous tissues, recent studies have also focused on identifying genes dysregulated specifically in metastatic cancer (83, 106, 107). *EZH2*, a member of the polycomb group family of transcriptional repressors, has emerged recently as a candidate gene that is specifically overexpressed in metastatic and aggressive localized PCAs (69, 106, 107). In addition to being overexpressed in PCA, *EZH2* is overexpressed or amplified in other cancers, which suggests that *EZH2* may act as an oncogene (108). Recently, *EZH2* expression in the content of a polycomb complex was examined during PCA progression in the $NKX3.1^{+/-}$; $PTEN^{+/-}$ mouse model described above. PIN lesions displayed moderate elevation in the number of cells expressing *EZH2*, and cancerous tissues displayed further elevation when assayed at the transcript and protein level (109).

Besides acting as a histone methyltransferase responsible for gene silencing, recent evidence demonstrates that EZH2 expression, controlled by the pRB/E2F pathway, is essential for proliferation in transformed and primary human cells, including PCA cells (107, 108, 110–112). EZH2 expression is also downregulated by activated p53 through p53/p21Waf1-mediated repression of the *EZH2* promoter, which results in inhibition of cell growth (110). These results, in addition to DNA microarray results demonstrating that *EZH2* transcripts are often increased in PCAs with increased proliferation as assessed by Ki67 staining (83, 106), have prompted speculation that EZH2 expression may be merely a marker of proliferation.

However, several lines of evidence suggest that EZH2 has a role in cancer pathogenesis aside from its role in controlling cell proliferation. In normal breast tissue sections examined with double immunoflourescence, EZH2 protein expression is found only in rare cells that are always Ki67 positive. However, in poorly differentiated ductal carcinoma in situ and carcinoma, the majority of EZH2-positive cells are not Ki67 positive (113). *EZH2* overexpression in immortalized normal breast cells has no effect on cell proliferation, however it causes increased invasion and promotes anchorage-independent growth (114). Finally, in the *NKX3.1*$^{+/-}$; *PTEN*$^{+/-}$ mouse model, increased EZH2 expression does not correlate with increased Ki67 levels (109). These results, in addition to the frequent amplification in various cancers, suggest that *EZH2* has functional roles in cancer pathogenesis aside from regulating proliferation, although further investigations are needed to determine the extent of its function in PCA pathogenesis and progression.

Gene Fusions of *TMPRSS2* and *ETS* Family Members

Candidate genes described in this section were identified by dividing samples into two classes (i.e., benign versus cancerous or localized versus metastatic) and looking for the most differentially expressed genes. However, many hematological malignancies are characterized by several exclusive chromosomal aberrations. For example, distinct groups of acute myeloid leukemia are characterized by inversion(16), which results in *CBFb:MYH11* fusion transcripts, and translocation(8;21), which results in *AML:ETO* fusion transcripts. Examination of gene expression data from acute myeloid leukemia samples reveals exclusive overexpression of *MYH11* and *ETO* in inversion(16) and translocation(8;21) cases, respectively (114a). If distinct subclasses of PCA exist, they will not be detected by current methods of gene expression analysis, which treat all PCAs as a single entity.

Tomlins and colleagues (80a) have recently developed a novel analysis method termed cancer outlier profile analysis (COPA) to identify and rank genes with marked overexpression in a subset of cases. Remarkably, in multiple independent data sets, COPA identified strong outlier profiles for v-ets erythroblastosis virus E26 oncogene like (*ERG*) and ets variant gene 1 (*ETV1*), two ETS family transcription factors in PCA. The outlier profiles of *ERG* and *ETV1* were mutually exclusive across multiple data sets. Through multiple analyses, Tomlins and colleagues demonstrated that fusions of the 5′ region of the androgen-regulated gene *TMPRSS2* with *ERG* or *ETV1* were characteristic of cases with aberrant expression of the respective ETS family member. The structure of the fusions is shown in **Figure 6**. In accordance with the hypothesis that the overexpression of the ETS members is driven by the androgen response elements in the *TMPRSS2* promoter, the authors demonstrated that *ERG* is androgen regulated in the PCA cell line VCaP (which expresses the *TMPRSS2:ERG* fusion) but not in PCA cell lines that do not express the fusion. Combining gene expression data across multiple studies with fluorescence in situ hybridization, the authors concluded that rearrangements in *ERG* or *ETV1* occur in the majority of all PCA cases (80a). Although additional studies are needed to determine the functional consequences of these fusions, the recurrent nature and exclusive overexpression of known oncogenes clearly suggest an important role for these fusions in PCA pathogenesis.

Integrative Analysis of Prostate Cancer Progression

As described above, thousands of genes dysregulated during PCA progression have been identified. In addition to the marked

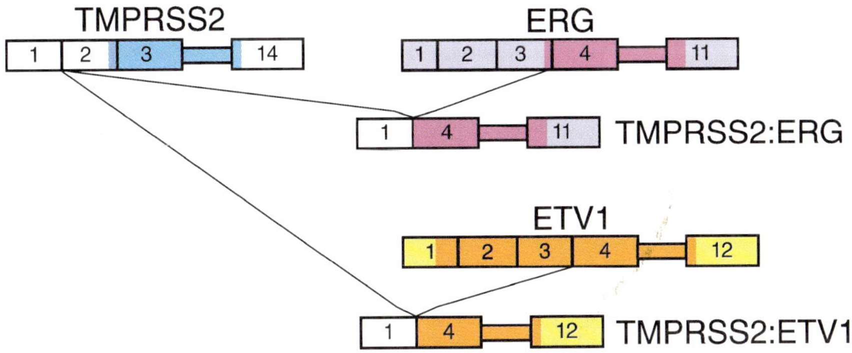

Figure 6

Structure of recurrent *TMPRSS2:ERG* and *TMPRSS2:ETV1* fusion transcripts in prostate cancer. Exons (*boxes*) of *TMPRSS2*, *ERG*, and *ETV1* were determined by aligning the GenBank reference sequence for each gene (NM_005656, NM_004449, and NM_004956, respectively) with the May 2004 assembly of the human genome using the University of California, Santa Cruz Genome Browser (**http://genome.ucsc.edu/cgi-bin/hgGateway**). Nontranslated regions are shown in lighter shades of color, and coding exons that are not depicted are indicated by the shorter boxes. Exon coloring for the fusion transcripts is from the original reference sequences.

difficulties in identifying which genes represent causal candidates rather than merely markers of the neoplastic state, technological and experimental differences also complicate the comparison of multiple data sets (115, 116). Rhodes and colleagues (117) have recently developed a Web site that catalogues expression profiling studies (**http://www.oncomine.org**) and a meta-analysis method to compare expression profiling studies from different platforms (85). Analyzing four of the earliest profiling studies, a cohort of genes, including *AMACR*, *Myc*, *FASN*, and *HPN*, were found to be significantly dysregulated across the data sets. Besides developing an improved way to identify candidate genes from profiling studies, bioinformatic approaches were also applied in an attempt to discover biologic pathways represented in the consistently dysregulated genes. Significant involvement of the polyamine biosynthesis pathway at a number of steps was identified, with enzymes directing substrates toward polyamines being overexpressed and the enzyme directing polyamine precursors toward an alternate pathway being underexpressed in PCA (85). Polyamines have been implicated in PCA biology, and enzymes involved in their biosynthesis are candidates for chemotherapeutic agents (118). As an update to Rhodes and colleague's previous work (85), we have performed a meta-analysis of eight studies profiling PCA versus benign prostate tissue and identified 216 genes present in six of eight studies that were dysregulated at a Q value (estimated false discovery rate) <0.10. A heatmap comparing the 69 overexpressed genes in PCA with benign tissue are shown in **Figure 7**. Taken together, these results indicate that bioinformatic mining of the massive amounts of data generated by microarray experiments can identify candidate genes and pathways involved in PCA progression

Other techniques that measure genome- or proteome-wide changes during the development of PCA are also used to identify candidate genes. Many of the candidate genes described above are identified by their consistent loss or amplification during PCA progression. Recently developed techniques, such as array comparative genomic hybridization (CGH) (119) and SNP arrays (120), allow for global monitoring of gains and losses, as well as LOH at increased resolutions. Although these studies have begun only

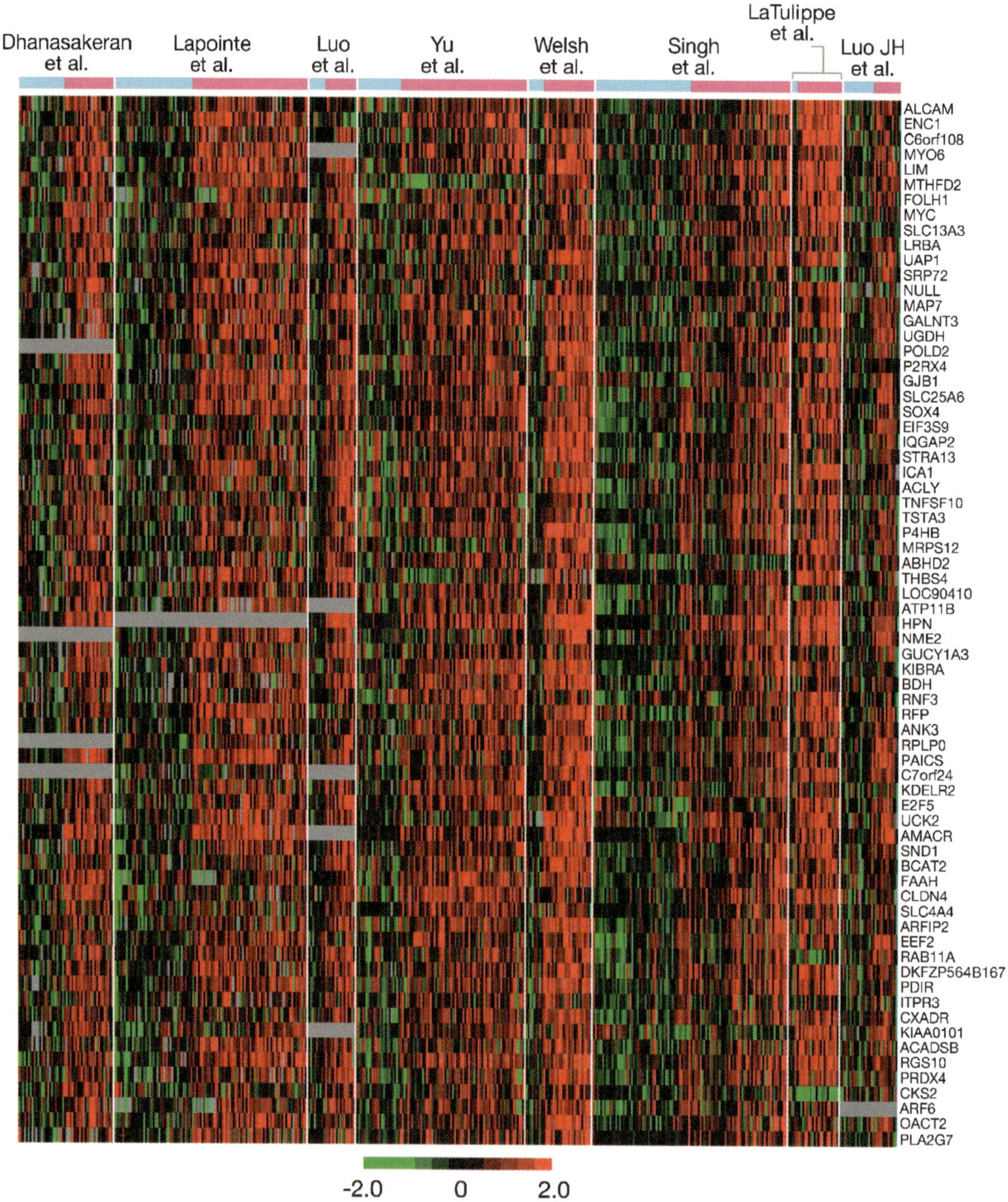

Figure 7

Meta-analysis of genes overexpressed in prostate cancer (PCA) compared with benign prostate tissue. A meta-analysis, as described in Reference 85, was performed on eight studies profiling PCA versus benign prostate tissue (70, 81, 83, 84, 106, 118a–118c). Two hundred and sixteen genes present in at least six of eight studies were identified at a significance threshold of Q (estimated false discovery rate) <0.10, and the 69 overexpressed genes are depicted. Rows represent the indicated genes, and columns represent individual profiled samples, with benign or PCA samples indicated in blue or magenta, respectively. Gray cells indicate missing values or genes that were not monitored in individual studies, and expression values are indicated by the color bar.

recently for PCA, they have confirmed previous studies and are identifying novel chromosomal regions that may harbor important genes involved in PCA pathogenesis. A recent study profiling 64 primary tumors using array CGH identified 8p21.2, the location of *NKX3.1*, as the most frequently lost locus in the data set (121). Interestingly, amplifications at 11q13.1 predicted PSA recurrence independent of other clinical parameters, which suggests that this region may harbor a gene or genes controlling tumor aggressiveness. Using SNP arrays, Lieberfarb and colleagues confirmed that LOH at 8p21 as well as 10q23, the locus of *PTEN*, were amongst the most consistently observed events in 50 PCA samples (122). Furthermore, they clustered the tumors on the basis of their patterns of LOH and identified distinct genetic subtypes amongst the cancers. The lack of overlapping regions of LOH between the different tumor samples suggests that many sets of genetic lesions, rather than progression through a defined series of events, may lead to PCA development. Although studies in this area are still in their infancy, these results support clinical and expression profiling results suggesting that PCA is a heterogeneous disease. Further technologic advances in these areas should also aid the search for candidate genes controlling various aspects of PCA progression.

As the ultimate effectors in most cellular processes are proteins, characterizing the PCA proteome should greatly facilitate understanding of the disease pathogenesis. Technological developments, including tissue microarrays (123) and reverse phase protein microarrays (124), have allowed for simultaneous high-throughput assaying of a single protein's expression across hundreds of samples and have been used extensively to validate PCA candidate genes. Alternatively, mass spectrometry (MS)-based profiling has enormous potential to characterize and quantify large numbers of proteins. Although MS has been applied recently to various aspects of PCA, it has yet to provide much insight into PCA pathogenesis (125). Much MS work has focused on identifying protein changes in serum for diagnostic and prognostic applications, and although these studies can differentiate patients with cancer from control patients, the identity of discriminatory peaks has not been determined (126, 127).

Studies have also quantified the secreted proteins generated from androgen stimulation of human PCA cells in culture in an attempt to discover biomarkers (128). Two recent studies profiling PCA tissue specimens demonstrate the potential of proteomics for characterizing PCA pathogenesis, similar to the role that DNA microarray technology has played recently (129, 130). Both studies generate protein profiles from benign and cancerous tissues by surface-enhanced laser desorption/ionization-time of flight (SELDI-TOF) MS. As this method does not identify the analyzed proteins, both studies used alternative techniques to identify and validate differentially expressed proteins between cancer and normal samples, although they did not characterize them functionally. Interestingly, the differential protein identified by Cheung and colleagues, growth differentiation factor 15, did not show differential expression at the transcript level using the same samples analyzed by MS (130). These results call attention to the fact that post-translational regulation can result in protein-expression changes during disease progression that cannot be measured by genomic or expression profiling studies, demonstrating the importance of characterizing the proteome for understanding PCA pathogenesis.

Other high-throughput techniques with the potential to identify underlying causes of PCA are developing at a rapid rate, including methods to analyze genome-wide methylation (131–134) and genome-wide RNA interference screens (135–137). Advances in these high-throughput techniques have the potential to revolutionize the understanding of PCA pathogenesis through cataloguing the PCA genome, transcriptome, and

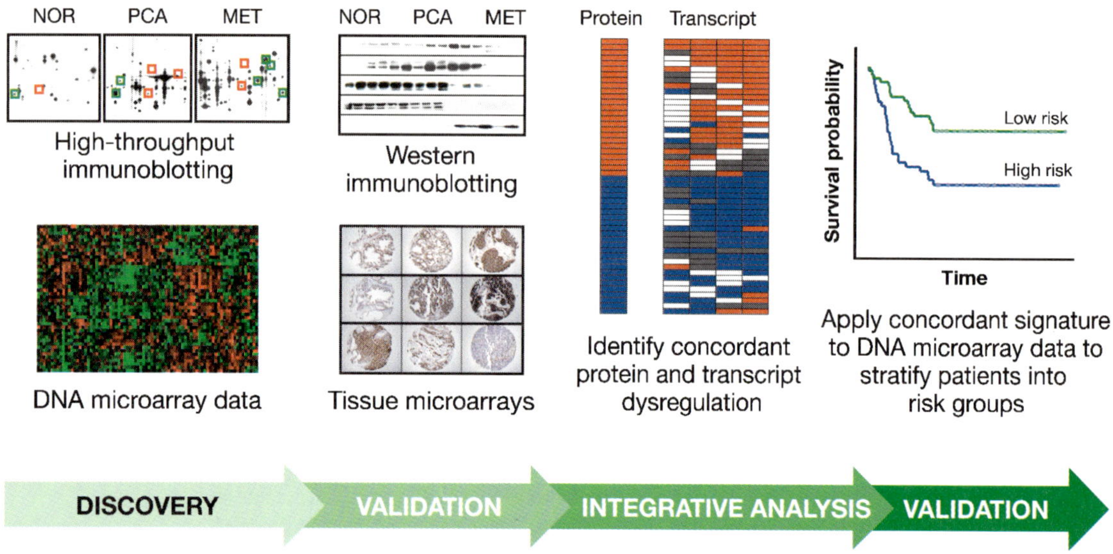

Figure 8

Schema of an integrative transcriptome and proteome analysis of prostate cancer (PCA). Steps in an integrative analysis combining high-throughput proteome and expression data to characterize PCA progression are presented. Varambally and colleagues (138a) used high-throughput immunoblotting to interrogate protein expression in benign prostate, localized PCA, and metastatic PCA tissue extracts. Proteins showing altered expression were validated using conventional immunoblotting and tissue microarrays. Protein-expression changes were then compared with transcript data from eight PCA profiling studies. The authors identified a signature of concordant transcript and protein changes between localized and metastatic PCA. This signature was able to identify localized tumors at increased risk for prostate-specific antigen (PSA) recurrence after surgical resection. NOR, normal prostate tissue; MET, metastatic disease.

proteome. Unfortunately, the problems inherent in comparing DNA microarray studies (differences in experimental conditions, platforms, and output formats) expand when attempting to integrate data from these different fields (138). In an attempt to understand PCA progression, Varambally and colleagues (138a) have recently conducted an integrative transcriptomic and proteomic analysis, as outlined in **Figure 8**. Using high-throughput immunoblotting employing antibodies against more than 1,300 proteins or post-translational modifications, the authors interrogated benign prostate and localized PCA and metastatic PCA tissue extracts. Sixty-four proteins were altered in localized PCA compared with benign tissue, and 156 additional proteins were dysregulated between localized and metastatic PCA. Candidate progression markers were then evaluated using conventional Western blotting and tissue microarrays. Finally, to combine these proteomic alterations with the wealth of PCA expression data, the authors performed an integrative analysis with eight PCA profiling studies. Interestingly, this analysis demonstrated only 60% concordance between transcript and protein levels. Most importantly, differential proteomic alterations between localized and metastatic PCA that were concordant with expression data served as predictors of clinical outcome in PCA. Thus, in addition to serving as attractive biomarker candidates, these genes and their encoded proteins may represent important candidates for understanding the clinical heterogeneity of PCA and disease progression.

CONCLUSIONS

Classical genetic techniques have identified several candidate genes involved in the pathogenesis of PCA, however a clear picture of PCA development has not emerged. As described in this review, high-throughput techniques have expanded our knowledge of the function of these genes, as well as identified thousands of other candidate genes, few of which have demonstrated a functional role in PCA development. To identify the most promising candidates from the wealth of genomic, transcriptomic, and proteomic data being generated, integrative methods must be developed. Clinical, histological, and genetic observations reveal PCA to be a heterogeneous disease. Future work should be able to identify whether the development and progression of PCA has a single underlying series of genetic events or whether PCA is really a group of genetically distinct subtypes that cannot be distinguished at the histological level. The development of high-throughput techniques and the careful integration of the data they produce should help to answer the unsolved etiology of PCA.

SUMMARY POINTS

1. PCA is a histologically, clinically, and genetically heterogeneous disease whose etiology is largely unknown.
2. Several lines of evidence point to the involvement of inflammation in the pathogenesis of PCA, including the loss of GSTP1 expression through promoter hypermethylation.
3. Classical genetic techniques have identified several genes in chromosomal regions that are frequently gained or lost in PCA, including *PTEN*, *NKX3.1*, and *Myc*. Subsequent experiments confirmed a functional role for these genes in PCA development and progression.
4. The transition to androgen independence is a crucial step in PCA progression, and recent evidence suggests that this transition is often controlled by modulation of the AR.
5. The SHH pathway is important for prostatic epithelial regeneration and the pathogenesis of advanced PCA, which supports the concept that prostate stem cells may drive PCA pathogenesis.
6. DNA microarrays have been used extensively to characterize the PCA transcriptome. *HPN*, *AMACR*, and *EZH2* are consistently dysregulated in multiple studies and may have functional roles in PCA progression. Fusion of *TMPRSS2* with *ETS* family members occurs in the majority of PCA and likely contributes to PCA pathogenesis.
7. High-throughput genomic, transcriptomic, and proteomic techniques are identifying thousands of candidates that are dysregulated in PCA progression, a small subset of which are involved mechanistically. Integrative approaches are needed to identify the most promising candidate genes.

UNRESOLVED ISSUES/FUTURE DIRECTIONS

1. The molecular characterization of PCA progression has yet to be accomplished. Distinguishing aggressive from indolent forms of PCA would have significant clinical implications, as it is estimated that nearly 20 men need to be treated to prevent one PCA-specific death.
2. High-throughput techniques demonstrate that the heterogeneity of PCA is reflected at the molecular level. Genomic and proteomic experiments demonstrate that tumors with expression and proteomic patterns similar to metastatic cancer are more likely to recur after prostatectomy. Presently it is unclear if tumors express these features at the earliest stages of carcinogenesis or if they develop them during PCA progression through a series of defined events. Being able to prospectively identify which tumors will demonstrate aggressive behavior at the PIN or early PCA stage will be crucial for treatment decisions.
3. Several lines of evidence suggest that chronic inflammation plays a role in PCA pathogenesis, possibly through SHH signaling in cancer stem cells. However, specific questions remain. Does PIA precede PIN or PCA in all cases? Can cells that exhibit stem cell–like behavior be identified and isolated from primary tumors? Does inflammation lead to expansion of these cells? Could the existence of cancer stem cells be the reason for the clinical response to androgen-ablation therapy?
4. Most DNA microarray studies have focused on identifying the genes that are differentially expressed most consistently between benign prostate and PCA. However, PCA consistently displays heterogeneity, which suggests that specific genetic events may drive subsets of PCA. The importance of *HER2/ERBB2* amplification in breast cancer, *EGFR* mutations in lung cancer, and *BCR-ABL* fusion in chronic myelogenous leukemia demonstrate the importance of identifying these subsets for understanding pathogenesis and identifying therapeutic targets in other cancers. Do *TMPRSS2:ETS* family member fusions define similar subsets in PCA? Do other subsets exist in PCA and can high-throughput studies identify them?

ACKNOWLEDGMENTS

We would like to thank Rohit Mehra for selecting the histopathology images used in **Figure 1**, as well as Jianjun Yu for carrying out the meta-analysis displayed in **Figure 2**. This work was supported by grants from the American Cancer Society (grant number RSG-02-179-01-MGO), the National Institutes of Health (grant numbers EDRN UO1 CA111275, R01 CA07063, RO1 AG0214104, and the University of Michigan Prostate SPORE P50 CA69568), and the Department of Defense (grant number PC020322). S.A.T. is a fellow of the Medical Scientist Training Program. A.M.C. is a Pew Biomedical Scholar.

LITERATURE CITED

1. Sakr WA, Ward C, Grignon DJ, Haas GP. 2000. Epidemiology and molecular biology of early prostatic neoplasia. *Mol. Urol.* 4:109–13

2. Rubin MA, De Marzo AM. 2004. Molecular genetics of human prostate cancer. *Mod. Pathol.* 17:380–88
3. Franks LM. 1954. Atrophy and hyperplasia in the prostate proper. *J. Pathol. Bacteriol.* 68:617–21
4. **De Marzo AM, Marchi VL, Epstein JI, Nelson WG. 1999. Proliferative inflammatory atrophy of the prostate: implications for prostatic carcinogenesis. *Am. J. Pathol.* 155:1985–92**
5. Nelson WG, De Marzo AM, Isaacs WB. 2003. Prostate cancer. *N. Engl. J. Med.* 349:366–81
6. Smith CJ, Gardner WA Jr. 1987. Inflammation-proliferation: possible relationships in the prostate. *Prog. Clin. Biol. Res.* 239:317–25
7. Gleason DF, Mellinger GT. 1974. Prediction of prognosis for prostatic adenocarcinoma by combined histological grading and clinical staging. *J. Urol.* 111:58–64
8. Nakayama M, Gonzalgo ML, Yegnasubramanian S, Lin X, De Marzo AM, Nelson WG. 2004. GSTP1 CpG island hypermethylation as a molecular biomarker for prostate cancer. *J. Cell. Biol.* 91:540–52
9. Lee WH, Morton RA, Epstein JI, Brooks JD, Campbell PA, et al. 1994. Cytidine methylation of regulatory sequences near the pi-class glutathione S-transferase gene accompanies human prostatic carcinogenesis. *Proc. Natl. Acad. Sci. USA* 91:11733–37
10. Lin X, Tascilar M, Lee WH, Vles WJ, Lee BH, et al. 2001. GSTP1 CpG island hypermethylation is responsible for the absence of GSTP1 expression in human prostate cancer cells. *Am. J. Pathol.* 159:1815–26
11. Nakayama M, Bennett CJ, Hicks JL, Epstein JI, Platz EA, et al. 2003. Hypermethylation of the human glutathione S-transferase-pi gene (GSTP1) CpG island is present in a subset of proliferative inflammatory atrophy lesions but not in normal or hyperplastic epithelium of the prostate: a detailed study using laser-capture microdissection. *Am. J. Pathol.* 163:923–33
12. Nelson CP, Kidd LC, Sauvageot J, Isaacs WB, De Marzo AM, et al. 2001. Protection against 2-hydroxyamino-1-methyl-6-phenylimidazo[4,5-b]pyridine cytotoxicity and DNA adduct formation in human prostate by glutathione S-transferase P1. *Cancer Res.* 61:103–9
13. Steck PA, Pershouse MA, Jasser SA, Yung WK, Lin H, et al. 1997. Identification of a candidate tumour suppressor gene, MMAC1, at chromosome 10q23.3 that is mutated in multiple advanced cancers. *Nat. Genet.* 15:356–62
14. Li DM, Sun H. 1997. TEP1, encoded by a candidate tumor suppressor locus, is a novel protein tyrosine phosphatase regulated by transforming growth factor beta. *Cancer Res.* 57:2124–29
15. Li J, Yen C, Liaw D, Podsypanina K, Bose S, et al. 1997. PTEN, a putative protein tyrosine phosphatase gene mutated in human brain, breast, and prostate cancer. *Science* 275:1943–47
16. Marsh DJ, Dahia PL, Zheng Z, Liaw D, Parsons R, et al. 1997. Germline mutations in PTEN are present in Bannayan-Zonana syndrome. *Nat. Genet.* 16:333–34
17. Liaw D, Marsh DJ, Li J, Dahia PL, Wang SI, et al. 1997. Germline mutations of the PTEN gene in Cowden disease, an inherited breast and thyroid cancer syndrome. *Nat. Genet.* 16:64–67

Characterizes PIA at the molecular level and proposes it as a candidate lesion for PIN and/or PCA.

18. Sansal I, Sellers WR. 2004. The biology and clinical relevance of the PTEN tumor suppressor pathway. *J. Clin. Oncol.* 22:2954–63
19. Suzuki H, Freije D, Nusskern DR, Okami K, Cairns P, et al. 1998. Interfocal heterogeneity of PTEN/MMAC1 gene alterations in multiple metastatic prostate cancer tissues. *Cancer Res.* 58:204–9
20. McMenamin ME, Soung P, Perera S, Kaplan I, Loda M, Sellers WR. 1999. Loss of PTEN expression in paraffin-embedded primary prostate cancer correlates with high Gleason score and advanced stage. *Cancer Res.* 59:4291–96
21. Di Cristofano A, Pesce B, Cordon-Cardo C, Pandolfi PP. 1998. Pten is essential for embryonic development and tumour suppression. *Nat. Genet.* 19:348–55
22. Podsypanina K, Ellenson LH, Nemes A, Gu J, Tamura M, et al. 1999. Mutation of Pten/Mmac1 in mice causes neoplasia in multiple organ systems. *Proc. Natl. Acad. Sci. USA* 96:1563–68
23. Suzuki A, de la Pompa JL, Stambolic V, Elia AJ, Sasaki T, et al. 1998. High cancer susceptibility and embryonic lethality associated with mutation of the PTEN tumor suppressor gene in mice. *Curr. Biol.* 8:1169–78
24. Kim MJ, Cardiff RD, Desai N, Banach-Petrosky WA, Parsons R, et al. 2002. Cooperativity of Nkx3.1 and Pten loss of function in a mouse model of prostate carcinogenesis. *Proc. Natl. Acad. Sci. USA* 99:2884–89
25. Abate-Shen C, Banach-Petrosky WA, Sun X, Economides KD, Desai N, et al. 2003. Nkx3.1; Pten mutant mice develop invasive prostate adenocarcinoma and lymph node metastases. *Cancer Res.* 63:3886–90
26. Kwabi-Addo B, Giri D, Schmidt K, Podsypanina K, Parsons R, et al. 2001. Haploinsufficiency of the Pten tumor suppressor gene promotes prostate cancer progression. *Proc. Natl. Acad. Sci. USA* 98:11563–68
27. Gao H, Ouyang X, Banach-Petrosky W, Borowsky AD, Lin Y, et al. 2004. A critical role for p27kip1 gene dosage in a mouse model of prostate carcinogenesis. *Proc. Natl. Acad. Sci. USA* 101:17204–9
28. Di Cristofano A, De Acetis M, Koff A, Cordon-Cardo C, Pandolfi PP. 2001. Pten and p27KIP1 cooperate in prostate cancer tumor suppression in the mouse. *Nat. Genet.* 27:222–24
29. Backman SA, Ghazarian D, So K, Sanchez O, Wagner KU, et al. 2004. Early onset of neoplasia in the prostate and skin of mice with tissue-specific deletion of Pten. *Proc. Natl. Acad. Sci. USA* 101:1725–30
30. Wang S, Gao J, Lei Q, Rozengurt N, Pritchard C, et al. 2003. Prostate-specific deletion of the murine Pten tumor suppressor gene leads to metastatic prostate cancer. *Cancer Cell* 4:209–21
31. Trotman LC, Niki M, Dotan ZA, Koutcher JA, Di Cristofano A, et al. 2003. Pten dose dictates cancer progression in the prostate. *PLoS Biol.* 1:E59
32. Majumder PK, Yeh JJ, George DJ, Febbo PG, Kum J, et al. 2003. Prostate intraepithelial neoplasia induced by prostate restricted Akt activation: the MPAKT model. *Proc. Natl. Acad. Sci. USA* 100:7841–46
33. Majumder PK, Febbo PG, Bikoff R, Berger R, Xue Q, et al. 2004. mTOR inhibition reverses Akt-dependent prostate intraepithelial neoplasia through regulation of apoptotic and HIF-1-dependent pathways. *Nat. Med.* 10:594–601
34. Davies MA, Kim SJ, Parikh NU, Dong Z, Bucana CD, Gallick GE. 2002. Adenoviral-mediated expression of MMAC/PTEN inhibits proliferation and metastasis of human prostate cancer cells. *Clin. Cancer Res.* 8:1904–14

35. Bandyopadhyay S, Pai SK, Hirota S, Hosobe S, Tsukada T, et al. 2004. PTEN up-regulates the tumor metastasis suppressor gene Drg-1 in prostate and breast cancer. *Cancer Res.* 64:7655–60
36. Freedland SJ, Seligson DB, Liu AY, Pantuck AJ, Paik SH, et al. 2003. Loss of CD10 (neutral endopeptidase) is a frequent and early event in human prostate cancer. *Prostate* 55:71–80
37. Sumitomo M, Iwase A, Zheng R, Navarro D, Kaminetzky D, et al. 2004. Synergy in tumor suppression by direct interaction of neutral endopeptidase with PTEN. *Cancer Cell* 5:67–78
38. Vocke CD, Pozzatti RO, Bostwick DG, Florence CD, Jennings SB, et al. 1996. Analysis of 99 microdissected prostate carcinomas reveals a high frequency of allelic loss on chromosome 8p12–21. *Cancer Res.* 56:2411–16
39. Emmert-Buck MR, Vocke CD, Pozzatti RO, Duray PH, Jennings SB, et al. 1995. Allelic loss on chromosome 8p12–21 in microdissected prostatic intraepithelial neoplasia. *Cancer Res.* 55:2959–62
40. He WW, Sciavolino PJ, Wing J, Augustus M, Hudson P, et al. 1997. A novel human prostate-specific, androgen-regulated homeobox gene (NKX3.1) that maps to 8p21, a region frequently deleted in prostate cancer. *Genomics* 43:69–77
41. Bhatia-Gaur R, Donjacour AA, Sciavolino PJ, Kim M, Desai N, et al. 1999. Roles for Nkx3.1 in prostate development and cancer. *Genes Dev.* 13:966–77
42. Chen H, Nandi AK, Li X, Bieberich CJ. 2002. NKX-3.1 interacts with prostate-derived Ets factor and regulates the activity of the PSA promoter. *Cancer Res.* 62:338–40
43. Abdulkadir SA, Magee JA, Peters TJ, Kaleem Z, Naughton CK, et al. 2002. Conditional loss of Nkx3.1 in adult mice induces prostatic intraepithelial neoplasia. *Mol. Cell. Biol.* 22:1495–503
44. Kim MJ, Bhatia-Gaur R, Banach-Petrosky WA, Desai N, Wang Y, et al. 2002. Nkx3.1 mutant mice recapitulate early stages of prostate carcinogenesis. *Cancer Res.* 62:2999–3004
45. Voeller HJ, Augustus M, Madike V, Bova GS, Carter KC, Gelmann EP. 1997. Coding region of NKX3.1, a prostate-specific homeobox gene on 8p21, is not mutated in human prostate cancers. *Cancer Res.* 57:4455–59
46. Bowen C, Bubendorf L, Voeller HJ, Slack R, Willi N, et al. 2000. Loss of NKX3.1 expression in human prostate cancers correlates with tumor progression. *Cancer Res.* 60:6111–15
47. Korkmaz CG, Korkmaz KS, Manola J, Xi Z, Risberg B, et al. 2004. Analysis of androgen regulated homeobox gene NKX3.1 during prostate carcinogenesis. *J. Urol.* 172:1134–39
48. Asatiani E, Huang WX, Wang A, Rodriguez Ortner E, Cavalli LR, et al. 2005. Deletion, methylation, and expression of the NKX3.1 suppressor gene in primary human prostate cancer. *Cancer Res.* 65:1164–73
49. Magee JA, Abdulkadir SA, Milbrandt J. 2003. Haploinsufficiency at the Nkx3.1 locus. A paradigm for stochastic, dosage-sensitive gene regulation during tumor initiation. *Cancer Cell* 3:273–83

Uses DNA microarrays elegantly to characterize the mechanism of NKX3.1 as a haploinsufficient tumor suppressor.

50. Koivisto P, Kolmer M, Visakorpi T, Kallioniemi OP. 1998. Androgen receptor gene and hormonal therapy failure of prostate cancer. *Am. J. Pathol.* 152:1–9
51. Feldman BJ, Feldman D. 2001. The development of androgen-independent prostate cancer. *Nat. Rev. Cancer* 1:34–45

52. Koivisto P, Kononen J, Palmberg C, Tammela T, Hyytinen E, et al. 1997. Androgen receptor gene amplification: a possible molecular mechanism for androgen deprivation therapy failure in prostate cancer. *Cancer Res.* 57:314–19
53. Linja MJ, Savinainen KJ, Saramaki OR, Tammela TL, Vessella RL, Visakorpi T. 2001. Amplification and overexpression of androgen receptor gene in hormone-refractory prostate cancer. *Cancer Res.* 61:3550–55
54. Latil A, Bieche I, Vidaud D, Lidereau R, Berthon P, et al. 2001. Evaluation of androgen, estrogen (ER alpha and ER beta), and progesterone receptor expression in human prostate cancer by real-time quantitative reverse transcription-polymerase chain reaction assays. *Cancer Res.* 61:1919–26
55. Linja MJ, Visakorpi T. 2004. Alterations of androgen receptor in prostate cancer. *J. Steroid Biochem. Mol. Biol.* 92:255–64
56. Han G, Buchanan G, Ittmann M, Harris JM, Yu X, et al. 2005. Mutation of the androgen receptor causes oncogenic transformation of the prostate. *Proc. Natl. Acad. Sci. USA* 102:1151–56
57. **Chen CD, Welsbie DS, Tran C, Baek SH, Chen R, et al. 2004. Molecular determinants of resistance to antiandrogen therapy. *Nat. Med.* 10:33–39**

A two- to fivefold increase in the AR is necessary and sufficient to confer androgen independence in a xenograft PCA model.

58. Sakr WA, Partin AW. 2001. Histological markers of risk and the role of high-grade prostatic intraepithelial neoplasia. *Urology* 57:115–20
59. Wang R, Xu J, Saramaki O, Visakorpi T, Sutherland WM, et al. 2004. PrLZ, a novel prostate-specific and androgen-responsive gene of the TPD52 family, amplified in chromosome 8q21.1 and overexpressed in human prostate cancer. *Cancer Res.* 64:1589–94
60. Rubin MA, Varambally S, Beroukhim R, Tomlins SA, Rhodes DR, et al. 2004. Overexpression, amplification, and androgen regulation of TPD52 in prostate cancer. *Cancer Res.* 64:3814–22
61. Saramaki O, Willi N, Bratt O, Gasser TC, Koivisto P, et al. 2001. Amplification of EIF3S3 gene is associated with advanced stage in prostate cancer. *Am. J. Pathol.* 159:2089–94
62. Edwards J, Krishna NS, Witton CJ, Bartlett JM. 2003. Gene amplifications associated with the development of hormone-resistant prostate cancer. *Clin. Cancer Res.* 9:5271–81
63. Nupponen NN, Kakkola L, Koivisto P, Visakorpi T. 1998. Genetic alterations in hormone-refractory recurrent prostate carcinomas. *Am. J. Pathol.* 153:141–48
64. Visakorpi T, Kallioniemi AH, Syvanen AC, Hyytinen ER, Karhu R, et al. 1995. Genetic changes in primary and recurrent prostate cancer by comparative genomic hybridization. *Cancer Res.* 55:342–47
65. Bernard D, Pourtier-Manzanedo A, Gil J, Beach DH. 2003. Myc confers androgen-independent prostate cancer cell growth. *J. Clin. Invest.* 112:1724–31
66. Zhang X, Lee C, Ng PY, Rubin M, Shabsigh A, Buttyan R. 2000. Prostatic neoplasia in transgenic mice with prostate-directed overexpression of the c-myc oncoprotein. *Prostate* 43:278–85
67. **Ellwood-Yen K, Graeber TG, Wongvipat J, Iruela-Arispe ML, Zhang J, et al. 2003. Myc-driven murine prostate cancer shares molecular features with human prostate tumors. *Cancer Cell* 4:223–38**

Demonstrates how DNA microarrays can be used to compare mouse PCA models to human prostate tumors.

68. van Lohuizen M, Verbeek S, Krimpenfort P, Domen J, Saris C, et al. 1989. Predisposition to lymphomagenesis in pim-1 transgenic mice: cooperation with c-myc and N-myc in murine leukemia virus-induced tumors. *Cell* 56:673–82

69. Rhodes DR, Sanda MG, Otte AP, Chinnaiyan AM, Rubin MA. 2003. Multiplex biomarker approach for determining risk of prostate-specific antigen-defined recurrence of prostate cancer. *J. Natl. Cancer Inst.* 95:661–68
70. Dhanasekaran SM, Barrette TR, Ghosh D, Shah R, Varambally S, et al. 2001. Delineation of prognostic biomarkers in prostate cancer. *Nature* 412:822–26
71. Taipale J, Beachy PA. 2001. The Hedgehog and Wnt signalling pathways in cancer. *Nature* 411:349–54
72. Walterhouse DO, Lamm ML, Villavicencio E, Iannaccone PM. 2003. Emerging roles for hedgehog-patched-Gli signal transduction in reproduction. *Biol. Reprod.* 69:8–14
73. Sanchez P, Hernandez AM, Stecca B, Kahler AJ, DeGueme AM, et al. 2004. Inhibition of prostate cancer proliferation by interference with SONIC HEDGEHOG-GLI1 signaling. *Proc. Natl. Acad. Sci. USA* 101:12561–66
74. Fan L, Pepicelli CV, Dibble CC, Catbagan W, Zarycki JL, et al. 2004. Hedgehog signaling promotes prostate xenograft tumor growth. *Endocrinology* 145:3961–70
75. Karhadkar SS, Bova GS, Abdallah N, Dhara S, Gardner D, et al. 2004. Hedgehog signalling in prostate regeneration, neoplasia and metastasis. *Nature* 431:707–12
76. Sheng T, Li C, Zhang X, Chi S, He N, et al. 2004. Activation of the hedgehog pathway in advanced prostate cancer. *Mol. Cancer* 3:29
77. Isaacs JT. 1999. The biology of hormone refractory prostate cancer. Why does it develop? *Urol. Clin. N. Am.* 26:263–73
78. Beachy PA, Karhadkar SS, Berman DM. 2004. Tissue repair and stem cell renewal in carcinogenesis. *Nature* 432:324–31
79. Pardal R, Clarke MF, Morrison SJ. 2003. Applying the principles of stem-cell biology to cancer. *Nat. Rev. Cancer* 3:895–902
80. Hudson DL. 2004. Epithelial stem cells in human prostate growth and disease. *Prostate Cancer Prostatic Dis.* 7:188–94
80a. Tomlins SA, Rhodes DR, Perner S, Dhanasekaran SM, Mehra R, et al. 2005. Recurrent fusion of TMPRSS2 and ETS transcription factor genes in prostate cancer. *Science* 310:644–48
81. Yu YP, Landsittel D, Jing L, Nelson J, Ren BG, et al. 2004. Gene expression alterations in prostate cancer predicting tumor aggression and preceding development of malignancy. *J. Clin. Oncol.* 22:2790–99
82. Glinsky GV, Glinskii AB, Stephenson AJ, Hoffman RM, Gerald WL. 2004. Gene expression profiling predicts clinical outcome of prostate cancer. *J. Clin. Invest.* 113:913–23
83. Lapointe J, Li C, Higgins JP, van de Rijn M, Bair E, et al. 2004. Gene expression profiling identifies clinically relevant subtypes of prostate cancer. *Proc. Natl. Acad. Sci. USA* 101:811–16
84. Singh D, Febbo PG, Ross K, Jackson DG, Manola J, et al. 2002. Gene expression correlates of clinical prostate cancer behavior. *Cancer Cell* 1:203–9
85. Rhodes DR, Barrette TR, Rubin MA, Ghosh D, Chinnaiyan AM. 2002. Meta-analysis of microarrays: interstudy validation of gene expression profiles reveals pathway dysregulation in prostate cancer. *Cancer Res.* 62:4427–33

Demonstrates how DNA microarray data from various platforms and bio-informatic techniques can be integrated to identify candidate genes involved in PCA pathogenesis.

86. Stephan C, Yousef GM, Scorilas A, Jung K, Jung M, et al. 2004. Hepsin is highly over expressed in and a new candidate for a prognostic indicator in prostate cancer. *J. Urol.* 171:187–91
87. Chen Z, Fan Z, McNeal JE, Nolley R, Caldwell MC, et al. 2003. Hepsin and maspin are inversely expressed in laser capture microdissectioned prostate cancer. *J. Urol.* 169:1316–19

88. Srikantan V, Valladares M, Rhim JS, Moul JW, Srivastava S. 2002. HEPSIN inhibits cell growth/invasion in prostate cancer cells. *Cancer Res.* 62:6812–16
89. Klezovitch O, Chevillet J, Mirosevich J, Roberts RL, Matusik RJ, Vasioukhin V. 2004. Hepsin promotes prostate cancer progression and metastasis. *Cancer Cell* 6:185–95
90. Rubin MA, Zhou M, Dhanasekaran SM, Varambally S, Barrette TR, et al. 2002. alpha-Methylacyl coenzyme A racemase as a tissue biomarker for prostate cancer. *JAMA* 287:1662–70
91. Luo J, Zha S, Gage WR, Dunn TA, Hicks JL, et al. 2002. Alpha-methylacyl-CoA racemase: a new molecular marker for prostate cancer. *Cancer Res.* 62:2220–26
92. Jiang Z, Woda BA, Rock KL, Xu Y, Savas L, et al. 2001. P504S: a new molecular marker for the detection of prostate carcinoma. *Am. J. Surg. Pathol.* 25:1397–404
93. Wu CL, Yang XJ, Tretiakova M, Patton KT, Halpern EF, et al. 2004. Analysis of alpha-methylacyl-CoA racemase (P504S) expression in high-grade prostatic intraepithelial neoplasia. *Hum. Pathol.* 35:1008–13
94. Sreekumar A, Laxman B, Rhodes DR, Bhagavathula S, Harwood J, et al. 2004. Humoral immune response to alpha-methylacyl-CoA racemase and prostate cancer. *J. Natl. Cancer Inst.* 96:834–43
95. Rogers CG, Yan G, Zha S, Gonzalgo ML, Isaacs WB, et al. 2004. Prostate cancer detection on urinalysis for alpha methylacyl coenzyme a racemase protein. *J. Urol.* 172:1501–3
96. Zielie PJ, Mobley JA, Ebb RG, Jiang Z, Blute RD, Ho SM. 2004. A novel diagnostic test for prostate cancer emerges from the determination of alpha-methylacyl-coenzyme a racemase in prostatic secretions. *J. Urol.* 172:1130–33
97. Xu JF, Thornburg T, Turner AR, Vitolins M, Case D, et al. 2005. Serum levels of phytanic acid are associated with prostate cancer risk. *Prostate* 63:209–14
98. Mobley JA, Leav I, Zielie P, Wotkowitz C, Evans J, et al. 2003. Branched fatty acids in dairy and beef products markedly enhance alpha-methylacyl-CoA racemase expression in prostate cancer cells in vitro. *Cancer Epidemiol. Biomark. Prev.* 12:775–83
99. Zha S, Ferdinandusse S, Hicks JL, Denis S, Dunn TA, et al. 2004. Peroxisomal branched chain fatty acid beta-oxidation pathway is upregulated in prostate cancer. *Prostate* 63:316–23
100. Baron A, Migita T, Tang D, Loda M. 2004. Fatty acid synthase: a metabolic oncogene in prostate cancer? *J. Cell. Biol.* 91:47–53
101. Moore S, Knudsen B, True LD, Hawley S, Etzioni R, et al. 2005. Loss of stearoyl-CoA desaturase expression is a frequent event in prostate carcinoma. *Int. J. Cancer* 114:563–71
102. Wiklund F, Gillanders EM, Albertus JA, Bergh A, Damber JE, et al. 2003. Genome-wide scan of Swedish families with hereditary prostate cancer: suggestive evidence of linkage at 5q11.2 and 19p13.3. *Prostate* 57:290–97
103. Hsieh CL, Oakley-Girvan I, Balise RR, Halpern J, Gallagher RP, et al. 2001. A genome screen of families with multiple cases of prostate cancer: evidence of genetic heterogeneity. *Am. J. Hum. Genet.* 69:148–58
104. Zheng SL, Chang BL, Faith DA, Johnson JR, Isaacs SD, et al. 2002. Sequence variants of alpha-methylacyl-CoA racemase are associated with prostate cancer risk. *Cancer Res.* 62:6485–88
105. Zha S, Ferdinandusse S, Denis S, Wanders RJ, Ewing CM, et al. 2003. Alpha-methylacyl-CoA racemase as an androgen-independent growth modifier in prostate cancer. *Cancer Res.* 63:7365–76

106. LaTulippe E, Satagopan J, Smith A, Scher H, Scardino P, et al. 2002. Comprehensive gene expression analysis of prostate cancer reveals distinct transcriptional programs associated with metastatic disease. *Cancer Res.* 62:4499–506

107. Varambally S, Dhanasekaran SM, Zhou M, Barrette TR, Kumar-Sinha C, et al. 2002. The polycomb group protein EZH2 is involved in progression of prostate cancer. *Nature* 419:624–29

108. Bracken AP, Pasini D, Capra M, Prosperini E, Colli E, Helin K. 2003. EZH2 is downstream of the pRB-E2F pathway, essential for proliferation and amplified in cancer. *EMBO J.* 22:5323–35

109. Kuzmichev A, Margueron R, Vaquero A, Preissner TS, Scher M, et al. 2005. Composition and histone substrates of polycomb repressive group complexes change during cellular differentiation. *Proc. Natl. Acad. Sci. USA* 102:1859–64

110. Tang X, Milyavsky M, Shats I, Erez N, Goldfinger N, Rotter V. 2004. Activated p53 suppresses the histone methyltransferase EZH2 gene. *Oncogene* 23:5759–69

111. Attwooll C, Oddi S, Cartwright P, Prosperini E, Agger K, et al. 2005. A novel repressive E2F6 complex containing the polycomb group protein, EPC1, that interacts with EZH2 in a proliferation-specific manner. *J. Biol. Chem.* 280:1199–208

112. Tonini T, Bagella L, D'Andrilli G, Claudio PP, Giordano A. 2004. Ezh2 reduces the ability of HDAC1-dependent pRb2/p130 transcriptional repression of cyclin A. *Oncogene* 23:4930–37

113. Raaphorst FM, Meijer CJ, Fieret E, Blokzijl T, Mommers E, et al. 2003. Poorly differentiated breast carcinoma is associated with increased expression of the human polycomb group EZH2 gene. *Neoplasia* 5:481–88

114. Kleer CG, Cao Q, Varambally S, Shen R, Ota I, et al. 2003. EZH2 is a marker of aggressive breast cancer and promotes neoplastic transformation of breast epithelial cells. *Proc. Natl. Acad. Sci. USA* 100:11606–11

114a. Valk PJ, Verhaak RG, Beijen MA, Erpelinck CA, Barjesteh van Waalwijk van Doorn-Khosrovani S, et al. 2004. Prognostically useful gene-expression profiles in acute myeloid leukemia. *N. Engl. J. Med.* 350:1617–28

115. Rhodes DR, Chinnaiyan AM. 2004. Bioinformatics strategies for translating genome-wide expression analyses into clinically useful cancer markers. *Ann. NY Acad. Sci.* 1020:32–40

116. Ghosh D, Barette TR, Rhodes D, Chinnaiyan AM. 2003. Statistical issues and methods for meta-analysis of microarray data: a case study in prostate cancer. *Funct. Integr. Genomics* 3:180–88

117. Rhodes DR, Yu JJ, Shanker K, Deshpande N, Varambally R, et al. 2004. ONCOMINE: a cancer microarray database and integrated data-mining platform. *Neoplasia* 6:1–6

118. Schipper RG, Romijn JC, Cuijpers VM, Verhofstad AA. 2003. Polyamines and prostatic cancer. *Biochem. Soc. Trans.* 31:375–80

118a. Luo J, Duggan DJ, Chen YD, Sauvageot J, Ewing CM, et al. 2001. Human prostate cancer and benign prostatic hyperplasia: molecular dissection by gene expression profiling. *Cancer Res.* 61:4683–88

118b. Welsh JB, Sapinoso LM, Su AI, Kern SG, Wang-Rodriguez J, et al. 2001. Analysis of gene expression identifies candidate markers and pharmacological targets in prostate cancer. *Cancer Res.* 61:5974–78

118c. Luo JH, Yu YP, Cieply K, Lin F, Deflavia P, et al. 2002. Gene expression analysis of prostate cancers. *Mol. Carcinog.* 33:25–35

Demonstrates the importance of EZH2 in PCA progression through control of proliferation and metastatic behavior.

119. Pinkel D, Segraves R, Sudar D, Clark S, Poole I, et al. 1998. High resolution analysis of DNA copy number variation using comparative genomic hybridization to microarrays. *Nat. Genet.* 20:207–11
120. Wang DG, Fan JB, Siao CJ, Berno A, Young P, et al. 1998. Large-scale identification, mapping, and genotyping of single-nucleotide polymorphisms in the human genome. *Science* 280:1077–82
121. Paris PL, Andaya A, Fridlyand J, Jain AN, Weinberg V, et al. 2004. Whole genome scanning identifies genotypes associated with recurrence and metastasis in prostate tumors. *Hum. Mol. Genet.* 13:1303–13
122. Lieberfarb ME, Lin M, Lechpammer M, Li C, Tanenbaum DM, et al. 2003. Genome-wide loss of heterozygosity analysis from laser capture microdissected prostate cancer using single nucleotide polymorphic allele (SNP) arrays and a novel bioinformatics platform dChipSNP. *Cancer Res.* 63:4781–85
123. Kononen J, Bubendorf L, Kallioniemi A, Barlund M, Schraml P, et al. 1998. Tissue microarrays for high-throughput molecular profiling of tumor specimens. *Nat. Med.* 4:844–47
124. Paweletz CP, Charboneau L, Bichsel VE, Simone NL, Chen T, et al. 2001. Reverse phase protein microarrays which capture disease progression show activation of pro-survival pathways at the cancer invasion front. *Oncogene* 20:1981–89
125. Wright ME, Han DK, Aebersold R. 2005. Mass spectrometry based expression profiling of clinical prostate cncer. *Mol. Cell Proteomics* 4:545–54
126. Semmes OJ, Feng Z, Adam BL, Banez LL, Bigbee WL, et al. 2005. Evaluation of serum protein profiling by surface-enhanced laser desorption/ionization time-of-flight mass spectrometry for the detection of prostate cancer: I. Assessment of platform reproducibility. *Clin. Chem.* 51:102–12
127. Ornstein DK, Rayford W, Fusaro VA, Conrads TP, Ross SJ, et al. 2004. Serum proteomic profiling can discriminate prostate cancer from benign prostates in men with total prostate specific antigen levels between 2.5 and 15.0 ng/ml. *J. Urol.* 172:1302–5
128. Martin DB, Gifford DR, Wright ME, Keller A, Yi E, et al. 2004. Quantitative proteomic analysis of proteins released by neoplastic prostate epithelium. *Cancer Res.* 64:347–55
129. Liu AY, Zhang H, Sorensen CM, Diamond DL. 2005. Analysis of prostate cancer by proteomics using tissue specimens. *J. Urol.* 173:73–78
130. Cheung PK, Woolcock B, Adomat H, Sutcliffe M, Bainbridge TC, et al. 2004. Protein profiling of microdissected prostate tissue links growth differentiation factor 15 to prostate carcinogenesis. *Cancer Res.* 64:5929–33
131. Yu YP, Paranjpe S, Nelson J, Finkelstein S, Ren B, et al. 2005. High throughput screening of methylation status of genes in prostate cancer using an oligonucleotide methylation array. *Carcinogenesis* 26:471–79
132. Costello JF, Fruhwald MC, Smiraglia DJ, Rush LJ, Robertson GP, et al. 2000. Aberrant CpG-island methylation has non-random and tumour-type-specific patterns. *Nat. Genet.* 24:132–38
133. Adorjan P, Distler J, Lipscher E, Model F, Muller J, et al. 2002. Tumour class prediction and discovery by microarray-based DNA methylation analysis. *Nucleic Acids Res.* 30: e21
134. Li LC, Carroll PR, Dahiya R. 2005. Epigenetic changes in prostate cancer: implication for diagnosis and treatment. *J. Natl. Cancer Inst.* 97:103–15
135. Zheng L, Liu J, Batalov S, Zhou D, Orth A, et al. 2004. An approach to genomewide screens of expressed small interfering RNAs in mammalian cells. *Proc. Natl. Acad. Sci. USA* 101:135–40

136. Paddison PJ, Silva JM, Conklin DS, Schlabach M, Li M, et al. 2004. A resource for large-scale RNA-interference-based screens in mammals. *Nature* 428:427–31
137. Berns K, Hijmans EM, Mullenders J, Brummelkamp TR, Velds A, et al. 2004. A large-scale RNAi screen in human cells identifies new components of the p53 pathway. *Nature* 428:431–37
138. Hood L, Heath JR, Phelps ME, Lin B. 2004. Systems biology and new technologies enable predictive and preventative medicine. *Science* 306:640–43
138a. Varambally S, Yu J, Laxman B, Rhodes DR, Mehra R, et al. 2005. Integrative genomic and proteomic analysis of prostate cancer reveals signatures of metastatic progression. *Cancer Cell* 8:393–406
139. Rossi S, Graner E, Febbo P, Weinstein L, Bhattacharya N, et al. 2003. Fatty acid synthase expression defines distinct molecular signatures in prostate cancer. *Mol. Cancer Res.* 1:707–15
140. Graner E, Tang D, Rossi S, Baron A, Migita T, et al. 2004. The isopeptidase USP2a regulates the stability of fatty acid synthase in prostate cancer. *Cancer Cell* 5:253–61
141. Shaffer DR, Viale A, Ishiwata R, Leversha M, Olgac S, et al. 2005. Evidence for a p27 tumor suppressive function independent of its role regulating cell proliferation in the prostate. *Proc. Natl. Acad. Sci. USA* 102:210–15
142. Freedland SJ, de Gregorio F, Sacoolidge JC, Elshimali YI, Csathy GS, et al. 2003. Predicting biochemical recurrence after radical prostatectomy for patients with organ-confined disease using p27 expression. *Urology* 61:1187–92
143. Ben-Izhak O, Lahav-Baratz S, Meretyk S, Ben-Eliezer S, Sabo E, et al. 2003. Inverse relationship between Skp2 ubiquitin ligase and the cyclin dependent kinase inhibitor p27Kip1 in prostate cancer. *J. Urol.* 170:241–45
144. Yang G, Ayala G, De Marzo A, Tian W, Frolov A, et al. 2002. Elevated Skp2 protein expression in human prostate cancer: association with loss of the cyclin-dependent kinase inhibitor p27 and PTEN and with reduced recurrence-free survival. *Clin. Cancer Res.* 8:3419–26
145. Osman I, Yee H, Taneja SS, Levinson B, Zeleniuch-Jacquotte A, et al. 2004. Neutral endopeptidase protein expression and prognosis in localized prostate cancer. *Clin. Cancer Res.* 10:4096–100

KSHV Infection and the Pathogenesis of Kaposi's Sarcoma

Don Ganem

Howard Hughes Medical Institute and Departments of Microbiology & Immunology and Medicine, University of California, San Francisco, San Francisco, California 94143; email: ganem@cgl.ucsf.edu

Annu. Rev. Pathol. Mech. Dis. 2006. 1:273–96

First published online as a Review in Advance on November 16, 2005

The *Annual Review of Pathology: Mechanisms of Disease* is online at pathmechdis.annualreviews.org

doi: 10.1146/annurev.pathol.1.110304.100133

1553-4006/06/0114-0273$20.00

Key Words

herpesviruses, Kaposi's sarcoma, human hepresvirus 8, latency

Abstract

Kaposi's sarcoma (KS) has long been suspected of having an infectious etiology on the basis of its unusual epidemiology, histopathology, and natural history. Nearly a decade ago, a novel herpesviral genome was discovered in KS biopsies, and since that time strong epidemiologic evidence has accumulated correlating infection with this KS-associated herpesvirus (KSHV, also known as human herpesvirus 8) with the development of the disease. Here we review the evidence linking KSHV infection to KS risk and discuss current notions of how KSHV gene expression promotes the development of this remarkable neoplasm. These studies show that both latent and lytic viral replicative cycles contribute significantly—but differently—to KS development. The studies also highlight mechanistic differences between oncogenesis caused by KSHV and that caused by its distant relative Epstein-Barr virus.

KAPOSI'S SARCOMA: AN OVERVIEW

Clinical KS. Kaposi's sarcoma (KS) is an unusual neoplasm first described by Kaposi in Eastern Europe in the nineteenth century (1), but later recognized to be endemic to the Mediterranean basin and Africa (2). This endemic or classical form of KS is typically an indolent disease, present most often in elderly males and usually affecting only the skin. In this form, it is rarely life-threatening. However, two other more aggressive clinical forms of KS are recognized—a lymphadenopathic variant seen in young children in the endemic zones and AIDS-related KS (3), occurring in immunodeficient subjects infected with HIV (a similar form exists among iatrogenically immunosuppressed transplant recipients). All forms share a common histology (see below), but the AIDS-related form is dramatically more aggressive; in addition to widespread and often disfiguring dermal involvement, there is frequent involvement of extracutaneous sites, most often of the lungs and gastrointestinal tract (3). In this form, there is extensive local edema, hemorrhage, and induration of the skin; gastrointestinal bleeding, abdominal pain, and respiratory failure are serious complications of visceral involvement. **Figure 1*a*** shows a typical dermal lesion from an AIDS-KS patient; **Figure 1*b*** shows a palatal KS lesion—a common site of involvement in the oral cavity. The reddish hue of the gross lesions is testament to their extensive angiogenesis, one of the signature features of KS.

Although the term sarcoma appears in its name, the clinical behavior and natural history of KS both suggest that analogies to classical forms of cancer are misplaced. KS lesions occur typically in a multifocal distribution rather than as solitary primary lesions followed later by metastases. Moreover, especially in the classical form of the disease, lesions do not usually display the relentless, inexorable progression that typifies many cancers. In classical KS, lesions often remain quiescent for long periods—indeed, spontaneous regression of KS lesions, though not particularly common, has been well documented. In forms of KS linked to immunosuppression, even partial restoration of immune competence leads to dramatic arrest and the gradual regression of many lesions. Not all cases of classical KS require chemotherapy, but such therapy is required more frequently to control AIDS KS.

Kaposi's sarcoma histology. Unlike most classical cancers, which arise from the clonal outgrowth of a single cell type, KS lesions are histologically complex (2, 4–9) (see **Figure 1*c***). The principal proliferating cell in advanced lesions is the so-called spindle cell, named for its dramatically elongated morphology; a high-power image of spindle cells is shown in **Figure 1*d***. Pathologists have argued about the origins of KS spindle cells for decades. Researchers have long thought that spindle cells are of endothelial lineage, and indeed they bear many endothelial markers, including CD31, CD34, CD36, factor XIII, En-4, and PAL-E (4–10). However, most spindle cells lack staining for factor VIII, a classical marker of differentiated vascular endothelium, and Weibel-Palade bodies are absent ultrastructurally. Confusion has been compounded by the finding that KS spindle cells display significant heterogeneity in marker expression. For example, a small number of cells in some biopsies do stain for factor VIII, whereas other cells stain for smooth muscle α-actin (4–6, 10), leading some researchers to speculate that spindle cells may arise from bipotential mesenchymal precursors of vascular cells. Another view, propounded initially by Beckstead et al. (19), is that the cells arise from lymphatic endothelium, a notion that has been encouraged further by the observation that clinical KS virtually never arises in tissues that lack lymphatics (e.g., the central nervous system) (2). Moreover, recently discovered molecular markers of lymphatic endothelium (VEGF-C, VEGF-R3, podoplanin, and LYVE-1) are also

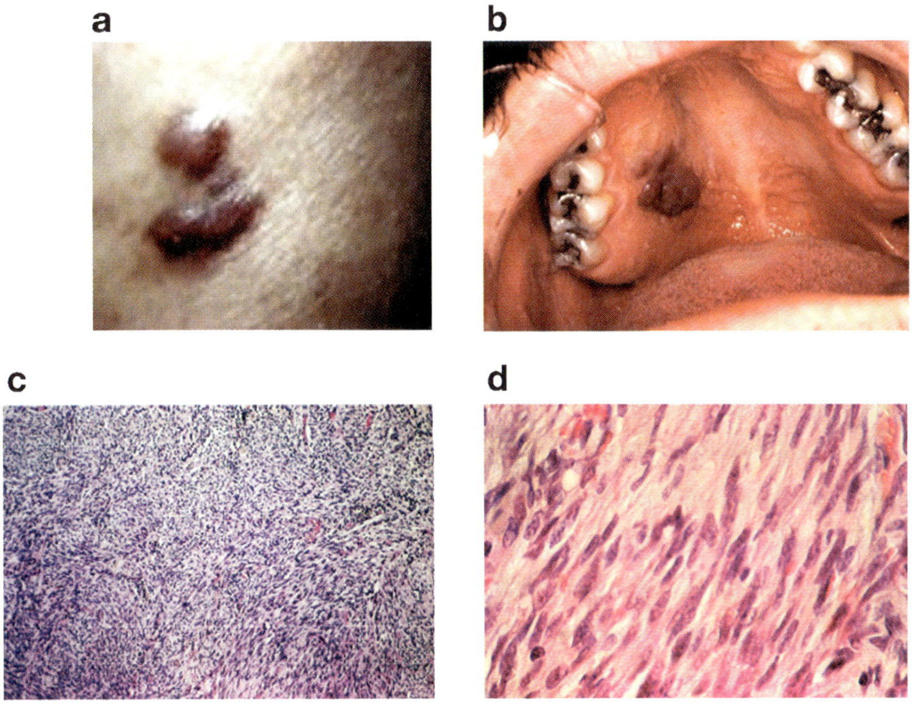

Figure 1

Kaposi's sarcoma (KS) lesions and their histopathology. (*a*) Cutaneous lesion of KS of an AIDS patient; this lesion depicts the nodular stage of KS. (*b*) KS lesion on the hard palate. (*c*) Low-power hematoxylin and eosin-stained section of dermal KS showing cords of spindle cells and slit-like neovascular spaces. (*d*) High-magnification view of KS spindle cells showing their dramatically elongated morphology. [All images courtesy of the Public Health Image Library of the U.S. Centers for Disease Control (**http://phil.cdc.gov**).]

expressed regularly by spindle cells in vivo (11–13).

Just as the field of pathology was beginning to accept that KS is derived from lymphatic endothelium, two recent papers have shown how tenuous such a conclusion may be (14, 15). These studies have examined the effects of KS-associated herpesvirus (KSHV) infection on the gene-expression programs of cultured vascular and lymphatic endothelium using DNA microarrays to profile host-gene transcription. They reveal that viral infection reprograms endothelial marker expression, which causes vascular endothelium to express certain lymphatic markers, whereas lymphatic endothelium shifts to a more vascular-like marker profile. Although these studies are conducted in vitro perforce, they may help explain the heterogeneity observed in marker expression in biopsies, and they certainly complicate attempts to discern the lineage of infected cells on the basis of patterns of marker expression alone.

Irrespective of their precise origin, spindle cells clearly represent the main proliferative element in KS. But analysis of spindle-cell clonality has shown that many KS lesions are oligo- or polyclonal—again reinforcing how different KS is from traditional cancer (16–18). Although this conclusion has been disputed by some research (20), even these dissenting studies have shown evidence of nonclonality in numerous tumors. What merits attention here is not the occasional tumor with clonality, but rather how different these results are from similar studies of classical tumors like breast or colon cancer, in which exceptions to monoclonality are almost never found.

Although spindle cells are considered the driving force behind KS histogenesis (see below), they are by no means the sole cell type in the tumor. All KS lesions also contain significant numbers of inflammatory cells (B and T cells, plasma cells, and monocytes) and a profusion of aberrant, slit-like neovascular spaces. These new vessels, the distinctive histologic signature of KS, are at least lined partially with KSHV-positive cells (21) and lack pericyte or smooth muscle accompaniment. Accordingly, they are prone to leakage and rupture, which is the presumed cause of the edema and hemorrhage so frequently observed in clinical KS.

From a pathogenetic point of view, it is useful to think of KS as being composed of three parallel processes: a proliferative component (involving chiefly spindle cells), an inflammatory component, and an angiogenic component. Although it is likely that these processes are interdependent and perhaps mutually reinforcing, thinking of them as individual entities allows the virologist to entertain different models for how viral gene expression may influence each component and thus affect the lesion as a whole (see below).

KS histology is not static, but varies considerably with the evolutionary state of the lesion. This has been studied most carefully in cutaneous KS because lesions of all stages can be easily observed and biopsied in this organ. Cutaneous KS involves the dermis exclusively and spares the overlying epidermis (22). Dermal KS begins as a so-called patch lesion, in which spindle cells are clearly demonstrable but are not necessarily the dominant element of the lesion. Inflammatory cells and neovascular elements are prominent at this stage—sometimes more prominent than the spindle-cell component (2). Neovascularization is well-established prior to the development of a nodule in contrast to more orthodox tumors, which undergo an angiogenic switch only when they outgrow their antecedent blood supply (23). Similarly, the inflammatory cells in KS are not late-stage elements recruited secondary to tumor necrosis or ischemia; rather, they are an integral part of the lesion, present from its earliest stages (2). As the lesion grows, the accumulation of spindle cells becomes more apparent. From its initial patch, KS progresses through a plaque-like stage to the nodular stage, in which masses of spindle cells generate macroscopically visible nodules (**Figure 1*a*** is a good example of a nodular lesion). In this state, the lesion often displays substantial local edema and induration, and hemorrhage from the slit-like vessels in the dermis is accompanied by phagocytosis of red blood cell debris with the generation of hemosiderin-laden macrophages (9).

KAPOSI'S SARCOMA CELL BIOLOGY AFFIRMS THAT KS IS NOT A TYPICAL CANCER

Classically, one criterion for malignant transformation in cell culture is the reduced dependence upon exogenous growth factors (this is often assayed by the ability of transformed cells to grow in reduced serum concentrations). However, cultured KS spindle cells, unlike classical tumor cells, remain highly dependent upon exogenous growth signals when cultured in vitro. Ensoli and colleagues were the first to grow KS spindle cells in culture and found them to be strongly dependent upon a cytokine-rich medium derived from supernatants of activated T cell cultures (6, 7, 24). To date, no less-complex medium that regularly allows spindle-cell outgrowth has been found, and certainly such lines do not grow in low-serum medium, nor do they display genetic instability, another hallmark of traditional cancers. KS spindle cells are generally diploid, and no characteristic chromosomal rearrangements are shared by multiple tumors. Classical KS lesions do not display microsatellite instability, although some advanced AIDS-KS lesions do (26). Cultured KS spindle cells also lack other markers of transformation: They do not form foci, nor grow in soft agar, nor form tumors in nude mice. However, an interesting phenotype is observed when the cells are injected subcutaneously in nude mice (27). Although they do not generate a tumor, they do survive for a brief interval, during which slit-like new vessels of murine origin appear in the surrounding tissue. When the human implant involutes, these vessels likewise disappear. This suggests a KS model in which spindle cells require growth factors from their microenvironment (perhaps from infiltrating inflammatory cells) for their survival and proliferation, but also produce angiogenic and proinflammatory substances to recruit the other components of the lesion. In this view, none of the partners in this process are fully autonomous; each depends upon the other (6, 7). Though these findings are derived necessarily from artificial experimental systems, they accord well with the known histology and clinical behavior of KS in vivo. All in all, most clinical and experimental observations about KS suggest that the differences between this disorder and classical cancers are at least as numerous as their similarities. It should then come as no surprise that the viral contributions to KS pathogenesis may be more variegated than those of other tumor viruses to more traditional cancers.

KAPOSI'S SARCOMA EPIDEMIOLOGY AND THE DISCOVERY OF KSHV

Not until the advent of epidemic, AIDS-related KS did large-scale epidemiologic studies produce strong evidence that KS may have an infectious etiology. KS was recognized early in the epidemic as a frequent complication of AIDS, with early estimates suggesting that untreated AIDS conferred a 20,000-fold increase in KS risk over the general population (28). Although first suspicions fell naturally on HIV as the etiologic culprit, it soon became clear that HIV infection alone could not account for KS development. Most cells (and all spindle cells) in an AIDS-KS biopsy do not harbor the HIV genome (29). More importantly, different AIDS populations often display staggering differences in KS risk, despite all being profoundly immunodeficient from their extensive HIV infection (28). In many studies, more than 20% of homosexual men with untreated AIDS developed KS, whereas KS developed in less than 2% of hemophiliacs with AIDS and virtually never in children with AIDS. Because most homosexual men acquired HIV primarily by a sexual route, whereas hemophiliacs and children acquired the virus principally from blood products or maternal hematogenous transmission, respectively, this suggested that a second, sexually transmitted cofactor was likely involved in KS pathogenesis. To search for this cofactor, Chang, Moore, and their collaborators examined KS tissue and normal tissue by representational difference analysis, looking for DNA sequences present in KS but absent in normal tissue. In a seminal paper, they reported the discovery of several novel fragments of DNA with distant homology to Epstein-Barr virus (EBV)—the first sighting of the KSHV genome (30). From this point, developing molecular clones of the entire viral genome was straightforward (31–34), and researchers could determine its complete DNA sequence (35). This facilitated the development of PCR tests for the presence of viral DNA in clinical samples, as well as expression of recombinant antigens for serologic testing (36). In 1996, Renne and colleagues (37) reported the development of a cell-culture system in which both latent and lytic infection could be observed; this set the stage for detailed analysis of the viral life cycle and also provided cells for immunofluorescence-based assays for antiviral antibodies. These reagents made it possible to study the distribution of KSHV infection in the human population, and within a matter of a few years the central features of KSHV epidemiology were established.

The epidemiology of KSHV points strongly to a critical role for this infection in KS pathogenesis. Viral DNA is always found in KS tumors, including HIV-negative forms of the disease (30, 36, 38, 39). Infection rates are high in groups in which KS is frequent and low in those in which it is rare (40, 41). This is also true globally: In societies in which classical KS is common, seroprevalence of KSHV is high (20%–25% of the population in the Mediterranean and up to 60% in parts of Africa; see Reference 36). In individual AIDS patients, infection with KSHV precedes the onset of KS and predicts an elevated risk of KS tumorigenesis (42, 43). Moreover, among male homosexuals in the United States, there is clear evidence of sexual transmission of KSHV (43), in accord with the epidemiologic predictions (28). These data, which are derived from the study of thousands of subjects, indicate strongly that KSHV infection is the sine qua non of KS; without it, clinical KS does not occur.

Although necessary for KS development, KSHV infection is not sufficient to engender KS. From 2%–7% of the U.S. population has serologic evidence of infection (36, 40, 41, 54), yet most of these individuals have no discernable KS risk, which clearly indicates that cofactors are required for tumorigenesis. In AIDS-related KS, that cofactor is obviously HIV infection [the identity of the cofactor(s) in classical KS remain unknown]. HIV's cofactor role in KS is strongly supported by (*a*) the dramatic reduction in KS incidence that has accompanied reduction of HIV viremia via antiretroviral therapy (44, 45) and (*b*) the remission of clinical KS in patients treated with HAART (highly active antiretroviral therapy) alone (46–48).

Exactly how HIV infection promotes KS development is still a matter of controversy. There is laboratory evidence that in certain settings HIV infection can augment KSHV replication in both cell-autonomous and paracrine fashions (49–52), but the in vivo relevance of these observations is unclear. (For instance, because dually infected cells are rare in vivo (29), cell-autonomous interactions between these viruses are unlikely to be critical.) Ensoli and colleagues have argued for a role for secreted HIV tat protein as a growth factor for KS spindle cells, again on the basis of experiments in cultured cells (reviewed in Reference 53). However, the interpretation of these data is complicated by the fact that cultured spindle cells tend to lose the KSHV genome (see below) and so cannot be relied upon to model faithfully all aspects of KS biology. Certainly, in the context of the whole organism, HIV infection is associated with cytokine upregulation, and such an environment should be conducive to sustaining spindle-cell survival and growth. Moreover, the T cell depletion and immunodeficiency induced by unchecked HIV replication is certain to be a factor in the progression of KS as it manifestly is in KS linked to iatrogenic immunosuppression. The controversy about HIV's role in KS development is unlikely to be resolved in the near future. However, it is worth pointing out that none of the models just summarized are mutually exclusive.

KSHV GENE EXPRESSION IN KAPOSI'S SARCOMA: AN OVERVIEW

As noted above, KSHV DNA is present in all KS tumors, irrespective of clinical type. Viral infection selectively targets spindle cells (21, 29, 55), with little or no infection of other cell types (though monocytes in the lesions may be infected) (55a).

Like all herpesviruses, KSHV can adopt either of two replicative programs, which are known as latency and lytic replication. In latency, viral gene expression is heavily restricted, with only a handful of viral genes being expressed; viral DNA is retained as a circular episome in the nucleus, and no progeny virions are produced. In most de novo KSHV infections of cultured cells, latency is the default pathway. In contrast, lytic replication involves the temporally regulated expression of virtually the entire viral genome, with viral DNA replication and production of infectious progeny, in the course of which the host cell dies. Lytic replication can be induced

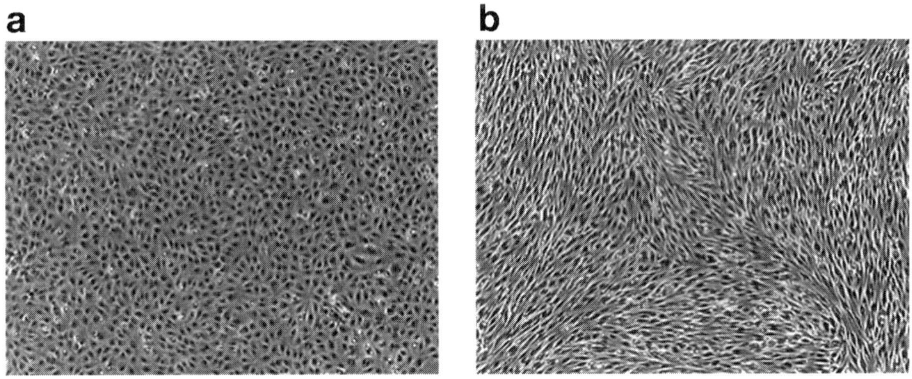

Figure 2

Latent KSHV infection causes endothelial cells to change to a spindle shape. Human umbilical vein endothelial cells in culture are depicted before (*left*) and after (*right*) latent infection by KSHV in cell culture.

from the latent state by the induction of the expression of a single viral gene, which encodes a transcription factor known as RTA (replication and transcription activator) (56, 57). In vitro, this can be achieved by the treatment of latently infected cells with phorbol esters or sodium butyrate or by transfection with constitutively active RTA alleles. The stimuli to KSHV lytic reactivation in vivo are unknown, but there is evidence that some cytokines can trigger such reactivation in culture (6, 7, 58).

Distinguishing between genes expressed in latency and those involved in lytic reactivation is important for a nuanced understanding of the viral contributions to KS pathogenesis. In traditional models of herpesviral oncogenesis, based largely on the role of Epstein-Barr virus (EBV) in Burkitt's lymphoma, the latency program is assigned the primary role in oncogenesis, by both promoting cell growth and impairing apoptosis. The lytic cycle, by contrast, has traditionally been thought not to contribute directly to oncogenesis because cells that enter this program invariably die. (Of course, it has long been acknowledged that lytic replication plays an important early role in viral oncogenesis by allowing the virus to spread throughout the host. This exposes many tissues to the virus and allows the establishment of many latent foci, which can then begin their long mutational march to cancer.)

By using known latency genes as probes in in situ hybridization studies, most KS spindle cells can be shown to be latently infected; only a small subpopulation of spindle cells (1%–3%) display lytic replicative markers (21, 29, 59, 60). This finding accords with conventional notions of the role of latency in tumors. Examination of early (patch) lesions of KS shows that only 10%–30% of spindle-like cells express latent genes (21), whereas in later lesions virtually all such cells are latently infected (21, 29). This clearly implies that latently infected cells have a growth or survival advantage in vivo. The nature of this advantage, however, has been difficult to assess in cell-culture systems. Although KSHV virions can infect many cell types in vitro (61–63), most established lines do not display alterations of morphology or growth properties. However, infection of primary endothelial cultures does yield a phenotype: Once latency is established, the cells undergo dramatic elongation to closely resemble spindle cells (**Figure 2**) (64–66). This rearrangement is accompanied by a dramatic reorganization of the actin cytoskeleton and has been traced to the expression of a single viral gene (v-FLIP) (Grossman & Ganem, unpublished observations). However, in most hands (65, 66, Grossman & Ganem, unpublished observations) this change is not associated with immortalization; the cells fail to grow in soft agar, and there have been no reports of tumorigenesis by such cells in nude mice. Note that there is one dissenting publication (67) in which immortalization of endothelia was reported following KSHV infection; however, in this study the cells that grew out largely lacked the KSHV genome. At a minimum, these studies suggest that the KSHV latency program may not be strongly immortalizing. This represents a clear difference from EBV latency (as studied in primary B cells), which is powerfully immortalizing in vitro (so much so that latent EBV infection is virtually the only reliable and efficient way to experimentally establish cultured B cell lines).

Nonetheless, the high prevalence of latent infection in the spindle-cell compartment and its escalating density as KS progresses clearly point to an important role for latent gene expression in KS pathogenesis. In the next section, we review the details of latent gene expression and focus on the functions of its key gene products.

THE KSHV LATENCY PROGRAM IN KAPOSI'S SARCOMA

Most of what we know about KSHV latency at the molecular level has not been derived from studying KS tumors. Rather, it is the product of the analysis of viral gene expression in cultured B cells from KSHV-related primary effusion lymphomas (PEL). These cells grow readily in culture, stably maintain latent KSHV genomes, and express latent transcripts and proteins in virtually all cells of the culture. In contrast, cultured KS cells usually segregate the viral genome during outgrowth (see below) and hence have been unusable for studies of the latency program. Fortunately, most transcripts identified in PEL cells can be shown by in situ hybridization or other methods to be expressed in primary KS tumors, although there is one exception: The protein know as vIRF3 is expressed in latent PEL cells but is not found in KS (68).

A more important problem concerns how these gene products function in KS development. At present, we have no animal model of KS, and no experimental animal can sustain a clinically evident infection following KSHV inoculation. There are simian relatives of KSHV, but the best-studied of these, rhesus rhadinovirus, does not induce a KS-like lesion (156). Furthermore, genetic manipulation of KSHV is still in its infancy. Although a few knockout mutations have been made in the genome via homologous recombination, this has proven to be an extremely difficult and labor-intensive endeavor with a high failure rate (61, 69, 70). Given these limitations, most studies have focused on the expression of the individual latency genes in heterologous cells—either immortalized epithelial cell lines (293 and HeLa cells), fibroblasts (either primary or established), or endothelial cells. Such cells can be assayed for phenotypic changes in their growth properties, for their sensitivity or resistance to apoptotic or other stimuli, or for interactions between the KSHV protein and host proteins of selected signaling or other pathways. However, conclusions drawn from such heterologous systems can be extrapolated to KS only with great caution. Despite these limitations, much has been learned about the individual gene products that have been expressed in KSHV latency. We will now focus on the six proteins known to be expressed in latently infected KS cells. Three of these [latency-associated nuclear antigen (LANA), v-cyclin, and v-FLIP] are encoded from one transcription unit and the others from a second, independent promoter.

Latency-associated nuclear antigen. LANA is a large, multifunctional protein that is the most widely used marker of KSHV latency. As the name implies, it is localized to the nucleus, where it accumulates in characteristic punctate foci (**Figure 3*b***) (40, 41). Although highly stereotypic, these structures do not correspond to any previously described nuclear subdomain. The protein itself comprises three major domains (**Figure 3*a***): a central region composed of variable numbers of highly acidic amino acid repeats, a C-terminal, more basic region involved in DNA binding and oligomerization, and an N-terminal region implicated in chromatin attachment and corepressor recruitment (71–73).

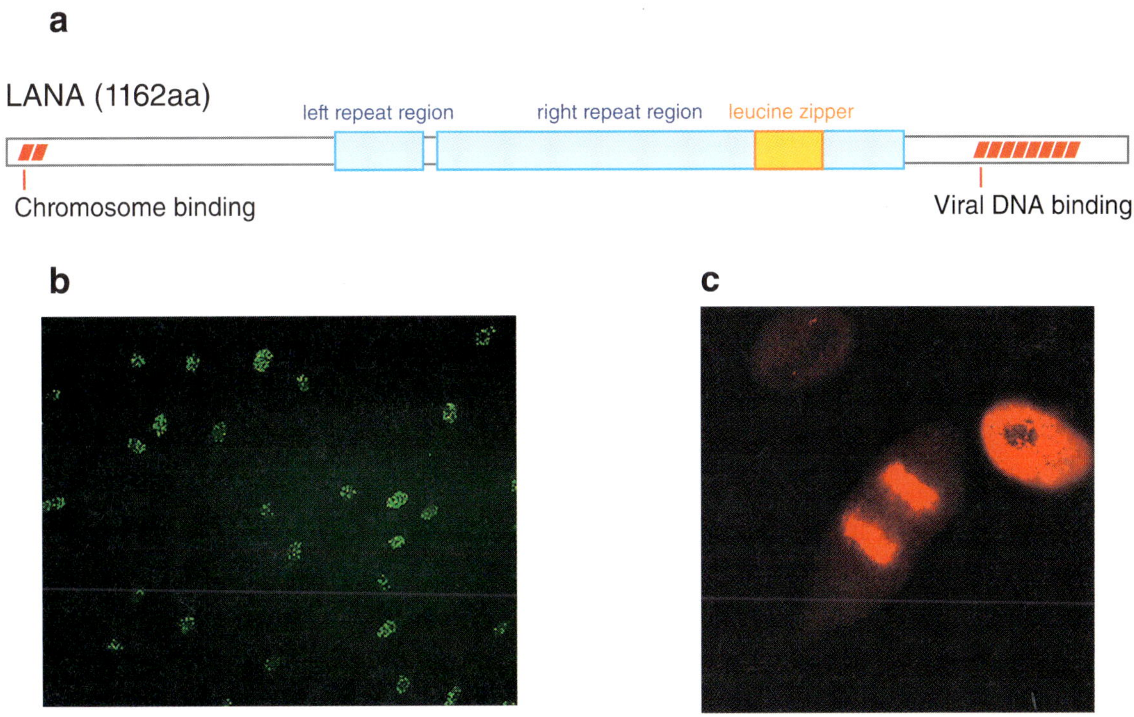

Figure 3

Latency-associated nuclear antigen (LANA) and its roles in KSHV latent episome maintenance. (*a*) Schematic depiction of coding organization of LANA with landmarks showing sites involved in binding to viral DNA and to host mitotic chromosomes. (*b*) Interphase nuclei of cells infected with KSHV in culture then stained for LANA by immunofluorescence. (*c*) LANA staining of a mitotic, cultured cell latently infected with KSHV; note LANA's association with mitotic chromosomes.

The best-characterized function of LANA is its involvement in the establishment and maintenance of the latent viral episome in the nucleus (74–75). As mentioned above, latency is established soon after viral entry in most infections. Incoming linear genomes are circularized in the nucleus, and the resulting plasmid-like DNA is replicated semiconservatively, likely in concert with the genome of its host cell. LANA's role in this process is severalfold. Its C-terminal domain can recognize a specific sequence in the viral genome [in its terminal repeat (TR) elements] (76–78); this binding allows it to mediate transient, semiconservative DNA replication (79–81). In addition, under certain laboratory conditions—usually employing a genetic selection for a drug-resistance marker on the viral plasmid—LANA and the TR sequences are all that are necessary for stable maintenance of the plasmid at a fixed copy number over many cell divisions. This activity appears to depend upon LANA's ability to bind mitotic chromosomes (**Figure 3*c***), thereby allowing passive segregation of viral genomes to the progeny of dividing cells (73, 74).

However, viral-episome maintenance is likely more complex than suggested by this simple scheme. Whereas LANA is necessary for plasmid maintenance, it is not always sufficient for it in many contexts that are less artificial than transfection followed by genetic selection. For example, when plasmids bearing LANA and the TRs are transfected into cells in the absence of a genetic selection, the resulting episomes are unstable and are lost rapidly following cell division (82). The same is true of viruses delivered by infection with authentic KSHV virions in culture. These findings suggest that genomic latency may be rather unstable under most conventional conditions. In some cell lines, as cells are passaged, a small subpopulation can stabilize the episome and go on to display permanent latency (82)—just as in PEL cell lines. It appears that in these sublines, the viral chromosome has undergone epigenetic changes in *cis* that allow episome stability; the biochemical nature of these changes, however, is not clear (82). Although these observations have by necessity been made in culture, there is strong reason to believe that they apply in vivo as well. Most telling, when KS spindle cells directly from a clinical lesion are placed in culture and stimulated to divide, they rapidly lose the viral episome that had been acquired in vivo (83–85). Thus, it appears that most KS spindle cells have not undergone the epigenetic events required for episome stabilization. This contrasts with PEL cells, which appear to efficiently stabilize latency in vivo. (What remains mysterious is why latency is stabilized in one situation but not the other.) The finding that spindle-cell latency is unstable has important pathogenetic implications that will be discussed later in this review.

LANA has other biochemical activities besides those involved in plasmid maintenance. In transfected cells, LANA binds p53, blocking its ability to act as a transcriptional activator and conferring increased resistance to p53-dependent apoptosis (86). Such an activity has obvious potential to promote cell survival, and this exact effect has been observed in primary endothelial cultures overexpressing LANA; although not immortalized, the cells' life span in vitro was prolonged (87). LANA has also been reported to bind to the tumor suppressor Rb (88); in transfected cells, this leads to enhanced expression of E2F-dependent reporter genes. This indicates that Rb binding by LANA is associated with loss of Rb function. However, other evidence (mostly in PEL cells) suggests that this inactivation of Rb is likely incomplete (89).

Another potential role for LANA in tumorigenesis derives from the fact that the protein interacts with GSK-3β, a kinase that inactivates β-catenin by targeting it for ubiquitination and degradation (90). When LANA binds GSK-3β, it relocates the kinase from the cytosol to the nucleus, which allows cellular accumulation of β-catenin. Oligomerization of that protein with the transcription factor LEF activates a proliferative program that includes expression of cyclin D, c-myc, and c-jun. Consistent with this, transient LANA expression in other cell types leads to enhanced S-phase entry (though not immortalization). These findings help define biochemical activities that make LANA-expressing cells more prone to survive and proliferate under the proper circumstances and also indicate that, unlike potent oncogenes like SV40 large T antigen, LANA expression by itself is not sufficient to trigger immortalization or transformation.

LANA can also act more directly on the program of host-gene expression. In cells expressing LANA stably, array-based expression profiling shows that many host genes are dysregulated, both positively and negatively (91). LANA's principal direct transcriptional activity appears to be repression. For example, LANA expression represses reporter genes linked to TR sequences, and when LANA is fused to the DNA-binding domain of GAL4 it inhibits expression of GAL4-dependent reporters (71, 72, 77, 92). This effect has been linked to the recruitment of the mSin3 corepressor complex via binding to the protein SAP30 (71). It is unknown if this activity is important pathogenetically in KS; it may have more to do with LANA's role in the establishment of latency, e.g., by leading to repression of lytic-cycle gene expression. LANA also binds to many other proteins that have a role in gene expression and chromatin structure; examples include the bromodomain-containing

RING3 protein, me-CpG-binding protein 2, heterochromatin protein 1, and various components of the transcription apparatus (72, 93–97). The biological roles of these activities in KS biogenesis are unknown.

v-cyclin. v-cyclin, a homolog of cellular cyclin D, is expressed principally from the LANA promoter via a spliced mRNA from which the upstream LANA gene has been removed (98–99). v-cyclin binds to and activates cdk6 (100), although this binding confers a slightly different substrate preference on cdk6 from that endowed by binding of cellular cyclin D (101, 102). v-cyclin overexpression induces S-phase entry in quiescent 3T3 cells and also overcomes an Rb-mediated growth arrest induced by cdk inhibitors (103). In fact, the v-cyclin/cdk6 complex is less sensitive to inhibition by cdk inhibitors like p27, p21, and p16. For p27, this resistance is enhanced by the fact that phosphorylation of the protein by v-cyclin/cdk6 targets p27 for proteasomal degradation (104, 105).

It has been difficult to assess how these activities relate to KS development in vivo. A major problem is the difficulty in obtaining cell lines that express v-cyclin stably. Such cells often undergo apoptosis, particularly if they express elevated levels of cdk6 (106). v-cyclin-induced apoptosis is associated with the phosphorylation (by v-cyclin/cdk6) and inactivation of the antiapoptotic factor bcl2 (107). It is unclear how this problem of apoptosis is mitigated in vivo, but the low levels of v-cyclin protein expressed in latency provides one explanation; the antiapoptotic effects of other latency proteins (e.g., LANA and v-FLIP) may represent another. Particularly relevant to the latter idea is the observation by Verschuren and colleagues (108) that loss of p53 allows cells to survive in the presence of elevated levels of v-cyclin.

v-FLIP. The third coding region expressed from the LANA promoter is a viral homolog of the FLICE inhibitory protein, v-FLIP. v-FLIP is the downstream gene in a spliced, bicistronic mRNA in which v-cyclin is the upstream gene; v-FLIP translation is made possible by the presence of an internal ribosome entry site (IRES) embedded within the v-cyclin coding region (109–111).

As a class, FLIPs contain death effector domains that allow them to bind adaptor proteins (TRADD and FADD) of the Fas/TNFR pathway (112). This interaction blocks the recruitment and activation of caspase 8, leading to blockade of Fas-induced, programmed cell death. Several herpesviruses encode v-FLIPs that employ this mechanism (112). Although some papers report that KSHV v-FLIP can also function in this fashion (113, 114), the findings have not been consistently replicated by all groups (Grundhoff & Ganem, unpublished observations), and there is growing evidence that the KSHV v-FLIP homolog may have additional or alternative functions. More recent reports suggest that KSHV v-FLIP can block cell death via induction of the antiapoptotic transcription factor NFκB (115). Consistent with this, v-FLIP is detected in cells complexed with NEMO (NFκB essential modulator; or IKKγ) (116,117). This complex activates IKK, which then leads to phosphorylation of IkB and release of active NFκB. Additionally, KSHV v-FLIP has been reported to bind TRAF2 and RIP upstream of IKK; TRAF binding also results in JNK (Jun N-terminal kinase) activation (118), although the import of the latter is not yet clear.

NFκB activation by v-FLIP has been linked to two biological activities in KSHV-mediated pathogenesis. In PEL, v-FLIP is the major factor promoting tumor cell survival; siRNA-mediated extinction of v-FLIP expression triggers cell death in cultured PEL cells (119). In primary endothelial cells, v-FLIP expression triggers the dramatic cellular elongation (spindling) traditionally associated with KSHV latency in this cell type (and KS tumors). Inhibitors of NFκB activation block this effect, which appears to reflect a major reorganization of the actin cytoskeleton (119a).

Apart from its role in extending cell survival and altering endothelial morphology, v-FLIP-mediated NFκB activation may also play a role in the maintenance of KSHV latency. Brown and colleagues (120) recently reported that activation of NFκB inhibits lytic-cycle gene expression and that inhibition of NFκB activation promotes lytic reactivation. If so, v-FLIP expression could help maintain the latent state by preventing inappropriate lytic induction owing to transient exposure to inducing stimuli.

The kaposin locus. The kaposin locus was identified initially in a screen for genes that are transcribed in latently infected PEL cells (31), but subsequent studies revealed that it is expressed at variable levels in latently infected KS spindle cells as well (29, 157). In addition, the promoter of the kaposin locus, which is separate from the LANA promoter, is strongly induced during lytic replication (121) owing to the presence of at least one high-affinity binding site for the lytic switch protein RTA (122–123). The single 1.4-kb kaposin mRNA encodes at least three proteins via differential initiation of translation (121). The 3′ end of of this transcript carries a small open reading frame (ORF) encoding kaposin A, a 60-amino-acid hydrophobic polypeptide found on the cell surface and on intracellular membranes (124). Interest in this protein was heightened when its overexpression in immortalized rodent fibroblasts triggered morphologic transformation in vitro and tumorigenesis in vivo (125). However, it is probably incorrect to think of transformation as its true purpose—KS spindle cells are not transformed, or even immortalized, by KSHV infection after all. Rather, transformation is probably a reflection of the fact that kaposin A has signaling activity that, when dialed to a very high level, can phenotypically alter a cell already immortalized as a result of other mutations. Subsequently it was found that in kaposin A–transformed cells kaposin A could bind cytohesin-1, a guanine nucleotide exchange factor for ARF GTPases and a regulator of integrin-mediated cell adhesion. Binding of kaposin A to cytohesin-1 stimulates GTP binding to ARF1, a process implicated in fibroblast transformation because the transformed phenotype can be reverted by expression of a cytohesin-1 mutant deficient in guanine nucleotide exchange (126). How these activities relate to KS pathogenesis is currently unknown.

Upstream of the kaposin A coding region is a series of tandemly repeated 23-nucleotide GC-rich elements of two families, termed direct repeat (DR) 1 and DR2. Although this region lacks AUG codons, at least two proteins can be translated from this region by initiation at CUG codons. (121). One of these proteins, kaposin B, is encoded predominantly by the repeat sequences; another, kaposin C, expresses the repeats fused in frame to the hydrophobic sequences of kaposin A. Kaposin B is currently known to function as an adapter protein in signal transduction by binding to and activating a kinase, MK2, that is normally a target of p38 phosphorylation (127). The activation mechanism is complex and not completely understood. Kaposin binds to a region of MK2 that is the binding target of a C-terminal autoinhibitory loop of the protein, which suggests that kaposin binding may displace this inhibitor. Kaposin binding may also sensitize MK2 to phosphorylation by p38 or shield active, phosphorylated MK2 from dephosphorylation. Consistent with the latter two models, inhibition of p38 kinase activity reduces (but does not entirely eliminate) MK2 activation, suggesting that upstream p38 activity plays an important role in MK2 activation.

What is the function of activated MK2? Recent studies establish that this kinase is a central regulator of a specialized pathway of mRNA stabilization. Many mRNAs for cytokines (e.g., IL1/3/4/6, TNF, and GM-CSF), growth factors (e.g.,VEGF), and oncoproteins (myc and fos) harbor AU-rich elements (AREs) in their 3′ untranslated regions that render the transcripts unstable (128). This instability is subject to regulation by MK2;

activated MK2 stabilizes these mRNAs, presumably by phosphorylating one or more of the effectors that recognize ARE (129). Consistent with this, kaposin B–expression blocks the degradation of ARE-containing mRNAs and substantially enhances cytokine release. This is an important result because KS lesions are replete with cytokines and growth factors and KS spindle cells both produce and require such cytokines. Post-transcriptional regulation by kaposin B is undoubtedly part of this cytokine production, but it is likely that transcriptional upregulation of cytokines (e.g., secondary to NFκB induction by v-FLIP) is also important in this regard.

A ROLE FOR THE LYTIC CYCLE IN KAPOSI'S SARCOMA PATHOGENESIS?

As noted above, precedents from other oncogenic herpesviruses led to an early focus on the latency program as a key factor driving KS pathogensis. However, the discovery that the KSHV latency program does not appear to be strongly immortalizing, whereas a negative result that is subject to all the usual caveats appertaining thereto, has raised questions about whether latency really suffices to drive KS pathogenesis unassisted. In fact, independent evidence from clinical studies suggests that lytic replication also plays a pivotal role in KS development. In patients with advanced AIDS, treatment with ganciclovir (GCV), a drug that blocks lytic but not latent KSHV infection, results in a prompt and dramatic decline in the incidence of new KS tumors (130). Because most of these patients have carried HIV and KSHV for many years, the impact of GCV is not attributable simply to the reduction of early dissemination to target cells. Rather, it appears that ongoing lytic replication is necessary throughout the entire natural history of KSHV infection to support lesion formation.

How might lytic replication contribute to KS tumor development? There are three nonexclusive possibilities:

1. If spindle cells are not immortalized in vivo, then in order for a tumor mass to expand, KSHV-positive cells that die must be replaced by new latently infected cells. The most obvious source of such cells would be from de novo infection of endothelia with viruses produced by lytic replication.

2. If, as noted above, KSHV latency is unstable, then as spindle cells proliferate, they would be expected to rapidly lose the viral genome. For KS to progress, cells that lose the KSHV genome must be replaced by cells newly recruited to latency by de novo infection with viruses produced by lytic replication.

3. The third manner by which lytic KSHV replication may contribute to KS pathogenesis harkens back to the view that KS is a composite of three processes: proliferation, inflammation, and angiogensis. Because lytically infected cells die, they cannot contribute significantly to the proliferative component of the disease. However, if lytically infected cells produce paracrine signaling molecules, they could promote both the inflammatory and angiogenic components of the lesion. In fact, examination of the KSHV genome (131) reveals numerous viral genes whose products are secreted signaling molecules—many of which are homologs of cellular cytokines or chemokines. The majority of these are lytic-cycle genes, including the three viral CC chemokines and v-IL6. Several of the viral chemokines are chemotactic for Th2 cells (132, 133), raising the possibility that these agents may blunt antiviral Th1 responses by favoring Th2 polarization of the local immune response. Other studies (134) report that the viral chemokines are chemotactic for endothelial cells, which suggests that KS lesions may be able to recruit more endothelial targets for infection. The v-IL6 protein has also been suggested to affect angiogenesis in model systems (135); in addition, v-IL6 signaling can block STAT2 phosphorylation by type I IFN receptors, possibly impairing antiviral responses to this important effector of innate immunity (136).

The KSHV lytic cycle (137, 138) also encodes a homolog of the 7 transmembrane G protein coupled receptors, a protein (termed v-GPCR) that clusters with the chemokine receptor subfamily of GPCRs (139). The protein displays constitutive signaling activity when expressed in the absence of known ligands (140, 141), which leads to the stimulation of the MAPK, PI3-kinase, and p38 pathways (142, 143), as well as the activation of NFκB activity (144). Cells experimentally transfected with v-GPCR display upregulation of many host genes, including VEGF—a major factor long suspected of playing an angiogenic role in KS histogenesis (142, 144, 145). Moreover, expression of v-GPCR in transgenic mice produces focal angioproliferative lesions that share some features with KS (146–148). Because this single viral gene product can be linked to both proliferation and angiogenesis, it has been proposed as key player in KS pathogenesis (144, 148). However, the restriction of v-GPCR expression to the lytic cycle complicates many of these inferences. First, v-GPCR's cell-autonomous, promitotic activity is likely to be negated by the direct cytotoxicity of the lytic cycle. Second, KSHV lytic replication imposes a strong and global block to de novo host-gene expression, mediated primarily by virus-induced turnover of host mRNA (149). In fact, few of the transcripts upregulated by v-GPCR transfection are found to be induced in a lytic infection of endothelial cells (150).

These studies do not entirely negate a role for v-GPCR in KS pathogenesis, but they do circumscribe its role. There is a brief window in infection between the onset of v-GPCR expression and the subsequent degradation of mRNA, during which very low levels of VEGF can be produced. For this to contribute significantly to KS progression in vivo, substantial levels of lytic replication would be required. In accord with this, clinical data suggest that KS is observed typically in patients with higher circulating KSHV loads (151–155).

CONCLUSIONS

The unusual histology and clinical behavior of KS suggests that its relationship to its causative herpesvirus may differ significantly from models of viral oncogenesis used to explain more canonical forms of cancer. Experimental studies suggest that the KSHV latency program is not as powerfully immortalizing as those of other oncogenic herpesviruses, and clinical data suggest that products of the lytic cycle make important and ongoing contributions to KS histogenesis. These notions have potentially important clinical implications because if they can be extrapolated to clinical KS, they suggest that sustained treatment of established KS lesions with antiviral drugs like ganciclovir may be of benefit. Beyond this, ongoing efforts to understand the relationship of viral gene expression to the proliferative, inflammatory, and angiogenic components of KS are sure to uncover many new viral regulators of fundamentally important host signaling pathways.

LITERATURE CITED

1. Kaposi M. 1872. Idiopathisches multiples pigmentsarkom her haut. *Arch. Dermatol. Shypilol.* 4:265–73
2. Herndier B, Ganem D. 2001. The biology of Kaposi's sarcoma. *Cancer Treat. Res.* 104:89–126
3. Mitsuyasu R. 1988. Kaposi's sarcoma in AIDS. *Inf. Dis. Clin. N. Am.* 2:511–20
4. Regezi JA, MacPhail LA, Daniels TE, Greenspan JS, Greenspan D, et al. 1993. Oral Kaposi's sarcoma: a 10-year retrospective histopathologic study. *J. Oral. Pathol. Med.* 22:292–97

5. Regezi JA, MacPhail LA, Daniels TE, DeSouza YG, Greenspan JS, Greenspan D. 1993. Human immunodeficiency virus-associated oral Kaposi's sarcoma. A heterogeneous cell population dominated by spindle-shaped endothelial cells. *Am. J. Pathol.* 143:240–49
6. Ensoli B, Sturzl M. 1998. Kaposi's sarcoma: a result of the interplay among inflammatory cytokines, angiogenic factors and viral agents. *Cytokine Growth Factor Rev.* 9:63–83
7. Ensoli B, Sgadari C, Barillari G, Sirianni MC, Sturzl M, Monini P. 2001. Biology of Kaposi's sarcoma. *Eur. J. Cancer* 37:1251–69
8. Sturzl M, Brandsetter H, Roth W. 1992. Kapois's sarcoma: review of gene expression and ultrastructure of KS spindle cells in vivo. *AIDS Res. Hum. Retrovir.* 8:1753–63
9. Cockerell CJ. 1991. Histopathologic features of Kaposi's sarcoma in HIV-infected individuals. *Cancer Surv.* 10:73–89
10. Kayaa EE, Parravicini C, Ordonez C, Gendelman R, Berti E, et al. 1995. Heterogeneity of spindle cells in Kaposi's sarcoma. *J. AIDS Hum. Retrovir.* 10:295–305
11. Weninger W, Partanen TA, Breiteneder-Geleff S, Mayer C, Kowalski H, et al. 1999. Expression of vascular endothelial growth factor receptor-3 and podoplanin suggests a lymphatic endothelial cell origin of Kaposi's sarcoma tumor cells. *Lab. Invest.* 79:243–51
12. Skobe M, Brown LF, Tognazzi K, Ganju RK, Dezube BJ, et al. 1999. Vascular endothelial growth factor-C (VEGF-C) and its receptors KDR and flt-4 are expressed in AIDS-associated Kaposi's sarcoma. *J. Invest. Dermatol.* 113:1047–53
13. Marchio S, Primo L, Pagano M, Palestro G, Albini A, et al. 1999. Vascular endothelial growth factor-C stimulates the migration and proliferation of Kaposi's sarcoma cells. *J. Biol. Chem.* 274:27617–22
14. Wang HW, Trotter MW, Lagos D, Bourboulia D, Henderson S, et al. 2004. Kaposi sarcoma herpesvirus-induced cellular reprogramming contributes to the lymphatic endothelial gene expression in Kaposi sarcoma. *Nat. Genet.* 36:687–93
15. Hong YK, Foreman K, Shin JW, Hirakawa S, Curry CL, et al. 2004. Lymphatic reprogramming of blood vascular endothelium by Kaposi sarcoma-associated herpesvirus. *Nat. Genet.* 36:683–85
16. Delabesse E, Oksenhendler E, Lebbe C, Verola O, Varet B, Turhan AG. 1997. Molecular analysis of clonality in Kaposi's sarcoma. *J. Clin. Pathol.* 50:664–68
17. Gill PS, Tsai YC, Rao AP, Spruck CH 3rd, Zheng T, et al. 1998. Evidence for multiclonality in multicentric Kaposi's sarcoma. *Proc. Natl. Acad. Sci. USA* 95:8257–61
18. Judde JG, Lacoste V, Briere J, Kassa-Kelembho E, Clyti E, et al. 2000. Monoclonality or oligoclonality of human herpesvirus 8 terminal repeat sequences in Kaposi's sarcoma and other diseases. *J. Natl. Cancer Inst.* 92:729–36
19. Beckstead JH, Wood GS, Fletcher V. 1995. Evidence for the origin of Kaposi's sarcoma from lymphatic endothelium. *Am. J. Pathol.* 119:294–300
20. Rabkin CS, Janz S, Lash A, Coleman AE, Musaba E, et al. 1997. Monoclonal origin of multicentric Kaposi's sarcoma lesions. *N. Engl. J. Med.* 336:988–93
21. Dupin NC, Fisher P, Kellam S, Ariad M, Tulliez N, et al. 1999. Distribution of human herpesvirus-8 latently infected cells in Kaposi's sarcoma, multicentric Castleman's disease, and primary effusion lymphoma. *Proc. Natl. Acad. Sci. USA* 96:4546–51
22. Parravicini C, Chandran B, Corbellino M, Berti E, Paulli M, et al. 2000. Differential viral protein expression in Kaposi's sarcoma-associated herpesvirus-infected diseases: Kaposi's sarcoma, primary effusion lymphoma, and multicentric Castleman's disease. *Am. J. Pathol.* 156:743–49

23. Hanahan D, Christofori G, Naik P, Arbeit J. 1996. Transgenic mouse models of tumour angiogenesis: the angiogenic switch, its molecular controls, and prospects for preclinical therapeutic models. *Eur. J. Cancer* 32A:2386–93
24. Ensoli BS, Nakamura SZ, Salahuddin P, Biberfeld L, Larsson B, et al. 1989. AIDS-Kaposi's sarcoma-derived cells express cytokines with autocrine and paracrine growth effects. *Science* 243:223–26
25. Miles SA, Rezai AR, Salazar-Gonzalez JF, Vander Meyden M, Stevens RH, et al. 1990. AIDS Kaposi sarcoma-derived cells produce and respond to interleukin 6. *Proc. Natl. Acad. Sci. USA* 87:4068–72
26. Bedi GC, Westra WH, Farzadegan H, Pitha PM, Sidransky D. 1995. Microsatellite instability in primary neoplasms from HIV+ patients. *Nat. Med.* 1:65–68
27. Salahuddin SZ, Nakamura S, Biberfeld P, Kaplan MH, Markham PD, et al. 1988. Angiogenic properties of Kaposi's sarcoma-derived cells after long-term culture in vitro. *Science* 242:430–33
28. Beral VT, Peterman A, Berkelman RL, Jaffe HW. 1990. Kaposi's sarcoma among persons with AIDS: a sexually transmitted infection? *Lancet* 335:123–28
29. Staskus KA, Zhong W, Gebhard K, Herndier B, Wang H, et al. 1997. Kaposi's sarcoma-associated herpesvirus gene expression in endothelial (spindle) tumor cells. *J. Virol.* 71:715–19
30. Chang YE, Cesarman MS, Pessin F, Lee J, Culpepper DM, et al. 1994. Identification of herpesvirus-like DNA sequences in AIDS-associated Kaposi's sarcoma. *Science* 266:1865–69
31. Zhong W, Wang H, Herndier B, Ganem D. 1996. Restricted expression of Kaposi sarcoma-associated herpesvirus (human herpesvirus 8) genes in Kaposi sarcoma. *Proc. Natl. Acad. Sci. USA* 93:6641–46
32. Moore PS, Boshoff C, Weiss RA, Chang Y. 1996. Molecular mimicry of human cytokine and cytokine response pathway genes by KSHV. *Science* 274:1739–44
33. Nicholas J, Ruvolo VR, Burns WH, Sandford G, Wan X, et al. 1997. Kaposi's sarcoma-associated human herpesvirus-8 encodes homologues of macrophage inflammatory protein-1 and interleukin-6. *Nat. Med.* 3:287–92
34. Neipel F, Albrecht JC, Fleckenstein B. 1997. Cell-homologous genes in the Kaposi's sarcoma-associated rhadinovirus human herpesvirus 8: determinants of its pathogenicity? *J. Virol.* 71:4187–92
35. Russo JJ, Bohenzky RA, Chien MC, Chen J, Yan MD, et al. 1996. Nucleotide sequence of the Kaposi sarcoma-associated herpesvirus (HHV8). *Proc. Natl. Acad. Sci. USA* 93:14862–67
36. Schulz TF. 1999. Epidemiology of Kaposi's sarcoma-associated herpesvirus/human herpesvirus 8. *Adv. Cancer Res.* 76:121–60
37. Renne R, Zhong W, Herndier B, McGrath M, Abbey ND, et al. 1996. Lytic growth of Kaposi's sarcoma-associated herpesvirus (human herpesvirus 8) in culture. *Nat. Med.* 2:342–46
38. Moore PS, Chang Y. 1995. Detection of herpesvirus-like DNA sequences in Kaposi's sarcoma in patients with and without HIV infection. *N. Engl. J. Med.* 332:1181–85
39. Huang YQ, Li JJ, Kaplan MH, Poiesz B, Katabira E, et al. 1995. Human herpesvirus-like nucleic acid in various forms of Kaposi's sarcoma. *Lancet* 345:759–61
40. Kedes DH, Operskalski E, Busch M, Kohn R, Flood J, Ganem D. 1996. The seroepidemiology of human herpesvirus 8 (Kaposi's sarcoma-associated herpesvirus):

distribution of infection in KS risk groups and evidence for sexual transmission. *Nat. Med.* 2:918–24
41. Gao SJ, Kingsley L, Li M, Zheng W, Parravicini C, et al. 1996. KSHV antibodies among Americans, Italians and Ugandans with and without Kaposi's sarcoma. *Nat. Med.* 2:925–28
42. Moore PS, Kingsley LA, Holmberg SD, Spira T, Gupta P, et al. 1996. Kaposi's sarcoma-associated herpesvirus infection prior to onset of Kaposi's sarcoma. *AIDS* 10:175–80
43. Martin JN, Ganem DE, Osmond DH, Page-Shafer KA, Macrae D, Kedes DH. 1998. Sexual transmission and the natural history of human herpesvirus 8 infection. *N. Engl. J. Med.* 338:948–54
44. Portsmouth S, Stebbing J, Gill J, Mandalia S, Bower M, et al. 2003. A comparison of regimens based on non-nucleoside reverse transcriptase inhibitors or protease inhibitors in preventing Kaposi's sarcoma. *AIDS* 17:F17–22
45. Gates AE, Kaplan LD. 2002. AIDS malignancies in the era of highly active antiretroviral therapy. *Oncology* 16:657–65
46. Cattelan AM, Calabro ML, Gasperini P, Aversa SM, Zanchetta M, et al. 2001. Acquired immunodeficiency syndrome-related Kaposi's sarcoma regression after highly active antiretroviral therapy: biologic correlates of clinical outcome. *J. Natl. Cancer Inst. Monogr.* 2001:44–49
47. Gill J, Bourboulia D, Wilkinson J, Hayes P, Cope A, et al. 2002. Prospective study of the effects of antiretroviral therapy on Kaposi sarcoma–associated herpesvirus infection in patients with and without Kaposi sarcoma. *J. AIDS* 31:384–90
48. Lebbe C, Blum L, Pellet C, Blanchard G, Verola O, et al. 1998. Clinical and biological impact of antiretroviral therapy with protease inhibitors on HIV-related Kaposi's sarcoma. *AIDS* 12:F45–49
49. Harrington W Jr, Sieczkowski L, Sosa C, Chan-a-Sue S, Cai JP, et al. 1997. Activation of HHV-8 by HIV-1 tat. *Lancet.* 349:774–75
50. Varthakavi V, Browning PJ, Spearman P. 1999. Human immunodeficiency virus replication in a primary effusion lymphoma cell line stimulates lytic-phase replication of Kaposi's sarcoma-associated herpesvirus. *J. Virol.* 73:10329–38
51. Varthakavi V, Smith RM, Deng H, Sun R, Spearman P. 2002. Human immunodeficiency virus type-1 activates lytic cycle replication of Kaposi's sarcoma-associated herpesvirus through induction of KSHV Rta. *Virology* 297:270–80
52. Huang LM, Chao MF, Chen MY, Shih HM, Chiang YP, et al. 2001. Reciprocal regulatory interaction between human herpesvirus 8 and human immunodeficiency virus type 1. *J. Biol. Chem.* 276:13427–32
53. Barillari G, Ensoli B. 2002. Angiogenic effects of extracellular human immunodeficiency virus type 1 Tat protein and its role in the pathogenesis of AIDS-associated Kaposi's sarcoma. *Clin. Microbiol. Rev.* 15:310–26
54. Pellett PE, Wright DJ, Engels EA, Ablashi DV, Dollard SC, et al. 2003. Multicenter comparison of serologic assays and estimation of human herpesvirus 8 seroprevalence among US blood donors. *Transfusion* 43:1260–68
55. Boshoff C, Schulz TF, Kennedy MM, Graham AK, Fisher CA, et al. 1995. Kaposi's sarcoma-associated herpesvirus infects endothelial and spindle cells. *Nat. Med.* 1:1274–78
55a. Blasig C, Zietz C, Haar B, Neipel F, Esser S, et al. 1997. Monocytes in Kaposi's sarcoma lesions are productively infected by human herpesvirus 8. *J. Virol.* 71:7963–68

56. Sun R, Lin SF, Gradoville L, Yuan Y, Zhu F, Miller G. 1998. A viral gene that activates lytic cycle expression of Kaposi's sarcoma-associated herpesvirus. *Proc. Natl. Acad. Sci. USA* 95:10866–71
57. Lukac DM, Renne R, Kirshner JR, Ganem D. 1998. Reactivation of Kaposi's sarcoma-associated herpesvirus infection from latency by expression of the ORF 50 transactivator, a homolog of the EBV R protein. *Virology* 252:304–12
58. Chang J, Renne R, Dittmer D, Ganem D. 2000. Induction of Kaposi's sarcoma-associated herpesvirus from latency by inflammatory cytokines. *Virology* 266:17–25
59. Sturzl M, Blasig C, Schreier A, Neipel F, Hohenadl C, et al. 1997. Expression of HHV-8 latency-associated T0.7 RNA in spindle cells and endothelial cells of AIDS-associated, classical and African Kaposi's sarcoma. *Int. J. Cancer* 72:68–71
60. Katano H, Sato Y, Kurata T, Mori S, Sata T. 2000. Expression and localization of human herpesvirus 8-encoded proteins in primary effusion lymphoma, Kaposi's sarcoma, and multicentric Castleman's disease. *Virology* 269:335–44
61. Vieira J, O'Hearn P, Kimball L, Chandran B, Corey L. 2001. Activation of Kaposi's sarcoma-associated herpesvirus (human herpesvirus 8) lytic replication by human cytomegalovirus. *J. Virol.* 75:1378–86
62. Lagunoff M, Bechtel J, Venetsanakos E, Roy AM, Abbey N, et al. 2002. De novo infection and serial transmission of Kaposi's sarcoma-associated herpesvirus in cultured endothelial cells. *J. Virol.* 76:2440–48
63. Bechtel JT, Liang Y, Hvidding J, Ganem D. 2003. Host range of Kaposi's sarcoma-associated herpesvirus in cultured cells. *J. Virol.* 77:6474–81
64. Ciufo DM, Cannon JS, Poole LJ, Wu FY, Murray P, et al. 2001. Spindle cell conversion by Kaposi's sarcoma-associated herpesvirus: formation of colonies and plaques with mixed lytic and latent gene expression in infected primary dermal microvascular endothelial cell cultures. *J. Virol.* 75:5614–26
65. Gao SJ, Deng JH, Zhou FC. 2003. Productive lytic replication of a recombinant Kaposi's sarcoma-associated herpesvirus in efficient primary infection of primary human endothelial cells. *J. Virol.* 77:9738–49
66. Tang J, Gordon GM, Muller MG, Dahiya M, Foreman KE. 2003. Kaposi's sarcoma-associated herpesvirus latency-associated nuclear antigen induces expression of the helix-loop-helix protein Id-1 in human endothelial cells. *J. Virol.* 77:5975–84
67. Flore O, Rafii S, Ely S, O'Leary JJ, Hyjek EM, Cesarman E. 1998. Transformation of primary human endothelial cells by Kaposi's sarcoma-associated herpesvirus. *Nature* 394:588–92
68. Rivas C, Thlick AE, Parravicini C, Moore PS, Chang Y. 2001. Kaposi's sarcoma-associated herpesvirus LANA2 is a B-cell-specific latent viral protein that inhibits p53. *J. Virol.* 75:429–38
69. Delecluse HJ, Kost M, Feederle R, Wilson L, Hammerschmidt W. 2001. Spontaneous activation of the lytic cycle in cells infected with a recombinant Kaposi's sarcoma-associated virus. *J. Virol.* 75:2921–28
70. Zhou FC, Zhang YJ, Deng JH, Wang XP, Pan HY, et al. 2002. Efficient infection by a recombinant Kaposi's sarcoma-associated herpesvirus cloned in a bacterial artificial chromosome: application for genetic analysis. *J. Virol.* 76:6185–96
71. Krithivas A, Young DB, Liao G, Greene D, Hayward SD. 2000. Human herpesvirus 8 LANA interacts with proteins of the mSin3 corepressor complex and negatively regulates Epstein-Barr virus gene expression in dually infected PEL cells. *J. Virol.* 74:9637–45

72. Krithivas A, Fujimuro M, Weidner M, Young DB, Hayward SD. 2002. Protein interactions targeting the latency-associated nuclear antigen of Kaposi's sarcoma-associated herpesvirus to cell chromosomes. *J. Virol.* 76:11596–604
73. Piolot T, Tramier M, Coppey M, Nicolas JC, Marechal V. 2001. Close but distinct regions of human herpesvirus 8 latency-associated nuclear antigen 1 are responsible for nuclear targeting and binding to human mitotic chromosomes. *J. Virol.* 75:3948–59
74. Ballestas ME, Chatis PA, Kaye KM. 1999. Efficient persistence of extrachromosomal KSHV DNA mediated by latency-associated nuclear antigen. *Science* 284:641–44
75. Cotter MA 2nd, Robertson ES. 1999. The latency-associated nuclear antigen tethers the Kaposi's sarcoma-associated herpesvirus genome to host chromosomes in body cavity-based lymphoma cells. *Virology* 264:254–64
76. Ballestas ME, Kaye KM. 2001. Kaposi's sarcoma-associated herpesvirus latency-associated nuclear antigen 1 mediates episome persistence through cis-acting terminal repeat (TR) sequence and specifically binds TR DNA. *J. Virol.* 75:3250–58
77. Garber AC, Shu MA, Hu J, Renne R. 2001. DNA binding and modulation of gene expression by the latency-associated nuclear antigen of Kaposi's sarcoma-associated herpesvirus. *J. Virol.* 75:7882–92
78. Garber AC, Hu J, Renne R. 2002. Latency-associated nuclear antigen (LANA) cooperatively binds to two sites within the terminal repeat, and both sites contribute to the ability of LANA to suppress transcription and to facilitate DNA replication. *J. Biol. Chem.* 277:27401–11
79. Hu J, Garber AC, Renne R. 2002. The Latency-associated nuclear antigen of Kaposi's sarcoma-associated herpesvirus supports latent DNA replication in dividing cells. *J. Virol.* 76:11677–87
80. Lim C, Sohn H, Lee D, Gwack Y, Choe J. 2002. Functional dissection of latency-associated nuclear antigen 1 of Kaposi's sarcoma-associated herpesvirus involved in latent DNA replication and transcription of terminal repeats of the viral genome. *J. Virol.* 76:10320–31
81. Grundhoff A, Ganem D. 2003. The latency-associated nuclear antigen of Kaposi's sarcoma-associated herpesvirus (KSHV) permits replication of terminal repeat-containing plasmids. *J. Virol.* 77:2779–83
82. Grundhoff A, Ganem D. 2004. The inefficient establishment of KSHV latency suggests an additional role for lytic viral replication in KS pathogenesis. *J. Clin. Invest.* 113:124–36
83. Aluigi MG, Albini A, Carlone S, Repetto L, De Marchi R, et al. 1996. KSHV sequences in biopsies and cultured spindle cells of epidemic, iatrogenic and Mediterranean forms of Kaposi's sarcoma. *Res. Virol.* 147:267–75
84. Dictor M, Rambech E, Way D, Witte M, Bendsoe N. 1996. Human herpesvirus 8 (Kaposi's sarcoma-associated herpesvirus) DNA in Kaposi's sarcoma lesions, AIDS Kaposi's sarcoma cell lines, endothelial Kaposi's sarcoma simulators, and the skin of immunosuppressed patients. *Am. J. Pathol.* 148:2009–16
85. Flamand L, Zeman RA, Bryant JL, Lunardi-Iskandar Y, Gallo RC. 1996. Absence of human herpesvirus 8 DNA sequences in neoplastic Kaposi's sarcoma cell lines. *J. AIDS Hum. Retrovirol.* 13:194–97
86. Friborg J Jr, Kong W, Hottiger MO, Nabel GJ. 1999. p53 inhibition by the LANA protein of KSHV protects against cell death. *Nature* 402:889–94

87. Watanabe T, Sugaya M, Atkins AM, Aquilino EA, Yang A, et al. 2003. Kaposi's sarcoma-associated herpesvirus latency-associated nuclear antigen prolongs the life span of primary human umbilical vein endothelial cells. *J. Virol.* 77:6188–96
88. Radkov SA, Kellam P, Boshoff C. 2000. The latent nuclear antigen of Kaposi sarcoma-associated herpesvirus targets the retinoblastoma-E2F pathway and with the oncogene Hras transforms primary rat cells. *Nat. Med.* 6:1121–27
89. Platt G, Carbone A, Mittnacht S. 2002. p16INK4a loss and sensitivity in KSHV associated primary effusion lymphoma. *Oncogene* 21:1823–31
90. Fujimuro M, Wu FY, ApRhys C, Kajumbula H, Young DB, et al. 2003. A novel viral mechanism for dysregulation of beta-catenin in Kaposi's sarcoma-associated herpesvirus latency. *Nat. Med.* 9:300–6
91. Renne R, Barry C, Dittmer D, Compitello N, Brown PO, Ganem D. 2001. Modulation of cellular and viral gene expression by the latency-associated nuclear antigen of Kaposi's sarcoma-associated herpesvirus. *J. Virol.* 75:458–68
92. Schwam DR, Luciano RL, Mahajan SS, Wong L, Wilson AC. 2000. Carboxy terminus of human herpesvirus 8 latency-associated nuclear antigen mediates dimerization, transcriptional repression, and targeting to nuclear bodies. *J. Virol.* 74:8532–40
93. Viejo-Borbolla A, Kati E, Sheldon JA, Nathan K, Mattsson K, et al. 2003. A Domain in the C-terminal region of latency-associated nuclear antigen 1 of Kaposi's sarcoma-associated Herpesvirus affects transcriptional activation and binding to nuclear heterochromatin. *J. Virol.* 77:7093–100
94. Platt GM, Simpson GR, Mittnacht S, Schulz TF. 1999. Latent nuclear antigen of Kaposi's sarcoma-associated herpesvirus interacts with RING3, a homolog of the Drosophila female sterile homeotic (fsh) gene. *J. Virol.* 73:9789–95
95. Mattsson K, Kiss C, Platt GM, Simpson GR, Kashuba E, et al. 2002. Latent nuclear antigen of Kaposi's sarcoma herpesvirus/human herpesvirus-8 induces and relocates RING3 to nuclear heterochromatin regions. *J. Gen. Virol.* 83:179–88
96. Lim C, Sohn H, Gwack Y, Choe J. 2000. Latency-associated nuclear antigen of Kaposi's sarcoma-associated herpesvirus (human herpesvirus-8) binds ATF4/CREB2 and inhibits its transcriptional activation activity. *J. Gen. Virol.* 81:2645–52
97. Lim C, Lee D, Seo T, Choi C, Choe J. 2003. Latency-associated nuclear antigen of Kaposi's sarcoma-associated herpesvirus functionally interacts with heterochromatin protein 1. *J. Biol. Chem.* 278:7397–405
98. Dittmer D, Lagunoff M, Renne R, Staskus K, Haase A, Ganem D. 1998. A cluster of latently expressed genes in Kaposi's sarcoma-associated herpesvirus. *J. Virol.* 72:8309–15
99. Sarid R, Wiezorek JS, Moore PS, Chang Y. 1999. Characterization and cell cycle regulation of the major Kaposi's sarcoma-associated herpesvirus (Human herpesvirus 8) latent genes and their promoter. *J. Virol.* 73:1438–46
100. Chang Y, Moore PS, Talbot SJ, Boshoff CH, Zarkowska T, et al. 1996. Cyclin encoded by KS herpesvirus. *Nature* 382:410–11
101. Godden-Kent D, Talbot S, Boshoff C, Chang Y, Moore P, et al. 1997. The cyclin encoded by Kaposi's sarcoma-associated herpesvirus stimulates cdk6 to phosphorylate the retinoblastoma protein and histone H1. *J. Virol.* 71:4193–98
102. Li M, Lee H, Yoon DW, Albrecht JC, Fleckenstein B, et al. 1997. Kaposi's sarcoma-associated herpesvirus encodes a functional cyclin. *J. Virol.* 71:1984–91
103. Swanton C, Mann DJ, Fleckenstein B, Neipel F, Peters G, Jones N. 1997. Herpes viral cyclin/Cdk6 complexes evade inhibition by CDK inhibitor proteins. *Nature* 390:184–87

104. Mann DJ, Child ES, Swanton C, Laman H, Jones N. 1999. Modulation of p27(Kip1) levels by the cyclin encoded by Kaposi's sarcoma-associated herpesvirus. *EMBO J.* 18:654–63
105. Ellis M, Chew YP, Fallis L, Freddersdorf S, Boshoff C, et al. 1999. Degradation of p27(Kip) cdk inhibitor triggered by Kaposi's sarcoma virus cyclin-cdk6 complex. *EMBO J.* 18:644–53
106. Ojala PM, Tiainen M, Salven P, Veikkola T, Castanos-Velez E, et al. 1999. Kaposi's sarcoma-associated herpesvirus-encoded v-cyclin triggers apoptosis in cells with high levels of cyclin-dependent kinase 6. *Cancer Res.* 59:4984–89
107. Ojala PM, Yamamoto K, Castanos-Velez E, Biberfeld P, Korsmeyer SJ, Makela TP. 2000. The apoptotic v-cyclin-CDK6 complex phosphorylates and inactivates Bcl-2. *Nat. Cell. Biol.* 2:819–25
108. Verschuren EW, Klefstrom J, Evan GI, Jones N. 2002. The oncogenic potential of Kaposi's sarcoma-associated herpesvirus cyclin is exposed by p53 loss in vitro and in vivo. *Cancer Cell* 2:229–41
109. Bieleski L, Talbot SJ. 2001. Kaposi's sarcoma-associated herpesvirus vCyclin open reading frame contains an internal ribosome entry site. *J. Virol.* 75:1864–69
110. Grundhoff A, Ganem D. 2001. Mechanisms governing expression of the v-FLIP gene of Kaposi's sarcoma-associated herpesvirus. *J. Virol.* 75:1857–63
111. Low W, Harries M, Ye H, Du MQ, Boshoff C, Collins M. 2001. Internal ribosome entry site regulates translation of Kaposi's sarcoma-associated herpesvirus FLICE inhibitory protein. *J. Virol.* 75:2938–45
112. Thome M, Schneider P, Hofmann K, Fickenscher H, Meinl E, et al. 1997. Viral FLICE-inhibitory proteins (FLIPs) prevent apoptosis induced by death receptors. *Nature* 386:517–21
113. Djerbi M, Screpanti V, Catrina AI, Bogen B, Biberfeld P, Grandien A. 1999. The inhibitor of death receptor signaling, FLICE-inhibitory protein defines a new class of tumor progression factors. *J. Exp. Med.* 190:1025–32
114. Belanger C, Gravel A, Tomoiu A, Janelle ME, Gosselin J, et al. 2001. Human herpesvirus 8 viral FLICE-inhibitory protein inhibits Fas-mediated apoptosis through binding and prevention of procaspase-8 maturation. *J. Hum. Virol.* 4:62–73
115. Chaudhary PM, Jasmin A, Eby MT, Hood L. 1999. Modulation of the NF-B pathway by virally encoded death effector domains-containing proteins. *Oncogene* 18:5738–46
116. Liu L, Eby MT, Rathore N, Sinha SK, Kumar A, Chaudhary PM. 2002. The human herpes virus 8-encoded viral FLICE inhibitory protein physically associates with and persistently activates the IB kinase complex. *J. Biol. Chem.* 277:13745–51
117. Field N, Low W, Daniels M, Howell S, Daviet L, et al. 2003. KSHV vFLIP binds to IKK-gamma to activate IKK. *J. Cell. Sci.* 116:3721–28
118. An J, Sun Y, Sun R, Rettig MB. 2003. Kaposi's sarcoma-associated herpesvirus encoded vFLIP induces cellular IL-6 expression: the role of the NF-kappaB and JNK/AP1 pathways. *Oncogene* 22:3371–85
119. Keller SA, Schattner EJ, Cesarman E. 2000. Inhibition of NF-B induces apoptosis of KSHV-infected primary effusion lymphoma cells. *Blood* 96:2537–42
119a. Grossman C, Podogrobskina S, Skobe M, Ganem D. 2005. Activation of NF-κB by the latent v-FLIP gene of KSHV is required for the spindle shape of virus-infected endothelial cells and contributes to their pro-inflammatory phenotype. *J. Virology*. Submitted
120. Brown HJ, Song MJ, Deng H, Wu TT, Cheng G, Sun R. 2003. NF-kappaB inhibits gammaherpesvirus lytic replication. *J. Virol.* 77:8532–40

121. Sadler R, Wu L, Forghani B, Renne R, Zhong W, et al. 1999. A complex translational program generates multiple novel proteins from the latently expressed kaposin (K12) locus of Kaposi's sarcoma-associated herpesvirus. *J. Virol.* 73:5722–30
122. Chang PJ, Shedd D, Gradoville L, Cho MS, Chen LW, et al. 2002. Open reading frame 50 protein of Kaposi's sarcoma-associated herpesvirus directly activates the viral PAN and K12 genes by binding to related response elements. *J. Virol.* 76:3168–78
123. Song MJ, Deng H, Sun R. 2003. Comparative study of regulation of RTA-responsive genes in Kaposi's sarcoma-associated herpesvirus/human herpesvirus 8. *J. Virol.* 77:9451–62
124. Tomkowicz B, Singh SP, Cartas M, Srinivasan A. 2002. Human herpesvirus-8 encoded Kaposin: subcellular localization using immunofluorescence and biochemical approaches. *DNA Cell Biol.* 21:151–62
125. Muralidhar S, Pumfery AM, Hassani M, Sadaie MR, Azumi N, et al. 1998. Identification of kaposin (ORF K12) as a human herpesvirus 8 (Kaposi's sarcoma associated herpesvirus) transforming gene. *J. Virol.* 72:4980–88
126. Kliche S, Nagel W, Kremmer E, Atzler C, Ege A, et al. 2001. Signaling by human herpesvirus 8 kaposin A through direct membrane recruitment of cytohesin-1. *Mol. Cell* 7:833–43
127. McCormick C, Ganem D. 2005. The kaposin B protein of KSHV activates the p38/MK2 pathway and stabilizes cytokine mRNAs. *Science* 307:739–41
128. Shaw G, Kamen R. 1986. A conserved AU sequence from the 3′ untranslated region of GM-CSF mRNA mediates selective mRNA degradation. *Cell* 46:659–67
129. Kotlyarov A, Gaestel M. 2002. Is MK2 (mitogen-activated protein kinase-activated protein kinase 2) the key for understanding post-transcriptional regulation of gene expression? *Biochem. Soc. Trans.* 30:959–63
130. Martin DF, Kuppermann BD, Wolitz RA, Palestine AG, Li H, Robinson CA. 1999. Oral ganciclovir for patients with cytomegalovirus retinitis treated with a ganciclovir implant. Roche Ganciclovir Study Group. *N. Engl. J. Med.* 340:1063–70
131. Nicholas J. 2003. Human herpesvirus-8-encoded signalling ligands and receptors. *J. Biomed. Sci.* 10:475–89
132. Sozzani S, Luini W, Bianchi G, Allavena P, Wells TN, et al. 1998. The viral chemokine macrophage inflammatory protein-II is a selective Th2 chemoattractant. *Blood* 92:4036–39
133. Stine JT, Wood C, Hill M, Epp A, Raport CJ, et al. 2000. KSHV-encoded CC chemokine vMIP-III is a CCR4 agonist, stimulates angiogenesis, and selectively chemoattracts TH2 cells. *Blood* 95:1151–57
134. Haque NS, Fallon JT, Taubman MB, Harpel PC. 2001. The chemokine receptor CCR8 mediates human endothelial cell chemotaxis induced by I-309 and Kaposi sarcoma herpesvirus-encoded vMIP-I and by lipoprotein(a)-stimulated endothelial cell conditioned medium. *Blood* 97:39–45
135. Aoki Y, Jaffe ES, Chang Y, Jones K, Teruya-Feldstein J, et al. 1999. Angiogenesis and hematopoiesis induced by Kaposi's sarcoma-associated herpesvirus-encoded interleukin-6. *Blood* 93:4034–43
136. Chatterjee M, Osborne J, Bestetti G, Chang Y, Moore PS. 2002. Viral IL-6-induced cell proliferation and immune evasion of interferon activity. *Science* 298:1432–35
137. Kirshner JR, Staskus K, Haase A, Lagunoff M, Ganem D. 1999. Expression of the open reading frame 74 (G-protein-coupled receptor) gene of Kaposi's sarcoma (KS)-associated herpesvirus: implications for KS pathogenesis. *J. Virol.* 73:6006–14

138. Chiou CJ, Poole LJ, Kim PS, Ciufo DM, Cannon JS, et al. 2002. Patterns of gene expression and a transactivation function exhibited by the vGCR (ORF74) chemokine receptor protein of Kaposi's sarcoma-associated herpesvirus. *J. Virol.* 76:3421–39
139. Cesarman E, Nador RG, Bai F, Bohenzky RA, Russo JJ, et al. 1996. Kaposi's sarcoma-associated herpesvirus contains G protein-coupled receptor and cyclin D homologs which are expressed in Kaposi's sarcoma and malignant lymphoma. *J. Virol.* 70:8218–23
140. Arvanitakis L, Geras-Raaka E, Varma A, Gershengorn MC, Cesarman E. 1997. Human herpesvirus KSHV encodes a constitutively active G-protein-coupled receptor linked to cell proliferation. *Nature* 385:347–50
141. Gershengorn MC, Geras-Raaka E, Varma A, Clark-Lewis I. 1998. Chemokines activate Kaposi's sarcoma-associated herpesvirus G protein-coupled receptor in mammalian cells in culture. *J. Clin. Invest.* 102:1469–72
142. Sodhi A, Montaner S, Patel V, Zohar M, Bais C, et al. 2000. The Kaposi's sarcoma-associated herpes virus G protein-coupled receptor up-regulates vascular endothelial growth factor expression and secretion through mitogen-activated protein kinase and p38 pathways acting on hypoxia-inducible factor 1 alpha. *Cancer Res.* 60:4873–80
143. Smit MJ, Verzijl D, Casarosa P, Navis M, Timmerman H, Leurs R. 2002. Kaposi's sarcoma-associated herpesvirus-encoded G protein-coupled receptor ORF74 constitutively activates p44/p42 MAPK and Akt via G(i) and phospholipase C-dependent signaling pathways. *J. Virol.* 76:1744–52
144. Schwarz M, Murphy PM. 2001. Kaposi's sarcoma-associated herpesvirus G protein-coupled receptor constitutively activates NF-kappa B and induces proinflammatory cytokine and chemokine production via a C-terminal signaling determinant. *J. Immunol.* 167:505–13
145. Bais C, Santomasso B, Coso O, Arvanitakis L, Raaka EG, et al. 1998. G-protein-coupled receptor of Kaposi's sarcoma-associated herpesvirus is a viral oncogene and angiogenesis activator. *Nature* 391:86–89
146. Polson AG, Wang D, DeRisi J, Ganem D. 2002. Modulation of host gene expression by the constitutively active G protein-coupled receptor of Kaposi's sarcoma-associated herpesvirus. *Cancer Res.* 62:4525–30
147. Yang TY, Chen SC, Leach MW, Manfra D, Homey B, et al. 2000. Transgenic expression of the chemokine receptor encoded by human herpesvirus 8 induces an angioproliferative disease resembling Kaposi's sarcoma. *J. Exp. Med.* 191:445–54
148. Guo HG, Sadowska M, Reid W, Tschachler E, Hayward G, Reitz M. 2003. Kaposi's sarcoma-like tumors in a human herpesvirus 8 ORF74 transgenic mouse. *J. Virol.* 77:2631–39
149. Montaner S, Sodhi A, Molinolo A, Bugge TH, Sawai ET, et al. 2003. Endothelial infection with KSHV genes in vivo reveals that vGPCR initiates Kaposi's sarcomagenesis and can promote the tumorigenic potential of viral latent genes. *Cancer Cell* 3:23–36
150. Glaunsinger B, Ganem D. 2004. Lytic KSHV infection inhibits host gene expression by accelerating global mRNA turnover. *Mol. Cell* 13:713–23
151. Glaunsinger B, Ganem D. 2004. Highly selective escape from Kaposi's sarcoma associated herpesvirus-mediated host shutoff: implications for the pathogenesis of Kaposi's sarcoma. *J. Exp. Med.* 200:391–98
152. Engels EA, Biggar RJ, Marshall VA, Walters MA, Gamache CJ, et al. 2003. Detection and quantification of Kaposi's sarcoma-associated herpesvirus to predict AIDS-associated Kaposi's sarcoma. *AIDS* 17:1847–51

153. Whitby D, Howard MR, Tenant-Flowers M, Brink NS, Copas A, et al. 1995. Detection of Kaposi sarcoma associated herpesvirus in peripheral blood of HIV-infected individuals and progression to Kaposi's sarcoma. *Lancet* 346:799–802
154. Campbell TB, Borok M, Gwanzura L, MaWhinney S, White IE, et al. 2000. Relationship of human herpesvirus 8 peripheral blood virus load and Kaposi's sarcoma clinical stage. *AIDS* 14:2109–16
155. Quinlivan EB, Zhang C, Stewart PW, Komoltri C, Davis MG, Wehbie RS. 2002. Elevated virus loads of Kaposi's sarcoma-associated human herpesvirus 8 predict Kaposi's sarcoma disease progression, but elevated levels of human immunodeficiency virus type 1 do not. *J. Infect. Dis.* 185:1736–44
156. Cannon MJ, Dollard SC, Black JB, Edlin BR, Hannah C, et al. 2003. Risk factors for Kaposi's sarcoma in men seropositive for both human herpesvirus 8 and human immunodeficiency virus. *AIDS* 17:215–22
157. Ruff K, Baskin GB, Simpson L, Murphey-Corb M, Levy LS. 2003. Rhesus rhadinovirus infection in healthy and SIV-infected macaques at Tulane National Primate Research Center. *J. Med. Primatol.* 32:1–6
158. Sturzl M, Blasig C, Schreier A, Neipel F, Hohenadl C, et al. 1997. Expression of HHV-8 latency-associated T0.7 RNA in spindle cells and endothelial cells of AIDS-associated, classical and African Kaposi's sarcoma. *Int. J. Cancer* 72:68–71

Inflammation and Atherosclerosis

Göran K. Hansson, Anna-Karin L. Robertson, and Cecilia Söderberg-Nauclér

Department of Medicine and Center for Molecular Medicine, Karolinska Institute, Stockholm SE-17176, Sweden; email: Goran.Hansson@ki.se, Anna-Karin.Robertson@yale.edu, cecilia.soderberg.naucler@ki.se

Annu. Rev. Pathol. Mech. Dis. 2006. 1:297–329

First published online as a Review in Advance on October 26, 2005

The *Annual Review of Pathology: Mechanisms of Disease* is online at pathmechdis.annualreviews.org

doi: 10.1146/annurev.pathol.1.110304.100100

1553-4006/06/0114-0297$20.00

Key Words

adaptive immunity, autoimmunity, hypercholesterolemia, innate immunity, myocardial infarction, stroke, thrombosis

Abstract

Atherosclerosis, the cause of myocardial infarction, stroke, and ischemic gangrene, is an inflammatory disease. The atherosclerotic process is initiated when cholesterol-containing low-density lipoproteins accumulate in the intima and activate the endothelium. Leukocyte adhesion molecules and chemokines promote recruitment of monocytes and T cells. Monocytes differentiate into macrophages and upregulate pattern recognition receptors, including scavenger receptors and toll-like receptors. Scavenger receptors mediate lipoprotein internalization, which leads to foam-cell formation. Toll-like receptors transmit activating signals that lead to the release of cytokines, proteases, and vasoactive molecules. T cells in lesions recognize local antigens and mount T helper-1 responses with secretion of pro-inflammatory cytokines that contribute to local inflammation and growth of the plaque. Intensified inflammatory activation may lead to local proteolysis, plaque rupture, and thrombus formation, which causes ischemia and infarction. Inflammatory markers are already used to monitor the disease process and anti-inflammatory therapy may be useful to control disease activity.

CAD: coronary artery disease

Plaque: mature atherosclerotic lesion, synonymous with atheroma

LDL: low-density lipoprotein

Atheroma: raised atherosclerotic lesion with a lipid core containing both foam cells and extracellular lipid, also a type IV lesion

Fatty streak (type II–III lesions): early lesions containing foam cells

INTRODUCTION

Atherosclerosis is the underlying cause of most cardiovascular diseases, including coronary artery disease (CAD), ischemic gangrene, abdominal aortic aneurysms, and many cases of heart failure and stroke. This group of diseases constitutes the main cause of death in the Western world today. In addition, the World Health Organization expects cardiovascular disease to be the major killer globally within 15 years owing to both its rapidly increasing prevalence in developing countries and Eastern Europe and an accumulation of metabolic risk factors, including obesity and diabetes, in the Western world. These facts underscore the need for intensified research in parallel with increased preventive measures against atherosclerotic diseases.

Nearly 20 years ago, activated T lymphocytes and HLA class II expression were detected in atherosclerotic plaques. At the same time, vascular cells were found to produce, as well as respond to, immune cytokines. Together, these findings strongly suggested that immune mechanisms are involved in atherosclerosis. Additional support came from the findings that auto-antibodies against oxidized low-density lipoprotein (oxLDL) and heat shock protein (HSP) 60 are associated with atherosclerotic cardiovascular disease.

In spite of all this, scientists were generally skeptical of the immune hypothesis of atherosclerosis. However, recent experimental, clinical, and epidemiological studies have confirmed that inflammation plays an important role in atherosclerosis, revealed cross-talk between inflammation and lipid metabolism, identified inflammatory molecules as markers of disease activity, and suggested inflammatory targets for possible future therapy.

HISTOPATHOLOGY OF ATHEROSCLEROSIS REVEALS AN IMMUNE/INFLAMMATORY PROCESS

Atherosclerotic lesions, termed atheromas or atherosclerotic plaques, typically present as asymmetric focal thickenings of the innermost layer of the artery, the intima. The lesions are composed of cells, connective tissue elements, lipids, and debris. Most of the cells found in atheromas are blood-borne inflammatory/immune cells, and the remainder are vascular endothelial and smooth muscle cells. The atheroma is preceded chronologically by so-called fatty streaks, which are sites of accumulation of lipid droplets and immune cells. Lipid-laden macrophages (termed foam cells because of the bubbly appearance of lipid droplets throughout their cytoplasm) dominate these fatty streaks, which also contain T cells, dendritic cells, and mast cells. Fatty streaks are prevalent in young individuals, never cause symptoms, and may either progress into atheromas or disappear with time.

The atheroma is structurally more complex than the fatty streak. In the center of the atheroma, macrophage foam cells, dead cells, and extracellular lipid droplets form a core region surrounded by a cap of smooth muscle cells and a collagen-rich matrix. Immunocompetent T cells and macrophages infiltrate throughout the lesion and are particularly abundant (*a*) in the shoulder region where the atheroma grows and (*b*) at the interface between cap and core. Many of the immune cells in the atheroma exhibit signs of activation and produce pro-inflammatory cytokines.

GENE-TARGETED MOUSE MODELS PERMIT DISSECTION OF MOLECULAR PATHOGENESIS

For studies of early phases of atherosclerosis, we have to rely on animal models. Previously, fat-fed rabbits, primates, and mice were often used as models. Now, however, these models have largely been replaced by two knockout mouse strains that develop hypercholesterolemia and atherosclerosis (1). The apolipoprotein E (*apoE*) homozygous knockout (−/−) mouse develops spontaneous atherosclerosis that culminates in myocardial infarction, stroke, and aneurysm (2, 3), whereas the LDL receptor (*Ldlr*) −/− mouse responds to fat feeding by hypercholesterolemia and lesion development. Crosses of these knockouts with mice that carry deletions in genes of the immune system have provided important information on the pathogenesis of atherosclerosis. In addition, bone marrow transplantation and adoptive cell transfer have offered insights into the role of specific populations of blood-borne cells in disease development.

ATHEROSCLEROSIS: AN INFLAMMATORY RESPONSE TO LIPOPROTEIN RETENTION

The early phase of atherosclerotic disease is best explained as an inflammatory response elicited by retention of lipoproteins in the arterial intima.

The Initiation Phase: Recruitment of Inflammatory Cells to the Artery Wall

Hypercholesterolemia and hypertension, two major risk factors for atherosclerosis, cause focal endothelial activation in large- and medium-sized arteries. When plasma levels of the cholesterol-rich very low-density lipoprotein (VLDL) and LDL rise, the lipoproteins infiltrate the artery wall to an extent that exceeds the capacity for elimination and are retained in the extracellular matrix (**Figure 1**) (4). This is an initiating step in atherosclerosis (5).

LDL modification, through enzymatic attack or non-enzymatic oxidation in the intima, leads to release of bioactive phospholipids that can activate endothelial cells (6) (**Figure 1**). Activated endothelial cells express several types of leukocyte adhesion molecules, which cause blood cells rolling on the vascular surface to adhere at the site of activation (7). As the vascular cell adhesion molecule-1 (VCAM-1) is typically upregulated in response to such stimuli, cells carrying counter-receptors for VCAM-1, i.e., monocytes and lymphocytes, preferentially adhere to these sites (8) (**Figure 1**). Several phospholipid species generated during lipoprotein oxidation can modulate endothelial functions (9, 10). Therefore, the precise spectrum of local phospholipids may be decisive for the extent of vascular inflammation at sites of lipoprotein oxidation. In addition to mononuclear leukocytes, platelets also adhere to activated endothelial cells. Inhibition of platelet adhesion reduces leukocyte infiltration and atherosclerosis in hypercholesterolemic mice (11).

Endothelial activation occurs preferentially at sites of hemodynamic strain (12). Hemodynamic flow patterns typical for atherosclerosis-prone segments (low average shear but high oscillatory shear stress) cause increased expression of adhesion molecules and inflammatory genes by endothelial cells (13) and may, like LDL accumulation, promote inflammation.

Once adherent to the endothelium, leukocytes migrate into the underlying intima in response to chemoattractant stimuli including chemokines (**Figure 1**). Several different categories of chemokines may participate in recruitment of distinct leukocyte classes to the atheroma. Monocyte chemoattractant protein-1 (MCP-1 or CCL2) attracts leukocytes bearing the chemokine receptor CCR2, i.e., monocytes and T and B cells (14, 15). RANTES or CCL5 (which binds

VCAM: vascular cell adhesion molecule

IFN: interferon

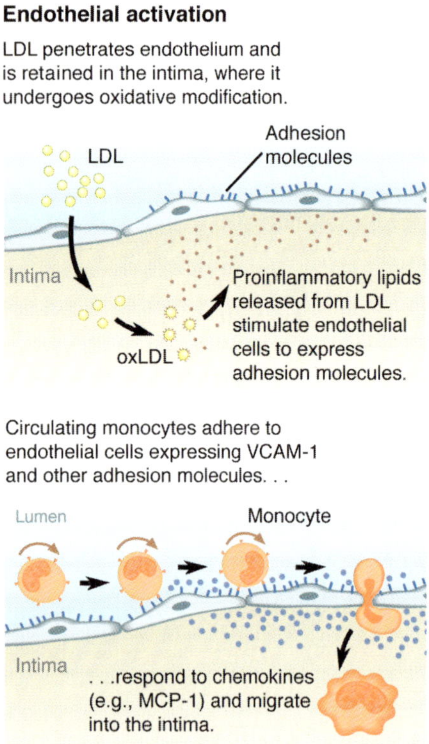

Figure 1

Recruitment and activation of macrophages in atheroma. Macrophages, which are abundant in atheroma, are recruited from blood monocytes that enter through the surface endothelium. In advanced lesions, plaque microvessels may also provide a route of entry for monocytes. Several leukocyte adhesion molecules and chemokines govern the recruitment process, which is followed by differentiation of the monocytes into macrophages. During this process, pattern recognition receptors, such as scavenger receptors (ScRs), are upregulated. ScRs mediate the uptake of oxidized low-density lipoprotein (oxLDL), and cause the accumulation of LDL-derived cholesterol and foam-cell formation. Other macrophages are primed for activation when stimulated by the T cell cytokine, interferon-γ (IFNγ). These macrophages are activated by pathogen-associated molecular patterns that ligate toll-like receptors (TLRs), as well as the pro-inflammatory cytokines interleukin (IL)-1 and tumor necrosis factor (TNF). As a result of activation, the macrophages release a host of pro-inflammatory mediators, including reactive oxygen and nitrogen species, pro-inflammatory cytokines, vasoactive molecules, and several kinds of proteases. Th1, T helper-1; MCP-1, monocyte chemoattractant protein-1; M-CSF, macrophage-colony-stimulating factor; VCAM-1, vascular cell adhesion molecule-1; HSP60, heat shock protein 60.

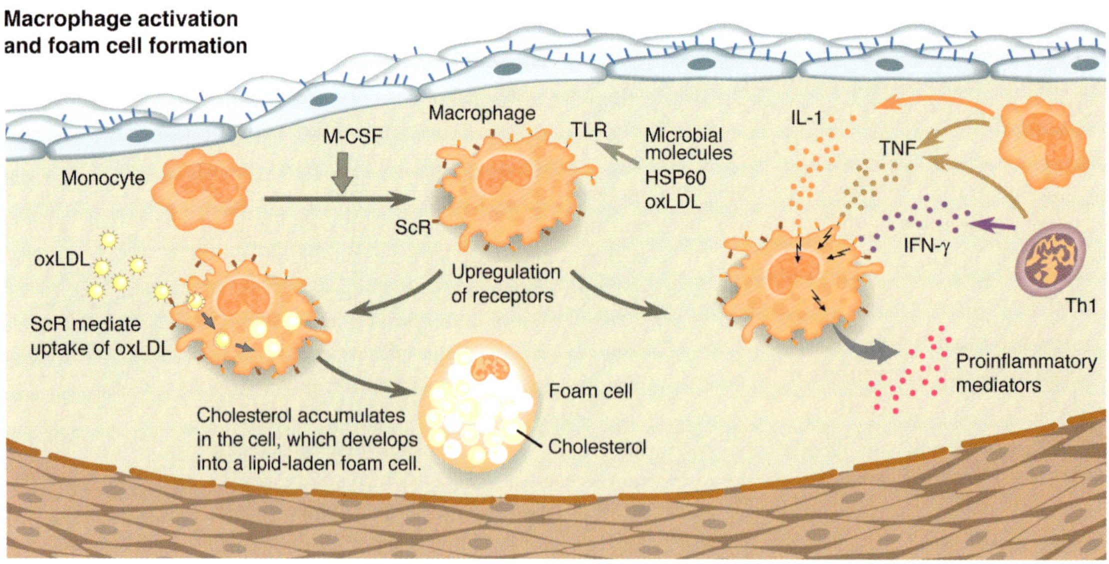

to CCR1 on T cells), IP-10 (or CXCL10), monokine induced by interferon (IFN)-γ (Mig or CXCL9), IFN-inducible T cell α-chemoattractant (I-TAC or CXCL11) [which all bind to CXCR3 on T cells (16)], and eotaxin (CCL11) [involved in the recruitment of CCR3+ eosinophils (17)] are all found in human and experimental lesions. Gene targeting of MCP-1 or CCR2 inhibits disease development (14, 15), as does pharmacological blockade of RANTES (18). The membrane-bound chemokine, fractalkine (CX3CL1), is also expressed and promotes recruitment of CX3CR1+ mononuclear cells to the forming lesion (19). Thus, a spectrum of different chemokines mediates chemotactic recruitment of adherent monocytes and lymphocytes to the forming lesion.

Macrophages Expressing Pattern Recognition Receptors Dominate the Forming Plaque

A cytokine/growth factor produced in the inflamed intima, macrophage-colony-stimulating factor (M-CSF), induces entering monocytes to differentiate into macrophages (**Figure 1**). Macrophage differentiation is a necessary step for atherosclerosis (20) and is associated with upregulation of pattern recognition receptors for innate immunity, including scavenger receptors (ScRs) and toll-like receptors (TLRs) (21).

ScRs internalize a broad range of molecules and particles carrying pathogen-like molecular patterns (22). Bacterial endotoxins, apoptotic cell fragments, and oxLDL particles are all taken up and degraded through this pathway. If cholesterol derived from uptake of oxLDL cannot be mobilized from the cell to a sufficient extent, it accumulates as cytosolic droplets. This process is augmented in inflammation because pro-inflammatory cytokines and endotoxins inhibit expression of ATP-binding cassette transporters ABCA1 and ABCG1, which export cholesterol from the cell (23, 24). Consequently, the macrophage transforms into a foam cell, the prototypic cell of atherosclerosis (**Figure 1**).

Unlike ScRs, TLRs do not mediate endocytosis; instead, when bound by ligands with pathogen-like molecular patterns, TLRs initiate a signal cascade that leads to macrophage activation (25) (**Figure 1**). Similar effects are observed in dendritic cells, mast cells, and endothelial cells, which also express TLR (26).

Bacterial toxins, stress proteins, and DNA motifs are all recognized by various TLRs (26). In addition, HSP60 and oxLDL may activate these receptors (27, 28). Cells in human atherosclerotic lesions display a spectrum of TLR types (29, 30). As many of these cells exhibit signs of nuclear factor (NF) κB activation (30), it is possible that plaque inflammation depends partly on this pathway (31). In support of this notion, targeted gene deletion of TLR4 or MyD88, a key molecule in the TLR signaling pathway, inhibits atherosclerosis in *apoE−/−* mice (32, 33).

Glycated macromolecules, which are produced in increased amounts in diabetics, promote inflammation by a similar mechanism as TLR ligands (34). Advanced glycation endproducts (AGE) bind to receptors for AGE on macrophages, endothelial cells, and smooth muscle cells. This triggers NFκB activation, promotes vascular inflammation, and increases atherosclerosis in hypercholesterolemic mice (35).

Macrophage activation in atheroma leads to release of vasoactive molecules such as nitric oxide, endothelins, and several eicosanoids (36, 37) (**Figure 1**). The activated macrophages also produce reactive oxygen species. This production has important consequences for lipoprotein oxidation and cytotoxicity (38). Finally, activated macrophages secrete proteolytic enzymes that may degrade matrix components. The loss of matrix components may subsequently lead to destabilization of plaques and an increased risk for plaque rupture and thrombosis (39–42).

Pattern recognition receptors: broad-specificity receptors that bind ligands with pathogen-associated molecular patterns

TLR: toll-like receptor

MHC: major histocompatibility complex

ACS: acute coronary syndrome

Activation of macrophages may take place not only after ligation of their pattern recognition receptors, but also as part of antigen-dependent activation of the adaptive arm of immunity (21). In the latter case, macrophages play a dual role by (*a*) presenting antigen to T cells and (*b*) subsequently responding to cytokines produced by activated T cells (**Figures 1** and **2**).

T Cells in Lesion Development and Progression

T cells are recruited to the forming lesion by mechanisms similar to monocyte recruitment (**Figure 2**). However, their pattern of activation differs, as T cell activation is dependent upon recognition of cognate antigens and simultaneous ligation of costimulatory receptors.

T cells infiltrate plaques. CD4+ T cells dominate over CD8+ cells in human atherosclerotic plaques (43). Most of the T cells bear antigen receptors of the T cell receptor (TCR) $\alpha\beta$ type (44, 45) and are often found in clusters in shoulder regions of the lesion (43, 46). Major histocompatibility complex (MHC) class II–expressing macrophages and dendritic cells can be detected close to these T cells. This observation suggests that there is an ongoing immune activation in atheromas (46–50).

T cells in atheromas display an activated/memory phenotype (44), and the proportion of activated T cells is particularly high in plaques that cause acute coronary syndrome (ACS) (51, 52). Recruitment of these cells depends upon the spectrum of adhesion molecules and chemokine receptors expressed by these cells (**Figure 2**) and follows the same principles as outlined above for monocytes.

Although T cells are recruited to tissues in an antigen-independent manner, antigen-induced activation initiates proliferation and expansion of antigen-specific clones (53–55). Therefore, antigen-specific expansion is likely to be important for plaque inflammation, growth, and activation.

Role of T and B cells in mouse models of disease. To study the role of lymphocytes in atherosclerosis, *Rag-1−/−*, *Rag-2−/−*, and *scid/scid* mice lacking mature T and B cells were crossed with *apoE−/−* or *Ldlr−/−* mice (56–59). Compared with immunocompetent *apoE−/−* mice, the immunodeficient ones develop much smaller lesions. Transfer of CD4+ T cells from older *apoE−/−* mice to *apoE−/− scid/scid* mice restored lesion development almost to the levels found in *apoE−/−* mice. This result indicates that CD4+ cells are pro-atherogenic in the context of hypercholesterolemia (58).

CD8+ T lymphocytes, although less abundant than CD4+ cells (43), may also contribute to atherosclerosis. For instance, activation of antigen-specific CD8+ cells by an artificial smooth muscle antigen in a transgenic model leads to severely accelerated atherosclerosis in the $apoE^{-/-}$ model (60). Different subsets of CD8+ cells may exert different effects in atherosclerosis, including direct cytotoxicity and secretion of proinflammatory cytokines.

Costimulation. Activation of naïve T cells requires two signals: (*a*) ligation of the antigen receptor by antigen/MHC and (*b*) ligation of the costimulatory molecule CD28 on T cells by CD80 or CD86 on the antigen-presenting cell (APC). In addition, interaction between CD40-ligand (CD40L or CD154) on T cells and CD40 on APC is important for T cell activation. Abrogation of either of these interactions inhibits atherosclerosis.

T cells, APC, platelets, macrophages, endothelial cells, and smooth muscle cells in atherosclerotic lesions can express CD40L as well as CD40 (61). Interruption of the CD40-CD40L pathway in hypercholesterolemic mice by treatment with anti-CD40L antibodies or targeted CD40L gene deletion results in

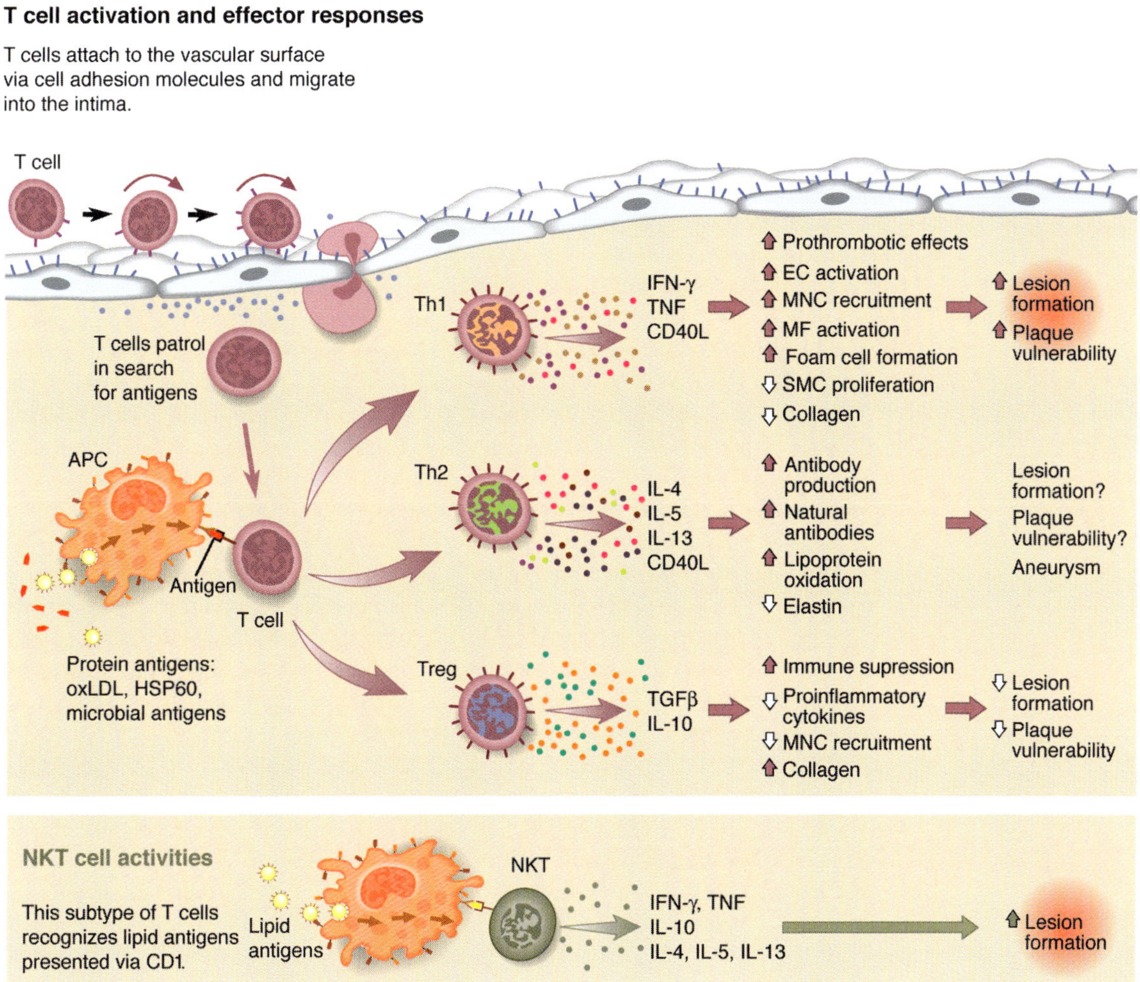

Figure 2

Recruitment and activation of T cells in atheromas. T cells enter the developing atheroma guided by adhesion molecules and chemokines. They respond to local peptide antigens [e.g., oxidized low-density lipoprotein (oxLDL), heat shock protein (HSP) 60, and microbial antigens] bound to major histocompatibility complex (MHC) molecules on the surface of antigen-presenting cells (APCs). T cell activation can lead to several types of effector responses, among which the T helper-1 (Th1) response is most prevalent in atheroma. The Th1 response involves several pro-inflammatory cytokines and promotes lesion formation and plaque vulnerability. Regulatory T cells (Treg) inhibit this process, whereas the role of Th2 cells remains controversial. Natural killer T (NKT) cells recognize lipid antigens presented by CD1 molecules and elicit effector responses similar to those of MHC-restricted T cells. IFN, interferon; TNF, tumor necrosis factor; EC, endothelial cell; MNC, mononuclear cells; MF, macrophages; SMC, smooth muscle cells; TFGβ, transforming growth factor beta; IL, interleukin.

TNF: tumor necrosis factor

MDA: malondialdehyde

reduction and stabilization of lesions (62–65). However, attempts to develop CD40 blockade as anti-atherosclerotic therapy has been hampered by thrombotic complications that probably depend on platelet expression of CD40L (66).

In human atherosclerotic lesions, CD80 and CD86 are detected on macrophages and CD28 is expressed by T cells (67). *Ldlr−/−* mice deficient in CD80 and CD86 exhibit reduced lesion development with decreased MHC class II expression (68). Cross-talk between the CD28-CD80/86 and CD40L-CD40 pathways may also be important for lesion development.

A third pair of costimulatory molecules for T cell activation, OX40 and its ligand (OX40L), were recently implicated in atherosclerosis in a genetic study (69). A genetic locus conferring susceptibility to atherosclerosis in mice, *Ath1*, was found to be identical to *OX40L*; the same gene was identified as a genetic risk factor for myocardial infarction in humans. OX40L is expressed in atherosclerotic lesions (69) and is important for the generation of memory/effector T cells (70). The T cell protein OX40 (CD134) is a member of the tumor necrosis factor (TNF) receptor superfamily, which contains several other molecules involved in immune activation (70); it is possible that other members of the family also contribute to atherosclerosis.

Antigens Implicated in Atherogenesis

Several antigens have been associated with atherosclerosis. Ten percent of CD4+ T cell clones derived from human plaques respond to oxLDL as an MHC class II–restricted antigen (53). Other plaque T cells react to *Chlamydia pneumoniae* (71, 72) and HSP65/60 derived from several pathogens (73, 74).

Molecular mimicry, a phenomenon in which cross-reactivity between self molecules and foreign molecules on pathogens can lead to antiself responses, can also cause T cell reactivity in atheromas. Immune responses to microbial HSP65/60 are also activated by human HSP60, which is expressed in human atherosclerotic lesions (45) and by macrophages exposed to oxLDL (75). Antibodies to HSP are increased in patients with atherosclerosis (76, 77), and parenteral immunization with HSP65/60 aggravates fatty streak formation in mice and rabbits (78, 79).

Altered self molecules may also elicit immune responses. Lipid peroxidation of polyunsaturated fatty acids in the phospholipids and cholesteryl esters of LDL during the formation of oxLDL also results in the production of reactive aldehydes that can create additional immunogenic neoepitopes by binding to lysine and histidine residues in the apolipoprotein B (ApoB) component of LDL (80). The increased antibody titers to oxLDL found in atherosclerotic patients and experimental animals (81) contain antibodies to both native and malondialdehyde (MDA)-modified peptide sequences of ApoB (82), as well as to the oxidized phospholipid components of LDL (83).

"Natural" antibodies to phospholipids such as phosphocholine are produced by B1 cells, a subset of B cells, even without immunization. These antibodies are produced in the absence of T cells, are usually of IgM type, increase upon immunization, and cross-react with phospholipids on apoptotic cells, oxLDL, and the capsule of *Streptococcus pneumoniae* (84). Interestingly, vaccination with *S. pneumoniae* reduces atherosclerosis in *apoE−/−* mice. This result suggests that phospholipid immunity is atheroprotective (see below) (83).

β2-glycoprotein I (β2GPI) is a phospholipid-binding protein found on platelets, on endothelial cells and in human atherosclerotic plaques (85). Auto-antibodies against β2GPI have been found in patients with different inflammatory disorders, including atherosclerosis (86). Immunization with human β2GPI accelerates atherosclerotic lesions in *LDLR−/−* mice (87). It is possible that some of the immune reactions to β2GPI are directed against phospholipids bound to this protein.

These data show that several T cell–dependent and –independent antigens are present in atherosclerotic plaques, elicit immune responses, and may contribute to disease progression. This contribution to disease progression probably occurs through stimulation of immune effector responses involving immune cytokines.

Predominance of T Helper-1 Effector Cells and Cytokines

CD4+ T cells differentiate into several subtypes, among them T helper-1 (Th1) effector cells (which produce IFNγ and TNF), Th2 cells (which secrete IL-4, IL-5, and IL-13), and several types of regulatory T cells (**Figure 2**). Th1 cells induce macrophage activation and delayed-type hypersensitivity, whereas Th2 cells promote eosinophilic inflammation and allergy-type reactions. Regulatory T cells suppress the effector functions of other immune cells.

Data from human and animal studies show a predominant Th1 pattern in atherosclerosis. The prototypic Th1 cytokine IFNγ is produced locally (53, 88), as are the Th1-stimulating cytokines IL-12 and IL-18 (89, 90). In contrast, only small amounts of IL-4 and IL-5 have been detected (91, 92). This contrasts with atherosclerotic aneurysms, in which Th2 cells dominate the infiltrates (93).

Th1 differentiation depends upon the transcription factor, T-bet. In its absence, Th1 effector cells do not develop; this leads to significant reduction of atherosclerosis in hypercholesterolemic mice (**Table 1**). Analogously, deletion of the Th1-inducing cytokines IL-12 and IL-18 (**Table 1**) or administration of either the Th1 inhibitory drug pentoxifyllin (94) or IL-18 binding protein (95) reduces disease, whereas administration of either IL-12 or IL-18 increases lesion size (96, 97).

IFNγ is a major pro-atherogenic Th1 cytokine. It promotes macrophage and endothelial activation with production of adhesion molecules, cytokines, chemokines, radicals, proteases, and coagulation factors. In addition, IFNγ inhibits cell proliferation, collagen production, and cholesterol efflux (**Table 2**). Targeted deletion of IFNγ or its receptor reduces disease (**Table 2**) whereas administration of recombinant IFNγ acclerates lesion development in hypercholesterolemic mice (98) as well as in allotransplanted arteries (99). Although Th1 cells are major sources of IFNγ, this cytokine can also be produced by CD8+ T cells, natural killer T (NKT) cells, NK cells, and IL-18 stimulated smooth muscle cells (100, 101).

TNF, also known as TNFα, is produced by Th1 cells, macrophages, and NK cells. It acts through NFκB, is pro-inflammatory and cytotoxic, and inhibits key metabolic enzymes including lipoprotein lipase. Gene targeting of TNF leads to reduced atherosclerosis, similar to the effects of IFNγ (101a, 231). The related cytokine lymphotoxin (TNFβ) is also produced by Th1 cells and exerts similar effects. IL-1, produced by vascular cells as well as macrophages, has a spectrum of action that overlaps partly with TNF and TLR ligands, with induction of metalloproteinases, nitric oxide synthase, and adhesion molecules.

Complex roles of T helper-2 cytokines. Th2 cytokines include IL-4, IL-5, and IL-13; however, Th2 cells also produce other cytokines including IL-3, IL-10, and granulocyte-monocyte-colony-stimulating factor (GM-CSF). IL-4 and IL-13 are major stimuli for antibody production, whereas IL-5 promotes eosinophilic inflammation as well as antibody secretion. The role of IL-4, which is important in allergic inflammation and stimulates both B cells and mast cells in atherosclerosis, has been investigated using fat-fed mice of the C57BL/6 strain. Unfortunately, these studies have yielded

Table 1 Effects of immune defects on atherosclerosis in gene-targeted mouse models

Immune function under study	Immune system gene deleted	Mouse model used	Effect of gene deletion on atherosclerosis	References
Adaptive immunity	*Rag-1*	*apoE−/−*	Reduced atherosclerosis (depending on diet)	(56, 57)
Adaptive immunity	*SCID*	*apoE−/−*	Reduced atherosclerosis	(58)
Antigen recognition	*TCRαβ*	*apoE−/−*	Reduced atherosclerosis	(224)
Antigen presentation	*CD1*	*apoE−/−*	Reduced atherosclerosis	(132–134)
Antigen recognition	*CD4*	*apoE−/−*	Varying effect	(224, 225)
Antigen recognition	*CD8*	*apoE−/−*	No effect	(224)
Costimulation	*CD80, CD86*	*Ldlr−/−*	Reduced atherosclerosis	(68)
Costimulation	*CD40L*	*apoE−/−*	Reduced atherosclerosis	(63)
Th1 polarization	*IL-12*	*apoE−/−*	Reduced atherosclerosis	(105)
Th1 polarization	*IL-18*	*apoE−/−*	Reduced atherosclerosis	(226)
Th1 polarization	*T-bet*	*Ldlr−/−*	Reduced atherosclerosis	(227)
Th1/IFNγ	*IFNγR*	*apoE−/−*	Reduced atherosclerosis	(228)
Th1/IFNγ	*IFNγ*	*apoE−/−*, *Ldlr−/−*	Reduced atherosclerosis	(229, 230)
Th1/inflammation	*TNF*	*apoE−/−*	Reduced atherosclerosis	(101a)
Anti-inflammatory cytokine	*IL-10*	*apoE−/−*	Increased atherosclerosis	(123)
Th2	*IL-4*	*apoE−/−*, *Ldlr−/−*	Decreased atherosclerosis	(104, 105)
Th2	*IL-5*	*Ldlr−/−*	Increased atherosclerosis	(108)
Anti-inflammatory cytokine	*TGFβ*	*apoE−/−*	Increased atherosclerosis	(118)
Downstream cytokine	*IL-6*	*apoE−/−*	Minor effect seen at late stage	(232, 233)

conflicting results (102, 103). However, studies in genetically hypercholesterolemic *apoE−/−* and *Ldlr−/−* mice point to a pro-atherogenic effect of IL-4 (104, 105). This effect may be due to the ability of IL-4 to upregulate CD36 and lipoxygenases (106, 107), while IL-4's capacity to activate mast cells may contribute to plaque destabilization and rupture. IL-4 also induces macrophages to secrete the elastolytic enzyme matrix metalloproteinase (MMP)-1, which causes matrix degradation and promotes aneurysm formation (93).

In contrast to IL-4, IL-5 is produced by mast cells as well as by Th2 cells and stimulates the growth and differentiation of eosinophils. Irradiated *Ldlr−/−* mice reconstituted with IL-5-deficient bone marrow display increased atherosclerosis (108). IL-5 also stimulates differentiation of B cells, including those producing natural antibodies such as IgM antiphosphocholine. IL-5-deficient mice have lower titers of antibody to phosphorylcholine; thus, increased natural antibody production may mediate the atheroprotective effect of IL-5.

Regulatory T cells and anti-inflammatory cytokines. Regulatory T cells are implicated in maintenance of self-tolerance and control

Table 2 Atherogenic effects of IFNγ

Indicator	Change in indicator
Th1 response	Increased
Expression of MHC class II, CD40, CD40L, CD80 and CD86 (MØ)	Increased
Expression of MHC class II (SMC[b] and EC[c])	Increased
Expression of VCAM-1 (SMC)	Increased
Expression of ICAM-1 (MØ)	Increased
Expression of CXCL16 (MØ), SRA[d] (SMC)	Increased
Expression of ABCA-1 (MØ)	Decreased
SMC proliferation	Decreased
SMC differentiation	Decreased
Collagen synthesis (SMC)	Decreased
EC proliferation	Decreased
EC fibrinolytic activity	Decreased
Synthesis of pro-inflammatory cytokines (MØ)	Increased
Procoagulant acitivity (MØ)	Increased
Production of reactive nitrogen and oxygen radicals (MØ)	Increased
Production of chemokines (EC, SMC, MØ)	Increased

[a]MØ, macrophages.
[b]SMC, smooth muscle cells.
[c]EC, endothelial cells.
[d]SRA, Scavenger Receptor-A.

of autoimmunity. Several types of regulatory T cells have been identified, including CD4+, CD25+, FoxP3+ regulatory T cells (Treg), IL-10-producing type 1 regulatory T cells (Tr1), and transforming growth factor beta (TGFβ)-producing Th3 cells (109). The suppressive effects of these regulatory T cells are mediated, at least partly, through production of TGFβ and/or IL-10 (110).

Recent reports suggest that regulatory T cells infiltrate lesions of *apoE−/−* mice (111) and that Tr1 cells may inhibit lesion growth (112). Although several studies have established a role for mediators produced by regulatory T cells, further studies will be needed to clarify the role of these cell types.

Transforming growth factor β. TGFβ is a pluripotent cytokine secreted by a number of cells, including regulatory T cells, macrophages, dendritic cells, platelets, endothelial cells, and smooth muscle cells (113). Many different cells carry TGFβ receptors and are thus sensitive to its effects. TGFβ is secreted in an inactive form and must be activated by proteolytic cleavage. It is immunosuppressive and plays an essential role in keeping the immune system in check (110, 114).

TGF: transforming growth factor

TGFβ is known to be atheroprotective, although the mechanism of this effect has been unclear (115–117). Two recent studies show that the T cell is a major target of TGFβ action in atherosclerosis. We crossed the *apoE−/−* mouse with a transgenic mouse that expresses a dominant-negative TGFβ type II receptor (dnTGFβRII) on CD4+ and CD8+ T cells (118). The offspring of this cross produces T cells that are insensitive to TGFβ, although all other aspects of TGFβ secretion and signaling remain intact. These mice exhibited a dramatic increase in atherosclerosis, with large, vulnerable lesions throughout the arterial system. In another study, Gojova and colleagues (119) transplanted bone marrow from mice that expressed dnTGFβRII under the control of the CD2 promoter into irradiated *LDLR−/−* mice (119). This treatment also led to vulnerable lesions after abrogation of TGFβ signaling in T cells, although no increase in lesion size was registered in the latter study. Taken together, these studies indicate that a major atheroprotective effect of TGFβ is due to its inhibition of T cells. Inhibition of T cell activation via the effects of TGFβ may therefore represent an important anti-atherosclerotic strategy.

Interleukin-10. IL-10 is produced by regulatory and Th2 CD4+ T cells, NK cells, macrophages, and dendritic cells. IL-10 is immunosuppressive and inhibits the secretion of other cytokines, including IFNγ, from T cells and macrophages (120). In wild-type C57Bl/6 mice, IL-10 deficiency results in increased development of fatty streaks (121, 122). Similarly, IL-10-deficient *apoE−/−* mice develop larger atherosclerotic lesions (123) (**Table 1**), as do irradiated *Ldlr−/−* mice receiving IL-10-deficient bone marrow (124). Conversely, IL-10 overexpression inhibits lesion formation in wild-type C57Bl/6, *apoE−/−*, and *LDLR−/−* mice (121, 125–127). In addition, IL-10 may promote plaque stability, with reduced pro-MMP activity, decreased collagen, reduced tissue factor activity, and lesser thrombogenicity (123, 124). As IL-10 enhances the production of TGFβ (and vice versa), these two cytokines may act in concert to stabilize atherosclerosis.

Natural killer T cells. Although all classical T cells recognize peptide fragments of protein antigens displayed on MHC molecules, a recently recognized cell type, the NKT cell, reacts to lipids displayed on CD1 molecules on the APC surface. CD1-dependent antigens include microbial glycolipids and possibly certain mammalian gangliosides (128, 129). NKT cells express TCR with α and β chains, which do not display the clonal heterogeneity typical for T cells. Therefore, the antigenic repertoire detected by CD1-dependent NKT cells is probably much smaller than that recognized by MHC-restricted T cells.

Recent data suggest that NKT cells contribute to atherosclerosis (**Figure 2**). NKT cell-specific TCR mRNA as well as CD1 molecules required for NKT cell activation are found in lesions (130, 131). CD1−/− × *apoE−/−* mice develop significantly smaller lesions than CD1+ littermates (132, 133). Conversely, activation of NKT cells by injection of a synthetic lipid antigen exacerbates lesion formation (132, 134). NKT cell activation is accompanied by elevated levels of IFNγ and other pro-inflammatory cytokines and results in increased plaque formation (135), and it is possible that NKT cell recognition of local lipid antigens is important in the initiation of atherosclerosis (**Figure 2**).

Natural killer cells. NK cells attack cells with reduced MHC expression, are not antigen-specific, and belong to the innate immune system (136). NK cells are important contributors to defense against tumors but recent studies suggest that these cells may also participate in atherosclerosis (137, 138). However, diverging results were obtained in bone marrow transfer studies employing different types of NK-cell defects. Further studies are therefore needed to clarify the role of NK cells in atherosclerosis.

Mast Cells

Mast cells, together with basophils and eosinophils, are effector cells of allergic reactions. They are activated when antigen-bound IgE cross-links their Fcε receptors. This leads to secretion of proteases (e.g., tryptase and chymase), histamine, lipid mediators (e.g., prostaglandin D_2, platelet-activating factor, and several leukotrienes), and cytokines [e.g., IL-3, TNF, macrophage inflammatory protein (MIP)-1α, IL-4, IL-5, and IL-13]. Mast cells are present in atherosclerotic lesions and are activated at sites of plaque rupture (139). Mast cells may be important in the pathology of atheromas because mast cell secretory products can modify lipoproteins, modulate the function of vascular and inflammatory cells, destroy matrix components, and impact the permeability, contractility, cell proliferation, and hemostatic properties of the vessel wall (140). Newly developed mouse models of mast cell deficiency should be helpful for clarifying the role of these cells in atherosclerosis.

B Cells and Antibodies

Only a few B cells are detected in atherosclerotic plaques (43), but substantial amounts of B cells and plasma cells are found in periadventitial lymphoid infiltrates surrounding advanced lesions (141). Several lines of evidence support the hypothesis that humoral immunity protects against atherosclerosis. Injections of intravenous immunoglobulin preparations inhibit atherosclerosis in *apoE−/−* mice (142). This effect is mediated by the Fc portion and is probably due to ligation of the inhibitory FcγRII-receptor (CD32) (143). Splenectomy (i.e., removal of the B cell–rich spleen) increases lesion development in *apoE−/−* mice, whereas B cell transfer from atherosclerotic to splenectomized *apoE−/−* mice ameliorates atherosclerosis (144). Similarly, transfer of bone marrow from *μMT* mice, which carry a targeted deletion in the transmembrane μ chain of IgM and lack mature B cells, into *Ldlr−/−* mice increases lesion growth in these animals (145). These effects may depend at least partly upon the production by B cells of antibodies against candidate antigens, including oxLDL (83, 144, 146).

Infections and Atherosclerosis

Pathogenic microorganisms may infect cells in the arterial wall, promote local inflammation, induce adaptive immune responses, and cause cellular alterations that may contribute to the development of atherosclerotic plaques. Certain common bacteria such as *C. pneumoniae*, *Mycoplasma pneumoniae*, and *Helicobacter pylori*, which cause chronic infections, as well as the herpes virus family members cytomegalovirus (CMV), Epstein-Barr virus, and herpes-simplex virus type I have all been implicated in atherosclerosis. If so, these pathogens could act either directly as the primary causative agents themselves or indirectly as contributors to the total pathogen burden that has been suggested to promote atherosclerosis (147). However, a meta-analysis supports a possible pathogenetic role in CAD only for *C. pneumoniae* and CMV (148).

C. pneumoniae and CMV are ubiquitous, with 50%–100% of the human population infected. Initial sero-epidemiological evidence for an association between *C. pneumoniae* and atherosclerosis (149) was supported by detection of this intracellular pathogen in (occasional cells of) atherosclerotic lesions (150). However, *C. pneumoniae* infection does not cause atherosclerosis in animals although it may stimulate disease progression and possibly activate plaques (151–153). This activation could be due either to direct action in plaques or to remote signaling via inflammatory mediators (154). Molecular mimicry between *C. pneumoniae* antigens and human molecules may conceivably contribute to such inflammatory activation (155). However, several secondary prevention trials that used antibiotics for the prevention of ACS (through the treatment of possible *C. pneumoniae* infections) met with limited success. This result suggests that *C. pneumoniae* infection is not a major cause of ACS (156, 157).

CMV seropositivity correlates with atherosclerosis, restenosis after coronary angioplasty, and transplant vascular sclerosis (TVS, also known as transplant arteriosclerosis or chronic vascular rejection of organ grafts) (158). CMV antigens and DNA have been detected both in TVS and atherosclerotic vessels (159–161). CMV infection in cardiac-transplant recipients doubles the rate of long-term graft failure because of accelerated TVS. CMV infection also accelerates experimental TVS (162). In addition, prophylactic administration of CMV-specific drugs decreases the risk of developing TVS (163).

CMV targets vascular endothelial and smooth muscle cells and causes endothelial expression of intercellular-adhesion molecule 1 (ICAM-1) and several chemokines (164, 165). Infected vascular smooth muscle cells express the CMV-encoded chemokine receptor homologue US28 and display increased migration in response to MCP-1 and RANTES (166). In animal studies, an atherosclerosis-like process is induced by infecting chickens with an avian herpesvirus, Marek's disease virus (167). CMV infection of *apoE−/−* mice increases lesion size, lesion T cell content, and systemic levels of IFNγ and TNF (168, 169). Although this result suggests that an immune response to CMV may aggravate early atherosclerosis, an inflammatory microenvironment in the atherosclerotic artery may also result in reactivation of virus. Viral reactivation could conceivably contribute to plaque activation and ACS. Indeed, seropositivity to CMV increases the risk of death in patients with CAD (170), and patients with acute myocardial infarction frequently develop CMV antigenemia (171).

ACUTE CORONARY SYNDROMES

Accumulating data suggest that inflammatory activation of plaques elicits coronary thrombosis, which leads to myocardial ischemia and infarction. A similar process probably leads to infarction in other vascular regions such as the cerebral circulation; however, the most comprehensive information is available from the coronary circulation.

Plaque Activation Elicits Thrombosis and Clinical Symptoms

Progressive reduction of luminal size can lead to clinical syndromes such as effort angina and intermittent claudication, but it is remarkable that even very large plaques may be completely asymptomatic (172). Acute clinical complications such as myocardial infarction and ischemic stroke are caused by the formation of a thrombus on the plaque. Thrombus formation, in turn, seems to require damage of the plaque surface. Thus, approximately 70% of coronary thrombi occur at sites of plaque fissuring, whereas 30% seem to be caused by superficial endothelial erosion (173, 174). Patients with ACS display signs of inflammation, with elevated levels of circulating cytokines, acute phase reactants, and activated T cells (175, 176). The elevated levels may reflect exacerbated plaque inflammation, which promotes or causes plaque rupture and thrombosis.

Mechanisms of Plaque Rupture

What causes a silent atherosclerotic lesion to rupture? Activated macrophages, T cells, and mast cells are found at sites of plaque rupture (51, 177, 178) and produce several types of molecules that can destabilize lesions: proinflammatory cytokines, proteases, coagulation factors, radicals, and vasoactive molecules (**Figure 3**). These agents inhibit the formation of stable fibrous caps, attack cap collagen, and initiate thrombus formation (179–182). All these reactions are likely to promote and possibly elicit plaque activation, rupture, thrombosis, and ischemia.

Three types of proteases have been implicated as key players in plaque activation: MMPs, cysteine proteases, and chymase (42, 140, 183). Several members of these families of enzymes are found in the plaque and may degrade its matrix. MMP activity is controlled at several levels. Inflammatory and immune cytokines induce the production of several MMPs, plasmin activates proforms of the enzymes, and inhibitor proteins (e.g., tissue inhibitor of metalloproteinase) suppress their action (183). Similarly, cysteine proteases are induced by certain cytokines and checked by inhibitors termed cystatins. Several of these molecules play decisive roles in aneurysm formation and cerebral hemorrhage (184, 185). However, mechanistic studies in models of atherosclerosis have yielded complex results: Certain MMPs reduce lesion size rather than increase it. At the same time, such studies show unequivocally that the activities of these enzymes impact plaque composition. Therefore, these enzymes may represent targets for future therapy. Animal models of plaque rupture will be important for determining the role of these proteases in plaque activation and myocardial infarction.

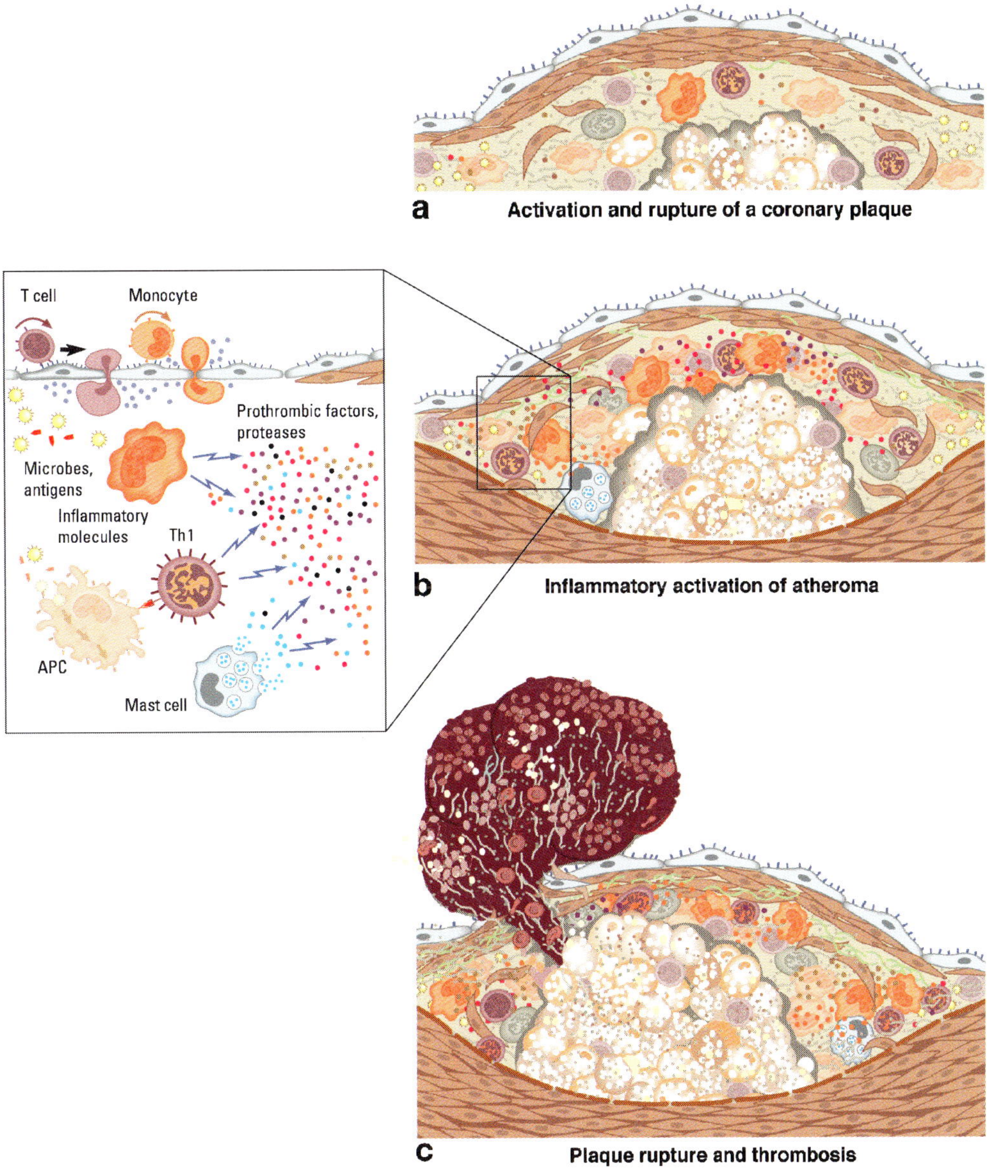

Figure 3

Activation and rupture of a coronary plaque. This process usually takes place at the shoulder of the plaque. (*a*) Advanced atheroma with a smooth muscle cap covering the lipid-rich core. Occasional inflammatory cells are present throughout the atheroma, which is clinically silent. (*b*) Inflammatory activation of atheroma. Macrophages, T cells, and mast cells respond to pro-inflammatory stimuli by producing proteases, cytokines, and prothrombotic factors. Proteolytic destruction of collagen and inhibition of smooth muscle growth leads to reduced thickness and strength of the cap. (*c*) Plaque rupture and thrombosis. The weakened cap, which cannot withstand the hemodynamic forces, fissures and, consequently, exposes thrombogenic plaque material. The subsequent precipitation of platelets and coagulation factors forms a thrombus. Ischemia ensues in the end organ (e.g., brain or myocardium). APC, antigen-presenting cell; Th1, T helper-1.

Table 3 Inflammatory markers in coronary artery disease

Analyte	Source	Use
CRP	Liver (+Plaque?)	ACS marker and risk factor
IL-6	Immune cells and vascular cells	ACS marker and risk factor
Pentraxin-3	Plaque	ACS marker and risk factor
Fibrinogen	Liver	Risk factor
s[a]CD40L	Immune cells, vascular cells and platelets	Risk factor
sIL-2 receptor	T cells	ACS marker
$CD4^{+}28^{null}$ T cells	T cells	ACS marker
sICAM-1	Endothelial cells and others	Risk factor
sVCAM-1	Endothelial and smooth muscle cells	Risk factor
sP-selectin	Endothelial cells and platelets	Risk factor

[a]s, soluble.

SYSTEMIC IMMUNE/ INFLAMMATORY ACTIVITY

The inflammatory process in the atherosclerotic artery may lead to detectable blood levels of pro-inflammatory cytokines and other acute phase reactants (**Table 3**). C-reactive protein (CRP) and IL-6 are elevated in patients with unstable angina and myocardial infarction; high levels of these factors predict a poor outcome (175, 186, 187). Other inflammatory markers are also elevated in these patients, including IL-7, IL-8, soluble CD40 ligand, and the CRP-related protein pentraxin-3 (188–190). Activated T cells are detected, and the proportion of $CD4{+}CD28^{null}$ subset of pro-inflammatory T cells is increased in the blood of these patients (176, 191). The immune repertoire of T cells is also perturbed in these patients: Certain T cell clones are expanded in preference to others, and there is increased reactivity to oxLDL (176). This observation suggests that an autoimmune response may be involved in ACS.

Recently published genetic studies support a role for immune mechanisms in atherosclerosis and CAD. Studies of *Ath1*, a quantitative trait locus for susceptibility to atherosclerosis in mice, revealed that OX40L, a transmembrane protein with costimulatory effects on T cells, is a genetic risk factor for disease in humans (see above) (69). Polymorphism in another immunoregulatory gene, the MHC class II transactivator MHC2TA, was found to be associated with increased risk for three inflammatory diseases, namely CAD, multiple sclerosis, and rheumatoid arthritis (192). These studies provide strong support for a pathogenic role of immune activation in human atherosclerosis.

Inflammatory Markers and the Risk of Coronary Artery Disease

Although inflammatory activity is increased significantly in activated plaques of ACS patients, a smouldering inflammation characterizes silent plaques. Such lesions may also release inflammatory mediators into the systemic circulation (**Table 3**). In addition, inflammatory mediators are released by adipose tissue in patients with metabolic syndrome (193–195). Therefore, elevated inflammatory markers may reflect metabolic risk factors for atherosclerosis as well as smoldering inflammation in existing atherosclerotic plaques.

Modestly elevated CRP detectable by a high-sensitive immunoassay is an independent risk factor for CAD in a healthy population (196, 197) and, independently of plasma cholesterol levels, predicts outcome after statin therapy (198). It is currently debated whether CRP analysis should be used in screens of asymptomatic individuals (197, 198). Other acute phase reactants (including erythrocyte sedimentation rate, fibrinogen, and other plasma proteins) also provide information about the inflammatory risk for CAD (199, 200). The fact that several different inflammatory markers with different biological activities contribute to the statistical risk for CAD makes it unlikely that CRP or any of the other markers actually causes the disease. Instead, these markers reflect the local inflammatory process in the artery and, perhaps, in other tissues and organs [e.g., adipose tissue (see above)]. Further research will be needed to clarify the role of these molecules as markers of risk as well as possible contributors to disease progression.

IMMUNOMODULATORY STRATEGIES TO PREVENT OR TREAT ATHEROSCLEROSIS

Our current understanding of the immunopathogenesis of atherosclerosis suggests that immunomodulatory strategies, including vaccination and pharmacologic immunomodulation, may be useful in the future to combat against this disease.

Immunization with Oxidized Low-Density Lipoprotein

Several groups have reported a reduction of atherosclerosis in hypercholesterolemic rabbits and mice after immunization with oxLDL (201–204). The increase in production of IgG against MDA-LDL after oxLDL immunization (203–205) implies that antigen-specific CD4+ T cells are activated by the immunization. Such an effect probably involves immune recognition of protein-derived peptide fragments. Indeed, immunization with native peptides from the LDL protein, apolipoprotein B100, reduced lesion development in *apoE−/−* mice (206). Immunization with MDA-LDL resulted in a Th2 bias, with reduced IFNγ production and elevated levels of IL-5 (108). This treatment may confer protection by inducing antibodies that inhibit uptake of oxLDL in macrophages.

All these findings suggest that T cell–dependent peptide/MHC/CD4 responses are important in atheroprotective immunization. However, recent studies show that nonpeptide, non-T cell–dependent responses may also play important roles. OxLDL immunization reduces atherosclerosis even in the absence of CD4 (207). This result emphasizes the importance of T cell–independent responses, which include natural antibodies to LDL lipids (83).

Neonatal and mucosal tolerance. Induction of neonatal tolerance to oxLDL reduces atherosclerosis in *apoE−/−* mice (208). This process involves clonal deletion of reactive cells but may also engage other tolerizing mechanisms. Oral and nasal tolerance can also reduce immune responses to foreign or self-antigens, probably by induction of regulatory T cells. Such mucosal tolerance to HSP65 (209, 210) and β2GPI (211) inhibits lesion development in *Ldlr−/−* mice. These effects may depend upon reduced production of IFNγ and/or increased production of anti-inflammatory cytokines (e.g., TGFβ and IL-10) in tolerized mice.

Pharmacological Approaches

The immunosuppressants cyclosporin A and sirolimus inhibit vascular repair (212, 213). Sirolimus is used clinically to coat stents that are used to prevent restenosis after angioplasty. The clinical effect of immunosuppressants may be due both to anti-inflammatory (e.g., reduced IL-12 and IFNγ and elevated TGFβ) and antiproliferative (e.g., attenuated platelet-derived growth factor responses) action.

Statins, which are inhibitors of 3-hydroxy-3-methylglutaryl coenzyme A (HMG-CoA) reductase, are commonly used for treatment of hypercholesterolemia and prevention of atherosclerotic diseases. In recent years, statins have also been found to modulate immune activation. This activation is possibly due to the fact that mevalonate, the product of HMG-CoA reductase, is the precursor of not only cholesterol but also isoprenoid compounds that regulate several cellular processes, including immune activation (214). In addition, reduced membrane cholesterol may impair receptor clustering and therefore antigen-dependent activation (215).

Finally, statins modulate lymphocyte function–associated antigen-1 (LFA-1) by binding to an allosteric domain in the integrin (216, 217); this can also inhibit T cell activation and suppress inflammation. Statins decrease IFNγ-inducible expression of MHC class II proteins in endothelial cells and monocytes/macrophages and MHC class II–dependent T cell proliferation (218). They also reduce CD40 expression in atherosclerotic lesions (219). Through their inhibitory effect on the expression of several adhesion molecules and chemokines, statins may decrease the recruitment of monocytes and T cells into the arterial wall (220, 221). In addition, statins contribute to plaque stabilization by reducing MMP expression and decreasing the risk for thrombotic events by inhibiting tissue factor (220, 221). Statin treatment attenuates experimental autoimmune encephalomyelitis, a model for multiple sclerosis, with attenuated MHC class II expression in the central nervous system concomitant with a shift from production of IL-2, IFNγ, IL-12, and TNFα to IL-4, IL-5, IL-10, and TGFβ (222). Therefore, statins may be beneficial for treatment of several inflammatory disorders, a notion that was validated recently when atorvastatin treatment was found to ameliorate rheumatoid arthritis in a clinical trial (223).

CONCLUSIONS

Atherosclerosis is an inflammatory disease. Immune cells—macrophages, T cells, NKT cells, dendritic cells, and mast cells—infiltrate lesions at all stages. Disease development is slowed by inhibition of immune-cell recruitment and accelerated by cytokines and antigens that activate immune cells. Pathogen-associated molecular patterns may activate lesional macrophages, and several antigens, including oxLDL, induce T cell activation, cellular immune responses, and antibody formation. Infections as well as autoimmune reactions may contribute to such activation. Inflammatory effector mechanisms operate largely through cytokine secretion and their activation may conceivably cause plaque rupture, thrombosis, and acute ischemic symptoms. Anti-inflammatory and immunosuppressive mechanisms (such as anti-inflammatory cytokines, protective antibodies, and regulatory T cells), which may be induced by immunization as well as by immunopharmacological methods, inhibit atherosclerosis and may be attractive targets for disease prevention and/or treatment. Interestingly, several drugs currently used to treat atherosclerotic patients operate at least partly through immune inhibitory mechanisms.

SUMMARY POINTS

1. Atherosclerosis is an inflammatory disease elicited at sites of lipoprotein accumulation and hemodynamic strain. It begins when monocytes and T cells enter the artery wall at such sites.
2. Pattern recognition receptors, including ScRs and TLRs on macrophages, are important mediators of intracellular cholesterol accumulation and innate immune activation in the atherosclerotic plaque.
3. T cells in plaques mount adaptive immune responses to local antigens and develop Th1 effector responses that lead to macrophage activation.
4. Pro-inflammatory cytokines released by Th1 cells and macrophages are major pro-atherogenic molecules.
5. Anti-atherosclerotic immune responses are mounted by B cells that produce antibodies to components of oxidized lipoproteins and by immune cells (e.g., regulatory T cells) that produce anti-inflammatory cytokines.

6. Activation of plaque inflammation leads to protease secretion, tissue destruction, and plaque rupture. In turn, thrombosis produces ischemia and infarction.
7. CRP, and perhaps also other markers of inflammation, may be used to monitor cardiovascular risk.
8. Statins, which lower the risk for myocardial infarction, reduce inflammation as well as plasma cholesterol levels.

FUTURE DIRECTIONS/UNRESOLVED ISSUES

1. How important are innate versus adaptive immune responses in the plaque?
2. Which antigens dominate the adaptive immune response in atherosclerosis?
3. Do infectious agents play a role in atherosclerosis, and if so, which?
4. Can we prevent or treat atherosclerosis by immunomodulatory or anti-inflammatory strategies?

DISCLOSURE STATEMENT

G.K.H. was a consultant for Bioinvent AB and owns Patent W001/68119A1.

ACKNOWLEDGMENTS

Our work is supported by the Swedish Research Council, Heart-Lung Foundation, Söderberg Foundation, AFA funds, European Union (Framework VI), and National Institutes of Health. We thank Annika Röhl for the preparation of color graphics.

LITERATURE CITED

1. Breslow JL. 1996. Mouse models of atherosclerosis. *Science* 272:685–88
2. Caligiuri G, Levy B, Pernow J, Thoren P, Hansson GK. 1999. Myocardial infarction mediated by endothelin receptor signaling in hypercholesterolemic mice. *Proc. Natl. Acad. Sci. USA* 96:6920–4
3. Carmeliet P, Moons L, Lijnen R, Baes M, Lemaitre V, et al. 1997. Urokinase-generated plasmin activates matrix metalloproteinases during aneurysm formation. *Nat. Genet.* 17:439–44
4. Camejo G, Hurt-Camejo E, Wiklund O, Bondjers G. 1998. Association of apo B lipoproteins with arterial proteoglycans: pathological significance and molecular basis. *Atherosclerosis* 139:205–22
5. Skålén K, Gustafsson M, Rydberg EK, Hulten LM, Wiklund O, et al. 2002. Subendothelial retention of atherogenic lipoproteins in early atherosclerosis. *Nature* 417:750–4
6. Kume N, Cybulsky MI, Gimbrone MA. 1992. Lysophosphatidylcholine, a component of atherogenic lipoproteins, induces mononuclear leukocyte adhesion molecules in cultured human and rabbit arterial endothelial cells. *J. Clin. Invest.* 90:1138–44

7. Eriksson EE, Xie X, Werr J, Thoren P, Lindbom L. 2001. Importance of primary capture and L-selectin-dependent secondary capture in leukocyte accumulation in inflammation and atherosclerosis in vivo. *J. Exp. Med.* 194:205–18
8. Cybulsky MI, Gimbrone MA. 1991. Endothelial expression of a mononuclear leukocyte adhesion molecule during atherosclerosis. *Science* 251:788–91
9. Watson AD, Leitinger N, Navab M, Faull KF, Hörkkö S, et al. 1997. Structural identification by mass spectrometry of oxidized phospholipids in minimally oxidized low density lipoprotein that induce monocyte/endothelial interactions and evidence for their presence in vivo. *J. Biol. Chem.* 272:13597–607
10. Leitinger N. 2003. Oxidized phospholipids as modulators of inflammation in atherosclerosis. *Curr. Opin. Lipidol.* 14:421–30
11. Massberg S, Brand K, Gruner S, Page S, Muller E, et al. 2002. A critical role of platelet adhesion in the initiation of atherosclerotic lesion formation. *J. Exp. Med.* 196:887–96
12. Nakashima Y, Raines EW, Plump AS, Breslow JL, Ross R. 1998. Upregulation of VCAM-1 and ICAM-1 at atherosclerosis-prone sites on the endothelium in the apoE-deficient mouse. *Arterioscler. Thromb. Vasc. Biol.* 18:842–51
13. Dai G, Kaazempur-Mofrad MR, Natarajan S, Zhang Y, Vaughn S, et al. 2004. Distinct endothelial phenotypes evoked by arterial waveforms derived from atherosclerosis-susceptible and -resistant regions of human vasculature. *Proc. Natl. Acad. Sci. USA* 101:14871–76
14. Boring L, Gosling J, Cleary M, Charo IF. 1998. Decreased lesion formation in CCR2−/− mice reveals a role for chemokines in the initiation of atherosclerosis. *Nature* 394:894–97
15. Gu L, Okada Y, Clinton SK, Gerard C, Sukhova GK, et al. 1998. Absence of monocyte chemoattractant protein-1 reduces atherosclerosis in low density lipoprotein receptor-deficient mice. *Mol. Cell.* 2:275–81
16. Mach F, Sauty A, Iarossi AS, Sukhova GK, Neote K, et al. 1999. Differential expression of three T lymphocyte-activating CXC chemokines by human atheroma-associated cells. *J. Clin. Invest.* 104:1041–50
17. Haley KJ, Lilly CM, Yang JH, Feng Y, Kennedy SP, et al. 2000. Overexpression of eotaxin and the CCR3 receptor in human atherosclerosis: using genomic technology to identify a potential novel pathway of vascular inflammation. *Circulation* 102:2185–89
18. Veillard NR, Kwak B, Pelli G, Mulhaupt F, James RW, et al. 2004. Antagonism of RANTES receptors reduces atherosclerotic plaque formation in mice. *Circ. Res.* 94:253–61
19. Lesnik P, Haskell CA, Charo IF. 2003. Decreased atherosclerosis in CX3CR1−/− mice reveals a role for fractalkine in atherogenesis. *J. Clin. Invest.* 111:333–40
20. Smith JD, Trogan E, Ginsberg M, Grigaux C, Tian J, Miyata M. 1995. Decreased atherosclerosis in mice deficient in both macrophage colony-stimulating factor (op) and apolipoprotein E. *Proc. Natl. Acad. Sci. USA* 92:8264–68
21. Hansson GK, Libby P, Schönbeck U, Yan ZQ. 2002. Innate and adaptive immunity in the pathogenesis of atherosclerosis. *Circ. Res.* 91:281–91
22. Peiser L, Mukhopadhyay S, Gordon S. 2002. Scavenger receptors in innate immunity. *Curr. Opin. Immunol.* 14:123–28
23. Panousis CG, Zuckerman SH. 2000. Interferon-γ induces downregulation of Tangier disease gene (ATP-binding-cassette transporter 1) in macrophage-derived foam cells. *Arterioscler. Thromb. Vasc. Biol.* 20:1565–71

24. Khovidhunkit W, Moser AH, Shigenaga JK, Grunfeld C, Feingold KR. 2003. Endotoxin down-regulates ABCG5 and ABCG8 in mouse liver and ABCA1 and ABCG1 in J774 murine macrophages: differential role of LXR. *J. Lipid. Res.* 44:1728–36
25. Janeway CA Jr., Medzhitov R. 2002. Innate immune recognition. *Annu. Rev. Immunol.* 20:197–216
26. Faure E, Thomas L, Xu H, Medvedev A, Equils O, Arditi M. 2001. Bacterial lipopolysaccharide and IFN-gamma induce Toll-like receptor 2 and Toll-like receptor 4 expression in human endothelial cells: role of NF-kappa B activation. *J. Immunol.* 166:2018–24
27. Xu Q. 2002. Role of heat shock proteins in atherosclerosis. *Arterioscler. Thromb. Vasc. Biol.* 22:1547–59
28. Miller YI, Chang MK, Binder CJ, Shaw PX, Witztum JL. 2003. Oxidized low density lipoprotein and innate immune receptors. *Curr. Opin. Lipidol.* 14:437–45
29. Xu XH, Shah PK, Faure E, Equils O, Thomas L, et al. 2001. Toll-like receptor-4 is expressed by macrophages in murine and human lipid-rich atherosclerotic plaques and upregulated by oxidized LDL. *Circulation* 104:3103–8
30. Edfeldt K, Swedenborg J, Hansson GK, Yan ZQ. 2002. Expression of toll-like receptors in human atherosclerotic lesions: a possible pathway for plaque activation. *Circulation* 105:1158–61
31. Monaco C, Andreakos E, Kiriakidis S, Mauri C, Bicknell C, et al. 2004. Canonical pathway of nuclear factor kappa B activation selectively regulates proinflammatory and prothrombotic responses in human atherosclerosis. *Proc. Natl. Acad. Sci. USA* 101:5634–39
32. Michelsen KS, Wong MH, Shah PK, Zhang W, Yano J, et al. 2004. *Proc. Natl. Acad. Sci. USA* 101:10679–84
33. Björkbacka H, Kunjathoor VV, Moore KJ, Koehn S, Ordija CM, et al. 2004. Reduced atherosclerosis in MyD88-null mice links elevated serum cholesterol levels to activation of innate immunity signaling pathways. *Nat. Med.* 10:416–21
34. Yan SF, Ramasamy R, Naka Y, Schmidt AM. 2003. Glycation, inflammation, and RAGE: a scaffold for the macrovascular complications of diabetes and beyond. *Circ. Res.* 93:1159–69
35. Park L, Raman KG, Lee KJ, Lu Y, Ferran LJ Jr, et al. 1998. Suppression of accelerated diabetic atherosclerosis by the soluble receptor for advanced glycation endproducts. *Nat. Med.* 4:1025–31
36. Zeiher AM, Goebel H, Schächinger V, Ihling C. 1995. Tissue endothelin-1 immunoreactivity in the active coronary atherosclerotic plaque. A clue to the mechanism of increased vasoreactivity of the culprit lesion in unstable angina. *Circulation* 91:941–47
37. Buttery LDK, Springall DR, Chester AH, Evans TJ, Standfield N, et al. 1996. Inducible nitric oxide synthase is present within human atherosclerotic lesions and promotes the formation and activity of peroxynitrite. *Lab. Invest.* 75:77–85
38. Sugiyama S, Okada Y, Sukhova GK, Virmani R, Heinecke JW, Libby P. 2001. Macrophage myeloperoxidase regulation by granulocyte macrophage colony-stimulating factor in human atherosclerosis and implications in acute coronary syndromes. *Am. J. Pathol.* 158:879–91
39. Shah PK, Falk E, Badimon JJ, Fernandez OA, Mailhac A, et al. 1995. Human monocyte-derived macrophages induce collagen breakdown in fibrous caps of atherosclerotic plaques. Potential role of matrix-degrading metalloproteinases and implications for plaque rupture. *Circulation* 92:1565–69

40. Jormsjö S, Wuttge DM, Sirsjö A, Whatling C, Hamsten A, et al. 2002. Differential expression of cysteine and aspartic proteases during progression of atherosclerosis in apolipoprotein E-deficient mice. *Am. J. Pathol.* 161:939–45
41. Libby P, Aikawa M. 2002. Stabilization of atherosclerotic plaques: new mechanisms and clinical targets. *Nat. Med.* 8:1257–62
42. Liu J, Sukhova GK, Sun JS, Xu WH, Libby P, Shi GP. 2004. Lysosomal cysteine proteases in atherosclerosis. *Arterioscler. Thromb. Vasc. Biol.* 24:1359–66
43. Jonasson L, Holm J, Skalli O, Bondjers G, Hansson GK. 1986. Regional accumulations of T cells, macrophages, and smooth muscle cells in the human atherosclerotic plaque. *Arteriosclerosis* 6:131–38
44. Stemme S, Holm J, Hansson GK. 1992. T lymphocytes in human atherosclerotic plaques are memory cells expressing CD45RO and the integrin VLA-1. *Arterioscl. Thromb.* 12:206–11
45. Kleindienst R, Xu Q, Willeit J, Waldenberger FR, Weimann S, Wick G. 1993. Immunology of atherosclerosis. Demonstration of heat shock protein 60 expression and T lymphocytes bearing α/β or γ/δ receptor in human atherosclerotic lesions. *Am. J. Pathol.* 142:1927–37
46. van der Wal AC, Das PK, Bentz van de Berg D, van der Loos CM, Becker AE. 1989. Atherosclerotic lesions in humans. In situ immunophenotypic analysis suggesting an immune mediated response. *Lab. Invest.* 61:166–70
47. Jonasson L, Holm J, Skalli O, Gabbiani G, Hansson GK. 1985. Expression of class II transplantation antigen on vascular smooth muscle cells in human atherosclerosis. *J. Clin. Invest.* 76:125–31
48. Kishikawa H, Shimokama T, Watanabe T. 1993. Localization of T lymphocytes and macrophages expressing IL-1, IL-2 receptor, IL-6 and TNF in human aortic intima. Role of cell-mediated immunity in human atherogenesis. *Virchows. Arch. A Pathol. Anat. Histopathol.* 423:433–42
49. Bobryshev YV, Lord RS. 1995. S-100 positive cells in human arterial intima and in atherosclerotic lesions. *Cardiovasc. Res.* 29:689–96
50. Yilmaz A, Lochno M, Traeg F, Cicha I, Reiss C, et al. 2004. Emergence of dendritic cells in rupture-prone regions of vulnerable carotid plaques. *Atherosclerosis* 176:101–10
51. van der Wal AC, Becker AE, van der Loos CM, Das PK. 1994. Site of intimal rupture or erosion of thrombosed coronary atherosclerotic plaques is characterized by an inflammatory process irrespective of the dominant plaque morphology. *Circulation* 89:36–44
52. Hosono M, de Boer OJ, van der Wal AC, van der Loos CM, Teeling P, et al. 2003. Increased expression of T cell activation markers (CD25, CD26, CD40L and CD69) in atherectomy specimens of patients with unstable angina and acute myocardial infarction. *Atherosclerosis* 168:73–80
53. Stemme S, Faber B, Holm J, Wiklund O, Witztum JL, Hansson GK. 1995. T lymphocytes from human atherosclerotic plaques recognize oxidized low density lipoprotein. *Proc. Natl. Acad. Sci. USA* 92:3893–97
54. Paulsson G, Zhou X., Törnquist E., Hansson GK. 2000. Oligoclonal T cell expansions in atherosclerotic lesions of apoE-deficient mice. *Arterioscl. Thromb. Vasc. Biol.* 20:10–17
55. Yamazaki K, Ohsawa Y, Itoh H, Ueki K, Tabeta K, et al. 2004. T-cell clonality to Porphyromonas gingivalis and human heat shock protein 60s in patients with atherosclerosis and periodontitis. *Oral. Microbiol. Immunol.* 19:160–67
56. Dansky HM, Charlton SA, Harper MM, Smith JD. 1997. T and B lymphocytes play a minor role in atherosclerotic plaque formation in the apolipoprotein E-deficient mouse. *Proc. Natl. Acad. Sci. USA* 94:4642–46

57. Daugherty A, Puré E, Delfel-Butteiger D, Leferovich J, Roselaar SE. 1997. The effects of total lymphocyte deficiency on the extent of atherosclerosis in apolipoprotein−/− mice. *J. Clin. Invest.* 100:1575–80
58. Zhou X, Nicoletti A, Elhage R, Hansson GK. 2000. Transfer of CD4(+) T cells aggravates atherosclerosis in immunodeficient apolipoprotein E knockout mice. *Circulation* 102:2919–22
59. Reardon CA, Blachowicz L, White T, Cabana V, Wang Y, et al. 2001. Effect of immune deficiency on lipoproteins and atherosclerosis in male apolipoprotein E-deficient mice. *Arterioscler. Thromb. Vasc. Biol.* 21:1011–16
60. Ludewig B, Freigang S, Jaggi M, Kurrer MO, Pei YC, et al. 2000. Linking immune-mediated arterial inflammation and cholesterol-induced atherosclerosis in a transgenic mouse model. *Proc. Natl. Acad. Sci. USA* 97:12752–57
61. Mach F, Schönbeck U, Sukhova GK, Bourcier T, Bonnefoy JY, et al. 1997. Functional CD40 ligand is expressed on human vascular endothelial cells, smooth muscle cells, and macrophages - implications for CD40-CD40 ligand signaling in atherosclerosis. *Proc. Natl. Acad. Sci. USA* 94:1931–36
62. Mach F, Schönbeck U, Sukhova GK, Atkinson E, Libby P. 1998. Reduction of atherosclerosis in mice by inhibition of CD40 signalling. *Nature* 394:200–3
63. Lutgens E, Gorelik L, Daemen MJ, de Muinck ED, Grewal IS, et al. 1999. Requirement for CD154 in the progression of atherosclerosis. *Nat. Med.* 5:1313–16
64. Lutgens E, Cleutjens KB, Heeneman S, Koteliansky VE, Burkly LC, Daemen MJ. 2000. Both early and delayed anti-CD40L antibody treatment induces a stable plaque phenotype. *Proc. Natl. Acad. Sci. USA* 97:7464–69
65. Schönbeck U, Sukhova GK, Shimizu K, Mach F, Libby P. 2000 Inhibition of CD40 signaling limits evolution of established atherosclerosis in mice. *Proc. Natl. Acad. Sci. USA* 97:7458–63
66. Henn V, Slupsky JR, Gräfe M, Anagnostopoulos I, Förster R, Müller-Berghaus G, Kroczek RA. 1998. CD40 ligand on activated platelets triggers an inflammatory reaction of endothelial cells. *Nature* 391:591–94
67. de Boer OJ, Hirsch F, van der Wal AC, van der Loos CM, Das PK, Becker AE. 1997. Costimulatory molecules in human atherosclerotic plaques: an indication of antigen specific T lymphocyte activation. *Atherosclerosis* 133:227–34
68. Buono C, Pang H, Uchida Y, Libby P, Sharpe AH, Lichtman AH. 2004. B7–1/B7–2 costimulation regulates plaque antigen-specific T-cell responses and atherogenesis in low-density lipoprotein receptor-deficient mice. *Circulation* 109:2009–15
69. Wang X, Ria M, Kelmenson PM, Eriksson P, Higgins DC, et al. 2005. Positional identification of TNFSF4, encoding OX40 ligand, as a gene that influences atherosclerosis susceptibility. *Nat. Genet.* 37: 365–72
70. Sugamura K, Ishii N, Weinberg AD. 2004. Therapeutic targeting of the effector T-cell co-stimulatory molecule OX40. *Nat. Rev. Immunol.* 4:420–31
71. de Boer OJ, van der Wal AC, Houtkamp MA, Ossewaarde JM, Teeling P, Becker AE. 2000. Unstable atherosclerotic plaques contain T-cells that respond to Chlamydia pneumoniae. *Cardiovasc. Res.* 48:402–8
72. Mosorin M, Surcel HM, Laurila A, Lehtinen M, Karttunen R, et al. 2000. Detection of Chlamydia pneumoniae-reactive T lymphocytes in human atherosclerotic plaques of carotid artery. *Arterioscler. Thromb. Vasc. Biol.* 20: 1061–67
73. Metzler B, Mayr M, Dietrich H, Singh M, Wiebe E, et al. 1999. Inhibition of arteriosclerosis by T-cell depletion in normocholesterolemic rabbits immunized with heat shock protein 65. *Arterioscler. Thromb. Vasc. Biol.* 19:1905–11

74. Choi JI, Chung SW, Kang HS, Rhim BY, Kim SJ. 2002. Establishment of Porphyromonas gingivalis heat-shock-protein-specific T-cell lines from atherosclerosis patients. *J. Dent. Res.* 81:344–48
75. Frostegård J, Kjellman B, Gidlund M, Andersson B, Jindal S, Kiessling R. 1996. Induction of heat shock protein in monocytic cells by oxidized low density lipoprotein. *Atherosclerosis* 121:93–103
76. Xu Q, Willeit J, Marosi M, Kleindienst R, Oberhollenzer F, et al. 1993. Association of serum antibodies to heat-shock protein 65 with carotid atherosclerosis. *Lancet* 341:255–59
77. Xu Q, Kiechl S, Mayr M, Metzler B, Egger G, et al. 1999. Association of serum antibodies to heat-shock protein 65 with carotid atherosclerosis: clinical significance determined in a follow-up study. *Circulation* 100:1169–74
78. Xu Q, Dietrich H, Steiner HJ, Gown AM, Schoel B, et al. 1992. Induction of arteriosclerosis in normocholesterolemic rabbits by immunization with heat shock protein 65. *Arterioscl. Thromb.* 12:789–99
79. George J, Shoenfeld Y, Afek A, Gilburd B, Keren P, et al. 1999. Enhanced fatty streak formation in C57BL/6J mice by immunization with heat shock protein-65. *Arterioscler. Thromb. Vasc. Biol.* 19:505–10
80. Palinski W, Rosenfeld ME, Ylä-Herttuala S, Gurtner GC, Socher SS, et al. 1989 Low density lipoprotein undergoes oxidative modification in vivo. *Proc. Natl. Acad. Sci. USA* 86:1372–76
81. Vaarala O. 2000. Antibodies to oxidised LDL. *Lupus* 9:202–5
82. Fredrikson GN, Hedblad B, Berglund G, Alm R, Ares M, et al. 2003. Identification of immune responses against aldehyde-modified peptide sequences in apoB associated with cardiovascular disease. *Arterioscler. Thromb. Vasc. Biol.* 23:872–78
83. Binder CJ, Hörkkö S, Dewan A, Chang MK, Kieu EP, et al. 2003. Pneumococcal vaccination decreases atherosclerotic lesion formation: molecular mimicry between Streptococcus pneumoniae and oxidized LDL. *Nat. Med.* 9:736–43
84. Chang MK, Binder CJ, Miller YI, Subbanagounder G, Silverman GJ, et al. 2004. Apoptotic cells with oxidation-specific epitopes are immunogenic and proinflammatory. *J. Exp. Med.* 200:1359–70
85. George J, Harats D, Gilburd B, Afek A, Levy Y, et al. 1999. Immunolocalization of β2-glycoprotein I (apolipoprotein H) to human atherosclerotic plaques: potential implications for lesion progression. *Circulation* 99:2227–30
86. Wu R, Nityanand S, Berglund L, Lithell H, Holm G, Lefvert AK. 1997. Antibodies against cardiolipin and oxidatively modified LDL in 50-year-old men predict myocardial infarction. *Arterioscler. Thromb. Vasc. Biol.* 17:3159–63
87. George J, Afek A, Gilburd B, Blank M, Levy Y, et al. 1998. Induction of early atherosclerosis in LDL-receptor-deficient mice immunized with β2-glycoprotein I. *Circulation* 98:1108–15
88. Hansson GK, Holm J, Jonasson L. 1989. Detection of activated T lymphocytes in the human atherosclerotic plaque. *Am. J. Pathol.* 135:169–75
89. Uyemura K, Demer L, Castle SC, Jullien D, Berliner JA, et al. 1996. Cross-regulatory roles of interleukin (IL)-12 and IL-10 in atherosclerosis. *J. Clin. Invest.* 97:2130–38
90. Benagiano M, Azzurri A, Ciervo A, Amedei A, Tamburini C, et al. 2003. T helper type 1 lymphocytes drive inflammation in human atherosclerotic lesions. *Proc. Natl. Acad. Sci. USA* 100:6658–63

91. Frostegård J, Ulfgren AK, Nyberg P, Hedin U, Swedenborg J, et al. 1999. Cytokine expression in advanced human atherosclerotic plaques: dominance of pro-inflammatory (Th1) and macrophage-stimulating cytokines. *Atherosclerosis* 145:33–43
92. Zhou X, Paulsson G, Stemme S, Hansson GK. 1998. Hypercholesterolemia is associated with a T helper (Th) 1/Th2 switch of the autoimmune response in atherosclerotic apo E-knockout mice. *J. Clin. Invest.* 101:1717–25
93. Shimizu K, Shichiri M, Libby P, Lee RT, Mitchell RN. 2004. Th2-predominant inflammation and blockade of IFN-γ signaling induce aneurysms in allografted aortas. *J. Clin. Invest.* 114:300–8
94. Laurat E, Poirier B, Tupin E, Caligiuri G, Hansson GK, et al. 2001. In vivo downregulation of T helper cell 1 immune responses reduces atherogenesis in apolipoprotein E-knockout mice. *Circulation* 104:197–202
95. Mallat Z, Corbaz A, Scoazec A, Graber P, Alouani S, et al. 2001. Interleukin-18/interleukin-18 binding protein signaling modulates atherosclerotic lesion development and stability. *Circ. Res.* 89:E41–45
96. Lee TS, Yen HC, Pan CC, Chau LY. 1999. The role of interleukin 12 in the development of atherosclerosis in ApoE-deficient mice. *Arterioscler. Thromb. Vasc. Biol.* 19:734–42
97. Whitman SC, Ravisankar P, Daugherty A. 2002. Interleukin-18 enhances atherosclerosis in apolipoprotein E(−/−) mice through release of interferon-γ. *Circ. Res.* 90:E34–38
98. Whitman SC, Ravisankar P, Elam H, Daugherty A. 2000. Exogenous interferon-γ enhances atherosclerosis in apolipoprotein E−/− mice. *Am. J. Pathol.* 157:1819–24
99. Tellides G, Tereb DA, Kirkiles-Smith NC, Kim RW, Wilson JH, et al. 2000. Interferon-γ elicits arteriosclerosis in the absence of leukocytes. *Nature* 403:207–11
100. Gerdes N, Sukhova G, Libby P, Reynolds RS, Young JL, Schönbeck U. 2002 Expression of interleukin (IL)-18 and functional IL-18 receptor on human vascular endothelial cells, smooth muscle cells, and macrophages: implications for atherogenesis. *J. Exp. Med.* 195:1–14
101. Tenger C, Sundborger A, Jawien J, Zhou X. 2005. IL-18 accelerates atherosclerosis accompanied by elevation of IFN-γ and CXCL16 expression independently of T cells. *Arterioscler. Thromb. Vasc. Biol.* 25:791–96
101a. Branen L, Hovgaard L, Nitulescu M, Bengtsson E, Nilsson J, Jovinge S. 2004. Inhibition of tumor necrosis factor-alpha reduces atherosclerosis in apolipoprotein E knockout mice. *Arterioscler. Thromb. Vasc. Biol.* 24:2137–42
102. George J, Shoenfeld Y, Gilburd B, Afek A, Shaish A, Harats D. 2000. Requisite role for interleukin-4 in the acceleration of fatty streaks induced by heat shock protein 65 or Mycobacterium tuberculosis. *Circ. Res.* 86: 1203–10
103. Huber SA, Sakkinen P, David C, Newell MK, Tracy RP. 2001. T helper-cell phenotype regulates atherosclerosis in mice under conditions of mild hypercholesterolemia. *Circulation* 103:2610–16
104. King VL, Szilvassy SJ, Daugherty A. 2002. Interleukin-4 deficiency decreases atherosclerotic lesion formation in a site-specific manner in female LDL receptor−/− mice. *Arterioscler. Thromb. Vasc. Biol.* 22:456–61
105. Davenport P, Tipping PG. 2003. The role of interleukin-4 and interleukin-12 in the progression of atherosclerosis in apolipoprotein E-deficient mice. *Am. J. Pathol.* 163:1117–25
106. Huang JT, Welch JS, Ricote M, Binder CJ, Willson TM, et al. 1999. Interleukin-4-dependent production of PPAR-γ ligands in macrophages by 12/15-lipoxygenase. *Nature* 400:378–82

107. Yesner LM, Huh HY, Pearce SF, Silverstein RL. 1996. Regulation of monocyte CD36 and thrombospondin-1 expression by soluble mediators. *Arterioscler. Thromb. Vasc. Biol.* 16:1019–25
108. Binder CJ, Hartvigsen K, Chang MK, Miller M, Broide D, et al. 2004. IL-5 links adaptive and natural immunity specific for epitopes of oxidized LDL and protects from atherosclerosis. *J. Clin. Invest.* 114:427–37
109. Fehervari Z, Sakaguchi S. 2004. CD4+ Tregs and immune control. *J. Clin. Invest.* 114:1209–17
110. Gorelik L, Flavell RA. 2002. Transforming growth factor-β in T-cell biology. *Nat. Rev. Immunol.* 2:46–53
111. Veillard NR, Steffens S, Burger F, Pelli G, Mach F. 2004. Differential expression patterns of proinflammatory and antiinflammatory mediators during atherogenesis in mice. *Arterioscler. Thromb. Vasc. Biol.* 24:2339–44
112. Mallat Z, Gojova A, Brun V, Esposito B, Fournier N, et al. 2003. Induction of a regulatory T cell type 1 response reduces the development of atherosclerosis in apolipoprotein E-knockout mice. *Circulation* 108:1232–37
113. Letterio JJ, Roberts AB. 1998. Regulation of immune responses by TGF-β. *Annu. Rev. Immunol.* 16:137–61
114. Kulkarni AB, Huh CG, Becker D, Geiser A, Lyght M, et al. 1993. Transforming growth factor β1 null mutation in mice causes excessive inflammatory response and early death. *Proc. Natl. Acad. Sci. USA* 90:770–74
115. Grainger DJ, Witchell CM, Metcalfe JC. 1995. Tamoxifen elevates transforming growth factor-β and suppresses diet-induced formation of lipid lesions in mouse aorta. *Nat. Med.* 1:1067–73
116. Mallat Z, Gojova A, Marchiol-Fournigault C, Esposito B, Kamate C, et al. 2001. Inhibition of transforming growth factor-β signaling accelerates atherosclerosis and induces an unstable plaque phenotype in mice. *Circ. Res.* 89:930–34
117. Lutgens E, Gijbels M, Smook M, Heeringa P, Gotwals P, et al. 2002. Transforming growth factor-β mediates balance between inflammation and fibrosis during plaque progression. *Arterioscler. Thromb. Vasc. Biol.* 22:975–82
118. Robertson AK, Rudling M, Zhou X, Gorelik L, Flavell RA, Hansson GK. 2003. Disruption of TGF-β signaling in T cells accelerates atherosclerosis. *J. Clin. Invest.* 112:1342–50
119. Gojova A, Brun V, Esposito B, Cottrez F, Gourdy P, et al. 2003. Specific abrogation of transforming growth factor-β signaling in T cells alters atherosclerotic lesion size and composition in mice. *Blood* 102:4052–58
120. Mocellin S, Marincola F, Rossi CR, Nitti D, Lise M. 2004. The multifaceted relationship between IL-10 and adaptive immunity: putting together the pieces of a puzzle. *Cytokine Growth Factor Rev.* 15:61–76
121. Pinderski Oslund LJ, Hedrick CC, Olvera T, Hagenbaugh A, Territo M, et al. 1999. Interleukin-10 blocks atherosclerotic events in vitro and in vivo. *Arterioscler. Thromb. Vasc. Biol.* 19:2847–53
122. Mallat Z, Besnard S, Duriez M, Deleuze V, Emmanuel F, et al. 1999. Protective role of interleukin-10 in atherosclerosis. *Circ. Res.* 85:E17–24
123. Caligiuri G, Rudling M, Ollivier V, Jacob MP, Michel JB, et al. 2003. Interleukin-10 deficiency increases atherosclerosis, thrombosis, and low-density lipoproteins in apolipoprotein E knockout mice. *Mol. Med.* 9:10–17

124. Potteaux S, Esposito B, van Oostrom O, Brun V, Ardouin P, et al. 2004. Leukocyte-derived interleukin 10 is required for protection against atherosclerosis in low-density lipoprotein receptor knockout mice. *Arterioscler. Thromb. Vasc. Biol.* 24:1474–78
125. Pinderski LJ, Fischbein MP, Subbanagounder G, Fishbein MC, Kubo N, et al. 2002. Overexpression of interleukin-10 by activated T lymphocytes inhibits atherosclerosis in LDL receptor-deficient mice by altering lymphocyte and macrophage phenotypes. *Circ. Res.* 90:1064–71
126. Von Der Thusen JH, Kuiper J, Fekkes ML, De Vos P, Van Berkel TJ, Biessen EA. 2001. Attenuation of atherogenesis by systemic and local adenovirus-mediated gene transfer of interleukin-10 in LDLr−/− mice. *Faseb. J.* 15:2730–32
127. Namiki M, Kawashima S, Yamashita T, Ozaki M, Sakoda T, et al. 2004. Intramuscular gene transfer of interleukin-10 cDNA reduces atherosclerosis in apolipoprotein E-knockout mice. *Atherosclerosis* 172:21–29
128. Zhou D, Mattner J, Cantu C III, Schrantz N, Yin N, et al. 2004. Lysosomal glycosphingolipid recognition by NKT cells. *Science* 306:1786–89
129. Mattner J, Debord KL, Ismail N, Goff RD, Cantu C III, et al. 2005. Exogenous and endogenous glycolipid antigens activate NKT cells during microbial infections. *Nature* 434:525–29
130. Melian A, Geng YJ, Sukhova GK, Libby P, Porcelli SA. 1999. CD1 expression in human atherosclerosis. A potential mechanism for T cell activation by foam cells. *Am. J. Pathol.* 155:775–86
131. Paulsson G, Zhou X, Törnquist E, Hansson GK. 2000. Oligoclonal T cell expansions in atherosclerotic lesions of apolipoprotein E-deficient mice. *Arterioscler. Thromb. Vasc. Biol.* 20:10–17
132. Tupin E, Nicoletti A, Elhage R, Rudling M, Ljunggren HG, et al. 2004. CD1d-dependent activation of NKT cells aggravates atherosclerosis. *J. Exp. Med.* 199:417–22
133. Major AS, Wilson MT, McCaleb JL, Ru Su Y, Stanic AK, et al. 2004. Quantitative and qualitative differences in proatherogenic NKT cells in apolipoprotein E-deficient mice. *Arterioscler. Thromb. Vasc. Biol.* 24:2351–57
134. Nakai Y, Iwabuchi K, Fujii S, Ishimori N, Dashtsoodol N, et al. 2004. *Blood* 104:2051–59
135. Aslanian AM, Chapman HA, Charo IF. 2005. Transient role for CD1d-restricted natural killer T cells in the formation of atherosclerotic lesions. *Arterioscler. Thromb. Vasc. Biol.* 25:628–32
136. Kärre K. 2002. NK cells, MHC class I molecules and the missing self. *Scand. J. Immunol.* 55:221–28
137. Schiller NK, Boisvert WA, Curtiss LK. 2002. Inflammation in atherosclerosis: lesion formation in LDL receptor-deficient mice with perforin and Lyst(beige) mutations. *Arterioscler. Thromb. Vasc. Biol.* 22:1341–46
138. Whitman SC, Rateri DL, Szilvassy SJ, Yokoyama W, Daugherty A. 2004. Depletion of natural killer cell function decreases atherosclerosis in low-density lipoprotein receptor null mice. *Arterioscler. Thromb. Vasc. Biol.* 24:1049–54
139. Kaartinen M, Penttilä A, Kovanen PT. 1994. Accumulation of activated mast cells in the shoulder region of human coronary atheroma, the predilection site of atheromatous rupture. *Circulation* 90:1669–78
140. Lindstedt KA, Kovanen PT. 2004. Mast cells in vulnerable coronary plaques: potential mechanisms linking mast cell activation to plaque erosion and rupture. *Curr. Opin. Lipidol.* 15:567–73
141. Parums D, Mitchinson MJ. 1981. Demonstration of immunoglobulin in the neighbourhood of advanced atherosclerotic plaques. *Atherosclerosis* 38:211–16

142. Nicoletti A, Kaveri S, Caligiuri G, Bariety J, Hansson GK. 1998. Immunoglobulin treatment reduces atherosclerosis in apo E knockout mice. *J. Clin. Invest.* 102:910–18
143. Yuan Z, Kishimoto C, Sano H, Shioji K, Xu Y, Yokode M. 2003. Immunoglobulin treatment suppresses atherosclerosis in apolipoprotein E-deficient mice via the Fc portion. *Am. J. Physiol. Heart Circ. Physiol.* 285:H899–906
144. Caligiuri G, Nicoletti A, Poirier B, Hansson GK. 2002. Protective immunity against atherosclerosis carried by B cells of hypercholesterolemic mice. *J. Clin. Invest.* 109:745–53
145. Major AS, Fazio S, Linton MF. 2002. B-lymphocyte deficiency increases atherosclerosis in LDL receptor-null mice. *Arterioscler. Thromb. Vasc. Biol.* 22:1892–98
146. Schiopu A, Bengtsson J, Söderberg I, Janciauskiene S, Lindgren S, et al. 2004. Recombinant human antibodies against aldehyde-modified apolipoprotein B-100 peptide sequences inhibit atherosclerosis. *Circulation* 110:2047–52
147. Libby P, Egan D, Skarlatos S. 1997. Roles of infectious agents in atherosclerosis and restenosis. An assessment of the evidence and need for future research. *Circulation* 96:4095–103
148. Danesh J, Collins R, Peto R. 1997. Chronic infections and coronary heart disease: is there a link? *Lancet* 350:430–36
149. Saikku P, Leinonen M, Mattila K, Ekman MR, Nieminen MS, et al. 1988. Serological evidence of an association of a novel Chlamydia, TWAR, with chronic coronary heart disease and acute myocardial infarction. *Lancet* 2:983–86
150. Kuo CC, Gown AM, Benditt EP, Grayston JT. 1993. Detection of chlamydia pneumoniae in aortic lesions of atherosclerosis by immunocytochemical stain. *Arterioscler. Thromb.* 13:1501–4
151. Hu H, Pierce GN, Zhong G. 1999. The atherogenic effects of Chlamydia are dependent on serum cholesterol and specific to Chlamydia pneumoniae. *J. Clin. Invest.* 103:747–53
152. Caligiuri G, Rottenberg M, Nicoletti A, Wigzell H, Hansson GK. 2001. Chlamydia pneumoniae infection does not induce or modify atherosclerosis in mice. *Circulation* 103:2834–38
153. Aalto-Setala K, Laitinen K, Erkkila L, Leinonen M, Jauhiainen M, et al. 2001. Chlamydia pneumoniae does not increase atherosclerosis in the aortic root of apolipoprotein E-deficient mice. *Arterioscler. Thromb. Vasc. Biol.* 21:578–84
154. Kalayoglu MV, Libby P, Byrne GI. 2002. Chlamydia pneumoniae as an emerging risk factor in cardiovascular disease. *JAMA* 288:2724–31
155. Perschinka H, Mayr M, Millonig G, Mayerl C, Van Der Zee R, et al. 2003. Cross-reactive B-cell epitopes of microbial and human heat shock protein 60/65 in atherosclerosis. *Arterioscler. Thromb. Vasc. Biol.* 23:1060–65
156. O'Connor CM, Dunne MW, Pfeffer MA, Muhlestein JB, Yao L, et al. 2003. Azithromycin for the secondary prevention of coronary heart disease events: the WIZARD study: a randomized controlled trial. *JAMA* 290:1459–66
157. Cercek B, Shah PK, Noc M, Zahger D, Zeymer U, et al. 2003. Effect of short-term treatment with azithromycin on recurrent ischaemic events in patients with acute coronary syndrome in the Azithromycin in Acute Coronary Syndrome (AZACS) trial: a randomised controlled trial. *Lancet* 361:809–13
158. Epstein SE, Zhou YF, Zhu J. 1999. Infection and atherosclerosis: emerging mechanistic paradigms. *Circulation* 100:E20–28
159. Hendrix MGR, Salimans MMM, Boven CPA, Bruggeman CA. 1990. High prevalence of latently present cytomegalovirus in arterial walls of patients suffering from grade III atherosclerosis. *Am. J. Pathol.* 136:23–28

160. Melnick JL, Adam E, Debakey ME. 1993. Cytomegalovirus and atherosclerosis. *Eur. Heart J.* 14:30–38
161. Zhou YF, Leon MB, Waclawiw MA, Popma JJ, Yu ZX, et al. 1996. Association between prior cytomegalovirus infection and the risk of restenosis after coronary atherectomy. *N. Engl. J. Med.* 335:624–30
162. Lemström K, Sihvola R, Bruggeman C, Häyry P, Koskinen P. 1997. Cytomegalovirus infection-enhanced cardiac allograft vasculopathy is abolished by DHPG prophylaxis in the rat. *Circulation* 95:2614–16
163. Valantine HA. 2004. The role of viruses in cardiac allograft vasculopathy. *Am. J. Transplant.* 4:169–77
164. Sedmak DD, Knight DA, Vook NC, Waldman JW. 1994. Divergent patterns of ELAM-1, ICAM-1, and VCAM-1 expression on cytomegalovirus-infected endothelial cells. *Transplant* 58:1379–85
165. Streblow DN, Kreklywich C, Yin Q, De La Melena VT, Corless CL, et al. 2003. Cytomegalovirus-mediated upregulation of chemokine expression correlates with the acceleration of chronic rejection in rat heart transplants. *J. Virol.* 77:2182–94
166. Streblow DN, Söderberg-Naucler C, Vieira J, Smith P, Wakabayashi E, et al. 1999. The human cytomegalovirus chemokine receptor US28 mediates vascular smooth muscle cell migration. *Cell* 99:511–20
167. Fabricant CG, Fabricant J. 1999. Atherosclerosis induced by infection with Marek's disease herpesvirus in chickens. *Am. Heart J.* 38:S465–68
168. Hsich E, Zhou YF, Paigen B, Johnson TM, Burnett MS, Epstein SE. 2001. Cytomegalovirus infection increases development of atherosclerosis in Apolipoprotein-E knockout mice. *Atherosclerosis* 156:23–28
169. Vliegen I, Duijvestijn A, Grauls G, Herngreen S, Bruggeman C, Stassen F. 2004. Cytomegalovirus infection aggravates atherogenesis in apoE knockout mice by both local and systemic immune activation. *Microbes Infect.* 6:17–24
170. Muhlestein JB, Horne BD, Carlquist JF, Madsen TE, Bair TL, et al. 2000. Cytomegalovirus seropositivity and C-reactive protein have independent and combined predictive value for mortality in patients with angiographically demonstrated coronary artery disease. *Circulation* 102:1917–23
171. Prosch S, Wendt CE, Reinke P, Priemer C, Oppert M, et al. 2000. A novel link between stress and human cytomegalovirus (HCMV) infection: sympathetic hyperactivity stimulates HCMV activation. *Virology* 272:357–65
172. Brown BG, Zhao XQ, Sacco DE, Albers JJ. 1993. Lipid lowering and plaque regression. New insights into prevention of plaque disruption and clinical events in coronary disease. *Circulation* 87:1781–91
173. Falk E, Shah PK, Fuster V. 1995. Coronary plaque disruption. *Circulation* 92:657–71
174. Davies MJ. 1996. Stability and instability: the two faces of coronary atherosclerosis. The Paul Dudley White lecture, 1995. *Circulation* 94: 2013–20
175. Liuzzo G, Biasucci LM, Gallimore JR, Grillo RL, Rebuzzi AG, et al. 1994. The prognostic value of C-reactive protein and serum amyloid a protein in severe unstable angina. *N. Engl. J. Med.* 331:417–24
176. Caligiuri G, Paulsson G, Nicoletti A, Maseri A, Hansson GK. 2000. Evidence for antigen-driven T-cell response in unstable angina. *Circulation* 102:1114–19
177. Moreno PR, Falk E, Palacios IF, Newell JB, Fuster V, Fallon JT. 1994. Macrophage infiltration in acute coronary syndromes. Implications for plaque rupture. *Circulation* 90:775–78

178. Kaartinen M, van der Wal AC, van der Loos CM, Piek JJ, Koch KT, et al. 1998. Mast cell infiltration in acute coronary syndromes: implications for plaque rupture. *J. Am. Coll. Cardiol.* 32:606–12
179. Hansson GK, Hellstrand M, Rymo L, Rubbia L, Gabbiani G. 1989. Interferon γ inhibits both proliferation and expression of differentiation-specific α-smooth muscle actin in arterial smooth muscle cells. *J. Exp. Med.* 170:1595–608
180. Amento EP, Ehsani N, Palmer H, Libby P. 1991. Cytokines and growth factors positively and negatively regulate interstitial collagen gene expression in human vascular smooth muscle cells. *Arterioscl. Thromb.* 11:1223–30
181. Sarén P, Welgus HG, Kovanen PT. 1996. TNF-α and IL-1β selectively induce expression of 92-kDa gelatinase by human macrophages. *J. Immunol.* 157:4159–65
182. Mach F, Schönbeck U, Bonnefoy JY, Pober JS, Libby P. 1997. Activation of monocyte/macrophage functions related to acute atheroma complication by ligation of CD40: induction of collagenase, stromelysin, and tissue factor. *Circulation* 96:396–99
183. Jones CB, Sane DC, Herrington DM. 2003. Matrix metalloproteinases: a review of their structure and role in acute coronary syndrome. *Cardiovasc. Res.* 59:812–23
184. Palsdottir A, Abrahamson M, Thorsteinsson L, Arnason A, Olafsson I, et al. 1988. Mutation in cystatin C gene causes hereditary brain haemorrhage. *Lancet* 2:603–4
185. Sukhova GK, Wang B, Libby P, Pan JH, Zhang Y, et al. 2005. Cystatin C deficiency increases elastic lamina degradation and aortic dilatation in apolipoprotein E-null mice. *Circ. Res.* 96:368–75
186. Biasucci LM, Vitelli A, Liuzzo G, Altamura S, Caligiuri G, et al. 1996. Elevated levels of interleukin-6 in unstable angina. *Circulation* 94:874–77
187. Lindahl B, Toss H, Siegbahn A, Venge P, Wallentin L. 2000. Markers of myocardial damage and inflammation in relation to long-term mortality in unstable coronary artery disease. FRISC Study Group. Fragmin during Instability in Coronary Artery Disease. *N. Engl. J. Med.* 343:1139–47
188. Aukrust P, Müller F, Ueland T, Berget T, Aaser E, et al. 1999. Enhanced levels of soluble and membrane-bound CD40 ligand in patients with unstable angina. *Circulation* 100:614–20
189. Peri G, Introna M, Corradi D, Iacuitti G, Signorini S, et al. 2000. PTX3, A prototypical long pentraxin, is an early indicator of acute myocardial infarction in humans. *Circulation* 102:636–41
190. Damås JK, Waehre T, Yndestad A, Otterdal K, Hognestad A, et al. 2003. Interleukin-7-mediated inflammation in unstable angina: possible role of chemokines and platelets. *Circulation* 107:2670–76
191. Liuzzo G, Goronzy JJ, Yang H, Kopecky SL, Holmes DR, et al. 2000. Monoclonal T-cell proliferation and plaque instability in acute coronary syndromes. *Circulation* 101:2883–88
192. Swanberg M, Lidman O, Padyukov L, Eriksson P, Åkesson E, et al. 2005. MHC2TA is associated with differential MHC molecule expression and susceptibility to rheumatoid arthritis, multiple sclerosis and myocardial infarction. *Nat. Genet.* 37:486–94
193. Arner P. 2003. The adipocyte in insulin resistance: key molecules and the impact of the thiazolidinediones. *Trends Endocrinol. Metab.* 14:137–45
194. Linton MF, Fazio S. 2003. Macrophages, inflammation, and atherosclerosis. *Int. J. Obes. Relat. Metab. Disord.* 27(Suppl 3):S35–40
195. Yudkin JS, Juhan-Vague I, Hawe E, Humphries SE, di Minno G, et al. 2004. Low-grade inflammation may play a role in the etiology of the metabolic syndrome in patients with coronary heart disease: the HIFMECH study. *Metabolism* 53:852–57

196. Ridker PM, Hennekens CH, Buring JE, Rifai N. 2000. C-reactive protein and other markers of inflammation in the prediction of cardiovascular disease in women. *N. Engl. J. Med.* 342:836–43
197. Danesh J, Wheeler JG, Hirschfield GM, Eda S, Eiriksdottir G, et al. 2004. C-reactive protein and other circulating markers of inflammation in the prediction of coronary heart disease. *N. Engl. J. Med.* 350:1387–97
198. Ridker PM, Cannon CP, Morrow D, Rifai N, Rose LM, et al. 2005. C-reactive protein levels and outcomes after statin therapy. *N. Engl. J. Med.* 352:20–28
199. Wilhelmsen L, Svärdsudd K, Korsan-Bengtsen K, Larsson B, Welin L, Tibblin G. 1984. Fibrinogen as a risk factor for stroke and myocardial infarction. *N. Engl. J. Med.* 311:501–5
200. Engström G, Hedblad B, Stavenow L, Tyden P, Lind P, et al. 2004. Fatality of future coronary events is related to inflammation-sensitive plasma proteins: a population-based prospective cohort study. *Circulation* 110:27–31
201. Palinski W, Miller E, Witztum JL. 1995. Immunization of low density lipoprotein (LDL) receptor-deficient rabbits with homologous malondialdehyde-modified LDL reduces atherogenesis. *Proc. Natl. Acad. Sci. USA* 92:821–25
202. Ameli S, Hultgårdh-Nilsson A, Regnström J, Calara F, Yano J, et al. 1996. Effect of immunization with homologous LDL and oxidized LDL on early atherosclerosis in hypercholesterolemic rabbits. *Arterioscler. Thromb. Vasc. Biol.* 16:1074–79
203. Freigang S, Hörkkö S, Miller E, Witztum JL, Palinski W. 1998. Immunization of LDL receptor-deficient mice with homologous malondialdehyde-modified and native LDL reduces progression of atherosclerosis by mechanisms other than induction of high titers of antibodies to oxidative neoepitopes. *Arterioscl. Thromb. Vasc. Biol.* 18:1972–82
204. Zhou X, Caligiuri G, Hamsten A, Lefvert AK, Hansson GK. 2001. LDL immunization induces T-cell-dependent antibody formation and protection against atherosclerosis. *Arterioscler. Thromb. Vasc. Biol.* 21:108–14
205. George J, Afek A, Gilburd B, Levkovitz H, Shaish A, et al. 1998. Hyperimmunization of apo-E-deficient mice with homologous malondialdehyde low-density lipoprotein suppresses early atherogenesis. *Atherosclerosis* 138:147–52
206. Fredrikson GN, Söderberg I, Lindholm M, Dimayuga P, Chyu KY, et al. 2003. Inhibition of atherosclerosis in apoE-null mice by immunization with apoB-100 peptide sequences. *Arterioscler. Thromb. Vasc. Biol.* 23:879–84
207. Zhou X, Robertson AK, Rudling M, Parini P, Hansson GK. 2005. Lesion development and response to immunization reveal a complex role for CD4 in atherosclerosis. *Circ. Res.* 96:427–34
208. Nicoletti A, Paulsson G, Caligiuri G, Zhou X, Hansson GK. 2000. Induction of neonatal tolerance to oxidized lipoprotein reduces atherosclerosis in ApoE knockout mice. *Mol. Med.* 6:283–90
209. Maron R, Sukhova G, Faria AM, Hoffmann E, Mach F, et al. 2002. Mucosal administration of heat shock protein-65 decreases atherosclerosis and inflammation in aortic arch of low-density lipoprotein receptor-deficient mice. *Circulation* 106:1708–15
210. Harats D, Yacov N, Gilburd B, Shoenfeld Y, George J. 2002. Oral tolerance with heat shock protein 65 attenuates Mycobacterium tuberculosis-induced and high-fat-diet-driven atherosclerotic lesions. *J. Am. Coll. Cardiol.* 40:1333–38
211. George J, Yacov N, Breitbart E, Bangio L, Shaish A, et al. 2004. Suppression of early atherosclerosis in LDL-receptor deficient mice by oral tolerance with β2-glycoprotein I. *Cardiovasc. Res.* 62:603–9

212. Jonasson L, Holm J, Hansson GK. 1988. Cyclosporin A inhibits smooth muscle proliferation in the vascular response to injury. *Proc. Natl. Acad. Sci. USA* 85:2303–6
213. Gallo R, Padurean A, Jayaraman T, Marx S, Roque M, et al. 1999. Inhibition of intimal thickening after balloon angioplasty in porcine coronary arteries by targeting regulators of the cell cycle. *Circulation* 99:2164–70
214. Mach F. 2003. Statins as novel immunomodulators: from cell to potential clinical benefit. *Thromb. Haemost.* 90:607–10
215. Janes PW, Ley SC, Magee AI, Kabouridis PS. 2000. The role of lipid rafts in T cell antigen receptor (TCR) signalling. *Semin. Immunol.* 12:23–34
216. Weitz-Schmidt G, Welzenbach K, Brinkmann V, Kamata T, Kallen J, et al. 2001. Statins selectively inhibit leukocyte function antigen-1 by binding to a novel regulatory integrin site. *Nat. Med.* 7:687–92
217. Weitz-Schmidt G, Welzenbach K, Dawson J, Kallen J. 2004. Improved lymphocyte function-associated antigen-1 (LFA-1) inhibition by statin derivatives: molecular basis determined by x-ray analysis and monitoring of LFA-1 conformational changes in vitro and ex vivo. *J. Biol. Chem.* 279:46764–71
218. Kwak B, Mulhaupt F, Myit S, Mach F. 2000. Statins as a newly recognized type of immunomodulator. *Nature Med.* 6:1399–402
219. Mulhaupt F, Matter CM, Kwak BR, Pelli G, Veillard NR, et al. 2003. Statins (HMG-CoA reductase inhibitors) reduce CD40 expression in human vascular cells. *Cardiovasc. Res.* 59:755–66
220. Schönbeck U, Libby P. 2004. Inflammation, immunity, and HMG-CoA reductase inhibitors: statins as antiinflammatory agents? *Circulation* 109:II18–26
221. Blanco-Colio LM, Tunon J, Martin-Ventura JL, Egido J. 2003. Anti-inflammatory and immunomodulatory effects of statins. *Kidney Int.* 63:12–23
222. Youssef S, Stuve O, Patarroyo JC, Ruiz PJ, Radosevich JL, et al. 2002. The HMG-CoA reductase inhibitor, atorvastatin, promotes a Th2 bias and reverses paralysis in central nervous system autoimmune disease. *Nature* 420:78–84
223. McCarey DW, McInnes IB, Madhok R, Hampson R, Scherbakov O, et al. 2004. Trial of Atorvastatin in Rheumatoid Arthritis (TARA): double-blind, randomised placebo-controlled trial. *Lancet* 363:2015–21
224. Elhage R, Gourdy P, Brouchet L, Jawien J, Fouque MJ, et al. 2004. Deleting TCR $\alpha\beta+$ or CD4+ T lymphocytes leads to opposite effects on site-specific atherosclerosis in female apolipoprotein E-deficient mice. *Am. J. Pathol.* 165:2013–18
225. Zhou X, Robertson AK, Rudling M, Parini P, Hansson GK. 2005. Lesion development and response to immunization reveal a complex role for CD4 in atherosclerosis. *Circ. Res.* 96:427–34
226. Elhage R, Jawien J, Rudling M, Ljunggren HG, Takeda K, et al. 2003. Reduced atherosclerosis in interleukin-18 deficient apolipoprotein E-knockout mice. *Cardiovasc. Res.* 59:234–40
227. Buono C, Binder CJ, Stavrakis G, Witztum JL, Glimcher LH, Lichtman AH. 2005. T-bet deficiency reduces atherosclerosis and alters plaque antigen-specific immune responses. *Proc. Natl. Acad. Sci. USA* 102:1596–601
228. Gupta S, Pablo AM, Jiang X-C, Wang N, Tall AR, Schindler C. 1997. IFN-γ potentiates atherosclerosis in apoE knock-out mice. *J. Clin. Invest.* 99:2752–61
229. Whitman SC, Ravisankar P, Daugherty A. 2002. IFN-γ deficiency exerts gender-specific effects on atherogenesis in apolipoprotein E−/− mice. *J. Interferon. Cytokine Res.* 22:661–70

230. Buono C, Come CE, Stavrakis G, Maguire GF, Connelly PW, Lichtman AH. 2003. Influence of interferon-γ on the extent and phenotype of diet-induced atherosclerosis in the LDLR-deficient mouse. *Arterioscler. Thromb. Vasc. Biol.* 23:454–60
231. Schreyer SA, Peschon JJ, LeBoeuf RC. 1996. Accelerated atherosclerosis in mice lacking tumor necrosis factor receptor p55. *J. Biol. Chem.* 271:26174–78
232. Elhage R, Clamens S, Besnard S, Mallat Z, Tedgui A, et al. 2001. Involvement of interleukin-6 in atherosclerosis but not in the prevention of fatty streak formation by 17β -estradiol in apolipoprotein E-deficient mice. *Atherosclerosis* 156:315–20
233. Song L, Schindler C. 2004. IL-6 and the acute phase response in murine atherosclerosis. *Atherosclerosis* 177:43–51

Lung Cancer Preneoplasia

Ignacio I. Wistuba[1] and Adi F. Gazdar[2]

[1]Departments of Pathology and Thoracic/Head and Neck Medical Oncology, M.D. Anderson Cancer Center, University of Texas, Houston, Texas 77030; email: iiwistuba@mdanderon.org

[2]Hamon Center for Therapeutic Oncology Research and Department of Pathology University of Texas Southwestern Medical Center, Dallas, Texas 75390; email: adi.gazdar@utsouthwestern.edu

Annu. Rev. Pathol. Mech. Dis. 2006. 1:331–48

First published online as a Review in Advance on October 26, 2005

The *Annual Review of Pathology: Mechanisms of Disease* is online at pathmechdis.annualreviews.org

doi: 10.1146/annurev.pathol.1.110304.100103

1553-4006/06/0114-0331$20.00

Key Words

smoking, bronchial dysplasia, atypical adenomatous hyperplasia, EGFR mutations

Abstract

From histological and biological perspectives, lung cancer is a complex neoplasm. Although the sequential preneoplastic changes have been defined for centrally arising squamous carcinomas of the lung, they have been poorly documented for the other major forms of lung cancers, including small cell lung carcinoma and adenocarcinomas. There are three main morphologic forms of preneoplastic lesions recognized in the lung: squamous dysplasias, atypical adenomatous hyperplasia, and diffuse idiopathic pulmonary neuroendocrine cell hyperplasia. However, these lesions account for the development of only a subset of lung cancers. Several studies have provided information regarding the molecular characterization of lung preneoplastic changes, especially for squamous cell carcinoma. These molecular changes have been detected in the histologically normal and abnormal respiratory epithelium of smokers. Two different molecular pathways have been detected in lung adenocarcinoma pathogenesis: smoking-associated activation of RAS signaling, and nonsmoking-associated activation of EGFR signaling; the latter is detected in histologically normal respiratory epithelium.

SCLC: small cell lung carcinoma

NSCLC: non-small cell lung carcinoma

CIS: carcinoma in situ

AAH: atypical adenomatous hyperplasia

INTRODUCTION

Lung cancer is the leading cause of cancer deaths in the United States and worldwide (1). The high mortality rate of this disease is due primarily to the fact that the majority of lung cancers are diagnosed at advanced stages when the options for treatment are mostly palliative. Experience with other epithelial tumors, such as uterine, cervical, esophageal, and colon carcinomas, has shown that if neoplastic lesions can be detected and treated at their intraepithelial stage the chances for survival can be improved significantly. Thus, to reduce the mortality rate of lung cancer, new techniques and approaches must be developed to diagnose and treat pre-invasive lesions. However, the early diagnosis of lung cancer represents an enormous challenge. From histopathological and biological perspectives, lung cancer is a highly complex neoplasm (2), probably having multiple preneoplastic pathways.

Lung cancer consists of several histological types, including small cell lung carcinoma (SCLC) and non-small cell lung carcinoma (NSCLC) types of squamous cell carcinoma, adenocarcinoma (including the noninvasive type of bronchioloalveolar carcinoma), and large cell carcinoma (3). Lung cancers may arise from the major bronchi (central tumors) or small bronchi, bronchioles, or alveoli (peripheral tumors) of the distant airway of the lung. Squamous cell carcinomas and SCLCs usually arise centrally, whereas adenocarcinomas and large cell carcinomas usually arise peripherally. However, the specific respiratory epithelial cell type from which each lung cancer type develops has not been established. As with other epithelial malignancies, researchers believe lung cancers arise after a series of progressive pathological changes, known as preneoplastic or premalignant lesions (4). Although the sequential preneoplastic changes have been defined for centrally arising squamous carcinomas of the lung, they have been poorly documented for the other major forms of lung cancers (4).

Although many molecular abnormalities have been described in clinically evident lung cancers (2), relatively little is known about the molecular events preceding the development of lung carcinomas and the underlying genetic basis of lung carcinogenesis. In the past decade, several studies have provided information regarding the molecular characterization of the preneoplastic changes involved in the pathogenesis of lung cancer, especially squamous cell carcinoma and adenocarcinoma (5, 6). Many of these molecular changes have been detected in the histologically normal respiratory mucosa of smokers (5).

The high-risk population targeted for early detection efforts are heavy smokers and patients who have survived a cancer of the upper aerodigestive tract. However, conventional morphologic methods for the identification of premalignant cell populations in the lung airways have important limitations. This has led to research in biological properties, including molecular and genetic changes, of the respiratory epithelium and its corresponding preneoplastic cells and lesions. Further research in this area may provide new methods for assessing the likehood of developing invasive lung cancer in smokers and allow for early detection and monitoring of their response to chemopreventive regimens.

In this review we will describe the recognized preneoplastic lesions for major types of lung cancers, such as bronchial squamous dysplasia and carcinoma in situ (CIS) for squamous cell carcinoma (7); atypical adenomatous hyperplasia (AAH), a putative preneoplastic lesion, for a subset of adenocarcinomas (6); and neuroendocrine cell hyperplasia for neuroendocrine lung carcinomas (7). In addition, we will review the current concepts of early pathogenesis and the progression of lung cancer.

OVERVIEW OF LUNG CANCER MOLECULAR PATHOLOGY

Several molecular and genetic studies have revealed that multiple genetic and epigentic changes are found in clinically evident lung cancers, involving known and putative recessive oncogenes (tumor suppressor genes, TSGs) as well as several dominant oncogenes (8). Most of the molecular and genetic studies of lung cancers have been performed on the major types of lung cancer (2). Many growth factors or regulatory peptides and their receptors are overexpressed by cancer cells and adjacent normal-appearing cells in the lung, and thus provide a series of autocrine and paracrine growth stimulatory loops in this neoplasm (9). The list of recessive oncogenes involved in lung cancer is likely to include as many as 10 to 15 known and putative genes (2), and possibly many more. Oncogenes that contribute to the pathogenesis of lung cancer include *CMYC*, mutated *KRAS* (10% to 20%, predominantly adenocarcinomas), overexpression of *Cyclin D1* and *BCL2*, and mutations in *ERBB* family genes such as *EGFR* (epidermal growth factor receptor) (10–12) and *HER2/neu* (12, 13). The latter two oncogenes occur almost exclusively in adenocarcinomas, patients of East Asian ethnic groups, and non- or light smokers (12). Several TSGs, such as *TP53* (17p13), *RB* (13q14), $p16^{INK4a}$ (9p21), and new candidate TSGs at several chromosomal regions, including the short arm of chromosomes 3 (3p12, *DUTT1* gene; 3p14.2, *FHIT* gene; 3p21, *RASFF1A* and *FUS-1* gene; 3p22–24, *BAP-1* gene), show frequent abnormalities in lung cancer (2). Recessive oncogenes are believed to be inactivated via a two-step process involving both alleles. Knudson has proposed that the first hit is frequently a point mutation, whereas the second allele is subsequently inactivated via a chromosomal deletion, translocation, or other event such as methylation of gene promoter regions (14). In addition to those specific genetic changes, other evidence indicates that genetic instability is concurrent with lung cancer. This evidence includes changes in the number of short-tandem DNA repeats (also known as microsatellites), which are frequently present in a wide variety of cancer types, including lung. Overall, an average of 35% (range 0%–76%) of SCLCs and 22% (range 2%–49%) of NSCLCs show some evidence of genetic instability at individual loci (8).

TSG: tumor suppressor gene

EGFR: epidermal growth factor receptor

Studies of many lung cancers have demonstrated different patterns of molecular alterations between the two major groups of lung carcinomas (SCLC and NSCLC) (15, 16) and among the two major histologic types of NSCLC (squamous cell carcinomas and adenocarcinomas) (17–20). Allelic loss analyses at different chromosomal regions and the methylation status of multiple genes have provided clear evidence, on a genome-wide scale, that SCLC and NSCLC differ significantly in the TSGs that are inactivated during their pathogenesis (21–24). In addition, a variety of studies on gene expression profiles have sought to identify specific profiles and new molecular markers for histologically different lung cancers, including adenocarcinomas (25, 26). Specifically, we have found different patterns of allelic loss involving the two major histologic types of NSCLC, with higher incidences of deletions at 17p13 (*TP53*), 13q14 (*RB*), 9p21 ($p16^{INK4a}$), 8p21–23, and several 3p regions in squamous cell carcinomas (17, 27, 28). Recently, differences in $p16^{INK4a}$, *APC*, and *H-cadherin* gene methylation frequencies have been detected between squamous cell and adenocarcinoma, suggesting that different gene methylation patterns characterize the two major histologic types of NSCLC (24). Recent findings indicate that mutations in three genes, *KRAS*, *EGFR*, and *Her2/neu*, occur almost exclusively in lung cancers of adenocarcinoma histology (12, 29). In lung adenocarcinoma, *KRAS* and *EGFR* mutations are mutually exclusive, which indicates two distinct pathways for lung adenocarcinoma development (12, 30). Whereas in smokers tobacco-related carcinogens favor *KRAS* mutations, in nonsmokers unidentified carcinogens induce *EGFR* mutations (30). We refer to nonsmokers as people who have never smoked.

LUNG CANCER PRENOPLASTIC LESIONS

Lung cancers are believed to arise after a series of progressive pathological changes (preneoplastic or precursor lesions) in the respiratory mucosa. Although the sequential preneoplastic changes have been defined for centrally arising squamous carcinomas, they have been poorly documented for large cell carcinomas, adenocarcinomas, and SCLCs (4, 7). Mucosal changes in the large airways that may precede invasive squamous cell carcinoma include squamous dysplasia and CIS (4, 7). Adenocarcinomas may be preceded by morphological changes including AAH (4, 6) in peripheral airway cells. For SCLC, no specific preneoplastic changes have been described in the respiratory epithelium. Current information suggests that preneoplastic lesions are frequently extensive and multifocal throughout the lung, indicating a field effect (field cancerization) by which much of the respiratory epithelium has been mutagenized, presumably from exposure to tobacco-related carcinogens (5).

The recent histological classification of pre-invasive lung lesions by the World Health Organization (WHO) lists three main morphologic forms of preneoplastic lesions (3): (*a*) squamous dysplasia and CIS, (*b*) AAH, and (*c*) diffuse idiopathic pulmonary neuroendocrine cell hyperplasia (DIPNECH). However, as we will explain in this review, these lesions account for the development of only a subset of lung cancers.

Squamous Cell Carcinoma Preneoplastic Lesions

Mucosal changes in the large airways that may precede or accompany invasive squamous cell carcinoma include hyperplasia, squamous metaplasia, squamous dysplasia, and CIS (**Figure 1**) (4, 7). Two types of bronchial epithelial hyperplasia that are thought to be reactive lesions, goblet cell hyperplasia and basal cell (reserve cell) hyperplasia, may occur. Dysplastic squamous lesions are considered true preneoplastic lesions and may vary in degree (i.e., mild, moderate, or severe); however, these lesions represent a continuum of cytologic and histologic atypical changes that may show some overlapping features between categories. Whereas mild squamous dysplasia is characterized by minimal architectural and cytological disturbance, moderate dysplasia exhibits more cytological irregularity, which is even higher in severe dysplasia and is accompanied by considerable cellular polymorphism. In a subset of squamous dysplastic changes, the basal membrane thickens and there is vascular budding in the subepithelial tissues that results in papillary protrusions of the epithelium, lesions that have been termed angiogenic squamous dysplasia (31). CIS demonstrates extreme cytological aberrations with almost complete architectural disarray, but with an intact basement membrane and absence of stromal invasion. Foci of CIS usually arise near bifurcations in the segmental bronchi, subsequently extending proximally into the adjacent lobar bronchus and distally into subsegmental branches. These lesions are often not detected by conventional white-light bronchoscopy or gross examination. However, the utilization of fluorescent bronchoscopy, such as lung-imaging fluorescent endoscopy (LIFE), greatly increases the sensitivity for detection of squamous dysplastic and CIS lesions (32–34). Little is known about the rate and risks of progression from squamous dysplasia to CIS and ultimately to invasive squamous cell carcinoma. Recently, a longitudinal study addressing the natural histopathologic course of squamous preneoplastic lesions in bronchial epithelium using white-light and fluorescent bronchoscopy examinations was reported (35). In this study, the progression rate to CIS and invasive carcinoma was significantly higher in lesions with severe dysplasia (32%) compared with squamous metaplasias (4%) and low-grade

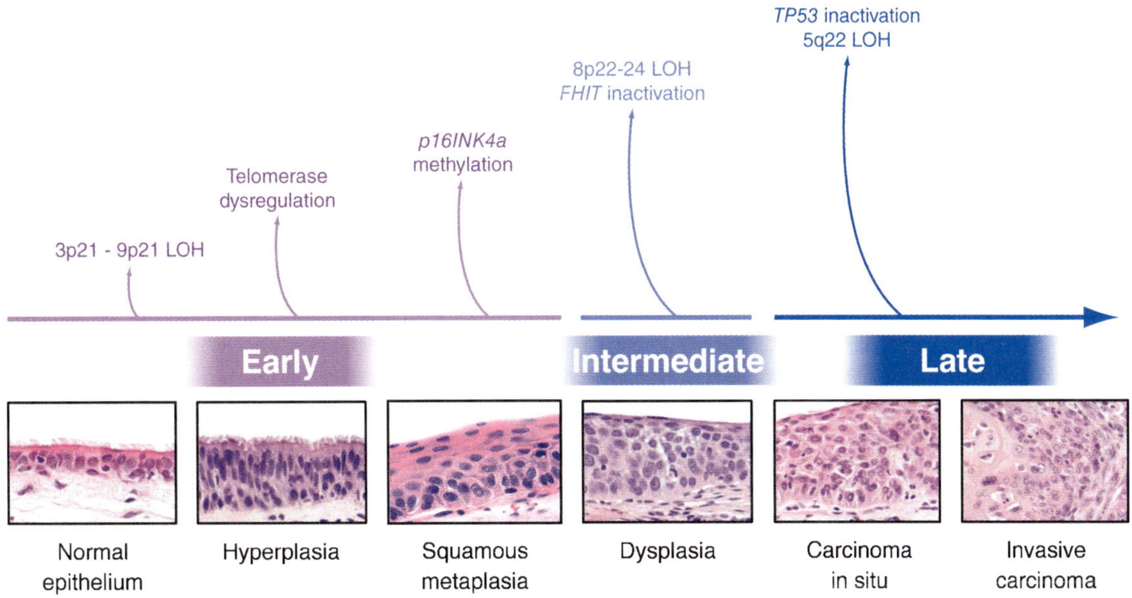

Figure 1

Histopatholological and molecular changes during the pathogenesis of squamous cell carcinoma of the lung with molecular changes commencing at early stages, and a histologically normal respiratory epithelium. There is stepwise molecular and histopathological sequence of events leading to dysplastic and invasive carcinoma stages. LOH, loss of heterozygosity.

dysplasias (9%). Somewhat striking, at the individual level, the rates of progression to squamous carcinoma were not significantly higher in individuals harboring high-grade dysplastic lesions (39%) compared with individuals having only lower-grade lesions (26%). In addition, the study detected the progression from squamous metaplasia and low-grade dysplasias (mild and moderate) to CIS and invasive carcinoma, suggesting that a stepwise histopathologic multistage development of lung squamous cell carcinoma does not always occur, or it is not always detected because of rapid progression. These findings suggest that the current histologic classification of preneoplastic squamous lesions of the bronchial epithelia may not be a reliable guide for risk assessment of lung cancer. Other types of biomarkers, including molecular and genetic markers, are needed.

There are no squamous cells in the normal airways. The progenitor or stem cells for the squamous metaplastic epithelium of the proximal airway is not known, but it is presumed that the basal cells represent a relatively quiescent zone that is the precursor of preneoplastic epithelium. In fact, squamous metaplasia usually precedes and accompanies basal cell hyperplasia. Interestingly, these cells express significant levels of Egfr protein and increased proliferative activity measured by Ki-67 staining (36, 37).

The current working model of the sequential molecular abnormalities in the pathogenesis of squamous cell lung carcinoma (**Figure 1**) indicates the following: (*a*) Genetic abnormalities commence in histologically normal epithelium and grow with increasing severity of histologic changes (27). (*b*) Mutations follow a sequence, with progressive allelic losses at multiple 3p (3p21, 3p14, 3p22–24, and 3p12) chromosome sites and 9p21 ($p16^{INK4a}$) as the earliest detectable changes. Later changes occur at 8p21–23, 13q14 (*RB*), and 17p13 (*TP53*) (17, 27, 28). $p16^{INK4a}$ methylation has also been detected at an early

BAC: bronchioloalveolar carcinoma

stage of squamous pre-invasive lesions with a frequency that increases during histopathologic progression (by 24% in squamous metaplasia and 50% in CIS) (38). (*c*) Molecular changes in the respiratory epithelium are extensive and multifocal throughout the bronchial tree of smokers and lung cancer patients, indicating a field cancerization effect by which much of the respiratory epithelium has been mutagenized, presumably from exposure to tobacco-related carcinogens (27, 28, 39, 40). (*d*) Multiple small patches of histologically normal and hyperplastic epithelium with clonal and subclonal molecular abnormalities, not much larger in size than the average bronchial biopsy obtained by fluorescent bronchoscopy and estimated to be approximately 40,000 to 360,000 cells, such as allelic loss (chromosome 3p and 9p21 regions) and genetic instability, can be detected in the normal and slightly abnormal bronchial epithelium of patients with lung cancer (41). These findings are consistent with evidence of numerous small monosomic and trisomic clonal and subclonal patches present in smoking-damaged upper aerodigestive epithelium as determined by fluorescent in situ hybridization (FISH) analyses (42).

Adenocarcinoma Precursor Lesions

In alveoli, type I pneumocytes are involved in respiratory gas exchange whereas type II cells produce surfactant proteins, essential for preventing alveoli from collapsing (43). In bronchioles, short, stubby ciliated cells and the secretory Clara cells are present. The Clara cells and the type II pneumocytes are believed to be the progenitor cells of the peripheral airways, and peripherally arising adenocarcinomas often express markers of these cell types (44, 45). Researchers suggest that adenocarcinomas may be preceded by AAH in peripheral airway cells (4, 6); however, the respiratory structures and the specific epithelial cell types involved in the origin of most lung adenocarcinomas are unknown. Although there is only one sequence of morphologic change identified so far for the development of invasive lung adenocarcinomas (AAH and bronchioloalveolar carcinoma, BAC), recent data indicate that at least two molecular pathways are involved, the *KRAS* and *EGFR* pathways in smoker and nonsmoker populations, respectively (**Figure 2**).

Atypical adenomatous hyperplasia. AAH is considered a putative precursor of adenocarcinoma (4, 6). AAH is a discrete parenchymal lesion arising in alveoli near terminal and respiratory bronchioles (**Figure 2**) and may be single or multiple lesions. These lesions maintain an alveolar structure lined by rounded, cuboidal, or low columnar cells. The alveolar walls may be slightly thickened by collagen, occasional fibroblasts, and lymphocytes. Cellularity and cytological atypia vary from minimal to high grade. The postulated progression of AAH to adenocarcinoma with BAC features, which is characterized by the growth of neoplastic cells along preexisting alveolar structures without evidences of stromal, pleural, or vascular invasion and without metastasis, is supported by morphometric, cytofluorometric, and molecular studies (6, 7). Distinction between highly atypical AAH and BAC is sometimes difficult. Somewhat arbitrarily, BAC are considered generally >10 mm in diameter, with more pleomorphism, mild stratification, packed cells, and abrupt transitions to adjacent alveolar lining cells. However, the distinction may, on occasion, be difficult. The differentiation phenotype derived from immunohistochemical and ultrastructural features indicates that AAHs originate from the progenitor cells of the peripheral airways (46, 47). Surfactant apoprotein and Clara cell–specific 10-kDd protein are expressed in almost all AAHs (46). As many as 25% of the cells show ultrastructural features of Clara cells and type II pneumocytes (47). Recent results from a study (48) performed in mice and lung cancer mouse models suggest that peripheral bronchioalveolar cells expressing Clara cell–specific protein and surfactant protein-C, and having in vitro stem

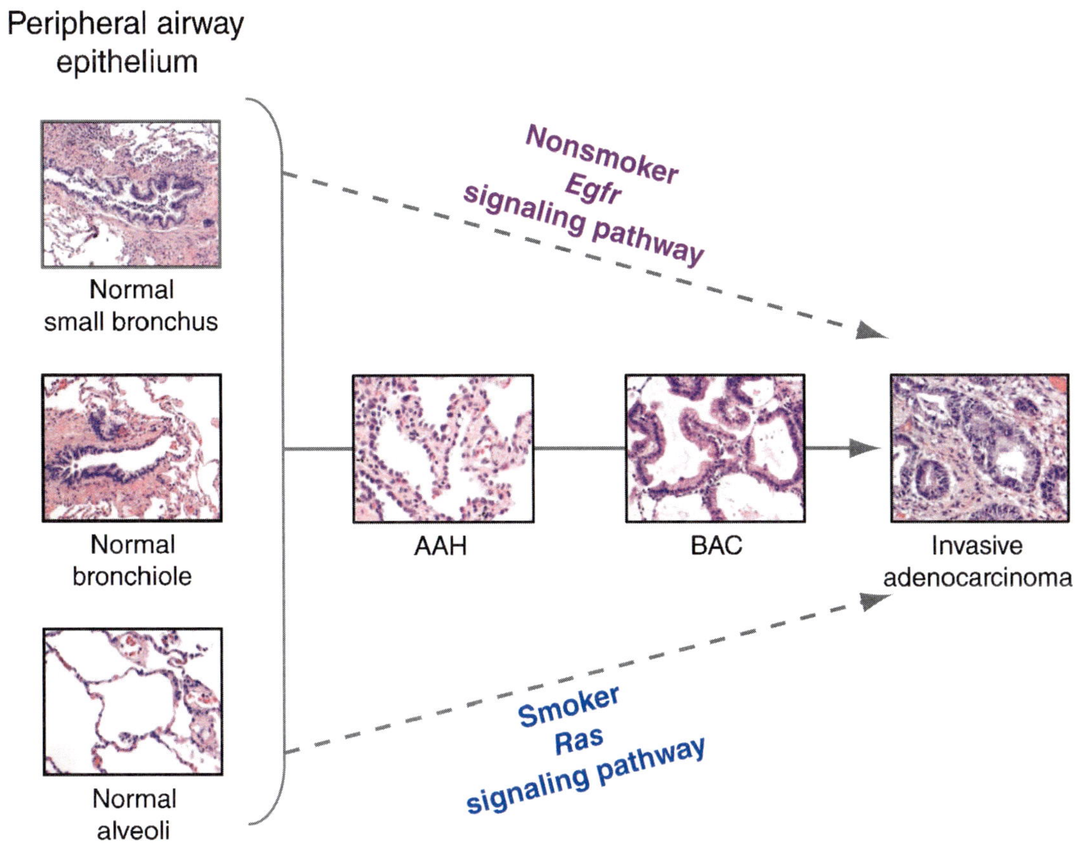

Figure 2

Two molecular pathways involved in the development of lung cancer have been recognized. AAH, atypical adenomatous hyperplasia; BAC, bronchioloalveolar carcinoma.

cell properties (termed bronchioalveolar stem cell, BASC), are the stem cell population that maintains the bronchiolar Clara cells and alveolar cells of the distal respiratory epithelium. In vitro studies performed in the same study indicated that the BASC-transformed counterpart gives rise to adenocarcinoma of the lung. BASCs expanded in response to oncogenic *KRAS* in culture and in precursors of mouse lung tumors in vivo (48).

An increasing body of evidence supports the concept of AAH as the precursor of at least a subset of adenocarcinomas. AAH is most frequently detected in lungs of patients bearing lung cancers (9%–20%), especially adenocarcinomas (as many as 40%), compared with squamous cell carcinomas (11%) (7, 49–52). In contrast, autopsy studies have reported AAH in ~3% of noncancer patients (53). Because inflation of the lungs prior to sectioning (a practice not common in the United States) aids identification, their true incidence may be higher than indicated. Some patients display a large number of AAH lesions (>40) in conjunction with multiple synchronous peripheral lung adenocarcinomas or BACs (51). However, it is extremely difficult to know the progression rate of AAH to lung adenocarcinoma, and it is also currently almost impossible to determine if AAHs may regress. Because they are air-filled structures, they may appear as ground glass opacities on computed tomography scans. However, AAH location, size, and relative invisibility to most imaging methods make longitudinal studies even more difficult than centrally located squamous preneoplastic lesions.

Several molecular changes frequently present in lung adenocarcinomas are also present in AAH lesions, and they are further evidence that AAH may represent true preneoplastic lesions (46). The most important finding is the presence of *KRAS* (codon 12) mutations in as many as 39% of AAHs, which are also a relatively frequent alteration in lung adenocarcinomas (6, 54). Other molecular alterations detected in AAH are overexpression of Cyclin D1 (~70%), p53 (ranging from 10% to 58%), survivin (48%), and HER2/neu (7%) proteins (6, 55, 56). Some AAH lesions have demonstrated loss of heterozygosity (LOH) in chromosomes 3p (18%), 9p ($p16^{INK4a}$, 13%), 9q (53%), 17q, and 17p (*TP53*, 6%), changes that are frequently detected in lung adenocarcinomas (57, 58). A study on lung adenocarcinoma with synchronous multiple AAHs showed frequent LOH of tuberous sclerosis complex (TSC)-associated regions (*TSC1* at 9q, 53%, and *TSC2* at 16p, 6%), suggesting that these are candidate loci for TSG in a subset of adenocarcinomas of the lung (58). Some cases of AAH have been monoclonal, suggesting that it may be a true preneoplastic lesion (59). Activation of telomerase, required for the perpetuation of cancer cells and expressed by human telomerase RNA component and telomerase reverse transcriptase mRNA, has been detected in 27% to 78% of AAH lesions, depending on their atypia level (60). Recently, it was shown that loss of *LKB1*, a serine/threonine kinase that functions as a TSG, is frequent in lung adenocarcinomas (25%) and AAH (21%) with severe cytological atypia, whereas it is rare in mild atypical AAH lesions (5%), suggesting that *LKB1* inactivation may play a role in the AAH progression to malignancy (61).

Bronchial and bronchiolar epithelium as precursors of adenocarcinomas. Despite evidence that AAH is a precursor lesion for peripheral lung adenocarcinomas, there is general consensus that the pathogenesis of many adenocarcinomas, especially those of central origin, is still unknown. The presence of *KRAS* mutations in bronchiolar epithelium with atypical changes raised the possibility that non-AAH lesions could also be the origin of lung adenocarcinomas (62). The recent findings of several distinct genetic changes specifically associated with lung adenocarcinoma, such as *EGFR* (10–12), *Her2/neu* (29), and *BRAF* (63) genes mutations, represent a unique opportunity to study further the pathogenesis of adenocarcinomas of the lung.

Somatic mutations of *EGFR*, a tyrosine kinase (TK) of the *ERBB* family, have been reported recently in a subset of lung adenocarcinomas (10–12, 64–67) (**Figure 3**). Those mutations are clinically relevant because most of them have been associated with sensitivity of lung adenocarcinoma to small molecule TK inhibitors (gefitinib and erlotinib) (10, 11, 64, 68). The mutations are associated significantly with adenocarcinoma histology, non- or light-smoker status, females, and East Asian ethnic groups (12). Data analysis from 13 (10, 12, 45, 65–67, 69–75) recently published studies on *EGFR* mutations in surgically resected specimens in more than 1600 lung cancers indicates that the incidence of mutations in adenocarcinomas is at least fourfold higher in East Asian populations (China, Japan, Korea, and Taiwan) compared with Western populations (Australia, Italy, and the United States) (**Figure 3*a***). Analysis of 721 *EGFR* mutations reported from surgically resected (12, 65–67, 69–71, 73–75) and small-biopsy lung cancer specimens (10, 11, 71, 76–82) demonstrated that more than 90% of the mutations detected in *EGFR* are in-frame deletions in exon 19, and there was a single missense mutation in exon 21 (L858R) (10–12, 64–67) (**Figure 3*b***). Researchers propose that lung cancer cells with mutant *EGFR* may become physiologically dependent on the continued activity of the gene for the maintenance of their malignant phenotype, which leads to accelerated development of lung adenocarcinoma (30). Recent studies indicate that

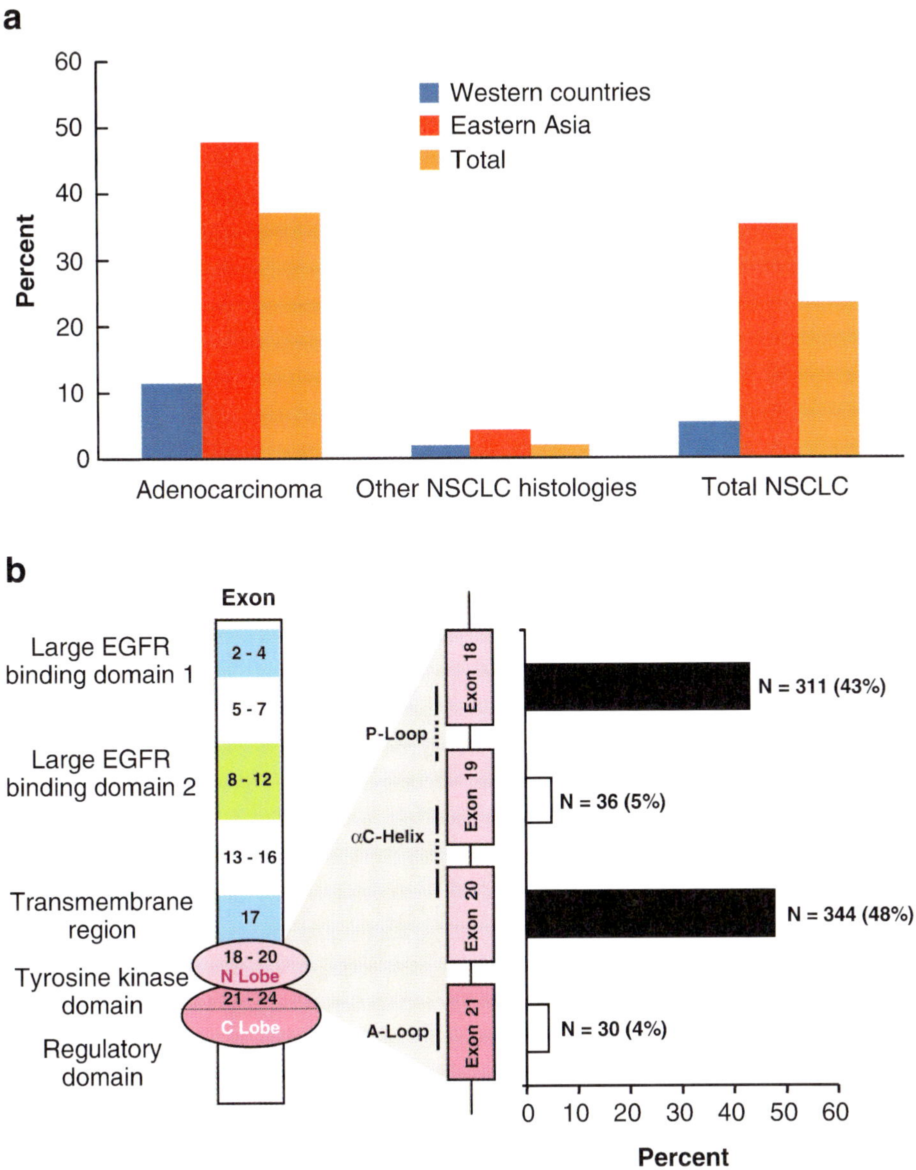

Figure 3

(*a*) Summary of epidermal growth factor receptor (*EGFR*) gene mutation frequency in lung cancer by histology and country of origin. Data analysis from 13 (10, 12, 45, 65–67, 69–75) recently published studies examining more than 1600 lung cancers have been summarized. (*b*) Summary of exon distribution of 721 *EGFR* mutations reported from surgically resected (12, 65–67, 69–71, 73–75) and small-biopsy (10, 11, 71, 76–82) lung cancer specimens.

tumor cell high *EGFR* copy number, identified by FISH technique and Egfr immunohistochemical expression, may also be effective predictors for EGFR TK inhibitors (76, 79, 83).

Some studies have investigated Egfr expression in centrally located bronchial preneoplastic lesions of the lung (36, 84), which are considered markers for squamous metaplasia (84). In lung adenocarcinoma, recent studies indicate that the recently identified TK domain of *EGFR* mutations is an early development in the pathogenesis of lung cancer, being identified in histologically normal epithelium of small bronchi and bronchioles adjacent to *EGFR* mutant adenocarcinomas (85). We have detected *EGFR* mutations in normal-appearing peripheral respiratory epithelium in 9 out of 21 (43%) adenocarcinoma patients (85), but not in patients without

DIPENECH: diffuse idiopathic pulmonary neuroendocrine cell hyperplasia

mutation in the tumor (85). Our finding of more frequent *EGFR* mutations in normal epithelium within the tumor (43%) than in adjacent sites (24%) suggests a localized field effect phenomenon for this abnormality in the respiratory epithelium of the lung. A higher frequency of mutations in cells obtained from small bronchi (35%) compared with bronchioles (18%) was detected. This finding may correlate with different cell types populating those epithelia, which could represent the site of the cell of origin for *EGFR* mutant adenocarcinomas of the lung. Although the cell type having those mutations is unknown, we hypothesize that stem or progenitor cells of the bronchial and bronchiolar epithelium bear such mutations. The finding of relatively infrequent *EGFR* mutations in AAH lesions (3 out of 40 examined) (45, 86) and the finding of no mutation (12) or relatively low frequency of mutation in true BACs of the lung (86) support the concept that genetic abnormalities of *EGFR* are not relevant in the pathogenesis of alveolar-type lung neoplasia.

The low frequency of molecular abnormalities detected in the centrally located bronchial respiratory epithelium in patients with peripheral lung adenocarcinomas, compared with specimens from patients with squamous cell carcinomas and SCLC (87), suggests the presence of two compartments in the lung with different degrees of smoking-related genetic damage. Thus, smokers who develop squamous cell carcinoma and SCLC have more smoking-related genetic damage in the respiratory epithelium of the central airway, whereas patients who develop adenocarcinoma have damage mainly in the peripheral airways (small bronchus, bronchioles, and alveoli).

Precursor Lesions of Neuroendocrine Tumors

As stated above, the precursor lesions for the most common type of neuroendocrine carcinoma of the lung, the SCLC, are unknown (4, 7). However, a rare lesion termed diffuse idiopathic pulmonary neuroendocrine cell hyperplasia (DIPENECH) has been associated with the development of other neuroendocrine tumors of the lung, typical and atypical carcinoids (4, 88, 89) (**Figure 4**). DIPENECH consists of a generalized proliferation of scattered single cells, small nodules, or linear proliferations of neuroendocrine cells present in the bronchial and bronchiolar epithelium. These lesions include local extraluminal proliferations in the form of tumorlets.

Small cell lung carcinoma precursors. As the development of epithelial cancers requires the stepwise accumulation of multiple mutations, which may represent a mutator phenotype, it is possible that those epithelial cell clones that have accumulated multiple mutations are at higher risk for developing malignant transformation (90). As stated before, no phenotypically identifiable epithelial lesion has been identified as a precursor for SCLC. We performed a study comparing the molecular changes (LOH at several chromosomal sites and microsatellite instability) occurring in histologically normal and mildly abnormal (hyperplastic), centrally located bronchial epithelium accompanying SCLCs and NSCLCs (squamous cell carcinomas and adenocarcinoma) (87). Normal and hyperplastic bronchial epithelium accompanying SCLC demonstrated a significantly higher incidence of genetic abnormalities than those adjacent to NSCLC tumor types (19). These findings indicate that more widespread and more extensive genetic damage is present in bronchial epithelium in patients with SCLC (**Figure 4**). The finding that some specimens of normal or mildly abnormal epithelia accompanying SCLCs have a high incidence of genetic changes (19) suggests that SCLC may arise directly from histologically normal or mildly abnormal epithelium, without passing through a more complex histologic sequence (parallel theory of cancer development).

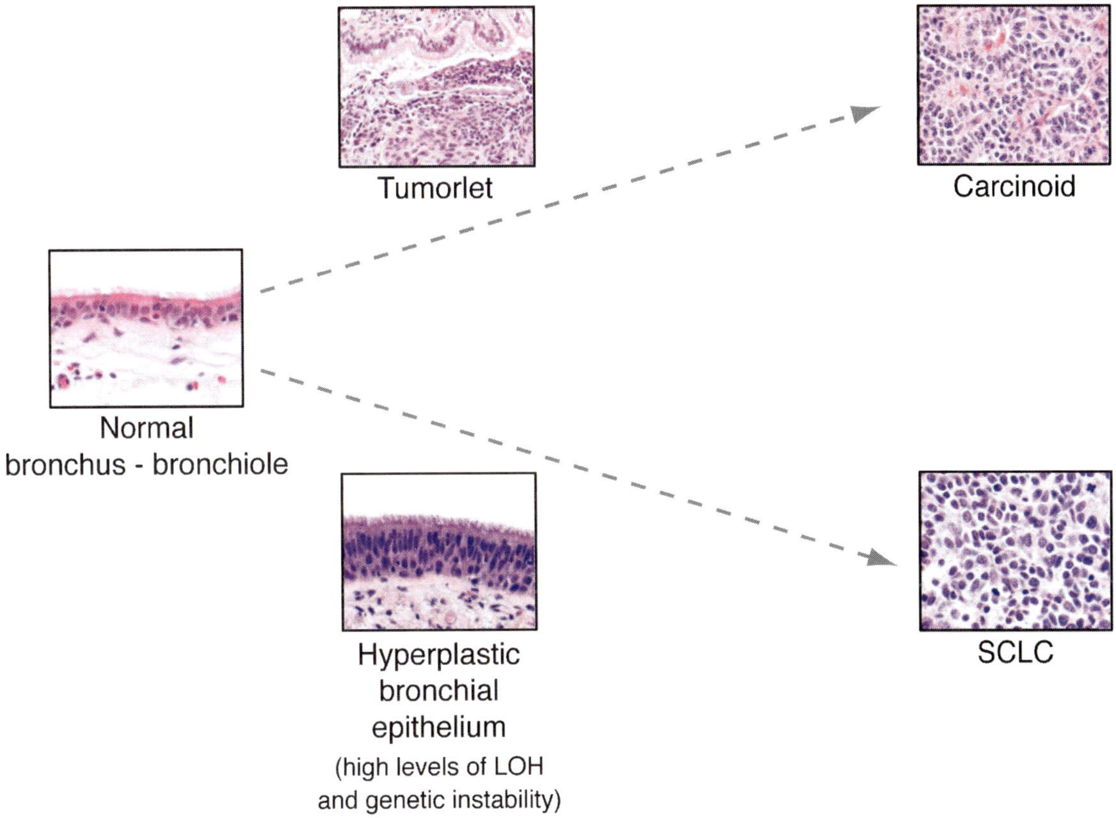

Figure 4

Although the molecular information is limited, available data suggest that tumorlet is the potential precursor for lung carcinoids, and small cell lung carcinoma (SCLC) may arise from molecularly altered, histologically normal, or hyperplastic bronchial epithelium. LOH, loss of heterozygosity.

SMOKING-DAMAGED BRONCHIAL EPITHELIUM

After smoking cessation, the risk of developing lung cancer decreases, but never reaches baseline levels of nonsmokers (91). Advanced lung preneoplastic changes occur more frequently in smokers than nonsmokers, and they increase in frequency with the amount of smoke exposure, adjusted by age (92). Risk factors that identify normal and premalignant bronchial tissue for malignant progression need to be better defined. However, only scant information is available regarding molecular changes in the respiratory epithelium of smokers without cancer. Two independent studies show that the genetic changes (loss of heterozygosity and microsatellite instability) found in invasive cancers and preneoplasia can also be identified in morphologically normal-appearing bronchial epithelium from current or former smokers, and they may persist for many years after smoking cessation (39, 40). In general, such genetic changes are not found in the bronchial epithelium from true nonsmokers. As has been observed in epithelial foci accompanying invasive lung carcinoma (27), allelic losses on chromosomes 3p and 9p are often present. These findings support the hypothesis that identifying genetic abnormalities, such as allelic losses, in biopsies may provide new methods for assessing the risk of smokers developing invasive lung cancer and monitoring their response to chemoprevention.

We have demonstrated that molecular changes (allelic loss and genomic instability) in the bronchial epithelium may persist long after smoking cessation (39, 40). Of interest, Lee and colleagues (37) reported that smoking appears to elicit a dose-related proliferative response in the bronchial epithelia of active smokers measured by the Ki-67 proliferation index. Although the proliferative response decreased gradually in former smokers, a subset of individuals had detectable proliferation for many years after quitting smoking (37).

Recent results on methylation analysis of several genes, including *RARβ-2*, *H-cadherin*, *APC*, *p16*^{INK4a}, and *RASFF1A*, indicate that abnormal gene methylation is a relatively frequent occurrence in oropharyngeal and bronchial epithelial cells in heavy smokers with evidence of sputum atypia (93). Methylation in one or more of three genes tested (*p16*^{INK4a}, *GSTP1*, and *DAPK*) has been demonstrated in bronchial brush specimens in approximately one third of smoker subjects (94). Aberrant promoter methylation of *p16*^{INK4a} was seen in at least one bronchial epithelial site from 44% of lung cancer patients and cancer-free smokers. No promoter methylation of these genes was detected in bronchial epithelium from nonsmokers. These results indicate that aberrant promoter hypermethylation of the *p16*^{INK4a} gene, and to a lesser extent, *DAPK*, occurs frequently in the bronchial epithelium of lung cancer patients and cancer-free smokers and persists after smoking cessation (95).

SUMMARY POINTS

1. Lung cancer results from the accumulation of multiple genetic and epigenetic changes. Different patterns of molecular alterations have been detected among the major lung cancer histology types.
2. Recent findings indicate that mutation of *KRAS*, *EGFR*, and *Her2/neu* genes occur almost exclusively in lung cancer of adenocarcinoma histology.
3. There are three main morphologic forms of preneoplastic lesions recognized in the lung: squamous dysplasias, atypical adenomatous hyperplasia, and diffuse idiopathic pulmonary neuroendocrine cell hyperplasia. However, these lesions account for the development of only a subset of lung cancers.
4. For squamous cell carcinoma of the lung, the current working model indicates a stepwise sequence of molecular and histopathological changes, with the molecular abnormalities starting in histologically normal and mildly abnormal epithelia.
5. AAH is considered a putative precursor of a subset of lung adenocarcinoma, and they demonstrate similar molecular changes than invasive tumors.
6. Two different molecular pathways have been detected in lung adenocarcinoma pathogenesis: smoking-related pathways associated with *KRAS* mutations and nonsmoking-related pathways associated with *EGFR* mutations; the latter are detected in histologically normal respiratory epithelium.
7. Molecular changes detected in lung tumors and associated preneoplastic lesions have been detected in smoking-damaged epithelium of smokers, including histologically normal bronchial epithelium.

8. Molecular changes in the respiratory epithelium are extensive and multifocal throughout the bronchial tree of smokers and lung cancer patients, indicating a field effect (i.e., field cancerization).

ACKNOWLEDGMENTS

The authors were supported by grant 5U01CA8497102, Specialized Program of Research Excellence (SPORE) in Lung Cancer grant P50CA70907 from the National Cancer Institute, Bethesda, MD (I.I.W. and A.F.G.), and the Department of Defense grant W81XWH-04-1-0142 (I.I.W).

LITERATURE CITED

1. Jemal A, Murray T, Ward E, Samuels A, Tiwari RC, et al. 2005. Cancer statistics, 2005. *CA Cancer J. Clin.* 55:10–30
2. Minna JD, Gazdar A. 2002. Focus on lung cancer. *Cancer Cell* 1:49–52
3. Travis WD, Brambilla E, Muller-Hermelink HK, Harris CC. 2004. Tumours of the lung. In *Pathology and Genetics: Tumours of the Lung, Pleura, Thymus and Heart*, ed. WD Travis, E Brambilla, HK Muller-Hermelink, CC Harris, pp. 9–124. Lyon: IARC
4. Colby TV, Wistuba II, Gazdar A. 1998. Precursors to pulmonary neoplasia. *Adv. Anat. Pathol.* 5:205–15
5. Wistuba II, Mao L, Gazdar AF. 2002. Smoking molecular damage in bronchial epithelium. *Oncogene* 21:7298–306
6. Westra WH. 2000. Early glandular neoplasia of the lung. *Respir. Med.* 1:163–69
7. Kerr KM. 2001. Pulmonary preinvasive neoplasia. *J. Clin. Pathol.* 54:257–71
8. Zochbauer-Muller S, Minna JD. 2000. The biology of lung cancer including potential clinical applications. *Chest Surg. Clin. N. Am.* 10:691–708
9. Viallet J, Sausville EA. 1996. Involvement of signal transduction pathways in lung cancer biology. *J. Cell Biochem. Suppl.* 24:228–36
10. Paez JG, Janne PA, Lee JC, Tracy S, Greulich H, et al. 2004. EGFR mutations in lung cancer: correlation with clinical response to gefitinib therapy. *Science* 304:1497–500
11. Lynch TJ, Bell DW, Sordella R, Gurubhagavatula S, Okimoto RA, et al. 2004. Activating mutations in the epidermal growth factor receptor underlying responsiveness of non-small-cell lung cancer to gefitinib. *N. Engl. J. Med.* 350:2129–39
12. Shigematsu H, Lin L, Takahashi T, Nomura M, Suzuki M, et al. 2005. Clinical and biological features associated with epidermal growth factor receptor gene mutations in lung cancers. *J. Natl. Cancer Inst.* 97:339–46
13. Stephens P, Hunter C, Bignell G, Edkins S, Davies H, et al. 2004. Lung cancer: intragenic ERBB2 kinase mutations in tumours. *Nature* 431:525–26
14. Knudson AG. 1989. Hereditary cancers disclose a class of cancer genes. *Cancer* 63:1888–91
15. Virmani AK, Fong KM, Kodagoda D, McIntire D, Hung J, et al. 1998. Allelotyping demonstrates common and distinct patterns of chromosomal loss in human lung cancer types. *Genes Chromosomes Cancer* 21:308–19
16. Girard L, Zochbauer-Muller S, Virmani AK, Gazdar AF, Minna JD. 2000. Genome-wide allelotyping of lung cancer identifies new regions of allelic loss, differences between small cell lung cancer and non-small cell lung cancer, and loci clustering. *Cancer Res.* 60:4894–906

17. Wistuba II, Behrens C, Virmani AK, Milchgrub S, Syed S, et al. 1999. Allelic losses at chromosome 8p21-23 are early and frequent events in the pathogenesis of lung cancer. *Cancer Res.* 59:1973–79
18. Shivapurkar N, Virmani AK, Wistuba II, Milchgrub S, Mackay B, et al. 1999. Deletions of chromosome 4 at multiple sites are frequent in malignant mesothelioma and small cell lung carcinoma. *Clin. Cancer Res.* 5:17–23
19. Wistuba II, Berry J, Behrens C, Maitra A, Shivapurkar N, et al. 2000. Molecular changes in the bronchial epithelium of patients with small cell lung cancer. *Clin. Cancer Res.* 6:2604–10
20. Wistuba II, Behrens C, Virmani AK, Mele G, Milchgrub S, et al. 2000. High resolution chromosome 3p allelotyping of human lung cancer and preneoplastic/preinvasive bronchial epithelium reveals multiple, discontinuous sites of 3p allele loss and three regions of frequent breakpoints. *Cancer Res.* 60:1949–60
21. Zochbauer-Muller S, Fong KM, Virmani AK, Geradts J, Gazdar AF, Minna JD. 2001. Aberrant promoter methylation of multiple genes in non-small cell lung cancers. *Cancer Res.* 61:249–55
22. Virmani AK, Rahti A, Zöchbauer-Muller S, Sacchi N, Fukuyama Y, et al. 2000. Promoter methylation and silencing of the retinoic acid receptor beta gene in lung carcinomas. *J. Natl. Cancer Inst.* 92:1303–7
23. Burbee DG, Forgacs E, Zochbauer-Muller S, Shivakumar L, Fong K, et al. 2001. Epigenetic inactivation of RASSF1A in lung and breast cancers and malignant phenotype suppression. *J. Natl. Cancer Inst.* 93:691–99
24. Toyooka S, Maruyama R, Toyooka KO, McLerran D, Feng Z, et al. 2003. Smoke exposure, histologic type and geography-related differences in the methylation profiles of non-small cell lung cancer. *Int. J. Cancer* 103:153–60
25. Bhattacharjee A, Richards WG, Staunton J, Li C, Monti S, et al. 2001. Classification of human lung carcinomas by mRNA expression profiling reveals distinct adenocarcinoma subclasses. *Proc. Natl. Acad. Sci. USA* 98:13790–95
26. Beer DG, Kardia SL, Huang CC, Giordano TJ, Levin AM, et al. 2002. Gene-expression profiles predict survival of patients with lung adenocarcinoma. *Nat. Med.* 8:816–24
27. Wistuba II, Behrens C, Milchgrub S, Bryant D, Hung J, et al. 1999. Sequential molecular abnormalities are involved in the multistage development of squamous cell lung carcinoma. *Oncogene* 18:643–50
28. Wistuba II, Behrens C, Virmani AK, Mele G, Milchgrub S, et al. 2000. High resolution chromosome 3p allelotyping of human lung cancer and preneoplastic/preinvasive bronchial epithelium reveals multiple, discontinuous sites of 3p allele loss and three regions of frequent breakpoints. *Cancer Res.* 60:1949–60
29. Shigematsu H, Takahashi T, Nomura M, Majmudar K, Suzuki M, et al. 2005. Somatic mutations of the HER2 kinase domain in lung adenocarcinomas. *Cancer Res.* 65:1642–46
30. Gazdar AF, Shigematsu H, Herz J, Minna JD. 2004. Mutations and addiction to EGFR: the Achilles 'heal' of lung cancers? *Trends Mol. Med.* 10:481–86
31. Keith RL, Miller YE, Gemmill RM, Drabkin HA, Dempsey EC, et al. 2000. Angiogenic squamous dysplasia in bronchi of individuals at high risk for lung cancer. *Clin. Cancer Res.* 6:1616–25
32. Lam S, Kennedy T, Unger M, Miller YE, Gelmont D, et al. 1998. Localization of bronchial intraepithelial neoplastic lesions by fluorescence bronchoscopy. *Chest* 113:696–702
33. Kennedy TC, Lam S, Hirsch FR. 2001. Review of recent advances in fluorescence bronchoscopy in early localization of central airway lung cancer. *Oncologist* 6:257–62

34. Hirsch FR, Prindiville SA, Miller YE, Franklin WA, Dempsey EC, et al. 2001. Fluorescence versus white-light bronchoscopy for detection of preneoplastic lesions: a randomized study. *J. Natl. Cancer Inst.* 93:1385–91
35. Breuer RH, Pasic A, Smit EF, van Vliet E, Vonk Noordegraaf A, et al. 2005. The natural course of preneoplastic lesions in bronchial epithelium. *Clin. Cancer Res.* 11:537–43
36. Hirsch FR, Franklin WA, Gazdar AF, Bunn PA Jr. 2001. Early detection of lung cancer: clinical perspectives of recent advances in biology and radiology. *Clin. Cancer Res.* 7:5–22
37. Lee JJ, Liu D, Lee JS, Kurie JM, Khuri FR, et al. 2001. Long-term impact of smoking on lung epithelial proliferation in current and former smokers. *J. Natl. Cancer Inst.* 93:1081–88
38. Belinsky SA, Nikula KJ, Palmisano WA, Michels R, Saccomanno G, et al. 1998. Aberrant methylation of p16(INK4a) is an early event in lung cancer and a potential biomarker for early diagnosis. *Proc. Natl. Acad. Sci. USA* 95:11891–96
39. Wistuba II, Lam S, Behrens C, Virmani AK, Fong KM, et al. 1997. Molecular damage in the bronchial epithelium of current and former smokers. *J. Natl. Cancer Inst.* 89:1366–73
40. Mao L, Lee JS, Kurie JM, Fan YH, Lippman SM, et al. 1997. Clonal genetic alterations in the lungs of current and former smokers. *J. Natl. Cancer Inst.* 89:857–62
41. Park IW, Wistuba II, Maitra A, Milchgrub S, Virmani AK, et al. 1999. Multiple clonal abnormalities in the bronchial epithelium of patients with lung cancer. *J. Natl. Cancer Inst.* 91:1863–68
42. Hittelman WN. 1999. Molecular cytogenetic evidence for multistep tumorigenesis: implications for risk assessment and early detection. In *Molecular Pathology of Early Cancer*, ed. S Srivastava, AF Gazdar, DE Henson, pp. 385–404. Van Demanstratt, Netherlands: IOS
43. Gartner LP, Hiatt JL. 2001. Respiratory system. In *Color Textbook of Histology*, ed. LP Gartner, JL Hiatt, pp. 343–64. Philadelphia: Saunders
44. Yatabe Y, Mitsudomi T, Takahashi T. 2002. TTF-1 expression in pulmonary adenocarcinomas. *Am. J. Surg. Pathol.* 26:767–73
45. Yatabe Y, Kosaka T, Takahashi T, Mitsudomi T. 2005. EGFR mutation is specific for terminal respiratory unit type adenocarcinoma. *Am. J. Surg. Pathol.* 29:633–39
46. Kitamura H, Kameda Y, Ito T, Hayashi H. 1999. Atypical adenomatous hyperplasia of the lung. Implications for the pathogenesis of peripheral lung adenocarcinoma. *Am. J. Clin. Pathol.* 111:610–22
47. Osanai M, Igarashi T, Yoshida Y. 2001. Unique cellular features in atypical adenomatous hyperplasia of the lung: ultrastructural evidence of its cytodifferentiation. *Ultrastruct. Pathol.* 25:367–73
48. Kim CF, Jackson EL, Woolfenden AE, Lawrence S, Babar I, et al. 2005. Identification of bronchioalveolar stem cells in normal lung and lung cancer. *Cell* 121:823–35
49. Weng SY, Tsuchiya E, Kasuga T, Sugano H. 1992. Incidence of atypical bronchioloalveolar cell hyperplasia of the lung: relation to histological subtypes of lung cancer. *Virchows Arch. A* 420:463–71
50. Nakanishi K. 1990. Alveolar epithelial hyperplasia and adenocarcinoma of the lung. *Arch. Pathol. Lab. Med.* 114:363–68
51. Chapman AD, Kerr KM. 2000. The association between atypical adenomatous hyperplasia and primary lung cancer. *Br. J. Cancer* 83:632–36
52. Koga T, Hashimoto S, Sugio K, Yonemitsu Y, Nakashima Y, et al. 2002. Lung adenocarcinoma with bronchioloalveolar carcinoma component is frequently associated with foci of high-grade atypical adenomatous hyperplasia. *Am. J. Clin. Pathol.* 117:464–70

53. Yokose T, Doi M, Tanno K, Yamazaki K, Ochiai A. 2001. Atypical adenomatous hyperplasia of the lung in autopsy cases. *Lung Cancer* 33:155–61
54. Westra WH, Baas IO, Hruban RH, Askin FB, Wilson K, et al. 1996. K-ras oncogene activation in atypical alveolar hyperplasias of the human lung. *Cancer Res.* 56:2224–28
55. Tominaga M, Sueoka N, Irie K, Iwanaga K, Tokunaga O, et al. 2003. Detection and discrimination of preneoplastic and early stages of lung adenocarcinoma using hmRNP B1, combined with the cell cycle-related markers p16, cyclin D1, and Ki-67. *Lung Cancer* 40:45–53
56. Nakanishi K, Kawai T, Kumaki F, Hiroi S, Mukai M, Ikeda E. 2003. Survivin expression in atypical adenomatous hyperplasia of the lung. *Am. J. Clin. Pathol.* 120:712–19
57. Kitaguchi S, Takeshima Y, Nishisaka T, Inai K. 1998. Proliferative activity, p53 expressin and loss of heterozygosity on 3p, 9 and 17p in atypical adenomatous hyperplasia of the lung. *Hiroshima J. Med. Sci.* 47:17–25
58. Takamochi K, Ogura T, Suzuki K, Kawasaki H, Kurashima Y, et al. 2001. Loss of heterozygosity on chromosome 9q and 16p in atypical adenomatous hyperplasia concomitant with adenocarcinoma of the lung. *Am. J. Pathol.* 159:1941–48
59. Niho S, Yokose T, Suzuki K, Kodama T, Nishiwaki Y, Mukai K. 1999. Monoclonality of atypical adenomatous hyperplasia of the lung. *Am. J. Pathol.* 154:249–54
60. Nakanishi K, Kawai T, Kumaki F, Hirot S, Mukai M, Ikeda E. 2002. Expression of human telomerase RNA component and telomerase reverse transcriptase mRNA in atypical adenomatous hyperplasia of the lung. *Hum. Pathol.* 33:697–702
61. Ghaffar H, Sahin F, Sanchez-Cespedes M, Su GH, Zahurak M, Sidransky D, et al. 2003. LKB1 protein expression in the evolution of glandular neoplasia of the lung. *Clin. Cancer Res.* 9:2998–3003
62. Sugio K, Kishimoto Y, Virmani A, Hung JY, Gazdar AF. 1994. K-*ras* mutations are a relatively late event in the pathogenesis of lung carcinomas. *Cancer Res.* 54:5811–15
63. Brose MS, Volpe P, Feldman M, Kumar M, Rishi I, et al. 2002. BRAF and RAS mutations in human lung cancer and melanoma. *Cancer Res.* 62:6997–7000
64. Pao W, Miller V, Zakowski M, Doherty J, Politi K, et al. 2004. EGF receptor gene mutations are common in lung cancers from "never smokers" and are associated with sensitivity of tumors to gefitinib and erlotinib. *Proc. Natl. Acad. Sci. USA* 101:13306–11
65. Huang SF, Liu HP, Li LH, Ku YC, Fu YN, et al. 2004. High frequency of epidermal growth factor receptor mutations with complex patterns in non-small cell lung cancers related to gefitinib responsiveness in Taiwan. *Clin. Cancer Res.* 10:8195–203
66. Kosaka T, Yatabe Y, Endoh H, Kuwano H, Takahashi T, Mitsudomi T. 2004. Mutations of the epidermal growth factor receptor gene in lung cancer: biological and clinical implications. *Cancer Res.* 64:8919–23
67. Tokumo M, Toyooka S, Kiura K, Shigematsu H, Tomii K, et al. 2005. The relationship between epidermal growth factor receptor mutations and clinicopathologic features in non-small cell lung cancers. *Clin. Cancer Res.* 11:1167–73
68. Amann J, Kalyankrishna S, Massion PP, Ohm JE, Girard L, et al. 2005. Aberrant epidermal growth factor receptor signaling and enhanced sensitivity to EGFR inhibitors in lung cancer. *Cancer Res.* 65:226–35
69. Sonobe M, Manabe T, Wada H, Tanaka F. 2005. Mutations in the epidermal growth factor receptor gene are linked to smoking-independent, lung adenocarcinoma. *Br. J. Cancer* 93:355–63
70. Sasaki H, Shimizu S, Endo K, Takada M, Kawahara M, et al. 2005. EGFR and erbB2 mutation status in Japanese lung cancer patients. *Int. J. Cancer.* In press

71. Mu XL, Li LY, Zhang XT, Wang MZ, Feng RE, et al. 2005. Gefitinib-sensitive mutations of the epidermal growth factor receptor tyrosine kinase domain in Chinese patients with non-small cell lung cancer. *Clin. Cancer Res.* 11:4289–94
72. Soung YH, Lee JW, Kim SY, Seo SH, Park WS, et al. 2005. Mutational analysis of EGFR and K-RAS genes in lung adenocarcinomas. *Virchows Arch.* 446:483–88
73. Yang SH, Mechanic LE, Yang P, Landi MT, Bowman ED, et al. 2005. Mutations in the tyrosine kinase domain of the epidermal growth factor receptor in non-small cell lung cancer. *Clin. Cancer Res.* 11:2106–10
74. Qin L, Tamasi J, Raggatt L, Li X, Feyen JH, et al. 2005. Amphiregulin is a novel growth factor involved in normal bone development and in the cellular response to parathyroid hormone stimulation. *J. Biol. Chem.* 280:3974–81
75. Marchetti A, Martella C, Felicioni L, Barassi F, Salvatore S, et al. 2005. EGFR mutations in non-small-cell lung cancer: analysis of a large series of cases and development of a rapid and sensitive method for diagnostic screening with potential implications on pharmacologic treatment. *J. Clin. Oncol.* 23:857–65
76. Tsao MS, Sakurada A, Cutz JC, Zhu CQ, Kamel-Reid S, et al. 2005. Erlotinib in lung cancer-molecular and clinical predictors of outcome. *N. Engl. J. Med.* 353:133–44
77. Zhang XT, Li LY, Mu XL, Cui QC, Chang XY, et al. 2005. The EGFR mutation and its correlation with response of gefitinib in previously treated Chinese patients with advanced non-small-cell lung cancer. *Ann. Oncol.* 16:1334–42
78. Chou TY, Chiu CH, Li LH, Hsiao CY, Tzen CY, et al. 2005. Mutation in the tyrosine kinase domain of epidermal growth factor receptor is a predictive and prognostic factor for gefitinib treatment in patients with non-small cell lung cancer. *Clin. Cancer Res.* 11:3750–57
79. Cappuzzo F, Hirsch FR, Rossi E, Bartolini S, Ceresoli GL, et al. 2005. Epidermal growth factor receptor gene and protein and gefitinib sensitivity in non-small-cell lung cancer. *J. Natl. Cancer Inst.* 97:643–55
80. Kim KS, Jeong JY, Kim YC, Na KJ, Kim YH, et al. 2005. Predictors of the response to gefitinib in refractory non-small cell lung cancer. *Clin. Cancer Res.* 11:2244–51
81. Mitsudomi T, Kosaka T, Endoh H, Horio Y, Hida T, et al. 2005. Mutations of the epidermal growth factor receptor gene predict prolonged survival after gefitinib treatment in patients with non-small-cell lung cancer with postoperative recurrence. *J. Clin. Oncol.* 23:2513–20
82. Han SW, Kim TY, Hwang PG, Jeong S, Kim J, et al. 2005. Predictive and prognostic impact of epidermal growth factor receptor mutation in non-small-cell lung cancer patients treated with gefitinib. *J. Clin. Oncol.* 23:2493–501
83. Hirsch FR, Varella-Garcia M, McCoy J, West H, Xavier AC, et al. 2005. Increased epidermal growth factor receptor gene copy number detected by fluorescence in situ hybridization associates with increased sensitivity to gefitinib in patients with bronchioloalveolar carcinoma subtypes: A Southwest Oncology Group Study. *J. Clin. Oncol.* 23: 6838–45
84. Kurie JM, Shin HJ, Lee JS, Morice RC, Ro JY, et al. 1996. Increased epidermal growth factor receptor expression in metaplastic bronchial epithelium. *Clin. Cancer Res.* 2:1787–93
85. Tang X, Shigematsu H, Bekele BN, Roth JA, Minna JD, et al. 2005. EGFR tyrosine kinase domain mutations are detected in histologically normal respiratory epithelium in lung cancer patients. *Cancer Res.* 65:7568–72
86. Yoshida Y, Shibata T, Kokubu A, Tsuta K, Matsuno Y, et al. 2005. Mutations of the epidermal growth factor receptor gene in atypical adenomatous hyperplasia and bronchioloalveolar carcinoma of the lung. *Lung Cancer* 50:1–8

87. Wistuba II, Berry J, Behrens C, Maitra A, Shivapurkar N, et al. 2000. Molecular changes in the bronchial epithelium of patients with small cell lung cancer. *Clin. Cancer Res.* 6:2604–10
88. Aguayo SM, Miller YE, Waldron JA Jr, Bogin RM, Sunday ME, et al. 1992. Brief report: idiopathic diffuse hyperplasia of pulmonary neuroendocrine cells and airways disease. *N. Engl. J. Med.* 327:1285–88
89. Armas OA, White DA, Erlanson RA, Rosai J. 1995. Diffuse idiopathic pulmonary neuroendocrine cell proliferation presenting as interstitial lung disease. *Am. J. Surg. Pathol.* 19:963–70
90. Loeb LA. 1991. Mutator phenotype may be required for multistage carcinogenesis. *Cancer Res.* 51:3075–79
91. Peto R, Darby S, Deo H, Silcocks P, Whitley E, Doll R. 2000. Smoking, smoking cessation, and lung cancer in the UK since 1950: combination of national statistics with two case-control studies. *Br. Med. J.* 321:323–29
92. Lam S, leRiche JC, Zheng Y, Coldman A, MacAulay C, et al. 1999. Sex-related differences in bronchial epithelial changes associated with tobacco smoking. *J. Natl. Cancer Inst.* 91:691–96
93. Zochbauer-Muller S, Lam S, Toyooka S, Virmani AK, Toyooka KO, et al. 2003. Aberrant methylation of multiple genes in the upper aerodigestive tract epithelium of heavy smokers. *Int. J. Cancer* 107:612–16
94. Soria JC, Rodriguez M, Liu DD, Lee JJ, Hong WK, Mao L. 2002. Aberrant promoter methylation of multiple genes in bronchial brush samples from former cigarette smokers. *Cancer Res.* 62:351–55
95. Belinsky SA, Palmisano WA, Gilliland FD, Crooks LA, Divine KK, et al. 2002. Aberrant promoter methylation in bronchial epithelium and sputum from current and former smokers. *Cancer Res.* 62:2370–77

Pathogenesis of Nonimmune Glomerulopathies

Christopher Kwoh,[1,2*] M. Brendan Shannon,[1*] Jeffrey H. Miner,[1] and Andrey Shaw[2]

[1]Renal Division, Department of Medicine, Washington University School of Medicine, St. Louis, Missouri 63113; email: ckwoh@im.wustl.edu, MShannon@wustl.edu, minerj@wustl.edu

[2]Department of Immunology and Pathology, Washington University School of Medicine, St. Louis, Missouri 63113; email: shaw@immunology.wustl.edu

Annu. Rev. Pathol. Mech. Dis. 2006. 1:349–74

First published online as a Review in Advance on October 28, 2005

The *Annual Review of Pathology: Mechanisms of Disease* is online at pathmechdis.annualreviews.org

doi: 10.1146/annurev.pathol.1.110304.100119

1553-4006/06/0114-0349$20.00

*First authorship

Key Words

slit diaphragm, podocyte, glomerulosclerosis, glomerular basement membrane, Alport syndrome

Abstract

Nonimmune glomerulopathies are an area of significant research. This review discusses the development of focal segmental glomerulosclerosis, with particular attention to the role of the podocyte in the initiation of glomerulosclerosis and the contribution to glomerulosclerosis from capillary hypertension and soluble factors such as transforming growth factor beta, platelet-derived growth factor, vascular endothelial growth factor, and angiotensin. The effects of these factors on endothelial and mesangial cells are also discussed. In addition, we review our current understanding of the slit diaphragm (a specialized cell junction found in the kidney), slit diaphragm–associated proteins (including nephrin, podocin, α-actinin-4, CD2-associated protein, and transient receptor potential channel 6), and the role of these proteins in glomerular disease. We also discuss the most recent research on the pathogenesis of collapsing glomerulosclerosis, human immunodeficiency virus associated nephropathy, Denys-Drash, diabetic nephropathy, Alport syndrome, and other diseases related to the interaction between the podocyte and the glomerular basement membrane.

INTRODUCTION

Focal segmental glomerulosclerosis (FSGS): a glomerular disease characterized by segmental regions of glomerular scar, with regions of uninvolved capillary loops

GBM: glomerular basement membrane

AS: Alport syndrome

When one examines the worldwide burden of kidney diseases, it is the nonimmunologic glomerular diseases, including hypertensive and diabetic nephropathy, that have the greatest social and economic impact (1). Additionally, as life expectancy increases, the role of nephron loss in normal aging will become an increasingly important factor in the progression of kidney insufficiency. Significant research has matured our understanding of the mechanisms of these nonimmune glomerular diseases and the pathways of progression.

Progressive sclerosis is a common finding in nearly all forms of nonimmune glomerular disease, regardless of the particular injury. Another commonality that is becoming increasingly apparent is that the podocyte, the visceral epithelial cell of the glomerulus, plays a critical role in the development and progression of most glomerular diseases and in all diseases presenting with glomerular proteinuria. Indeed, recent evidence has made it clear that podocyte injury is the cause of nearly all presentations of focal segmental glomerulosclerosis (FSGS), the most common primary glomerular diagnosis resulting in end-stage renal disease. Likewise, nearly all podocyte injuries, if they do not recover, may lead to podocyte loss and eventually glomerulosclerosis.

In the following discussion, we first review the pertinent anatomy and physiology of the glomerulus to lay a foundation for understanding the pathogenesis of glomerular disease. We then discuss the underlying mechanisms of the pathway from podocyte injury to progressive sclerosis. Following are discussions of the mechanisms by which specific diseases induce glomerular sclerosis and the role of soluble factors in the progression of glomerular disease. Lastly, the importance of the interactions of the podocyte with the glomerular basement membrane (GBM) are described in a discussion of our current understanding of Alport syndrome (AS) and related diseases. The focus of this review is on areas of recent research, with particular attention paid to the burgeoning field of the study of the slit diaphragm (a specialized cell junction found in the kidney) and its role in podocyte physiology and injury. In the interest of space, other diseases of podocyte injury, such as Fabry's disease, mitochondrial podocytopathy, and toxic injuries, are not discussed.

ANATOMIC STRUCTURE AND THE PHYSIOLOGY OF THE GLOMERULUS

Approximately 600,000 to 1 million glomeruli are present in each human kidney. Each glomerulus contains clusters of capillaries, which are lined by endothelial cells; blood traverses the glomerulus through these capillaries (**Figure 1*a*** and **Figure 2**). Clusters of capillary loops are bound together into distinct tufts by mesangial cells. Mesangial cells help to establish the structural integrity and organization of both the individual tufts and the glomerulus. The fenestrated endothelial cells rest on a GBM, which forms an incomplete cylinder with the open end held together by the mesangial cell. On the opposing side of the GBM are the glomerular epithelial cells or podocytes. These large, postmitotic, octopus-like cells have extensions, known as foot processes, that interdigitate with the foot processes of neighboring podocytes like the fingers of clasping hands. These foot processes, approximately 120 nm wide, are maintained by a complex arrangement of actin filaments. Adjacent foot processes are joined by a type of specialized cell junction known as the slit diaphragm, a 40-nm-wide structure that serves as the only indication of podocyte cell-cell contact. Beyond the interdigitations of the podocytes is Bowman's space, the area in which the primary urine first collects. Surrounding Bowman's space is Bowman's capsule, which demarcates the glomerulus and consists of parietal epithelial cells that lie on a basement membrane.

The endothelial cell, the GBM, and the podocyte foot processes comprise the

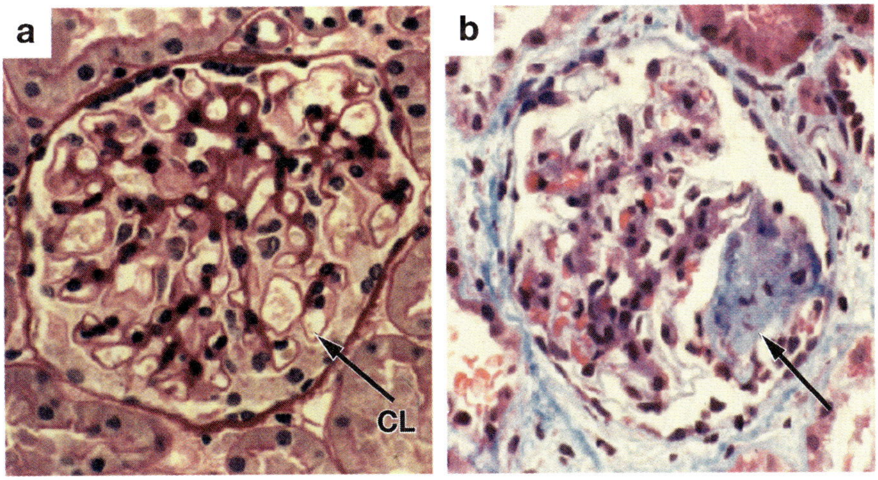

Figure 1

(*a*) Normal glomerulus. CL, capillary loop. (*b*) Focal segmental glomerulosclerosis. Arrow indicates area of sclerosis. [Images courtesy of Rosa Davila, M.D. (*a*) and Helen Liapis, M.D. (*b*).]

glomerular filtration barrier. The task of this barrier is to allow the bulk flow of fluid and small ions while preventing large-molecular-weight plasma components and proteins from passing into the urine. In addition, the GBM and podocyte are negatively charged; thus, anionic serum proteins are also repelled by the filtration barrier. Disruption of any of the components of the glomerular filtration barrier results in the loss of its protein-exclusion properties.

THE COMMON PATH: FROM PODOCYTE INJURY TO FOCAL SEGMENTAL GLOMERULOSCLEROSIS

Injury and death of the podocyte initiates a sequence of events that results ultimately in the pathologic finding of FSGS, a pattern of glomerular histology characterized by segmental areas of scarring in the perihilar regions, the tubular pole (tip lesion), or in a random distribution (classic FSGS), in addition to areas of uninvolved capillary loops (**Figure 1*b***). The various podocyte injuries that lead eventually to FSGS are discussed below. It is important to note that a variant of FSGS, termed collapsing FSGS and most often associated with human immunodeficiency virus (HIV), is thought to stem from dysregulation of podocyte differentiation rather than podocyte loss and therefore does not follow the common pathway.

The core observations and theories of the progression to glomerulosclerosis have been developed primarily by Kriz and colleagues, although many researchers have contributed. A large portion of the research into the mechanisms of FSGS has come from careful examination of histologic cross sections of rodent models of hypertension and nephron reduction with either rat uninephrectomy (the removal of one kidney) or five-sixths nephrectomy (uninephrectomy with vascular ablation of two thirds of the remaning kidney) (2–7). The pathway to glomerulosclerosis is diagramed in **Figure 2**.

HIV: human immunodeficiency virus

CD2AP: CD2-associated protein

PODOCYTE INJURY INITIATES GLOMERULOSCLEROSIS

Current dogma suggests that podocyte injury and subsequent loss initiates FSGS. Genetic defects in podocyte-specific proteins such as podocin (8), α-actinin-4 (9), and CD2-associated protein (CD2AP) (10) in mouse or human can result in a pattern of FSGS. In rodents with glomerulosclerosis from uninephrectomy, a decrease in podocyte number is one of the earliest changes (11). In agreement with these animal models, podocyte number has been shown to be a powerful predictor of progression and proteinuria

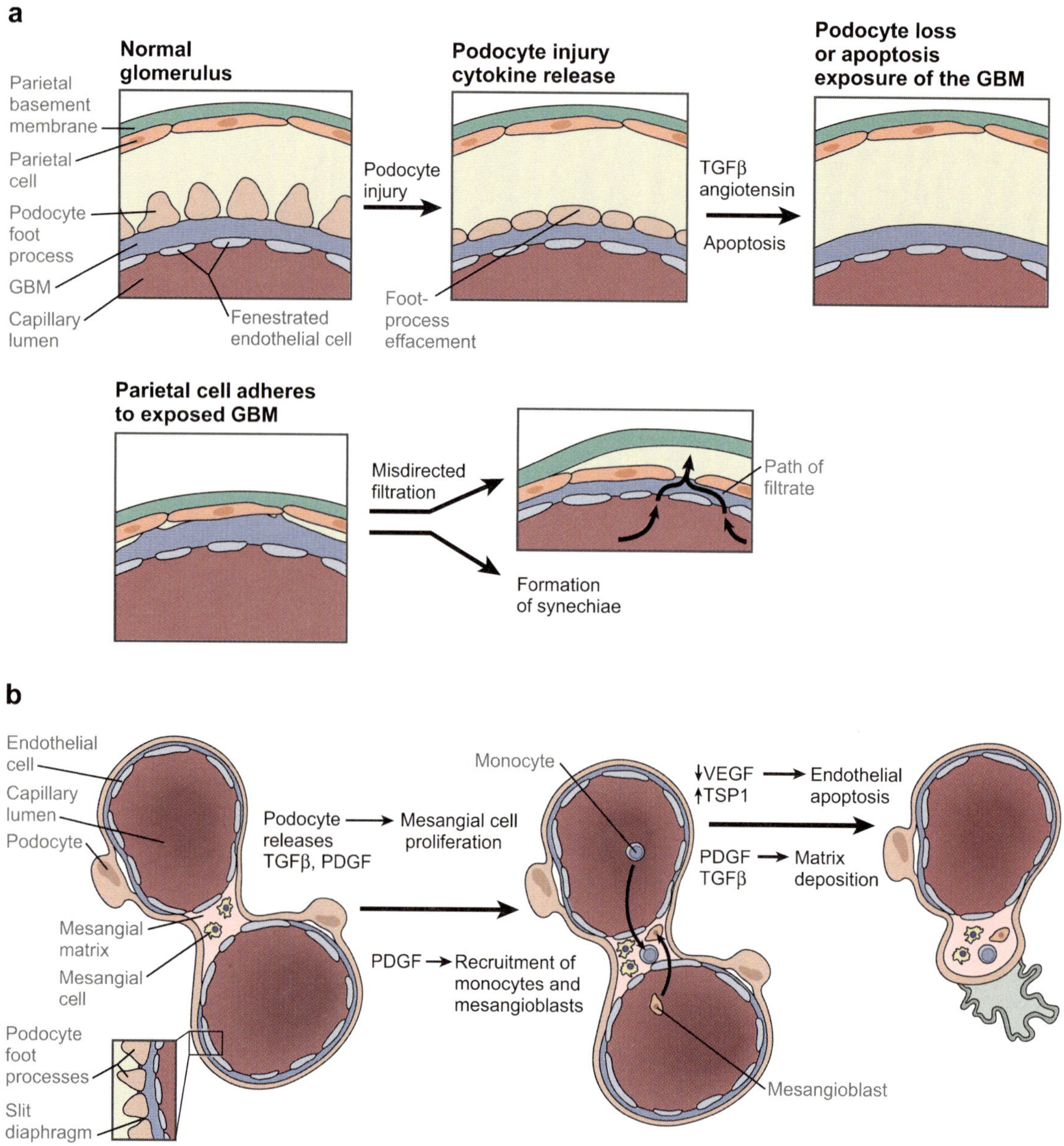

Figure 2

The progression of glomerulosclerosis. (*a*) Podocyte injury and loss, or apoptosis, results in glomerular basement membrane (GBM) exposure, parietal-cell adhesion to the GBM, and formation of synechiae or sclerosis from misdirected filtration. (*b*) A summary of the progression of sclerosis in the mesangial space and the role of cytokines released by the podocyte in response to injury. TGFβ, transforming growth factor beta; PDGF, platelet-derived growth factor; VEGF, vascular endothelial growth factor; TSP1, thrombospondin 1.

in sclerosing kidney diseases, including types I and II diabetic nephropathy and immunoglobulin A nephropathy (12, 13).

Several characteristics of the podocyte make it especially susceptible to injury. The podocyte plays an important role in maintaining the filtration barrier by ensuring that it is patent and permeable. Maintenance of the components of the filtration barrier, including the foot processes, slit diaphragm, and GBM, is likely to be a very dynamic and complex process. Indeed, one of the earliest responses to podocyte injury is rapid effacement of the foot processes. The podocyte also experiences very high transmural pressures [as much as 60 mm of Hg (14)], which exert significant mechanical stress. As we discuss, genetic predisposition may impair the ability of the podocyte to respond to injury. Importantly, the podocyte is terminally differentiated and therefore cannot divide (2). Thus, podocyte death or apoptosis is an irrevocable loss that can result in a state of permanent podocyte insufficiency.

Podocyte injury stimulates reactive changes that are likely to contribute to the process of glomerular injury. It is also becoming clear that, in addition to the well-known response to injury of podocyte foot-process fusion (through which interpodocyte foot-process spaces are lost), the release of cytokines, such as transforming growth factor beta (TGFβ), vascular endothelial growth factor (VEGF), and platelet-derived growth factor (PDGF), also play important roles in the development of sclerosis after podocyte injury (4, 7, 15, 16).

FORMATION OF SYNECHIAE

As the podocyte dies, the region of the GBM that would normally be covered by the podocyte becomes exposed (2). According to the model developed by Kriz and colleagues, areas of exposed GBM may then make contact with the parietal epithelial cell. This contact results in the formation of adhesions or synechiae as the parietal cell adheres to the GBM. These synechiae are thought to be some of the earliest signs of segmental glomerulosclerosis seen on microscopy (2, 17). Extension of the synechiae leads to collapse and sclerosis of the associated capillary tuft. Misdirected filtration at sites of the adhesion is thought to instigate the process of sclerosis. Tracer studies in uninephrectomized rats reveal passage of the tracer into the space between the parietal cell and the basement membrane of Bowman's capsule (3). Collapse of the capillary may be caused by locally accumulated protein debris (19). As the misdirected filtration also extends between the parietal epithelium and the GBM, it may eventually reach the vascular pole, occluding it and causing complete glomerular obscolescence (17).

In Kriz's model, GBM exposure rather than foot-process effacement is the critical factor in progression to FSGS. In support of this model, although minimal change disease (MCD) presents with diffuse foot-process effacement and electron-microscopic findings essentially identical to those in FSGS, progression to sclerosis is unusual, and MCD may be readily reversed with treatment. Indeed, GBM denudation is a rare finding in MCD (20). Varying degrees of podocyte loss or basement membrane exposure may explain the differences in the natural history of these two diseases.

TGFβ: transforming growth factor β

VEGF: vascular endothelial growth factor

PDGF: platelet-derived growth factor

CAPILLARY HYPERTENSION

The most common contributor of glomerulosclerosis, or capillary hypertension, is also likely the result of podocyte injury and GBM exposure (2). Capillary hypertension may occur as a result of either systemic hypertension or hyperfiltration and glomerular hypertrophy by various stimuli such as nephron loss, obesity, or sickle cell disease (21). Although endothelial and mesangial cells proliferate during glomerular hypertrophy, there is no corresponding increase in podocyte number to maintain the larger glomerulus because podocytes cannot divide (17). The mesangial cell must also continue to provide sufficient

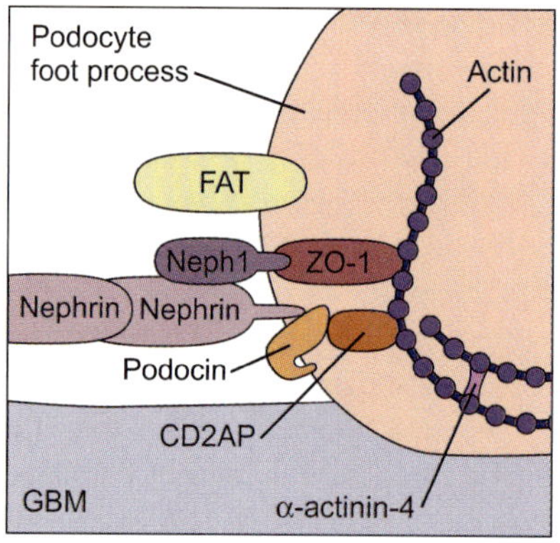

Figure 3

The arrangement of pertinent proteins at the slit diaphragm. Nephrin, Neph1, and FAT are in the extracellular domain, whereas zona occludins-1 (ZO-1), CD2-associated protein (CD2AP), and podocin are intracellular. A nephrin molecule from an adjacent foot process is also diagrammed. ZO-1 and CD2AP link slit-diaphragm components to actin, while α-actinin-4 crosslinks actin filaments. GBM, glomerular basement membrane.

mechanical strength to hold together the open end of the expanding capillary loop. If there is a failure of the mesangial cell to resist the forces of increased intraluminal pressure, the result is a massively enlarged loop and an even more dramatic increase in the GBM surface area. If the podocyte is unable to cover this increased surface area, portions of the basement membrane become exposed, foot-process detachment may occur, and synechiae will form.

THE SLIT DIAPHRAGM

The focus on the critical role of the podocyte in recent years has also been associated with renewed interest in the slit diaphragm. First identified by Karnovsky in the early 1970s, the slit diaphragm was defined as an electron-dense bridge between the podocyte foot processes seen by transmission electron microscopy (22). Although the slit diaphragm was proposed to function as the filtration barrier, progress in the study of the slit diaphragm was delayed owing to a lack of information at the molecular and genetic levels. The discovery that mutations in genes that encode two podocyte proteins, nephrin and CD2AP, could lead to nephrotic syndrome (10, 23) unleashed new interest in the podocyte and the slit diaphragm.

On the basis of the presence of a cytoskeletal linker protein, zona occludins-1 (ZO-1), the slit diaphragm is considered to be a modified tight junction that bridges neighboring podocyte foot processes (**Figure 3**). Specialized adhesion proteins not only hold the foot processes together, but also keep the space between the foot processes open. Nephrin, a member of the immunoglobulin superfamily of proteins, was the first extracellular component of the slit diaphragm identified. Database searching uncovered a family of nephrin-related molecules expressed in podocytes, such as Neph1 (24), which are also components of the slit diaphragm and indispensable for the integrity of the filtration barrier (25).

The current model suggests that the slit diaphragm is formed via the interactions of nephrin and neph family members with membrane proteins from adjacent foot processes; these protein interactions form a zipper-like structure (**Figure 3**) (26). Electron-micrographic tomography reveals that there may be multiple levels of slit diaphragms that form a layered weave with pores slightly smaller than the diameter of albumin; this observation suggests that these pores may play a role in the exclusion of albumin from the primary urine (26).

Whereas nephrin, neph family members, p-cadherin, and FAT are thought to compose the extracellular parts of the slit diaphragm, intracellular components of the slit diaphragm, such as CD2AP (10), ZO-1, podocin (8, 27), and α-actinin-4 (9), have also been identified (**Figure 3**). The exact functions of these proteins are unclear, but at least one function must be to anchor the transmembrane components of the slit to the cytoskeleton. CD2AP, a cytoplasmic scaffold protein, binds to nephrin and interacts with a variety of actin regulators in the cytoskeleton; this observation suggests that CD2AP may play a role in linking membrane proteins with the cytoskeleton (10, 28). Similarly, α-actinin-4 is an actin-binding protein. Although α-actinin-4 is expressed ubiquitously, mutations in the *ACTN4* gene uniquely affect the podocyte (9, 29). Podocin, a membrane-bound protein of the stomatin family (30), is a component of a specialized membrane compartment known as a lipid raft. One function of podocin may be to bind components of the slit diaphragm and recruit them to lipid rafts (27). The reason lipid rafts would be important for slit diaphragms is not known, although the rafts may help to organize proteins within the plasma membrane.

SLIT-DIAPHRAGM PROTEINS INVOLVED IN GLOMERULAR DISEASE

Nephrin

Mutations in the gene *NPHS1*, which encodes nephrin, cause congenital nephrotic syndrome of the Finnish type, a relatively common cause of nephrotic syndrome that presents in the neonatal period and has an estimated incidence of 1 in 10,000 live births in Finland (23). Clinically, this disease manifests as severe proteinuria and edema that appears typically within the first week of life, sometimes in utero, and almost always before three months (31). Without renal transplantation, death occurs before two years of age (31).

As of the present time, nearly 60 different *NPHS1* mutations have been identified in Finnish congenital nephrotic syndrome. Mutations of all types have been identified, including nonsense, frameshift, deletions, insertions, promoter, intron splicing, and missense mutations. Although approximately half of all cases worldwide are found in Finland, families with *NPHS1* mutations and congenital nephrotic syndrome have been identified in other geographical areas. More than 94% of patients of Finnish origin have one of two mutations (32). The more common, present in approximately 80% of Finnish cases, is the Fin major mutation, which is a 2-base-pair deletion that causes an early translational stop signal and no apparent protein expression. The second most common mutation, present in approximately 20% of cases, is the Fin minor mutation, which is a nonsense mutation resulting in a truncated protein. Outside of Finland these mutations are far less common, and other mutations predominate (32). Most of the missense mutations result in misfolded proteins that do not escape the endoplasmic reticulum (34), but some can be rescued by exogenous chaperones (35). With rare exceptions, however, it does not appear that the type of mutation results in any significant difference in clinical presentation (32, 33). In addition, several families have no identifiable *NPHS1* mutations (32). The syndrome in these families may be due to mutations in genes that encode other nephrin family members, in regulatory proteins required for proper nephrin expression, or in regulatory regions of *NPHS1*.

Lipid rafts: plasma membrane microdomains that have a unique lipid composition and are enriched in specific proteins

Mice deficient in nephrin develop severe neonatal nephrotic syndrome with death usually within the first day of life (36). It is not clear why the mouse phenotype is more severe than the human disease, but it is possible that most humans with congential nephrotic syndrome of the Finnish type retain some residual nephrin activity. As observed by electron microscopy, slit diaphragms are absent in these patients, although some podocyte foot processes and the spaces between adjacent foot processes (termed slit spaces) are preserved. Even though nephrin is an indispensable component of the slit diaphragm, the development of foot processes and slit spaces is not completely dependent upon nephrin. However, the slit spaces, which are 40 nm wide in the healthy kidney, range from 15–20 nm (in most cases) up to 120 nm in patients with nephrin deficiency (26).

Podocin

Through the use of traditional genetics in combination with positional cloning, a mutation in *NPHS2*, which encodes podocin, was identified as the cause of a case of familial FSGS (8). Mutations in *NPHS2* are now known to be associated with a wide range of presentations of FSGS. The strongest association is with idiopathic steroid-resistant nephrotic syndrome in children. In one study, 10% of examined cases had mutations in *NPHS2* (37). Further studies have revealed high frequencies of autosomal-recessive *NPHS2* mutations in both adult FSGS (38) and steroid-sensitive FSGS with frequent relapses (37).

The most common disease-causing *NPHS2* mutations, *R138Q* and *R138X*, encode misfolded proteins that do not traffic to lipid rafts and result in the mislocalization of nephrin in vitro; this observation demonstrates podocin's role in organizing the proteins at the slit diaphragm (39, 40). One common podocin variant, *R229Q*, is present in 1.5%–4% of the population, has decreased binding to nephrin in vitro, and may have a role in kidney disease (38). Although not clearly disease causing, *R229Q* is more frequent among adult proteinuric patients in comparison with the general population. This observation suggests that additional mutations or environmental factors contribute to FSGS. For example, childhood nephrotic syndrome patients with a single *R229Q* variant may have other secondary *NPHS2* mutations or mutations in the gene for nephrin in addition to the *R229Q* variant (37).

NPHS2-knockout mice present with nephrotic syndrome at birth and die between 1–3 weeks of age (41). Nephrin expression is dramatically decreased, and slit diaphragms are absent. Although this phenotype is much more severe than the phenotype of patients with *NPHS2* mutations, the difference in the severity of the phenotypes probably reflects the effect of complete protein absence versus that of a hypomorphic protein. The difference may also explain why the pathology of the mice more strongly resembles diffuse mesangial sclerosis than FSGS. The strong mesangial phenotype in a knockout of a podocyte-specific protein highlights the important influence that damage to the podocyte has on the other glomerular cells. *NPHS2*-haploinsufficient mice develop a phenotype six months after birth, at which time proteinuria is more common in the haploinsufficient mice than in their littermates.

Alpha-Actinin-4

ACTN4, which encodes α-actinin-4, was identified by positional cloning as the gene responsible for an autosomal-dominant form of FSGS. α-actinin-4 is a 100-kDa protein that forms homodimers and crosslinks actin filaments (9). α-actinin-4 is also implicated in macropinocytosis, an actin-mediated process for the internalization of large amounts of fluid (42). Although α-actinin-4 is expressed in many tissues in the body, immunofluorescence in the kidney demonstrates strong expression in the podocyte and little staining elsewhere, except in the endothelium (9).

Three families were originally identified as having mutations in *ACTN4*. Those persons affected with the mutation developed FSGS and hypertension as early as their teenage years, and many progressed to end-stage renal disease (9). Evaluation of the *ACTN4* mutation *K256E* revealed aberrant actin binding, as well as a tendency for the mutant α-actinin-4 molecules to aggregate. Mutant α-actinin-4 binds filamentous actin more strongly as compared with wild-type actinin; this observation suggests that mutations in α-actinin-4 may cause abnormalities in actin filament assembly and disassembly (9). In addition, overexpression of mutant *ACTN4* results in localized cytoplasmic aggregates that may, like aggregates of mutant proteins in diseases such as Huntington's disease, be toxic (especially to podocytes). Lastly, mutant α-actinin-4 has a shorter half-life than the wild-type proteins (43). These data suggest that the dominant mechanism in the pathology resulting from mutations in *ACTN4* is mediated via either toxicity or haploinsufficiency (43).

α-actinin-4-deficient mice develop a severe nephrotic syndrome and live only a few months; this observation confirms the podocyte-specific function of this widely expressed protein. To prove whether the mutant gene functions dominantly, a knockin mouse that replaces the normal *ACTN4* gene with the mutant *K256E* allele was developed (43). Mice homozygous for the mutation have a phenotype similar to the knockout, but heterozygous mice appear normal. Although this data does not support the hypothesis that *K256E* is a dominant mutation, the fact that multiple forms of α-actinin are expressed in mouse podocytes (unlike human podocytes) complicates the interpretation.

CD2-ASSOCIATED PROTEIN

CD2AP was initially identified as a protein involved in organizing the immunologic synapse, the site of T-lymphocyte attachment to antigen-presenting cells. This protein's vital role in the kidney was revealed by reverse genetics when *CD2AP*-knockout mice were found to develop nephrotic syndrome shortly after birth (10). As in the podocin-deficient mice, the primary glomerular pathology in *CD2AP*-knockout mice is global; expansion of the mesangium with mesangial deposits is the most prominent finding before progression to glomerulosclerosis. To prove that podocyte deficiency is the cause of the kidney phenotype, researchers showed that the glomerular disease in the *CD2AP*-knockout mouse can be rescued by podocyte-specific CD2AP expression (43a). In contrast to CD2AP-deficient mice, *CD2AP*-heterozygous mice are born with normal kidney function but develop pathological changes reminiscent of FSGS at approximately six months of age (44). Screening of patients with FSGS identified *CD2AP* DNA variants suggesting that *CD2AP* haploinsufficiency may play a role in the pathogenesis of the disease (44).

The exact function of CD2AP in the podocyte is unclear. As CD2AP may function to regulate the actin cytoskeleton and can bind to nephrin, initial ideas proposed that CD2AP may function to anchor the slit diaphragm to the actin cytoskeleton (10). Impaired anchoring of slit-diaphragm components may lead to slit-diaphragm damage, as the capillary pressure increases after birth. However, CD2AP also interacts with endophilin and synaptojanin, proteins important in endocytosis; this observation implicates CD2AP in regulation of the trafficking and sorting of internalized proteins (45). *CD2AP*-haploinsufficient mice have impaired formation of multivesicular bodies and accumulate immunoglobulin in the GBM (44). This observation suggests that the turnover of slit-diaphragm proteins may function to clear those proteins that can enter the GBM but are too large to pass through (44). Podocyte injury and GBM damage may develop because the accumulation of immunoglobulin increases the probability of immune-mediated damage over time.

On the basis of its interaction with phosphoinositide 3 (PI3) kinase, CD2AP is also potentially involved in the regulation of cell survival. CD2AP-deficient podocytes exhibit increased apoptosis that is especially apparent when they are not allowed to adhere to a surface (anoikis) (28). CD2AP has also been implicated in potentiating podocyte apoptosis mediated by TGFβ (45). *CD2AP*-knockout mice exhibit elevated TGFβ levels and increased podocyte apoptosis in vivo and in vitro; the results from this observation provide another potential mechanism for progressive glomerulosclerosis (45).

TRANSIENT RECEPTOR POTENTIAL CHANNEL 6

The newest addition to the list of proteins associated with FSGS is transient receptor potential channel 6 (TRPC6), a cation-selective ion channel. The association was identified initially in a New Zealand family with adult onset autosomal-dominant FSGS with complete penetrance (45a). Subsequent screening of other families with apparent autosomal-dominant FSGS identified five other unique

TRPC6 mutations (45b). Increases in the amplitude of triggered calcium influx and alterations of resting membrane potential were demonstrated in some, but not all of the mutated channels (45a,b). Although the mechanisms whereby TRPC6 mutations result in podocyte disease are not yet elucidated, they may involve alterations in slit diaphragm–associated calcium signaling, apoptosis, and cytoskeletal organization.

The Role of Slit-Diaphragm Loss in Podocyte Injury

How does damage to the slit diaphragm result in injury and eventual loss of the podocyte? Recent work suggests that the slit diaphragm may have functions in addition to the putative role as a component of the filtration barrier (**Figure 4**). These additional functions may include maintenance of cell polarity, removal of protein trapped in the GBM, and signaling to promote cell survival. The slit diaphragm may play an important role in the maintenance of cell polarity, as it is the only structure that participates in a cell-cell interaction. Loss of polarity may allow proteins normally localized to one area to become freely distributed across the podocyte membrane. The resulting protein disarray may disrupt the nature of the slit-diaphragm contact and contribute to the disorganized architecture and foot-process effacement seen in proteinuria. Given the growing knowledge about how cells maintain polarity, it will be interesting to see whether proteins involved in cell polarity are active in podocytes and whether defects in these proteins are linked with disease. Slit-diaphragm loss may also lead to increased fluid flow that would precipitate podocyte detachment from the GBM.

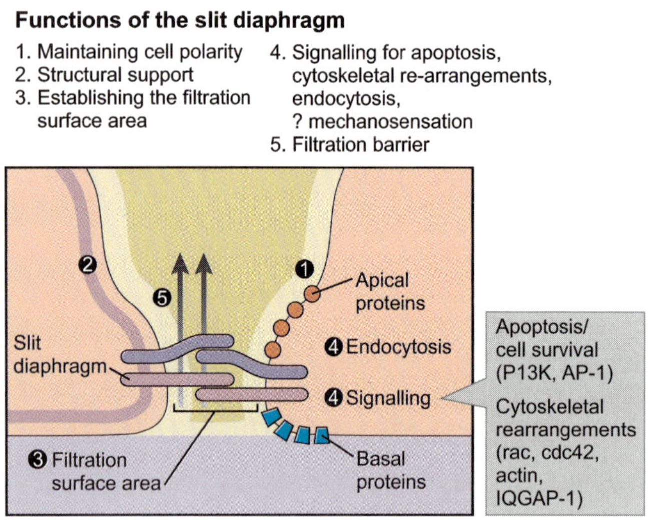

Figure 4

Functions of the slit diaphragm complex. The slit diaphragm (*1*) maintains cell polarity, (*2*) provides structural support by organizing the actin cytoskeleton, (*3*) establishes the size and architecture of the filtration surface area to control glomerular filtration rates, (*4*) signals for apoptosis, cytoskeletal rearrangements, and possibly endocytosis and mechanosensation, and (*5*) contributes to the size selective properties of the filtration barrier.

Recent information suggests that the slit diaphragm is a highly dynamic complex. Like other adhesion complexes, newer components of the complex are constitutively added while older components are removed. This dynamism may be important to keep the slit-diaphragm patent by providing a mechanism to remove proteins that may become trapped in the slit diaphragm. This hypothesis could potentially explain the observed linkage between slit-diaphragm components, the actin cytoskeleton, and intracellular trafficking pathways.

Growing evidence suggests that the slit diaphragm is likely to also have signaling functions. Recent work has shown that tyrosine phosphorylation of nephrin occurs both in vivo and in vitro and is correlated with the activation of signaling pathways (28, 47–50). In vitro, nephrin phosphorylation has multiple downstream effects, including the activation of transcription factors such as AP-1 and small G proteins such as Rac 1 and Cdc42 (49, 50). The involvement of Rac and Cdc42 suggests that nephrin signaling directly regulates the actin cytoskeleton. The Src family tyrosine kinase Fyn has been shown to bind to and phosphorylate nephrin in vitro (46, 47) and regulate the activity of TRPC6 channels (50a). In support of this, Fyn-deficient mice develop proteinuria and FSGS (47). Interestingly, phosphorylation of nephrin can be augmented by up to twentyfold by nephrin's interaction with podocin and CD2AP (49). Members of the Tec family of tyrosine kinases have also been implicated in the phosphorylation of Neph1 (24). FSGS caused by mutations in TRPC6 likely involves alterations in calcium signaling (45a,b). These intriguing associations have led to speculations that the slit diaphragm has important signaling functions in vivo.

The stimulus for nephrin phosphorylation and the function of signals mediated by the slit diaphragm are as yet unclear but may include the maintenance of polarity and the regulation of cell survival. The homology between podocin and the *Caenorhabditis elegans* mechanosensory protein mechanosensory channel complex-2 (MEC-2) has introduced the possibility that the slit diaphragm may also sense and respond to changes in intracapillary pressure. It may also be important to allow the podocyte to respond to increased protein load. These responses may include regulating the size of the slit-diaphragm opening as well as turnover of slit-diaphragm components. Signaling by nephrin via CD2AP/PI3-kinase complexes may be important to maintain cell viability (23). Increased apoptosis from slit-diaphragm loss may be the crucial link connecting slit-diaphragm dysfunction to podocyte loss.

Proteinuria and Podocyte Injury

Proteinuria has long been recognized as a strong predictor of the decline of kidney function in both humans and animal models (51). Whereas the degree of proteinuria may represent the degree of podocyte injury, it is also possible that proteinuria itself contributes to progression. Electron-microscopic studies demonstrate that proteinuria is associated with the presence of large numbers of protein droplets in the cell (52). The significance of these protein droplets is unclear, but the droplets probably represent pinocytotic and macropinocytotic vesicles. The presence of these vesicles suggests that proteinuria triggers pathological changes in the podocyte.

Experimental models in which large amounts of albumin are injected have been used to test the reaction of podocytes and tubular cells to protein overload and proteinuria (52). It is clear now that increased tubular uptake of albumin can result in interstitial inflammation and fibrosis (51). Exogenous administration of albumin is also associated with podocyte damage, foot-process effacement, and eventual podocyte death (52). Similar changes are seen in mice deficient for laminin $\alpha 5$, a GBM component; in these mice, podocytes first appear healthy but podocyte injury becomes readily apparent after prolonged proteinuria. These data support a mechanism where increased protein load leads to increased protein uptake by podocytes and tubular epithelium, which results in cellular toxicity.

SOLUBLE FACTORS AND THE RESPONSE TO GLOMERULAR INJURY

Glomerular injury appears to initiate a series of responses that may contribute to the development of glomerular sclerosis. These responses, for the most part, consist of the production of secreted factors that have a wide-ranging effect on cells within and outside the glomerulus. Although many of these factors are best described in inflammatory glomerulopathies, it is becoming more evident that they also play a critical role in the development of nonimmune glomerular diseases (**Figure 2**). Accumulating evidence suggests that inhibition of the action of some of these secreted factors can slow the progression to glomerulosclerosis.

Transforming Growth Factor Beta and Smads

TGFβ appears to be the most important secreted factor involved in the progression to sclerosis. Glomerulosclerosis develops in animal models of systemic (54) or kidney-specific (55) overexpression of TGFβ. In addition, in nearly all glomerular diseases there is an early increase in podocyte TGFβ expression (53). The release of TGFβ from podocytes may activate the mesangial-cell response to glomerular injury. As glomerular injury extends centrally, additional TGFβ is subsequently released by mesangial cells and inflammatory cells that infiltrate the glomerulus. TGFβ has numerous effects on the glomerulus, including increased extracellular-matrix production (56), hypertrophy, and podocyte apoptosis (52).

TGFβ may also play a role in the differentiation of mesangial cells from the immature mesangioblast to the mature mesangiocyte. The disruption of this transdifferentiation by the misexpression of TGFβ following glomerular injury may be critical in the progression of irreversible sclerosis (57). Normal mesangial cells secrete collagen type IV as the primary collagen in the mesangial matrix. Mesangioblasts, however, secrete collagens type I and type III (55). Whereas collagen type IV promotes mesangial cell survival in tissue culture via integrin-mediated signaling, collagens type I and III do not (58). In addition, the glomerulus lacks the appropriate metalloproteases to break down collagens type I and III. Thus, a disruption of mesangial cell differentiation by TGFβ may cause a permanent shift in glomerular collagen expression that may underlie the irreversibility of sclerotic changes (59).

In addition, evidence suggests that TGFβ enhances podocyte apoptosis. Transgenic mice expressing high levels of circulating TGFβ develop glomerulosclerosis at an early age (53). Podocyte apoptosis is the earliest detectable change, followed in several weeks by mesangial expansion. In vitro studies have implicated p38 mitogen-activated protein kinase, smad-7, and nuclear factor κB in TGFβ-induced apoptosis (52, 53). The glomerular expression of the proapoptotic smad-7 appears to be highest in podocytes (53). There is significant excitement about the potential to prevent glomerulosclerosis by blocking TGFβ and p38 activities.

Platelet-Derived Growth Factor

In response to injury and increased transmural hydrostatic pressure during glomerular hypertrophy, the endothelial cell releases PDGF family members that recruit mesangioblasts and macrophages to the mesangial space, promote mesangial proliferation, and increase extracellular-matrix deposition (60). Podocytes and mesangial cells also secrete PDGFs in response to injury. In the rat remnant-kidney model, increased PDGF expression and an increase in mesangial cellularity precede mesangial sclerosis; this observation suggests that PDGFs may be important early regulators in the response to glomerular injury (7). Mice with local kidney expression of PDGF-B develop glomerulosclerosis associated with mesangial transdifferentiation (55). Adenoviral expression of PDGFs B and D also induces glomerulosclerosis in animal models (60). In addition, neutralization of the PDGF-B receptor significantly decreases the degree of glomerulosclerosis, as well as the percentage of glomerular mesangial cells of bone marrow origin (61).

Vascular Endothelial Growth Factor

There is evidence that progressive glomerulosclerosis also occurs in association with progressive loss of endothelial cells, a loss that is mediated by changes in VEGF and thrombospondin 1 (TSP1). VEGF is expressed primarily by the podocyte and is indispensable for proper development of the capillary loop (62). VEGF can also stimulate endothelial cell proliferation, whereas TSP1 antagonizes cell proliferation and promotes apoptosis instead (11).

In the remnant-kidney rat model, hypertrophy and proliferation of endothelial cells (5) are correlated with upregulation of VEGF (11). However, this proliferation is followed by endothelial apoptosis, which occurs in association with increased production of TSP1 and loss of VEGF expression (11, 16). Some models have suggested that endothelial cell loss may in some cases be the initiating event in sclerosis. However, although administration of VEGF in the remnant-kidney model limits late endothelial cell loss, it does not prevent sclerosis (4).

Angiotensin

Clinicians and scientists alike are coming to appreciate the important role of the renin-angiotensin system on progression of glomerulosclerosis. Numerous clinical trials have demonstrated that blocking angiotensin can decrease proteinuria, nephron loss, and podocyte apoptosis (63). Early investigators attributed the benefits of angiotensin blockade to decreased glomerular capillary pressure, which would reduce the mechanical damage from transmural pressure on the glomerular components. However, further comparative studies demonstrate that the efficacy of angiotensin blockade is superior to blood pressure reductions via other agents; this result suggests that angiotensin blockade invokes additional protective mechanisms. Recent research has identified some of these additional effects.

The podocyte is both a critical source and target of angiotensin. Hyperfiltration and increased capillary pressure may result in stimulation of the angiotensin system in podocytes (64). Angiotensin has many effects on the podocyte including depolarization (65), cytoskeletal rearrangements possibly contributing to foot-process effacement (66), and stimulation of TGFβ secretion (67). That the podocyte is a crucial target for angiotensin was shown by the development of glomerulosclerosis in transgenic animals that overexpress the angiotensin receptor type I in podocytes (68). Angiotensin also increases TGFβ expression and response in mesangial cells.

PROLIFERATIVE PODOCYTE DISEASES

Human Immunodeficiency Virus–Associated Nephropathy and Collapsing Focal Segmental Glomerulosclerosis

HIV infection is associated with a glomerular disease known as collapsing FSGS. This nephropathy may result from the direct effects of HIV on the differentiation and proliferation of podocytes and presents with severe proteinuria in the setting of advanced HIV disease. Collapsing FSGS in response to HIV infection is characterized by the so-called collapsing pattern of the glomerular tuft: The tuft does not adhere to the Bowman's capsule but instead is drawn in toward the vascular pole.

HIV particles have been repeatedly identified within the glomerular visceral epithelial cell in HIV infection (69). Studies on the ability of HIV to infect mesangial cells have produced conflicting results, and the role of HIV virions in the mesangial cell is not clear (70, 71). Results from animal models point to alterations from specific HIV proteins as the etiology of the dysregulated podocyte. A direct toxic effect on podocytes is supported by a transgenic model in which expression of HIV proteins without virion formation is sufficient to cause nephropathy (72). Although several HIV-encoded proteins are thought to have a role in nephropathy, the mechanisms have not been established (73, 74).

In both collapsing FSGS due to HIV infection (75) and idiopathic collapsing FSGS (76), the podocytes lose their primary processes. This contrasts with classic FSGS in which the primary processes are maintained, and only the secondary foot processes are effaced. In both types of collapsing FSGS, the podocytes lose their characteristic actin-cytoskeleton architecture and also regain the ability to proliferate. In late stages these dysmorphic podocytes may detach and can be found floating in the urinary space. The

GBM becomes wrinkled and collapses under a crowded layer of proliferating podocytes. Sometimes there is the development of pseudocrescents, which are masses of proliferating podocytes that arise between the GBM and the Bowman's capsule and form a cobblestone appearance (**Figure 5**). In normal glomeruli, the podocyte foot processes may provide tensile strength that maintains patency of the capillary lumen. The combination of compression of the capillary loop by the enlarging mass of dysregulated podocytes as well as loss of the supportive foot processes results in an inward folding and collapse of the capillary loop.

If the podocyte loses its adherence to the GBM, classic FSGS may ensue. More often, however, the net gain of podocytes causes the epithelial cells to crowd over the exposed GBM. The pathway to classic FSGS is not entered, and instead the capillary tufts are drawn away from Bowman's capsule and sclerose inward. Soluble factors also contribute to progression of sclerosis. TGFβ levels are elevated in the setting of HIV nephropathy to levels that exceed those found in classic FSGS (77).

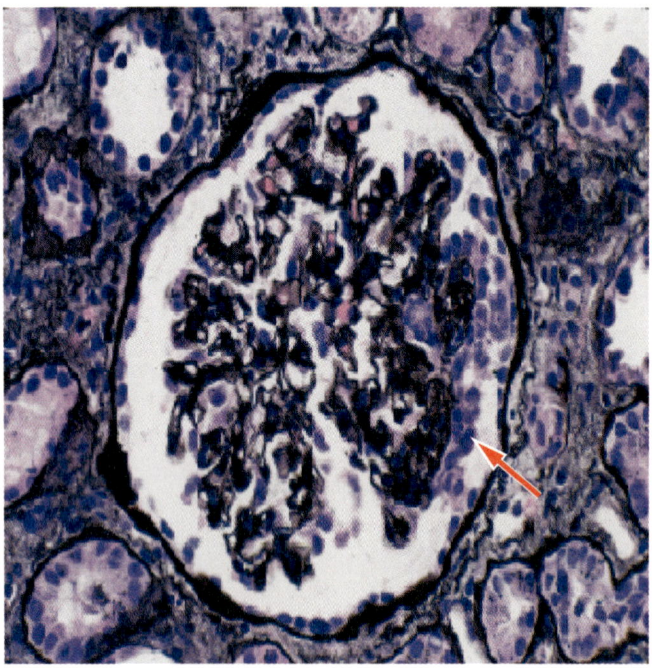

Figure 5

Collapsing focal segmental golmerulsclerosis. Red arrow indicates pseudocrescent formation with proliferating podocytes. (Courtesy of Helen Liapis, M.D.)

These phenotypic changes of the podocyte have been suggested to represent dedifferentiation to a more immature state (78). The cells lose expression of podocyte markers, including Wilm's tumor 1 (WT-1), synaptopodin, and podocalyxin (78). In addition, non-podocyte markers, such as the macrophage markers CD-68 and M-130, have also been identified (76). These data suggest that these dysmorphic podocytes may have acquired new functions.

Denys-Drash Syndrome

Denys-Drash is a rare type of familial nephrotic syndrome that results from mutations in the podocyte protein WT-1, a transcription factor involved in embryonic renal development (79). Although the precise mechanisms that underlie this syndrome are unclear, the podocytes in Denys-Drash proliferate abnormally and eventually slough; thus, this syndrome bears some resemblance to collapsing FSGS (80). In contrast to the other podocyte-associated diseases, Denys-Drash does not present with FSGS but rather with diffuse mesangial sclerosis and an absence of mesangial hypercellularity.

DIABETIC NEPHROPATHY

Diabetic nephropathy shares many of the same features as classic FSGS; however the disease is likely initiated in multiple components of the glomerulus, including the endothelium, the mesangium, and the podocyte. Some of the earliest changes are glomerular hypertrophy, hyperfiltration, and capillary hypertension, which promote podocyte loss via the mechanisms described above. Expansion of the mesangial matrix is prominent, as are areas of sclerosis. The effects of soluble mediators are similar to those in classic FSGS;

however, in diabetic nephropathy there are additional influences from hyperglycemia and advanced glycation end products (AGEs).

Hyperfiltration and hypertrophy may be mediated by several factors, including VEGF (81), insulin-like growth factor 1 (82), and AGEs (83). High glucose conditions can stimulate mesangial hypertrophy and expansion in vitro (84). Hyperglycemia has both direct and indirect effects on cellular activities that may contribute to diabetic nephropathy. High glucose concentrations stimulate the release of TGFβ and angiotensin II (85) and increase matrix deposition (86) by the mesangial cell (85). Hyperglycemia also results in the formation of AGEs, which are the products of nonenzymatic modifications formed by the reaction of glucose with proteins, lipids, and nucleic acids.

AGEs and the AGE receptor (RAGE), a multiligand receptor of the immunoglobulin family, have been implicated in diabetic nephropathy. Podocytes have the highest expression of RAGE in the glomerulus and expression is dramatically increased in diabetic kidneys (87). In vitro, activation of RAGE results in TGFβ induction (87), VEGF release (81), and activation of smad transcription factors independent of TGFβ. Overexpression of RAGE in mice results in glomerulosclerosis (88), whereas *RAGE*-knockout mice with diabetes do not develop glomerulosclerosis, matrix expansion, or GBM thickening (81).

Loss of podocytes in the urine has been associated with the progression of diabetic nephropathy (88a). Podocyte detachment may be mediated by decreased expression of α3β1 integrin, the principal protein involved in attaching podocytes to the GBM, in diabetic patients and animal models of diabetic nephropathy (88b). Decreased GBM contact decreases the threshold for apoptosis and detachment, further contributing to the podocytopenia of diabetic nephropathy.

Recent research has emphasized the presence of macrophages and monocytes in the mesangium in diabetic glomeruli. The presence of these cells is believed to enhance mesangial sclerosis as well as tissue destruction. High serum glucose stimulates secretion of the chemokine monocyte chemoattractant protein-1, which stimulates the recruitment of inflammatory cells (such as macrophages) to the mesangium (89). RAGE may also directly recruit leukocytes (90). There is also evidence of endothelial dysfunction in diabetic nephropathy. Microvascular hyalinosis is prominent in kidney biopsies and is mediated by elevated levels of angiotensin II in the setting of hyperglycemia (91). The result is severe narrowing of the arterioles and subsequent nephron ischemia.

Advanced glycation end products (AGEs): molecules formed from the nonenzymatic reaction of reducing sugars with proteins, lipids, and nucleic acids

RAGE: receptor for advanced glycation end products (AGEs)

ALPORT SYNDROME AND OTHER GENETIC DISORDERS OF THE GLOMERULAR BASEMENT MEMBRANE

In addition to the cellular components of the glomerulus, the integrity of the GBM and its interaction with the podocyte are also indispensable for proper glomerular development and function. This is demonstrated by a number of diseases of GBM components that result in proteinuria, podocyte foot-process effacement, and renal failure. The most common and best understood of these diseases is AS.

Alport Syndrome

AS is a developmental disorder of basement membranes. Its most common X-linked form is caused by mutations in the gene encoding the α5 chain of collagen type IV (92). Autosomal-recessive and, rarely, autosomal-dominant forms are caused by mutations in the genes encoding the α3 or α4 chains (93, 94). Effects on the GBM dominate the clinical picture, which is characterized by hematuria, proteinuria, and progressive renal failure in all cases. Some patients also suffer

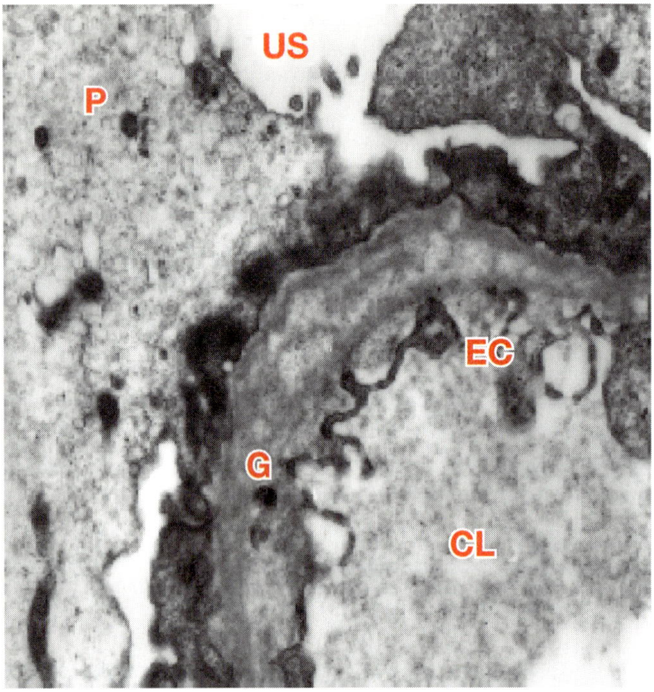

Figure 6

Alport syndrome. The characteristic "basket-weave" appearance of a multilamellated lamina densa interspersed with electron-lucent flocculent material in the glomerular basement membrane (G) (20,000x magnification). Podocyte (P) foot-process fusion is present overlying the lesion. EC, endothelial cell; US, urinary space; CL, capillary lumen. (Courtesy of Helen Liapis, M.D.)

from sensorineural hearing loss and ocular defects. The GBM was identified as the defective structure in X-linked AS in the 1970s (95). By electron microscopy, AS GBM contains thickened areas that exhibit either splitting of the lamina densa, or "basket-weaving," where the lamina densa appears multilayered with interspersed flocculent material (95) (**Figure 6**). Alport glomeruli have been described as having a fetal appearance, both at the light-microscopic level, where glomeruli appear small (96) and at the electron-microscopic level, where podocyte cell bodies have a more rounded appearance with large nuclei and small amounts of cytoplasm (97). Subsequently, it has become clear that the AS GBM is fetal in a biochemical sense as well.

The Glomerular Collagen Network in Alport Syndrome

There are six α chains that compose collagen type IV. Individual chains assemble to form trimeric protomers, and they do so in only specific ways. Thus, there are α1α1α2, α3α4α5, and α5α5α6 protomers, which make up the collagen type IV network in basement membranes. A mutation in one chain results in loss of all the chains in a given protomer from the basement membrane. Thus, in AS, mutations in the α5 chain prevent basement membrane expression of the α3 and α4 chains as well (98).

In the developing kidney, the embryonic precursors of the GBM are composed of α1α1α2 networks. As the glomerulus proceeds through embryonic development, however, the α1α1α2 network is gradually replaced by a network composed of α3α4α5 protomers (99, 100). These are the only collagen type IV protomers found in mature human GBM (101). In AS GBM, however, this isotype switching of collagen IV protomers does not occur, and there is persistence of the fetal α1α1α2 network (100–102) (**Figure 7**).

Detailed studies of animal models have shown that the α1α1α2 network is sufficient for the development of a normal GBM, and that, initially, renal function is normal. In a canine model of X-linked AS, GBM splitting and multilamellation occur by one month, whereas proteinuria is not present until two months of age (100). *COL4A3*-knockout mouse models of autosomal-recessive AS exhibit proteinuria by one to five months of age (depending on the genetic background) (103–105).

Several hypotheses have been proposed to explain how the persistence of the α1α1α2 network leads to the characteristic structural defects and subsequent renal failure in AS. When visualized by rotary-shadowing electron microscopy, the α3α4α5 network has a more complex superstructure as compared with the more rod-like superstructure of α1α1α2 protomers. Triple-helical domains of the $\alpha3\alpha4\alpha5$protomers are characterized by looping and supercoiling (106). The molecular superstructure of the $\alpha3\alpha4\alpha5$network is stabilized by disulfide crosslinks between triple helices as well as between noncollagenous domain-1 domains of adjacent protomers (106). Thus, the mechanical stability of an $\alpha3\alpha4\alpha5$-containing GBM may be inherently more resistant to the forces encountered during the passage of the glomerular filtrate through the GBM. In addition to mechanical forces of flow and stretch, the GBM may also be exposed to circulating endopeptidases. As the filtrate passes into the urinary space, one would expect the concentration of endopeptidases within the glomerular capillary lumen to be relatively higher than in the vascular space of other tissues. Kalluri and colleagues showed that total basement membrane extracts from AS kidney were digested more easily by collagenase, elastase, and a variety of cathepsins as compared with preparations of normal kidney basement membranes. Thus, the $\alpha3\alpha4\alpha5$ network may provide more protection against endoproteolysis. The characteristic splitting and multilamellation of the GBM in AS may be a result of endoproteolysis (101).

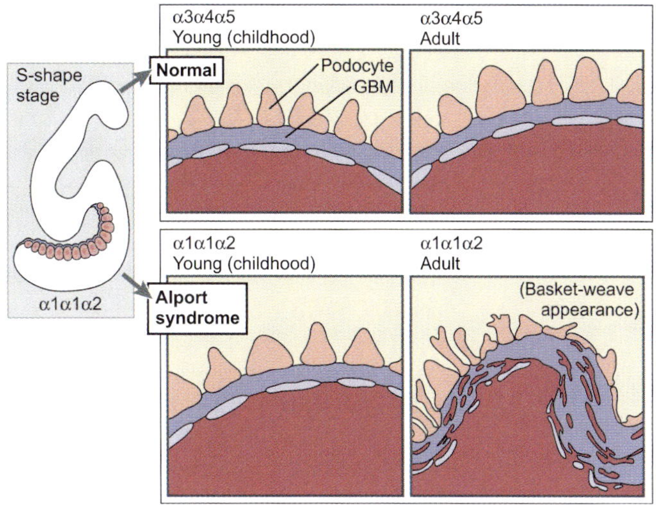

Figure 7

A developmental switch in collagen IV isoforms occurs in the glomerular basement membrane (GBM). The $\alpha1\alpha1\alpha2$ network of S-shape stage GBM is replaced by an $\alpha3\alpha4\alpha5$ network in mature glomeruli (*top panels*). In Alport glomeruli, however, the $\alpha1\alpha1\alpha2$ network persists. Over time the structural integrity of the GBM is compromised, manifest by the appearance of thickening, multilamellation and the characteristic "basket-weave" appearance (*lower right panel*).

Laminin Proteins in Alport Syndrome

The molecular composition of AS GBM differs not only in its collagen component, but in the aberrant expression of laminins as well (105, 107, 109). Mature GBM contains only the laminin-11 trimer (composed of laminin $\alpha5\beta2\gamma1$ chains). However, laminin $\alpha1$, $\alpha2$, and $\beta1$ chains have also been found in Alport GBM. As with collagen type IV, there is a developmental switch in the laminin composition of the GBM. Laminin $\alpha1$ and $\beta1$ chains are found in the developing glomerulus, but are replaced by $\alpha5$ and $\beta2$ chains by the capillary-loop stage of development. In Alport GBM, however, $\alpha1$ and $\beta1$ chains reappear, and this reappearance coincides with the onset of the ultrastructural lesions of GBM splitting. Ectopic laminin $\alpha1$ and $\beta1$ chains have in fact been localized by immuno-electron microscopy to the areas of GBM splitting (108). One possibility is that the presence of the fetal $\alpha1\alpha1\alpha2$ collagen network permits the re-expression of fetal laminin isoforms. Therefore, aberrant laminin composition may contribute as well to the observed ultrastructural abnormalities in Alport GBM. The presence of fetal isoforms of collagen and laminin, as well as ectopic laminins not normally found in the GBM, may contribute to the foot-process effacement seen in AS.

Other Genetic Disorders of the Glomerular Basement Membrane

Thin basement membrane nephropathy (TBMN) is inherited as an autosomal-dominant trait. Its clinical characteristics include persistent hematuria with minimal to no proteinuria and, in the majority of cases, the maintenance of normal renal function. The

GBM in TBMN is diffusely thinned, on average, to less than 200–250 nm (as compared with 350 nm in normal GBM) (110). Both *COL4A4* and *COL4A3* mutations have been shown to cause TBMN (111, 112). Patients that have such mutations have been described as potential carriers of autosomal-recessive AS (111).

Disruption of the interaction between the podocyte and the GBM may also cause glomerulopathy. CD151 is a member of the tetraspanin superfamily that is expressed in podocytes, where it interacts with integrin $\alpha3\beta1$ and other laminin-binding proteins (113). Mutations in CD151 have recently been identified as causing sensorineural hearing loss and renal failure, and cause a kidney phenotype similar to that seen in AS, (e.g., splitting and multilamellation of the GBM) (114).

Mutations in laminin $\beta2$, which encodes a key GBM component, have recently been described in humans that have congenital nephrotic syndrome together with mesangial sclerosis and eye defects (115). The ultrastructure of the GBM in the human disease has not been described, but a murine model develops a variably irregular and thickened GBM that has diffuse podocyte foot-process effacement (116).

Nail-patella syndrome, a congenital disorder that comprises hypoplastic patella and other skeletal features, dysplastic nails, and, in 30% of cases, kidney disease caused by mutations in the gene encoding the transcription factor LMX1B (117). The renal phenotype includes thickening and splitting of the GBM, foot-process effacement, and intramembranous deposition of collagen bundles. Identified targets of LMX1B include the genes *COL4A4*, *COL4A3*, *NPHS2*, and *CD2AP*. In an animal model, there is reduced expression of these proteins in GBM and podocytes (116–118).

CONCLUSIONS

Nonimmune glomerular diseases have been an area of great research interest. We discuss above a variety of mechanisms of glomerular disease and emphasize the central role that podocytes have in the initiation and progression of FSGS. Although many mechanisms of podocyte injury have been described, we focus above on the effects of altered slit-diaphragm components, diabetes, podocyte proliferation, and altered GBM-podocyte interaction. Although the initiation of these diseases is nonimmune, this fact does not mean there is no inflammation; the expression of various soluble inflammatory mediators as well as infiltration of the glomerulus with immune cells are critical in the development of glomerulosclerosis.

SUMMARY POINTS

1. FSGS is a disease of the podocyte, and podocyte loss is the critical event that initiates sclerosis.
2. Loss or disruption of the components of the podocyte and slit diaphragm may result in glomerulosclerosis. Nephrin, podocin, CD2AP, TRPC6, and α-actinin-4 have all been implicated in glomerular disease.
3. The pathogenesis of collapsing FSGS and HIV nephropathy involves an abnormal proliferation of podocytes and altered control of the cell cycle.
4. Diabetic nephropathy involves the effects of glucose and AGEs on several components of the glomerulus, including podocytes, mesangial cells, and endothelial cells.

5. The interaction between the GBM and the podocyte is critical for podocyte maintenance, as is evidenced by podocyte damage in diseases caused by defects in the GBM (such as AS and laminin disorders) and by defects in molecules involved in the interactions between the GBM and podocytes (such as integrins).

FUTURE DIRECTIONS/UNRESOLVED ISSUES

1. Future research may explore the therapeutic potential of blocking various soluble factors (such as TGFβ) or signaling molecules (such as p38) in slowing the progression of glomerulosclerosis.
2. Future research will also elucidate the role of signaling by the slit diaphragm and may provide insights into the pathophysiology and potential therapies of glomerular disease and hypertension.

ACKNOWLEDGMENTS

Special thanks to Tobias Huber, M.D., Helen Liapis, M.D., and Anita Vijayan, M.D. for critical peer review. Also special thanks to Helen Liapis, M.D. and Rosa Davila, M.D. for providing the histology images.

LITERATURE CITED

1. Collins AJ, Kasiske B, Herzog C, Chavers B, Foley R, et al. 2005. USRDS 2004 Annual data report. *Am. J. Kidney Dis.* 45:A5–7
2. **Kriz W, Elger M, Nagata M, Kretzler M, Uiker S, et al. 1994. The role of podocytes in the development of glomerular sclerosis. *Kidney Int.* 45:S64–S72**
3. Kriz W, Hartmann I, Hosser H, Hahnel B, Kranzlin B, et al. 2001. Tracer studies in the rat demonstrate misdirected filtration and peritubular filtrate spreading in nephrons with segmental glomerulosclerosis. *J. Am. Soc. Nephrol.* 12:496–506
4. Kang DH, Joly AH, Oh SW, Hugo C, Kerjaschki D, et al. 2001. Impaired angiogenesis in the rat remnant kidney model. *J. Am. Soc. Nephrol.* 12:1434–47
5. Lee LK, Meyer TW, Pollock AS, Lovett DH. 1995. Endothelial cell injury initiates glomerular sclerosis in the rat remnant kidney. *J. Clin. Invest.* 96:953–64
6. Kitamura H, Shimizu A, Masuda Y, Ishikazi M, Sugisaki Y, et al. 1998. Apoptosis in glomerular endothelial cells during the development of glomerulosclerosis in the remnant kidney model. *Exp. Nephrol.* 6:328–36
7. Floege J, Burns MW, Alpers CE, Yoshimura A, Pritzl P, et al. 1992. Glomerular cell proliferation and PDGF expression precede glomerular sclerosis in the rat remnant kidney model. *Kidney Int.* 41:297–309
8. **Boute N, Gribouval O, Boute N, Sich M, Benessy F, et al. 2000. NPHS2, encoding the glomerular protein podocin, is mutated in autosomal recessive steroid resistant nephrotic syndrome. *Nat. Genet.* 24:349–54**

Outlines of some of Kriz's early hypotheses on the role of the podocyte in glomerulosclerosis.

The original identification of podocin and its connection to autosomal-recessive familial FSGS.

9. Kaplan JM, Kim SH, North KN, Rennke H, Correia LA, et al. 2001. Mutations in ACTN4, encoding alpha actinin 4, cause familial focal segmental glomerulosclerosis. *Nat. Genet.* 24:251–56

The first description of α-actinin-4 involvement in autosomal-dominant familial FSGS.

10. Shih NY, Li J, Karpitskii V, Nguyen A, Dustin ML, et al. 1999. Congenital nephrotic syndrome in mice lacking CD2-associated protein. *Science* 286:312–15

An outline of the discovery that CD2AP is indispensable in glomerular filtration and health.

11. Kang DH, Hughes J, Mazzali M, Schreiner GF, Johnson RJ. 2001. Impaired angiogenesis in the rat remnant kidney model. Administration of VEGF reduces renal fibrosis and stabilizes renal function. *J. Am. Soc. Nephrol.* 12:1448–57
12. Meyer TW, Bennett PH, Nelson RG. 1999. Podocyte number predicts long term urinary albumin excretion in Pima Indians with type II diabetes and microalbuminuria. *Diabetilogia* 42:1341–44
13. Pagtalunan ME, Miller PL, Jumping-Eagle S, Nelson RG, Meyers BD, et al. 1997. Podocyte loss and progressive glomerular injury in Type II diabetes. *J. Clin. Invest.* 99:342–48
14. Brenner BM. 1985. Nephron adaptation to renal injury or ablation. *Am. J. Physiol. Renal Physiol.* 249:F324–F337
15. Abbate M, Zoja C, Morigi M, Rottoli D, Angioletti S, et al. 2002. Transforming growth factor beta is upregulated by podocytes in response to excess intraglomerular passage of proteins: a central pathway in progressive glomerulosclerosis. *Am. J. Pathol.* 161:2179–93
16. Shulman K, Rosen S, Tognazzi K, Manseau EJ, Brown LF. 1996. Expression of vascular permeability factor (VEGF) is altered in many glomerular diseases. *J. Am. Soc. Nephrol.* 7:661–66
17. Kriz W, Hosser H, Hahnel B, Gretz N, Provoost AP. 1998. From segmental glomerulosclerosis to total nephron degeneration and interstitial fibrosis: A histopathological study in rat models and human glomerulopathies. *Nephrol. Dial. Transplant.* 13:2781–98
18. Deleted in proof
19. Rennke HG. 1994. How does glomerular epithelial cell injury contribute to progressive glomerular damage? *Kidney Int.* 45:S58–S63
20. Lahdenkari AT, Lounatmaa K, Patrakka J, Holmberg C, Wartiovaara J, et al. 2004. Podocytes are firmly attached to glomerular basement membrane in kidneys with heavy proteinuria. *Am. Soc. Nephrol.* 15:2611–18
21. Saborio P, Scheinman JI. 1999. Sickle cell nephropathy. *J. Am. Soc. Nephrol.* 10:187–92
22. Rodewald R. 1974. Porous substructure of the glomerular slit diaphragm in the rat and mouse. *J. Cell Biol.* 60:423–33

23. Kestila M, Lenkkeri U, Mannikko M, Lamerdin J, McCready P, et al. 1998. Positionaly cloned gene for a novel glomerular protein "nephrin" is mutated in congenital nephrotic syndrome. *Mol. Cell.* 1:575–82

The first description of nephrin and its involvement in congenital nephritic syndrome of the Finnish type.

24. Sellin L, Huner TB, Gerke P, Quack I, Pavenstadt H, et al. 2003. NEPH1 defines a novel family of podocin interacting proteins. *FASEB J.* 17:115–17
25. Donoviel DB, Freed DD, Vogel H, Potter DG, Hawkins E, et al. 2001. Proteinuria and perinatal lethality in mice lacking NEPH1, a novel protein with homology to nephrin. *Mol. Cell. Biol.* 21:4829–36
26. Wartiovaara J, Ofverstedt LG, Khoshnoodi J, Zhang J, Makela E, et al. 2004. Nephrin strands contribute to a porous slit diaphragm scaffold as revealed by electron tomography. *J. Clin. Invest.* 10:475–1483
27. Schwarz K, Simons M, Reiser J, Saleem MA, Faul C, et al. 2001. Podocin, a raft-associated component of the glomerular slit diaphragm, interacts with CD2AP and nephrin. *J. Clin. Invest.* 108:1621–29

28. Huber TB, Hartleben B, Kim J, Schmidts M, Schermer B, et al. 2003. Nephrin and CD2AP associate with phosphoinositide 3-OH kinase and stimulate AKT-dependent signaling. *Mol. Cell. Biol.* 23:4917–28
29. Kos C, Le TC, Sinha S, Henderson JM, Kim SH, et al. 2003. Mice deficient in alpha-actinin 4 have severe glomerular disease. *J. Clin. Invest.* 111:1683–90
30. Roselli S, Gribouval O, Boute N, Sich M, Benessy F, et al. 2002. Podocin localizes in the kidney to the slit diaphragm area. *Am. J. Pathol.* 160:131–39
31. Holmberg C, Antikainen M, Ronnholm K, Ala Houhala M, Jalanko H. 1995. Management of congenital nephrotic syndrome of the Finnish type. *Pediatr. Nephrol.* 9:87–93
32. Lenkkeri U, Mannikko M, McCready P, Lamerdin J, Gribouval O, et al. 1999. Structure of the gene for congenital nephrotic syndrome of the Finnish type (NPHS1) and characterization of mutations. *Am. J. Hum. Genet.* 64:51–61
33. Pattrakka J, Kestila M, Wartiovaara J, Ruotsalainen V, Tissari P, et al. 2000. Congenital nephrotic syndrome (NPHS1): Features resulting from different mutations in Finnish patients. *Kidney Int.* 58:972–80
34. Liu L, Done SC, Khoshnoodi J, Bertorello A, Wartiovaara J, et al. 2001. Defective nephrin trafficking caused by missense mutations in the NPHSI gene: Insight into the mechanisms of congenital nephrotic syndrome. *Hum. Mol. Genet.* 10:2637–34
35. Liu XL, Done SC, Yan K, Kilpelainen P, Pikkarainen T, Tryggvason K. 2004. Defective trafficking of nephrin missense mutants rescued by a chemical chaperone. *J. Am. Soc. Nephrol.* 15:1731–38
36. Putaala H, Soininen R, Kilpelainen P, Wartiovaara J, Tryggvason K. 2001. The murine nephrin gene is specifically expressed in kidney, brain, and pancreas. Inactivation of the gene leads to massive proteinuria and neonatal death. *Hum. Mol. Genet.* 10:1–8
37. Caridi G, Bertelli R, DiDuca M, Dagnino M, Emma F, et al. 2003. Broadening the spectrum of diseases related to podocin mutations. *J. Am. Soc. Nephrol.* 14:1278–86
38. Tsukaguchi H, Sudhakar A, Le TC, Nguyen T, Yao J, et al. 2002. NPHS2 mutations in late onset focal segmental glomerulosclerosis: R229Q is a common disease associated allele. *J. Clin. Invest.* 110:1654–66
39. Huber TB, Simons M, Hartleben B, Semetz L, Schmidts M, et al. 2003. Molecular basis of the functional podocin-nephrin complex: mutations in the NPHS2 gene disrupt nephrin targeting to the lipid raft microdomains. *Hum. Mol. Genet.* 12:3397–3405
40. Nishibori Y, Liu L, Hosoyamada M, Endou H, Kudo A, et al. 2004. Disease-causing missense mutations in NPHS2 gene alter normal nephrin trafficking to the plasma membrane. *Kidney Int.* 66:1755–65
41. Roselli S, Heidet L, Sich M, Henger A, Kretzler M, et al. 2004. Early glomerular filtration defect and severe renal disease in podocin deficient mice. *Mol. Cell. Biol.* 24:550–60
42. Araki N, Hatae T, Yamada T, Hirohashi S. 2000. Actinin-4 is preferentially involved in circular ruffling and macropinocytosis in mouse macrophages. *J. Cell. Sci.* 113:3329–40
43. Yao J, Le TC, Kos CH, Henderson JM, Allen PG, et al. 2004. Alpha actinin 4 mediated FSGS: An inherited kidney disease caused by an aggregated and rapidly degraded cytoskeletal protein. *PLoS Biol.* 2:787–94
43a. Grunkemeyer J, Kwoh C, Huber T, Shaw A. 2005. CD2AP expression in podocytes rescues lethality of CD2AP deficiency. *J. Biol. Chem.* 280(33):29677–81
44. Kim JM, Wu H, Green G, Winkler CA, Kopp JB, et al. 2003. CD2-associated protein haploinsufficiency is linked to glomerular disease susceptibility. *Science* 300:1298–1300

The first paper to propose the novel class of glomerular disease that involves defective clearance of protein from the GBM.

45. Schiffer M, Mundel P, Shaw AS, Bottinger EP. 2004. A novel role for the adapter molecule CD2 associated protein in TGF-B induced apoptosis. *J. Biol. Chem.* 279:37004–37012
45a. Winn MP, Conlon PJ, Lynn KL, Farrington MK, Creazzo T, et al. 2005. A mutation in the TRPC6 cation channel causes familial segmental glomerulosclerosis. *Science* 308:1801–4
45b. Reiser J, Polu KR, Moller CC, Kenlan P, Altintas MM, et al. 2005. TRPC6 is a glomerular slit diaphragm-associated channel required for normal renal function. *Nat. Genet.* 37:739–44
46. Soubeyran P. 2002. Cbl-CIN85-endophilin complex mediates ligand-induced downregulation of EGF receptors. *Nature* 416:183–87
47. Verma R, Wharram B, Kovari I, Kunkel R, Nihalani D, et al. 2003. Fyn binds to and phosphorylates the slit diaphragm component nephrin. *J. Biol. Chem.* 278:20716–23
48. Li H, Lemay S, Aoudjit L, Kawachi H, Takano T. 2004. Src-family kinase fyn phosphorylates the cytoplasmic domain of nephrin and modulates it interaction with podocin. *J. Am. Soc. Nephrol.* 15:3006–15
49. Huber TB, Kottgen M, Schilling B, Walz G, Benzing T. 2001. Interaction with podocin facilitates nephrin signaling. *J. Biol. Chem.* 276:41543–46

One of the earliest papers to describe signaling through nephrin and the importance of the podocin-nephrin interaction.

50. Liu XL, Kilpelainen P, Hellman U, Sun Y, Wartiovaara J, et al. 2005. Characterization of the interactions of the nephrin intracellular domain: Evidence that the scaffolding protein IQGAP1 associates with nephrin. *FEBS J.* 272:228–43
50a. Hisatsune C, Kuroda Y, Nakamura K, Inoue T, Nakamura T, et al. 2003. Regulation of TRPC6 channel activity by tyrosine phosphorylation. *J. Biol. Chem.* 278:20716–23
51. Remuzzi G, Chiurchiu C, Ruggenenti P. 2004. Proteinuria predicting outcome in renal disease. *Kidney Int.* 92:S90–96
52. Davies D, Messina A, Thumwood CM, Ryan GB. 1985. Glomerular podocytic injury in protein overload proteinuria. *Pathology* 17:412–19
53. Schiffer M, Schiffer LE, Gupta A, Shaw AS, Roberts IS, et al. 2002. Inhibitory Smads and TGF-B signaling in glomerular cells. *J. Am. Soc. Nephrol.* 13:2657–66
54. Schiffer M, Bitzer M, Roberts IS, Kopp JB, ten Dijke P, et al. 2001. Apoptosis in podocytes induced by TGF-B and Smad 7. *J. Clin. Invest.* 108:807–16
55. Imai E, Isaka Y, Fujiwara Y, Kaneda Y, Kamada T, Ueda N. 1994. Introduction of a foreign gene into the kidney in vivo: Development of glomerulosclerosis by the transfection of gene for PDGF and TGF-β. *Contrib. Nephrol.* 107:205–15
56. Schnaper H, Hayashida T, Hubchak SC, Poncelet AC. 2003. TGF β signal induction and mesangial cell fibrogenesis. *Am. J. Physiol. Renal. Physiol.* 284:243–52
57. Ito T, Suzuki A, Imai E, Okabe M, Hori M. 2001. Bone marrow is a reservoir of repopulating mesangial cells during glomerular remodeling. *J. Am. Soc. Nephrol.* 12:2625–35
58. Mooney A, Jackson K, Bacon R, Streuli C, Edwards G, et al. 1999. Type IV collagen and laminin regulate glomerular mesangial cell susceptibility to apoptosis via beta-1 integrin mediated survival signals. *Am. J. Pathol.* 155:599–606
59. Essawy M, Soylemezoglu O, Muchaneta-Kubara EC, Shortland J, Brown CB, el Nahas AM. 1997. Myofibroblasts and the progression of diabetic nephropathy. *Nephrol. Dial. Transplant.* 12:43–50
60. Hudkins KL, Gilbertson DG, Carling M, Taneda S, Hughes SD, et al. 2004. Exogenous PDGF-D is a potent mesangial cell mitogen and causes a severe mesangial proliferative glomerulopathy. *J. Am. Soc. Nephrol.* 15:286–98

61. Suzuki A, Iwatani H, Ito T, Imai E, Okabe M, et al. 2004. Platelet derived growth factor plays a critical role to convert bone marrow cells into glomerular mesangial-like cells. *Kidney Int.* 65:15–24
62. Eremina V, Sood M, Haigh J, Nagy A, Lajoie G, et al. 2003. Glomerular specific alterations of VEGF-A expression lead to congenital and acquired glomerular disease. *J. Clin. Invest.* 111:707–16
63. Ruggenenti P. 2004. ACE inhibition and AT II antagonism in nondiabetic chronic nephropathies. *Semin. Nephrol.* 24:158–167
64. Durvasula RV, Petermann AT, Hiromura K, Blonski M, Pippin J, et al. 2004. Activation of a local tissue angiotensin system in podocytes by mechanical strain. *Kidney Int.* 65:30–39
65. Gloy J, Henger A, Fischer KG, Nitschke R, Mundel P, et al. 1997. Angiotensin II depolarizes podocyte in the intact glomerulus of the rat. *J. Clin. Invest.* 99:2772–81
66. Sharma R, Lovell HB, Wiegmann TB, Savin VJ. 1992. Vasoactive substances induce cytoskeletal changes in cultured rat glomerular epithelial cells. *J. Am. Soc. Nephrol.* 3:1131–38
67. Ding G, Reddy K, Kapasi AA, Franki N, Gibbons N, et al. 2002. Angiotensin II induces apoptosis in rat glomerular epithelial cells. *Am. J. Physiol. Renal Physiol.* 283:F173–F180
68. Hoffmann S, Podlich D, Hahnel B, Kriz W, Gretz N. 2004. Angiotensin II type I receptor overexpression in podocytes induces glomerulosclerosis in transgenic rats. *J. Am. Soc. Nephrol.* 15:1475–87
69. Marras D, Bruggeman LA, Gao F, Tanji N, Mansukhani MM, et al. 2002. Replication and compartmentalization of HIV-1 in kidney epithelium in patients with HIV-associated nephropathy. *Nat. Med.* 8:522–26
70. Alpers C, McClure J, Bursten SL. 1992. Human mesangial cells are resistant to multiple strains of human immuno deficiency virus strains 1 and 2. *Am. J. Kidney Dis.* 19:126–30
71. Green DF, Resnick L, Bourgoignie JJ. 1992. HIV infects glomerular endothelial and mesangial cells, but not epithelial cells in vitro. *Kidney Int.* 41:1956–60
72. Dickie P, Felser J, Eckhaus M, Bryant J, Silver J, et al. 1991. HIV associated nephropathy in transgenic mice expressing HIV-1 genes. *Virology* 185:109–19
73. Dickie P, Roberts A, Uwiera R, Witmer J, Sharma K, Kopp JB. 2004. Focal glomerulosclerosis in proximal and c-fms transgenic mice links Vpr expression to HIV associated nephropathy. *Virology* 322:69–81
74. He JC, Husain M, Sunamoto M, D'Agati VD, Klotman ME, et al. 2004. Nef stimulates proliferation of glomerular podocytes through activation of src dependent Stat3 and MAPK1,2 pathways. *J. Clin. Invest.* 114:643–51
75. **Barisoni L, Kriz W, Mundel P, D'Agati V. 1999. The dysregulated podocyte phenotype: a novel concept in the pathogenensis of collapsing idiopathic focal segmental glomerulosclerosis and HIV associated nephropathy. *J. Am. Soc. Nephrol.* 10:51–61**

The original proposal of podocyte phenotypic change in the pathogenesis of collapsing FSGS.

76. Bariety J, Nochy D, Mandet C, Jacquot C, Glotz D, Meyrier A. 1998. Podocytes undergo phenotypic change and express macrophage-associated markers in idiopathic collapsing glomerulopathy. *Kidney Int.* 53:918–25
77. Bodi I, Kimmel PL, Abraham AA, Svetkey LP, Klotman PE, Kopp JB. 1997. Renal TGF-B in HIV-associated kidney disease. *Kidney Int.* 51:1568–77
78. Barisoni L, Kopp JB. 2002. Modulation of podocyte phenotype in collapsing glomerulopathy. *Microsc. Res. Tech.* 57:254–62
79. Mrowka C, Schedl A. 2000. Wilm's tumor suppressor gene WT-1: From structure to renal pathophysiologic features. *J. Am. Soc. Nephrol.* 11:S106–S115

80. Yang AH, Chen JY, Chen BF. 2004. The dysregulated glomerular cell growth in Denys-Drash syndrome. *Virchows Arch.* 445:305–14
81. Wendt TM, Tanji N, Guo J, Kislinger TR, Qu W, et al. 2003. RAGE drives the development of glomerulosclerosis and implicates podocyte activation in the pathogenesis of diabetic nephropathy. *Am. J. Pathol.* 162:1123–37
82. Hirschberg R, Brunori G, Kopple JD, Guler HP. 1993. Effects of IGF-1 on renal function in normal men. *Kidney Int.* 43:387–97
83. Sabbatini M, Sansone G, Uccello F, Giliberti A, Conte G, Andreucci VE. 1992. Early glycosylation products induce glomerular hyperfiltration in diabetes mellitus. *Kidney Int.* 42:875–81
84. Wolf G, Schroeder R, Ziyadeh FN, Thaiss F, Zahner G, Stahl RA. 1997. High glucose stimulates expression of p27 in cultured mouse mesangial cells: Relationship to hypertrophy. *Am. J. Physiol.* 273:348–56
85. Hoffman BB, Sharma K, Zhu Y, Ziyadeh FN. 1998. Transcriptional activation of TGF-B in mesangial cell culture by high glucose concentration. *Kidney Int.* 58:1107–16
86. Singh R, Alavi N, Singh AK, Leehey DJ. 1994. Role of angiotensin II in glucose mediated inhibition of mesangial matrix degradation. *Diabetes* 48:2066–73
87. Yan SF, Ramasamy R, Naka Y, Schmidt AM. 2003. Glycation, inflammation, and RAGE. *Circ. Res.* 93:1159–69
88. Yamamoto Y, Kato I, Doi T, Yonekura H, Ohashi S, et al. 2001. Development and prevention of diabetic nephropathy in RAGE overexpressing mice. *J. Clin. Invest.* 108:261–68
88a. Nakamura T, Ushiyama C, Suzuki S, Hara M, Shimada N, et al. 2000. Urinary excretion of podocytes in patients with diabetic nephropathy. *Nephrol. Dial. Transplant.* 15:1379–83
88b. Regoli M, Bendayan M. 1997. Alterations in the expression of the alpha 3 beta 1 integrin in certain membrane domains of the glomerular epithelial cells (podocytes) in diabetes mellitus. *Diabetologia* 40:15–22
89. Ihm C, Park JK, Hong SP, Lee TW, Cho BS, et al. 1998. High glucose stimulates MCP-1 in human mesangial cells. *Nephron* 79:33–37
90. Chavakis T, Bierhaus A, Al-Fakhri N, Schneider D, Witte S, et al. 2003. The pattern recognition receptor (RAGE) is a counter receptor for leukocyte integrins: a novel pathway for inflammatory cell recuritment. *J. Exp. Med.* 198:1507–15
91. Adler S. 2004. Diabetic nephropathy: Linking histology, cell biology, and genetics. *Kidney Int.* 66:2095–2106
92. Barker D, Hostikka S, Zhou J, Chow LT, Oliphassnt AR, et al. 1990. Identification of mutations in the COL4A5 collagen gene in Alport syndrome. *Science* 248:1224–26
93. Mochizuki T, Lemmink H, Mariyama M, Antignac C, Gubler MC, et al. 1994. Identification of mutations in the α3(IV) and α4(IV) collagen genes in autosomal recessive Alport syndrome. *Nature Genet.* 8(1):77–82
94. van der Loop F, Heidet L, Timmer ED, van den Bosch BJ, Leinonen A, et al. 2000. Autosomal dominant Alport syndrome caused by a *COL4A3* splice site mutation. *Kidney Int.* 58(5):1870–75
95. Spear G, Slusser R. 1972. Alport's syndrome: emphasizing electron microscopic studies of the glomerulus. *Am. J. Pathol.* 69(2):213–24
96. Rumpelt H. 1987. Alport's syndrome: specificity and pathogenesis of glomerular basement membrane alterations. *Pediatr. Nephrol.* 1(3):422–27
97. Antonovych T, Deasy P, Tina LU, D'Albora JB, Hollerman CE, Calcagno PL. 1969. Hereditary nephritis: early clinical, functional and morphological studies. *Pediatr. Res.* 3(6):545–56

98. Hudson B, Tryggvason K, Sundaramoorthy M, Neilson EG. 2003. Alport's syndrome, Goodpasture's syndrome, and type IV collagen. *N. Engl. J. Med.* 348(25):2543–56
99. Miner J, Sanes J. 1994. Collagen IV alpha 3, alpha 4, and alpha 5 chains in rodent basal laminae: sequence, distribution, association with laminins, and developmental switches. *J. Cell Biol.* 127(3):879–91
100. Harvey S, Zheng K, Sado Y, Naito I, Ninomiya Y, et al. 1998. Role of distinct type IV collagen networks in glomerular development and function. *Kidney Int.* 54(6):1857–66
101. Kalluri R, Shield C, Todd P, Hudson BG, Neilson EG. 1997. Isoform switching of type IV collagen is developmentally arrested in X-linked Alport syndrome leading to increased susceptibility of renal basement membranes to endoproteolysis. *J. Clin. Invest.* 99(10): 2470–78
102. Nakanishi K, Yoshikawa N, Iijima K, Kitagawa K, Nakamura H, et al. 1994. Immunohistochemical study of α1–5 chains of type IV collagen in hereditary nephritis. *Kidney Int.* 46(5):1413–21
103. Miner J, Sanes J. 1996. Molecular and functional defects in kidneys of mice lacking collagen α3(IV): Implications for Alport syndrome. *J. Cell. Biol.* 135(5):1403–13
104. Cosgrove D, Meehan DT, Grunkemeyer JA, Kornak JM, Sayers R, et al. 1996. Collagen COL4A3 knockout: a mouse model for Alport syndrome. *Genes Dev.* 10(23):2981–92
105. Andrews K, Mudd J, Li C, Miner JH. 2002. Quantitative trait loci influence renal disease progression in a mouse model of Alport syndrome. *Am. J. Pathol.* 160(2):721–30
106. Gunwar S, Ballester F, Noelken ME, Sado Y, Ninomiya Y, Hudson BG. 1998. Glomerular basement membrane. Identification of a novel disulfide-cross-linked network of α3, α4 and α5 chains of type IV collagen and its implications for the pathogenesis of Alport syndrome. *J. Biol. Chem.* 273(15):8767–75
107. Abrahamson D, Prettyman A, Robert B, St John PL. 2003. Laminin-1 reexpression in Alport mouse glomerular basement membranes. *Kidney Int.* 63(3):826–34
108. Kashtan C, Kim Y, Lees GE, Thorner PS, Virtanen I, Miner JH. 2001. Abnormal glomerular basement membrane laminins in murine, canine and human Alport syndrome: Aberrant laminin α2 deposition is species independent. *J. Am. Soc. Nephrol.* 12(2):252–60
109. Savige J, Rana K, Tonna S, Buzza M, Dagher H, Wang YY. 2003. Thin basement membrane nephropathy. *Kidney Int.* 64(4):1169–78
110. Lemmink H, Nillesen W, Mochizuki T, Schroder CH, Brunner HG, et al. 1996. Benign familial hematuria due to mutation of the type IV collagen α4 gene. *J. Clin. Invest.* 98(5):1114–18
111. Buzza M, Wilson D, Savige J. 2001. Segregation of hematuria in thin basement membrane disease with haplotypes at the loci for Alport syndrome. *Kidney Int.* 59(5):1670–76
112. Sterk LMT, Geuijen CA, van den Berg JG, Claessen N, Weening JJ, Sonnenberg A. 2002. Association of the tetraspanin CD151 with the laminin-binding integrins {alpha}3{beta}1, {alpha}6{beta}1, {alpha}6{beta}4 and {alpha}7{beta}1 in cells in culture and in vivo. *J. Cell. Sci.* 115(6):1161–73
113. Karamatic Crew V, Burton N, Kagan A, Green CA, Levene C, et al. 2004. CD151, the first member of the tetraspanin (TM4) superfamily detected on erythrocytes, is essential for the correct assembly of human basement membranes in kidney and skin. *Blood* 104:2217–23
114. Zenker M, Aigner T, Wendler O, Tralau T, Muntefering H, et al. 2004. Human laminin {beta}2 deficiency causes congenital nephrosis with mesangial sclerosis and distinct eye abnormalities. *Hum. Mol. Genet.* 13:2625–32

115. Noakes P, Miner J, Gautam M, Cunningham JM, Sanes JR, Merlie JP. 1995. The renal glomerulus of mice lacking s-laminin/laminin B2: nephrosis despite molecular compensation by laminin B1. *Nature Genet.* 10(4):400–406
116. Dreyer S, Zhou G, Baldini A, Winterpacht A, Zabel B, et al. 1998. Mutations in LMX1B cause abnormal skeletal patterning and renal dysplasia in nail patella syndrome. *Nat. Genet.* 19(1):47–50
117. Morello R, Zhou G, Dreyer SD, Harvey SJ, Ninomiya Y, et al. 2001. Regulation of glomerular basement membrane collagen expression by *LMX1B* contributes to renal disease in nail patella syndrome. *Nature Genet.* 27(2):205–208

Proposes a link between the slit diaphragm and nail-patella syndrome.

118. **Miner JH, Morello R, Andrews KL, Li C, Antignac C, et al. 2002. Transcriptional induction of slit diaphragm proteins by Lmx1b is required in podocyte differentiation. *J. Clin. Invest.* 109(8):1065–72**

RELATED RESOURCES

Benzing T. 2004. Signaling at the slit diaphragm. *J. Am. Soc. Nephrol.* 15:1382–91

Spectrum of Epstein-Barr Virus–Associated Diseases

J.L. Kutok and F. Wang

Departments of Pathology and Medicine, Brigham and Women's Hospital, Harvard Medical School, Boston, Massachusetts 02115; email: jkutok@partners.org, fwang@rics.bwh.harvard.edu

Annu. Rev. Pathol. Mech. Dis. 2006. 1:375–404

First published online as a Review in Advance on October 28, 2005

The *Annual Review of Pathology: Mechanisms of Disease* is online at pathmechdis.annualreviews.org

doi: 10.1146/annurev.pathol.1.110304.100209

1553-4006/06/0114-0375$20.00

Key Words

gamma herpesvirus, infectious mononucleosis, Burkitt lymphoma, B lymphocyte, latent infection

Abstract

The association between Epstein-Barr virus (EBV) and a large number of benign and malignant diseases is unique among DNA viruses. Within infected tissues, proteins that are expressed during the normal lytic and latent viral life cycle lead to cellular alterations that contribute to these EBV-associated diseases. Although the early events of EBV infection are poorly understood, increasing knowledge of the viral processes that govern viral latency has shed light upon the potential mechanisms by which EBV infection can lead to cellular transformation. Our current understanding of the role of EBV in the development of Burkitt lymphoma, Hodgkin lymphoma, nasopharyngeal carcinoma, and other EBV-associated diseases is discussed.

INTRODUCTION

EBV: Epstein-Barr virus

BL: Burkitt lymphoma

IM: infectious mononucleosis

AIDS: acquired immunodeficiency syndrome

HL: Hodgkin lymphoma

Epstein-Barr virus (EBV) is one of the most extensively characterized members of the gamma subfamily of herpesviruses. This subfamily includes two genera. EBV belongs to the gamma-1 herpesviruses, or lymphocryptoviridae (LCV). LCV are found only in primates, with EBV representing the only LCV that infects humans. The gamma-2 herpesviruses, or rhadinoviridae (RV), infect both primates and a range of subprimate mammals. Kaposi sarcoma–associated herpesvirus (KSHV) is the only known RV that infects humans.

Although most viruses are identified initially as the cause of an acute illness, EBV was discovered because of its isolation within a tumor cell, the Burkitt lymphoma (BL) cell. Denis Burkitt, a British surgeon working in equatorial Africa, first described this aggressive B cell lymphoma in the late 1950s and early 1960s (1, 2). On the basis of the climatic and geographical distribution of this lymphoma, as well as its increased incidence in African children, Burkitt had long suspected an environmental or infectious etiology of the disease but was unsuccessful in identifying a candidate agent (3, 4). It was not until several years later in 1964 that Anthony Epstein, along with colleagues Yvonne Barr and Bert Achong, succeeded in culturing lymphoma cells from BL patients and identified herpesvirus particles in these cells by electron microscopy (5, 6).

After this initial discovery, epidemiological studies made it clear that BL is a rare neoplasm relative to the large pool of EBV-infected individuals. EBV is present in all populations, infecting more than 95% of human beings within the first decades of life. In developing countries, certain cultural practices often lead to EBV exposure in early childhood, and primary EBV infection in young children is typically associated with an unremarkable acute syndrome. In more developed countries, however, infection is often delayed, and acute primary EBV infection occurring in adolescence or adulthood can result in a self-limiting lymphoproliferative disorder known as infectious mononucleosis (IM) (7). The development of an EBV-specific immune response controls primary infection, but it is unable to purge the body completely of infection because the virus can hide within long-lived memory B cells. Thus, EBV infection persists asymptomatically during the host's life, maintaining a perpetual equilibrium between the immune response and a stealthy virus infection that results in no harm to the host. A low level of active viral replication continues asymptomatically in EBV carriers, leading to virus shedding via oral secretions and transmission of EBV from one individual to another.

Although EBV infection is benign and uneventful in the majority of humans, the link between EBV infection and human tumors is undeniable. EBV was detected in tissues from patients with nasopharyngeal carcinoma in the 1970s (8), non-Hodgkin lymphoma (NHL) in patients with acquired immunodeficiency syndrome (AIDS) in the early 1980s (9), and T cell and Hodgkin lymphomas (HL) in the late 1980s (10–12). EBV is currently associated with more than a dozen lymphoid and solid tissue malignancies in both immunocompetent and immunocompromised individuals (**Table 1**). Association with a common human pathogen does not necessarily implicate that pathogen's causal role in oncogenic transformation. However, the tight epidemiological linkage—clonal virus infection in early dysplastic and tumor cells, the presence of EBV infection in every malignant cell within a tumor, and viral genes capable of usurping normal cellular growth control—all suggest that EBV infection plays a causal role in the development of these associated malignancies.

Why has EBV, which has infected humans since their divergence from early subhuman primates, evolved to initiate tumor formation? Perhaps the simple answer is that EBV evolution has been driven by virus survival, not by disease. Persistence and reactivation are hallmarks of EBV and other herpesviruses survival. Because most humans are infected in adulthood, EBV infection must persist until new generations of susceptible hosts are born, and then the virus must reactivate to produce infectious viruses that can be transmitted to naïve hosts, thereby propagating itself over time. All LCV have evolved a unique set of viral genes that are absent in other herpesviruses and that exploit the normal physiology of B cells so that viruses can persist successfully in B cells. Because nonhuman primate LCV infection is also associated with tumor formation, it appears that the viral manipulation of cellular growth processes required for LCV persistence are inexorably linked to the potential for malignant transformation in a small but significant number of instances.

Table 1 Epstein-Barr virus–associated diseases

Nonmalignant disease
Infectious mononucleosis
Chronic active infection
Oral hairy leukoplakia
Malignant disease
Immunocompromised host
B cell malignancies
Acquired immunodeficiency
AIDS-associated B cell lymphomas
Post-transplantation lymphoproliferative disorder
Lymphomatoid granulomatosis
Methotrexate-associated B cell lymphoma
Congenital immunodeficiency
Severe combined immunodeficiency–associated B cell lymphomas
Wiskott-Aldrich syndrome–associated B cell lymphomas
X-linked lymphoproliferative disorder–associated B cell lymphomas
Mesenchymal malignancies
Leiomyosarcoma
Immunocompetent host
B cell malignancies
Burkitt lymphoma
Classical Hodgkin lymphoma
T cell malignancies
Extranodal NK/T cell lymphoma, nasal type
Virus-associated hemophagocytic syndrome T cell lymphomas
Epithelial cell malignancies
Nonglandular nasopharyngeal carcinoma
Lymphoepithelioma-like carcinoma (salivary, thymus, lungs, stomach)
Breast carcinoma
Hepatocellular carcinoma
Mesenchymal malignancies
Follicular dendritic cell sarcoma

PROPERTIES OF EBV

EBV has a toroid-shaped protein core wrapped within its linear, double-stranded, approximately 184-kb DNA genome. Details of the genomic structure have been described extensively in other reviews (13). Its structure is characterized by short and long unique sequence domains (U_S and U_L) that contain almost all the genome coding capacity, as well as internal (IR1) and terminal (TR) tandem and reiterated direct repeats. The virus contains a linear genome, and upon EBV infection of a cell (typically by a single virion), the linear termini are joined intracellularly to form circular, episomal DNA (14–16). Heterogeneity in the number of joined TR can distinguish clonal infection events. The number of TR present in a given linear genome is highly variable owing to the random TR cleavage that creates full-length genomes from the linear concatamers synthesized during viral replication. When a virus infects a cell, the linear genome is circularized into an episome, creating a signature number of TRs. The TR number remains constant during episomal replication in dividing, latently infected host cells; therefore, all daughter cells derived from a single infected cell share episomes with identical numbers of TR. This constitutes a marker that can determine the clonality of latently infected host cells in tissues. Southern blot analysis, which uses probes to detect DNA fragments containing EBV terminal repeat sequences, is an important clinical test for determining whether a patient's neoplasm is derived from a clonal population of EBV-infected cells (**Figure 1**) (17).

The virus gains entry into the B cell via interaction of the viral envelope protein gp350/220 with the B cell surface molecule CD21 (the receptor for the C3d component of complement) (18) (**Figure 2**). EBV can

CD21: complement C3d and Epstein-Barr virus receptor that complexes with CD19 and CD81; present on B lymphocytes, follicular dendritic cells, and a subset of T cells

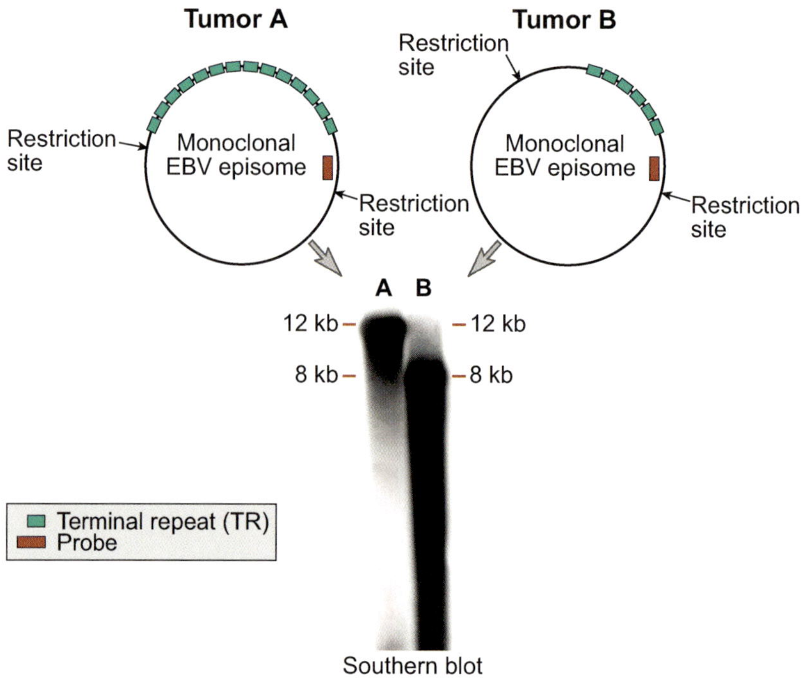

Figure 1

Epstein-Barr virus (EBV)-clonality assay by Southern blotting. Two monoclonal EBV-associated B cell lymphomas (tumors A and B) are depicted, each with a unique number of tandem terminal repeat sequences within the EBV episome. DNA is cut with *Bam*HI restriction endonuclease, whose cleavage sites flank the terminal repeats, and the DNA is electrophoresed and hybridized with an EBV-specific probe. In this example, tumor A gives a band at 12 kb, a size related directly to the number of terminal repeats in the EBV episome within that tumor (*left*). Fewer repeats are present in tumor B, which gives a band of ~8 kb upon Southern blotting (*right*).

Acyclovir: synthetic purine nucleoside analog, $C_8H_{10}N_5O_3$, derived from guanine that competes for DNA polymerase and is used in the treatment of gamma herpesvirus infections

also infect other cell types, such as epithelial cells, mesenchymal cells, and T cells [as evidenced by the association of EBV with tumors derived from these cell types (see **Table 1**)]; however, the EBV receptor on CD21-negative cells is unknown. Genetically engineered viruses that do not express gp350/220 can infect both B cells and epithelial cells (albeit at a reduced level), which indicates that additional cellular molecules besides CD21 can also allow virus entry into these cells (19). $\alpha_5\beta_1$ integrin may be a surface molecule that contributes to EBV infection of epithelial cells (20). Once EBV adsorption takes place, CD21 aggregates within the membrane and the virus is internalized within cytoplasmic vesicles (21, 22). Activation of B cell signal transduction pathways by virus binding may increase the efficiency of viral gene expression (23).

Infectious viruses are produced during the lytic phase of the EBV viral life cycle (**Figure 3**). Approximately 80 viral proteins are expressed during lytic viral replication, including transcriptional activators, DNA replication factors, and structural proteins such as viral capsid antigens. BZLF1 and BRLF1 proteins are the key mediators in the switch from latency to the lytic cycle and are the earliest indicators of lytic infection. These proteins are potent transactivators of other lytic cycle–related genes leading to the expression of the viral DNA polymerase that replicates the viral DNA as linear concatamers. Acyclovir, an antiviral drug, can inhibit lytic EBV infection by terminating viral DNA

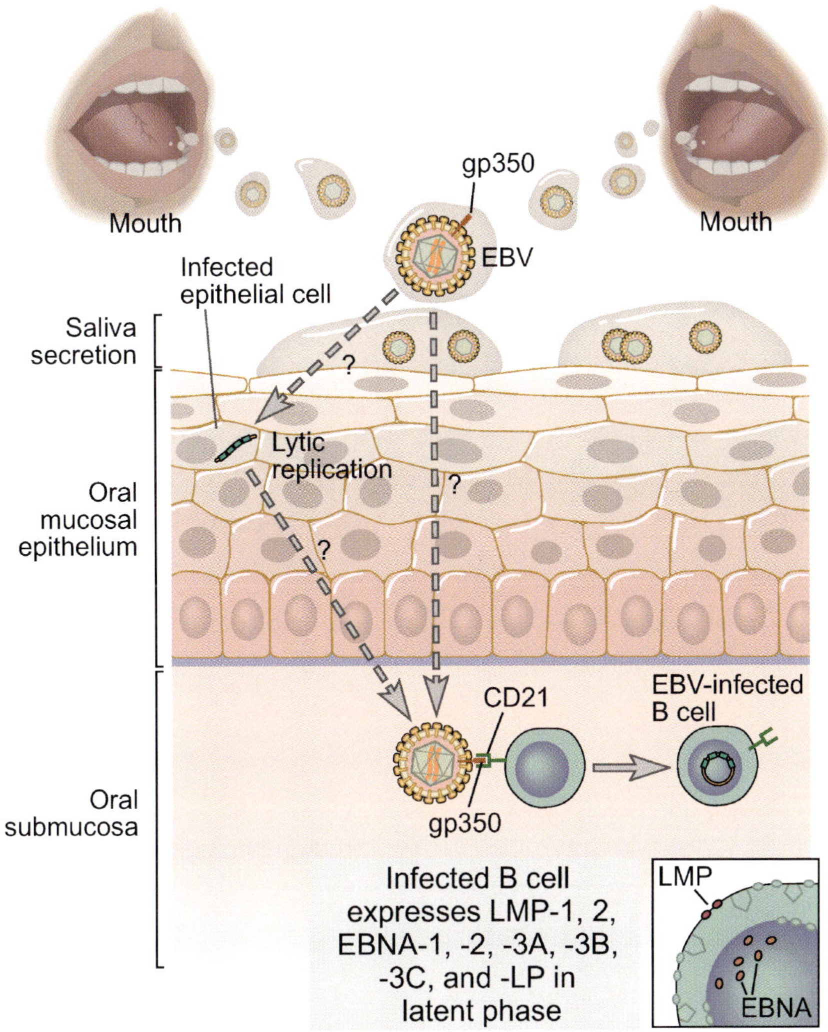

Figure 2

Schematic of the early steps in Epstein-Barr virus (EBV) infection. After close contact, viral particles present in the saliva of infected individuals enter into the oral cavity. Viruses enter into the underlying lymphoid tissue, which is rich in B lymphocytes [controversy remains as to whether viruses infect epithelial cells and replicate within the oral epithelium or pass directly into the underlying lymphoid tissue (depicted by *dashed arrows*)]. Once contact with the CD21-expressing B cell target is made via EBV gp350, the virus enters the B cell and expresses genes of the viral latency III program. LMP, latent membrane protein; EBNA, Epstein-Barr virus nuclear antigen.

synthesis when it is phosphorylated by viral kinases and incorporated into the viral DNA. Linear viral genomes are cleaved at the terminal repeats, packaged into viral capsids, and the enveloped virus is released from infected cells that are then destined to die (24–32). Some of the other viral proteins involved in lytic replication and their functions are listed in **Table 2**.

During the latent phase of the EBV viral life cycle, there is no production of infectious viruses and a highly restricted number of

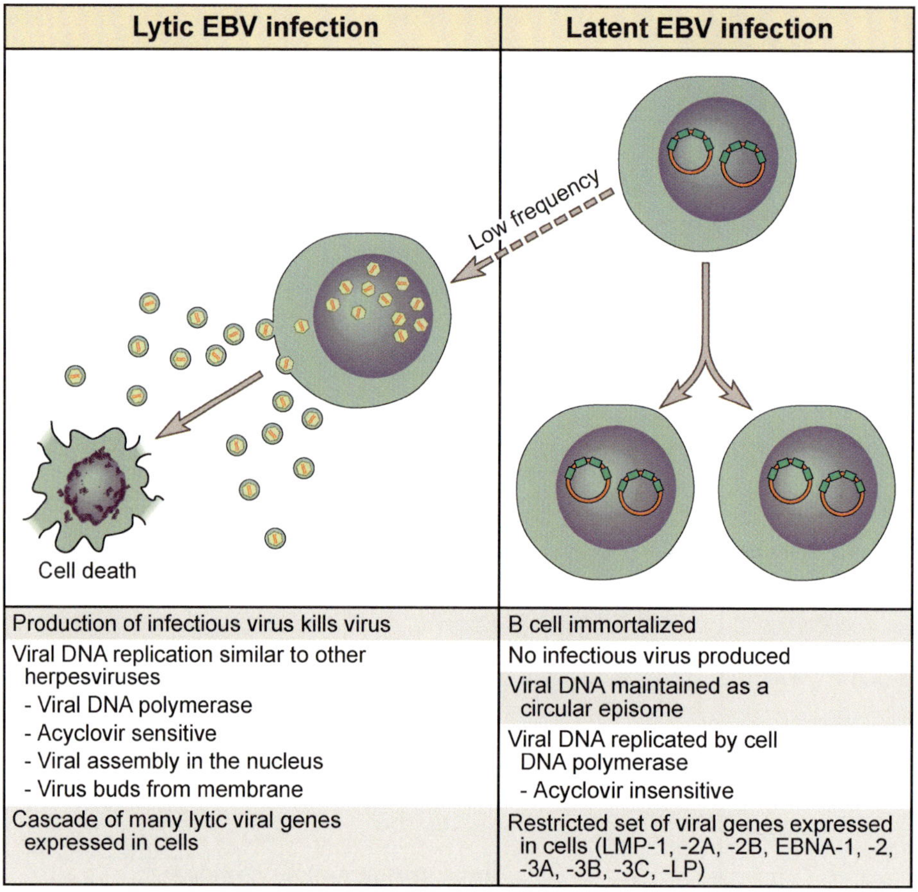

Figure 3

Comparison of major features of the lytic and latent cycles of Epstein-Barr virus (EBV) infection. EBV infection is latent in most cells, and transition into lytic infection occurs in a small percentage of latently infected cells (*dashed arrow*). LMP, latent membrane protein; EBNA, Epstein-Barr virus nuclear antigen.

EBNA: Epstein-Barr virus nuclear antigen

EBER: Epstein-Barr Virus–encoded RNAs

LMP: latent membrane protein

latent infection genes are expressed (**Table 3**) (**Figure 3**). Acyclovir is not an effective antiviral drug for inhibiting latent EBV infection because the viral kinases required to phosphorylate acyclovir are not expressed in latently infected cells. EBV genes expressed during latent infection can usurp normal B cell growth mechanisms, which leads to virus-induced immortalization of B cells and the establishment of lymphoblastoid cell lines (LCL). During latent infection, the viral genome is maintained as a circular episome, is replicated by cell DNA polymerase, and is equally distributed to daughter cells when the EBV-infected cell divides during the course of cellular growth.

Latent infection in EBV-immortalized B cells is associated with the expression of six nuclear antigens [Epstein-Barr virus nuclear antigen 1 (EBNA1), EBNA2, EBNA3A, EBNA3B, EBNA3C, and EBNA leader protein (LP)], three membrane proteins [latent membrane protein 1 (LMP1), LMP2A, and LMP2B], two small nonpolyadenylated Epstein-Barr virus–encoded small RNAs (EBER1 and EBER2), and transcripts from the *Bam*HI A region (BARTs). Different patterns of latent infection gene expression have been described in vivo and in vitro, and expression of this full repertoire of latent viral genes is referred to as latency III (**Table 4**).

Genetic studies with recombinant EBV demonstrate that EBNA2, EBNA3A, EBNA3C, and LMP1 are essential for B cell immortalization in vitro. EBNA2 is a transcriptional transactivator of viral and cellular genes that are important for growth transformation, and LMP1 activates nuclear factor kappa B (NFκB) by mimicking cell signaling through the proliferation- and survival-promoting B cell molecule CD40. The major functions of these and other latent infection gene products are listed in **Table 3**. LCLs have many of the properties of tumor cells in experimental systems, which include the ability to propagate indefinitely in culture medium and form solid tumors in nude or severe combined immunodeficiency (SCID) mice (33, 34).

PRIMARY INFECTION: INFECTIOUS MONONUCLEOSIS

The majority of primary EBV infections are clinically unremarkable, with symptoms that are indistinguishable from other acute viral syndromes. In some individuals, however, particularly those exposed to EBV in adolescence, primary EBV infection can result in the more distinctive IM syndrome (**Figure 4**). This is a self-limiting lymphoproliferative disease characterized by sore throat, fever, adenopathy, and splenomegaly. IM has thus served as a marker for primary EBV infection and has provided investigators with a means for studying the early events following exposure to the virus. However, this is not a perfect system for this purpose as it is not clear whether IM truly mirrors the same events that occur in all primary EBV infections. In addition, because IM is not detected clinically until after a several week incubation period, the earliest events after initial oropharyngeal contact with saliva containing cell-free EBV are mostly unknown. Once symptoms of IM are detected, high titers of cell-free infectious viruses are present in patient throat washings and saliva, indicating a significant degree of active viral replication (35).

Early studies indicate that viral replication within oropharyngeal epithelial cells is a potentially important early step in primary EBV infection, with viruses subsequently passing to subepithelial B cells through direct contact (36–38). It is well known that EBV infection and replication can occur within certain epithelial cell types. This is particularly evident in immunosuppressed AIDS patients with oral hairy leukoplakia, a lytic EBV infection of lingual epithelial cells (see **Table 1**). However, more recent studies showing an inability to detect EBV infection in the tonsillar epithelium of IM patients (39–41) has raised the possibility that EBV infection of epithelial cells is not critical for primary EBV infection and that viruses may initially bypass epithelial cells and instead directly infect B cells.

Despite ambiguity regarding the role of the oropharyngeal epithelial cells for EBV amplification during primary infection, it is clear that the B cell is the critical target for EBV infection. At the clinical peak of IM, between 0.1% to 1% of peripheral blood B cells can contain viruses (42), and these EBV-infected B cells from IM patients express the latency III program

Table 2 Selected Epstein-Barr virus–encoded lytic infection gene products

Lytic-associated genes	Proposed function
BZLF1 / BRLF1	Key transactivators of lytic EBV gene expression, coordinately upregulating expression from early EBV promoters (24–28, 31, 32)
BHRF1	Colinear homology with BCL-2, prevents apoptotic cell death in lytic EBV infection (124); nonessential for growth transformation of B cells and for virus replication in culture (125)
BCRF1	Homology to human interleukin-10; may downregulate the host immune response during viral replication (126)
BALF5	Replication factor; core DNA polymerase (127)
BALF2	Replication factor; single-strand DNA binding protein (127)
BMRF1	Replication factor; processivity factor (127)
BSLF1 and BBLF4	Replication factor; primase and helicase complex (127)
BBLF2/3	Replication factor; spliced primase helicase complex component (127)
BKRF3	Replication factor; uracil DNA glycosylase (127)
BLLF1 (gp350/220)	Mediates adsorption between EBV and CD21

Nuclear factor kappa B (NFκB): family of heterodimeric transcription factors implicated in the regulation of many genes that code for mediators of the immune, acute phase and inflammatory responses

Table 3 Selected Epstein-Barr virus–encoded latent infection gene products

Latency-associated genes	Proposed function
Epstein-Barr virus nuclear antigen 1 (EBNA1)	Binds EBV genome to chromosomes mediating episomal persistence and maintenance (128); may inhibit apoptosis in Burkitt lymphoma cells (129); Gly-Ala repeat inhibits processing of EBNA1 through protesomes, precluding presentation of antigenic peptides with MHC-I at the cell surface, thus avoiding detection by CD8+ T cells (54)
Epstein-Barr virus nuclear antigen 2 (EBNA2)	Transactivator of several viral genes (LMP1 and LMP2A) (130–132) and cellular genes (CD21, *c-FGR*, *c-MYC*, CD23) (133, 134) essential for cellular transformation (135); interacts with transcription factor RBP-JK to promote conversion of resting B lymphocytes into lymphoblastoid B cells (136)
Epstein-Barr virus nuclear antigen 3C (EBNA3C)	Essential for EBV-mediated transformation of primary B lymphocytes and interacts with RBP-Jk (137, 138); EBNA3C promotes LMP1 expression in the presence of EBNA2 (139, 140)
Epstein-Barr virus nuclear antigen leader protein (EBNA-LP)	Key role in upregulating cell gene expression critical for lymphoblastoid B cell outgrowth (141) and augments the ability of EBNA2 to transactivate LMP1 (142)
Latent membrane protein 1 (LMP1)	Mimics signaling through CD40, a B cell activation and differentiation receptor (143, 144), and in turn activates NFκB pathways to promote cell survival (145); promotes B cell lymphoma formation in transgenic mice expressing the gene (146)
Latent membrane protein 2A (LMP2A)	Constitutive dominant negative modulator of B cell receptor signaling by sequestering tyrosine kinases through interactions with its immunoreceptor tyrosine-based activation motifs (147), preventing entry into the lytic cycle by antigenic stimulation; promotes B cell survival through activation of the same sequestered tyrosine kinases in an antigen- and B cell receptor-independent manner (148, 149)
Epstein-Barr virus–encoded RNAs 1 and 2 (EBER1 and 2)	Small nonpolyadenylated RNAs that represent the most abundant RNAs in latently infected cells; role in EBV infection still unclear

Table 4 Patterns of latent infection gene expression in Epstein-Barr virus–infected cells

Latency program	Genes expressed
0	EBERs, (LMP2A)
I	EBERs, EBNA1
II	EBERs, EBNA1, LMP2A, LMP1
III	EBERs, EBNA1, LMP2A, LMP1, EBNA2, EBNA3s, EBNA-LP

of EBV gene expression, which suggests that virus-induced B cell proliferation contributes to the growth of virus-infected cells (43). These activated and proliferating EBV-infected B lymphocytes also commonly infiltrate lymphoid tissues. Lymph node or tonsillar biopsy during acute IM shows scattered reactive secondary follicles with a marked paracortical diffuse expansion of proliferating B immunoblasts (44) (**Figure 5**). Large, sometimes bizarre, mononuclear or binuclear immunoblasts, which may resemble the Reed-Sternberg (RS) cells of HL, are frequently noted (45, 46). Differentiating this diffuse immunoblastic proliferation in IM from lymphoma can be difficult on the basis of morphological findings alone.

The invasion of the immune system by EBV infection of B cells stimulates a vigorous CD8+ T cell response. These activated T cells are the characteristic atypical lymphocytes seen in peripheral blood smears of IM patients (**Figure 6**). Peripheral lymphocytosis, lymphadenopathy, and splenomegaly are more directly a result of this nonspecific T cell proliferation than the proliferation of EBV-infected B cells. The standard for diagnosing primary EBV infection is to identify the characteristic humoral response to primary EBV infection, an early IgG and IgM antibody response to viral capsid antigens coupled with a more delayed seroconversion to antibodies against the EBNAs. However, it is unclear to what extent humoral immunity contributes to overall control of the infection.

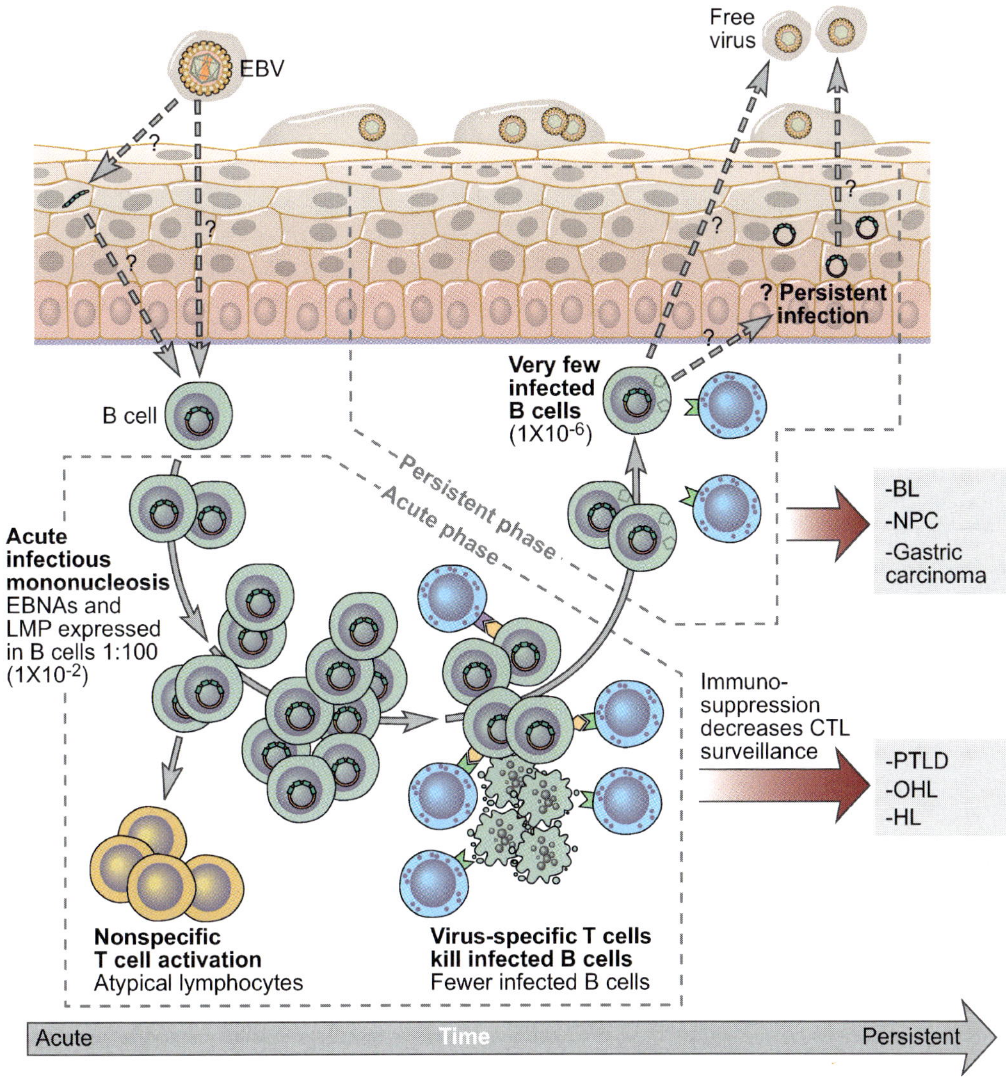

Figure 4

Schematic of the major events that occur during acute and persistent infection with Epstein-Barr virus (EBV). Once the target B cell is infected, EBV infection drives B lymphoid proliferation, which stimulates a nonspecific T cell activation. The activated T cells cause the appearance of atypical lymphocytes in the peripheral blood and, if sufficiently vigorous, T cell activation leads to infectious mononucleosis (IM) syndrome. Over time, EBV-specific T cell immunity develops, which reduces the number of infected B lymphocytes. Under normal conditions, the infection is controlled and enters into a latent phase where EBV infection is present in only a very few infected B cells (1×10^{-6}). Lytic replication, either in oral epithelial cells or B cells near the oral epithelium, results in the shedding of infectious viruses via oral secretions and renewal of the virus life cycle in a new host. Immunosuppression can result in decreased cytotoxic T cell (CTL) surveillance, which leads to an increased risk of developing certain EBV-associated diseases such as post-transplantation lymphoproliferative disorder (PTLD), oral hairy leukoplakia (OHL), and Hodgkin lymphoma (HL). Other EBV-related diseases [Burkitt lymphoma (BL), nasopharyngeal carcinoma (NPC), and gastric carcinoma] are not typically associated with overt immunosuppression, but likely arise as a result of other cofactors acting in concert with persistent EBV infection. EBNA, Epstein-Barr virus nuclear antigen; LMP, latent membrane protein.

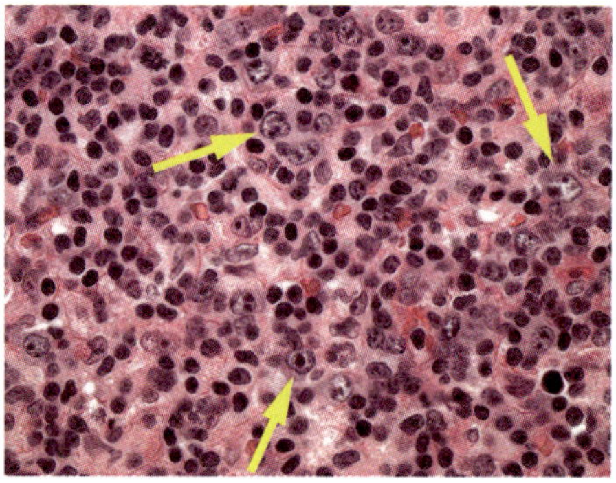

Figure 5

Tonsillar biopsy during acute infectious mononucleosis showing a diffuse paracortical expansion of proliferating B immunoblasts among reactive T cells with small hyperchromatic nuclei. Representative large, mononuclear B immunoblasts with prominent central nucleoli are identified by yellow arrows (hematoxylin and eosin stain; original magnification 400x).

Genetic diseases highlight the important role of the immune system in controlling acute primary EBV infection. X-linked lymphoproliferative disorder (XLP) is a rare condition in which affected young males are able to control infections with most pathogens, but are uniquely susceptible to EBV infection. Some patients die of uncontrolled B cell proliferation during acute EBV infection, which suggests that their immune system response is ineffective. However, other patients develop fulminant IM, pancytopenia, or hypogammaglobulinemia, which suggests an excessive and overactive immune system response. The clinical phenotypes may be consistent with a regulatory disorder of the EBV immune response. Most XLP patients have mutations in a gene known as SAP, or SLAM (signaling lymphocyte activation molecule)–associated protein (47, 48). SAP is expressed in T cells, natural killer (NK) cells, and NK/T cells, and it is an adapter molecule that regulates signaling through several members of the CD2 subfamily of cell surface receptors including SLAM. The role and mechanism by which SAP regulates cell signaling and immune system responses, let alone why SAP mutations result in an extreme sensitivity to EBV infection, remain unclear. The regulatory role in cell signaling, expression in a variety of cell types, and wide variety of mutations associated with XLP may contribute to the different clinical presentations of a genetic immunodeficiency with a common genetic target.

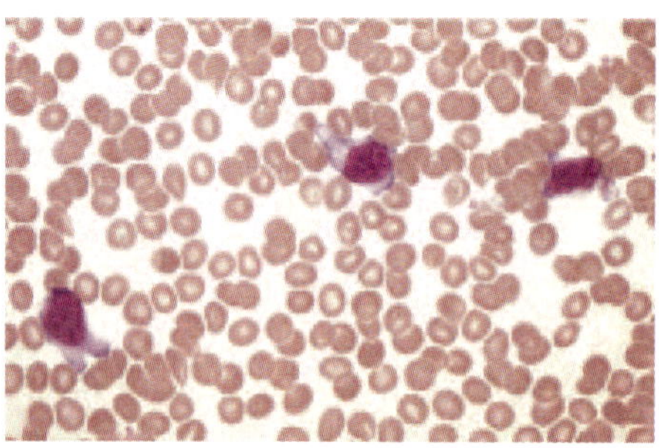

Figure 6

Several large, activated CD8+ T cells (atypical lymphocytes) in the peripheral blood smear of a patient with acute infectious mononucleosis (wright-giemsa stain; original magnification 400x).

Establishment of Persistent Infection

Eventually a virus-specific, HLA-restricted cytotoxic CD8+ T cell response that predominantly targets epitopes from the EBNA3A, -3B, and -3C subset of latent infection proteins (49) and the lytic infection protein BZLF1 develops. Presumably the development of a virus-specific adaptive immune response contributes to the control of EBV infection by reducing the number of EBV-infected B cells (**Figure 4**). However, the immune response fails to completely eliminate EBV infection in the body. Persistent EBV infection can be detected as a latent infection in peripheral blood lymphocytes and as a lytic infection in the oral cavity, which results in the shedding of infectious viruses via oral secretions. B cells are thought to be essential for persistent EBV infection because patients with X-linked agammaglobulinemia who lack B cells do not have evidence for persistent EBV infection (50). Maintenance of persistent infection does not appear to require active viral replication because peripheral blood EBV viral loads remain stable in healthy individuals receiving acyclovir (51). Thus, the ultimate goal during primary EBV infection appears to be the latent infection of B cells in order to achieve persistent infection.

How EBV infection persists for life in B cells and evades immune elimination remains elusive. One hypothesis is that EBV infects a naïve B cell, and expression of the latency III program drives the EBV-infected B cell to differentiate into a memory B cell so that viral persistence results from the intrinsic long-lived properties of the memory B cell (52). Alternatively, the latent infection genes may act directly to promote more long-lived B cells through their growth-deregulating and antiapoptotic functions (53). In either case, the pattern of latent EBV gene expression is markedly restricted in persistently infected, peripheral blood lymphocytes. At most there is evidence for expression of EBNA1, LMP2A, EBERs, and BARTs. It is unknown whether expression of the full latency III program is required or even occurs after primary infection. However, CD8+ cytotoxic T cells (CTLs) specific for epitopes from the EBNA3 family of proteins continue to dominate the immune response to latent infection proteins in persistently infected individuals, suggesting that a more complete repertoire of latent infection proteins may be expressed periodically. Thus, the ability to downregulate latent infection gene expression to a more restricted, i.e., non-EBNA3-expressing, pattern by switching transcriptional promoter usage may be one important mechanism for EBV immune evasion. The ability of the EBNA1 glycine-alanine repeat region to inhibit proteosomal degradation and presentation of EBNA1 peptide epitopes to CD8+ CTL may be another mechanism by which persistently infected B cells that still express EBNA1 may evade elimination by the immune system (54). These mechanisms and models can be difficult to prove by observational studies in EBV-infected humans. Animal models for experimental infection with closely related LCV-infected nonhuman primates may provide experimental systems to test these hypotheses for EBV infection (55).

EBV-ASSOCIATED DISEASES IN THE IMMUNOCOMPROMISED HOST

In a general sense, other EBV-associated diseases can be categorized by those that occur in immunosuppressed individuals versus those that occur in individuals without overt evidence of immunosuppression. The importance of the immune response for controlling persistent EBV infection is demonstrated by the emergence of EBV-driven B lymphocyte proliferations or lymphomas in patients with genetic or acquired immunosuppression. EBV-related lymphoproliferative disorders arise mostly in the setting of iatrogenic immunosuppression in organ transplantation or in AIDS, and similar disorders can cause complications for patients with genetic immunodeficiencies such as Severe Combined Immunodeficiciency, Wiskott-Aldrich syndrome, and Ataxia-Telangiectasia.

Post-Transplantation Lymphoproliferative Disorders

PTLDs: post-transplantation lymphoproliferative disorders

Post-transplantation lymphoproliferative disorders (PTLDs) comprise a varied group of almost exclusively B cell proliferations that range from spontaneously regressing, polytypic lymphoplasmacytoid B cell expansions that resemble inflammatory reactions to lethal clonal B cell proliferations that are indistinguishable from NHL (**Figure 7*a***). The majority of PTLDs are associated with EBV infection; however, the association appears to weaken in lesions that occur long after transplantation. These lymphoid proliferations have been divided into four main categories according to the current World Health Organization (WHO) classification: (*a*) reactive, plasmacytic hyperplasias or IM-like lymphoid hyperplasias, (*b*) polymorphic

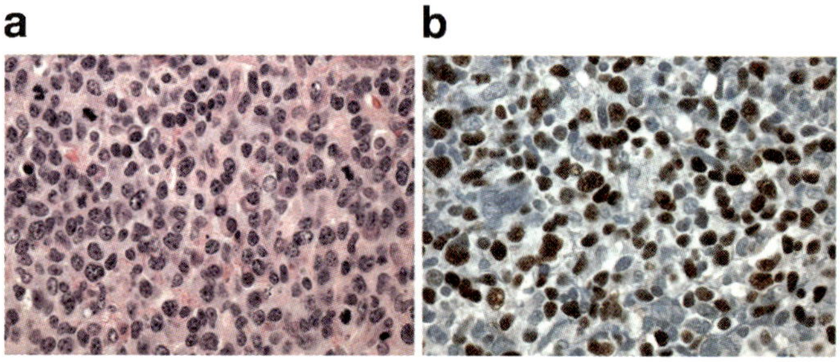

Figure 7

(*a*) Post-transplantation lymphoproliferative disorder (PTLD) within a lymph node showing a relatively monomorphous population of large B cells demonstrating some degree of plasmacytic differentiation (hematoxylin and eosin stain; original magnification 400X). (*b*) Immunohistochemical stains for Epstein-Barr virus nuclear antigen 2 (EBNA2) in the same case consistent with latency III program of viral gene expression (diaminobenzidine chromogen with hematoxylin counterstain; original magnification 400x).

PTLD, (*c*) monomorphic PTLD corresponding to B and T cell (rare) NHL, and (*d*) HL and HL-like PTLD (rare). A distinction between these lymphoid proliferations, however, is not distinct. Rather than occurring in nodal tissues, these tumors are found generally as multifocal lesions in extranodal sites, frequently involving the transplanted organ or gastrointestinal tract. PTLDs can occur in solid-organ or bone-marrow transplantation with an incidence related directly to the amount and duration of immunosuppressive therapy. Because immunosuppressive regimens are often more intensive and prolonged following solid organ transplantation, the incidence of PTLDs in this patient group is relatively high (ranging from 1% in renal transplant patients to as many as 3%–8% in heart and lung transplant recipients). PTLDs associated with bone-marrow transplantation are less common, occurring in approximately 1% of patients (56). These lymphoproliferations arise mostly from donor-derived EBV-infected B cells, as the pretransplant myeloablative conditioning regimens empty the host of persistent EBV-infected lymphoid cells.

The EBV-positive B cells in these disorders demonstrate most frequently the latency III program pattern of EBV gene expression, although other patterns of latent gene expression have been reported. Latency III program includes the expression of genes such as LMP1 and EBNA2, which are critical for cellular growth transformation (**Figure 7*b***). Without sufficient cytotoxic T cell function, there is uninhibited growth of EBV-infected B cells. Initially, this expanded EBV-infected B cell pool represents a polyclonal proliferation, and Southern blotting for both EBV terminal repeats or immunoglobulin gene rearrangements confirms the polyclonal nature of these early lesions. Additional empirical evidence for the role of T cell immunity in this process comes from the observation that if immunosuppresion is withdrawn or reduced or if the patient is infused with EBV-specific cytotoxic T cells from the allogeneic donor at this stage, these polyclonal EBV-driven expansions will often regress. In some cases, additional genetic defects may occur in EBV-infected cells that act either in concert with or obviate the need for virus-driven cell growth. These can include genes encoding *p53* (57), *c-MYC* (58), or *BCL-6* (59). These may be more aggressive clonal lymphoproliferations with a more restricted pattern of EBV latent gene expression that are unresponsive to reductions in immunosuppressive regimens.

EBV-Associated Lymphomas in AIDS

AIDS-associated lymphomas are a heterogenous group that includes primary central nervous system (CNS) lymphomas, diffuse large B cell lymphomas, HL, BL or BL-like lymphomas, and primary effusion lymphomas. The frequency of EBV infection in AIDS-related lymphomas is much more variable and depends on the subtype of tumor involved. For example, AIDS-associated CNS lymphomas are EBV infected in all cases. One potential explanation for this finding is that HIV-induced immunodeficiency may increase the trafficking of EBV-infected B cells into the brain, or the combined immunodeficiency and immunoprivileged nature of the CNS favors EBV-driven B lymphoproliferations. Most cases of diffuse, large B cell lymphomas with immunoblastic morphology and HL in AIDS patients are EBV related. These cases appear in the final stage of AIDS when the patient is severely immunocompromised. In contrast, Burkitt or Burkitt-like lymphomas in AIDS patients are associated with EBV infection in only 30%–50% of cases (60–62). In these cases, EBV infection and immunosuppression may increase the pool of B cells at risk for a *c-MYC* translocation (see below) and may not be the primary mechanism for driving malignant proliferation. EBV infection can be detected in some primary effusion lymphomas, but these B cell lymphoproliferations are linked consistently to KSHV infection, which suggests that the gamma-2 herpesvirus is more important for this malignancy than EBV infection.

Immunodeficiency-Related Leiomyosarcomas

In rare cases, immunocompromised patients have developed smooth muscle neoplasms that harbor clonal EBV genomes (63–65). These tumors arise typically in children in the setting of organ transplantation or AIDS and are most commonly located within the gastrointestinal tract or pulmonary tree. The pattern of EBV latent gene expression appears similar to that of the PTLDs corresponding to the latency III program type with specific expression of EBNA1, EBNA2, LMP1, and LMP2A genes (66). It is unclear how EBV contributes to this malignancy and how EBV gets into these cells. Smooth muscle cells are not believed to be a normal target for EBV infection, but variable degrees of staining for the EBV receptor, CD21, have been noted in these tumor cells (64, 65). No evidence of EBV infection has been noted in normal smooth muscle adjacent to EBV-positive leiomyosarcomas, and EBV infection has not been found to infect leiomyosarcomas in immunocompetent patients. Immunosuppression may somehow allow the rare, abnormal entry of EBV into smooth muscle cells, leading to a risk of malignant transformation.

Oral Hairy Leukoplakia

Oral hairy leukoplakia is a proliferative, hyperkeratotic, squamous mucosal epithelial cell lesion seen characteristically in immunocompromised patients. This disorder is noteworthy because it is the only EBV-associated disorder associated primarily with lytic replication. Lytic viral gene expression is demonstrated easily in lesions, and more advanced stages of viral replication are found in the more differentiated epithelial cell layers (**Figure 8**). It is unclear whether these lesions arise from persistently infected epithelial cells that become more permissive for lytic replication with immunosuppression, or if immunosuppression allows these lingual epithelial cells to be infected abnormally whereupon they are susceptible to excessive lytic replication and cell proliferation. Lesions regress with acyclovir treatment but reoccur frequently when treatment is stopped. This may be consistent with clearance and reinfection or an inability of acyclovir to clear persistent, latently infected epithelial cells.

EBV-ASSOCIATED MALIGNANCIES IN THE IMMUNOCOMPETENT HOST

BL, HL, and nasopharyngeal carcinoma are three of the most important EBV-associated malignancies in immunocompetent hosts. They typically occur many years after primary EBV infection so that EBV infection appears to be just one factor in what is actually a complex multistep process of malignant transformation.

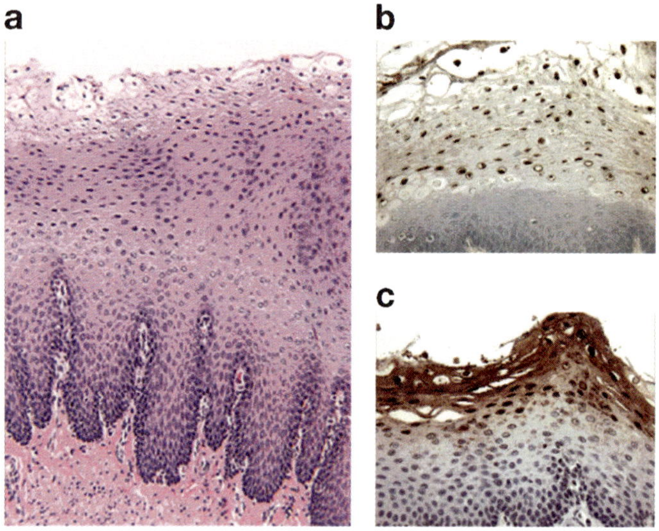

Figure 8

(*a*) Hyperkeratotic, destructive lesion of oral hairy leukoplakia showing viral cytopathic changes in the superficial epithelial cells (hematoxylin and eosin stain; original magnification 100x). (*b*) In situ hybridization for Epstein-Barr virus (EBV) DNA in oral hairy leukoplakia reveals active viral replication in the upper differentiated layers of the squamous mucosa in these patients, without involvement of the lower basal cell layers (diaminobenzidine chromogen with hematoxylin counterstain; original magnification 200x). (*c*) Immunohistochemical stain for the EBV viral capsid protein (VCA) in oral hairy leukoplakia shows cytoplasmic and nuclear staining also present in the upper layers of the squamous mucosa (diaminobenzidine chromogen with hematoxylin counterstain; original magnification 200x).

Somatic hypermutation: a process of affinity maturation within germinal center B cells in which the rearranged immunoglobulin gene is mutated, altering the antigen-binding properties of the molecule

Ig: immunoglobulin

Burkitt Lymphoma

There are three clinical variants of BL that differ in respect to their presentation, biology, and association with EBV. These are the endemic-, sporadic-, and immunodeficiency-associated variants. The endemic form of BL is the type described originally by Burkitt that occurs frequently (in 50–100 cases per 1,000,000 individuals) in the equatorial regions of Africa and Papua, New Guinea. There is almost 100% correspondence of endemic BL with the presence of EBV in the tumor cells. In contrast, the sporadic form of BL is seen mainly in young adults and children with no specific geographic distribution. Its incidence is much lower than the endemic disease, with 2–3 cases per 1,000,000 individuals (67). In the United States and Europe, where sporadic BL cases are uncommon, the association with EBV is low (15–30% of cases) (67–69).

The most common histological appearance of BL is as a diffuse, monomorphic infiltrate of intermediate-sized atypical lymphoid cells with round to slightly irregular nuclei, clumped chromatin, 1–3 distinct centrally placed nucleoli, and moderate amounts of deeply basophilic, often vacuolated cytoplasm (**Figure 9*a***). These cells are highly proliferative, showing frequent mitotic figures and apoptotic cell bodies. Coinciding with the high rate of apoptotic cell death is the presence of numerous intermixed phagocytic histiocytes (tingible-body macrophages) that impart the so-called starry sky low-power appearance of involved tissues (**Figure 9*b***).

The WHO classification scheme defines BL by the invariant presence of a *c-MYC* translocation resulting in the deregulation of c-MYC protein expression. This translocation involves the exchange of genetic material between the *c-MYC* oncogene at chromosome band 8q24 and either the immunoglobulin heavy chain gene (*IGH*) on chromosome 14 at band q32 [t(8;14)] (80% of cases), the kappa light chain loci at 2p11 [t(2;8)] (15% of cases), or the lambda light chain loci at 22q11 [t(8;22)] (5% of cases). The majority of work in studying the breakpoints has focused on the t(8;14) breakpoints. In endemic BL, the breakpoints on chromosome 8 occur in noncoding regions 5′ to *c-MYC* exon 1, and the breakpoints on chromosome 14 occur usually in the *IGH* joining regions at sites that are possible targets for somatic hypermutation, which occurs during germinal center B cell development. In sporadic and AIDS-associated BL, the t(8:14) breakpoints fall predominantly between *c-MYC* exons 1 and 2 on chromosome 8 and within the *IGH* switch region on chromosome 14 (68), which are involved in immunoglobulin (Ig) isotype class switching during germinal center B cell development. The presence of translocations within regions that undergo chromosome breakage during the maturation of germinal center B cells strengthens the argument that these translocations are mistakes that occur during normal B cell development. These translocations deregulate c-MYC expression, driving cells through the cell cycle and activating antiapoptotic pathways.

Despite the strong association between EBV infection and BL, EBV infection appears to be neither sufficient nor necessary for the development of BL. What, then, is the role for EBV in this process that must clearly involve *c-MYC* translocations during the germinal center B cell reaction? One model is that EBV is a potentiator of tumor formation and has little role in maintaining the tumor-cell phenotype. This model has EBV acting early in the lymphomagenic process by increasing the frequency of genomic instability within the infected B cell population (**Figure 10**). This could increase the probability that a *c-MYC* translocation is acquired, thus resulting in Burkitt lymphoma.

Alternatively, EBV infection could contribute to BL development by increasing the lymphomagenic potential of a *c-MYC* translocation-positive cell (**Figure 10**). This mechanism may explain why EBV infection remains present in every BL cell, i.e., EBV continues to provide a biological advantage for the tumor cell. Despite the downregulation of the common growth-promoting gene products that results from the latency I program of viral gene expression seen in most BL tumors, it is possible that some of these latency I program genes may provide a growth advantage. Even though EBNA1 and EBERs are not essential for B cell immortalization in tissue, there is data that EBNA1 or EBERs can have an effect on cell growth in some experimental systems.

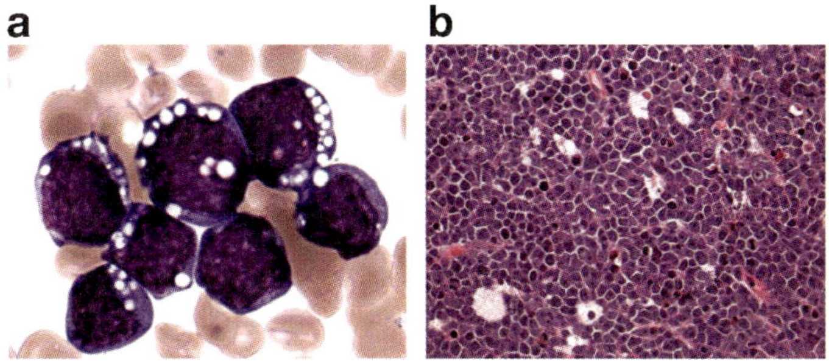

Figure 9

(*a*) Cytological appearance of Burkitt lymphoma (BL) showing intermediate-sized atypical lymphoid cells with round to slightly irregular nuclei, clumped chromatin, 1–3 distinct, centrally placed nucleoli, and moderate amounts of deeply basophilic and vacuolated cytoplasm (wright-giemsa stain; original magnification 400x). (*b*) Tissue section appearance of BL showing a mosaic tile–like appearance of the lymphoma cells and a high proliferative rate with frequent mitotic figures, apoptotic cell bodies, and numerous intermixed phagocytic histiocytes (tingible-body macrophages) that impart the so-called starry sky low-power appearance (hematoxylin and eosin stain; original magnification 200x).

Hodgkin Lymphoma

Classical HL (cHL) is an unusual neoplasm characterized by the presence of clonal, malignant multinucleated RS cells in a background of reactive inflammatory cells that includes granulocytes, lymphocytes, plasma cells, and histiocytes (**Figure 11*a***). The lymph nodes, spleen, bone marrow, and liver are most frequently involved in cHL. The bulk of the proliferation within these tissues is attributable to the reactive inflammatory cells that accompany the RS cells; the RS cells themselves comprise typically less than 1% of the cellularity. When present, EBV infection is clonal and present in the RS cells. A more restricted pattern of type II latent infection gene products is expressed, i.e., EBERs, EBNA1, LMP1, and LMP2A (**Figure 11*b***).

cHL is subdivided by histological criteria into mixed-cellularity, nodular-sclerosis, lymphocyte-rich, and lymphocyte-depleted subtypes. These so-called classical forms of the disease are distinct from lymphocyte-predominant HL, which is a unique clinicopathological entity not associated with EBV. cHL is a complex, multifactorial disease. EBV infection is associated with approximately 40% of cHL cases, most frequently with the mixed-cellularity subtype. This subtype is more common in males and demonstrates a bimodal age distribution (<10 and >50 years of age). EBV-negative cHL is most common in adolescents and young

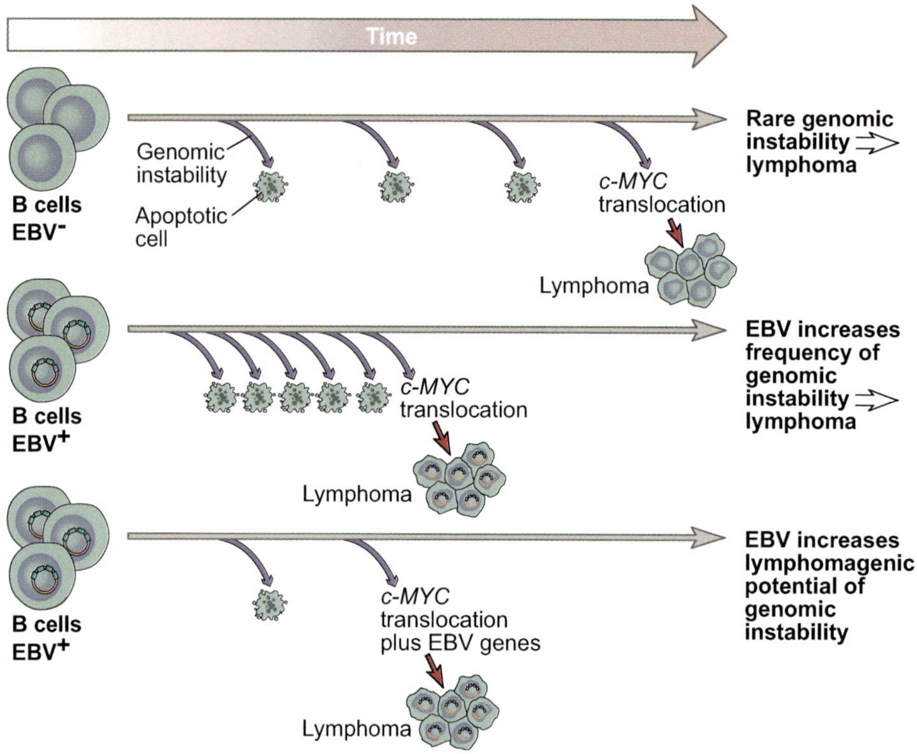

Figure 10

Hypothetical models for the role of Epstein-Barr virus (EBV) in Burkitt lymphoma (BL) tumorigenesis. BL is intrinsically linked to the presence of a *c-MYC* translocation, which is the result of rare genomic instability within a germinal center B cell (*top*). EBV could contribute to BL tumorigenesis by either increasing the frequency with which this rare translocation event occurs in the EBV-infected B cell population (*middle*) or by potentiating lymphomagenesis in an EBV-infected cell once it acquires a *c-MYC* translocation (*bottom*).

Apoptosis: programmed cell death that can occur when a cell is damaged beyond repair or infected with a virus

adults, does not show a gender predisposition, and is associated with a high standard of living in childhood.

Most investigators agree that RS cells are derived from germinal center B cells that have acquired crippling mutations in their Ig genes (70–72). Mutation of the Ig sequences (somatic hypermutation) is a normal process that B cells undergo in the germinal center in an effort to create Ig with increased affinity for antigen. A high-affinity Ig receptor is required to rescue a B cell from apoptosis in the germinal center. B cells with mutations that produce low-affinity or nonfunctional Ig are eliminated by apoptosis. So if RS cells acquire Ig mutations during affinity maturation that results in a nonfunctional Ig molecule, how do they escape apoptosis? In many cases, there is a high level of NFκB expressed in the RS cells, suggesting that these B cells with crippled Ig mutations can be rescued by activation of this transcription factor and subsequent induction of antiapoptotic cell genes (**Figure 12**). The discovery of RS cells with mutations in IκB (73, 74) is one nonviral mechanism whereby abnormal, constitutive NFκB activation may contribute to the development of HL. The EBV LMP1 is a potent activator of NFκB, and the activation of NFκB is an important step for EBV-induced B cell immortalization (**Figure 11*c***). In addition, the EBV LMP2A can mimic signaling effectively through the Ig

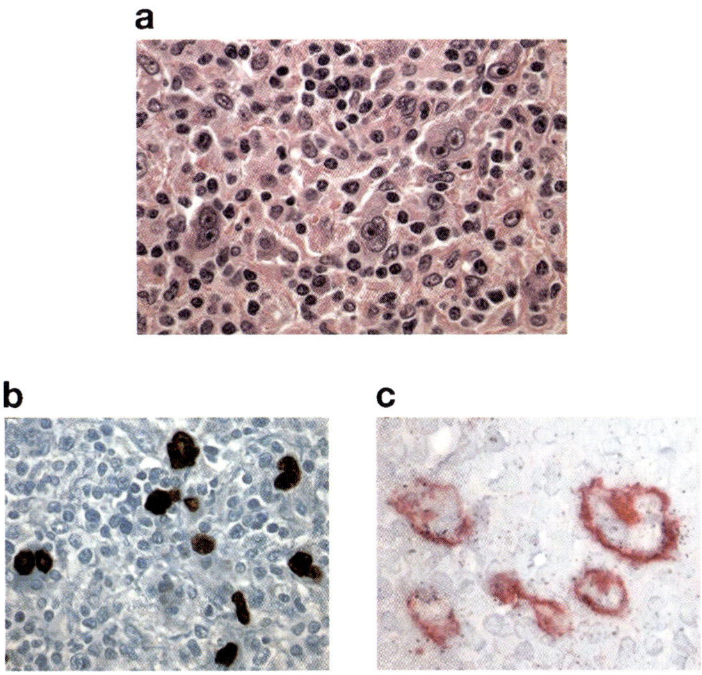

Figure 11

(*a*) Lymph node biopsy of classical Hodgkin lymphoma (cHL), mixed-cellularity type, showing malignant multinucleated Reed-Sternberg (RS) cells in a background of reactive inflammatory cells that includes granulocytes, lymphocytes, plasma cells, and histiocytes (hematoxylin and eosin stain; original magnification 400X). (*b*) In situ hybridization for Epstein-Barr virus–encoded small RNAs (EBERs) in cHL, mixed-cellularity type, showing prominent nuclear staining (diaminobenzidine chromogen with hematoxylin counterstain; original magnification 400x). (*c*) Immunohistochemical stains for latent membrane protein 1 in the RS cells of cHL, mixed-cellularity type (new fuchsin chromogen with methyl green counterstain; original magnification 400x).

receptor (75, 76). Thus, EBV infection may provide alternative mechanisms for rescuing abnormal B cells from apoptosis and illustrates how EBV gene products can substitute for specific molecular changes that are critical for tumorigenesis.

Nasopharyngeal Carcinoma

Nasopharyngeal carcinomas (NPC) are classified broadly into two major subtypes: (*a*) nonkeratinizing and (*b*) keratinizing nasopharyngeal carcinoma. The nonkeratinizing type is by far the most frequent, and nearly 100% of these tumors show evidence of EBV infection (**Figure 13**) (77, 78). The nonkeratinizing type can be poorly differentiated or undifferentiated, and the tumor cells are cytologically uniform with round to oval vesicular nuclei and distinct, medium-sized nucleoli. This subtype is often associated with a florid, reactive T lymphoid response that can even obscure the epithelial neoplasm. In these cases the term lymphoepithelioma has been applied. Clonal EBV infection is present in every tumor cell, and the lymphoid component present in the so-called lymphoepithelioma does not show evidence of EBV infection. These tumors are relatively rare worldwide, but there is a high incidence in Southeast Asian, Artic native, and North African populations where the vast majority of lesions are EBV related (79, 80). Potential explanations for the increased risk in

NPC: nasopharyngeal carcinoma

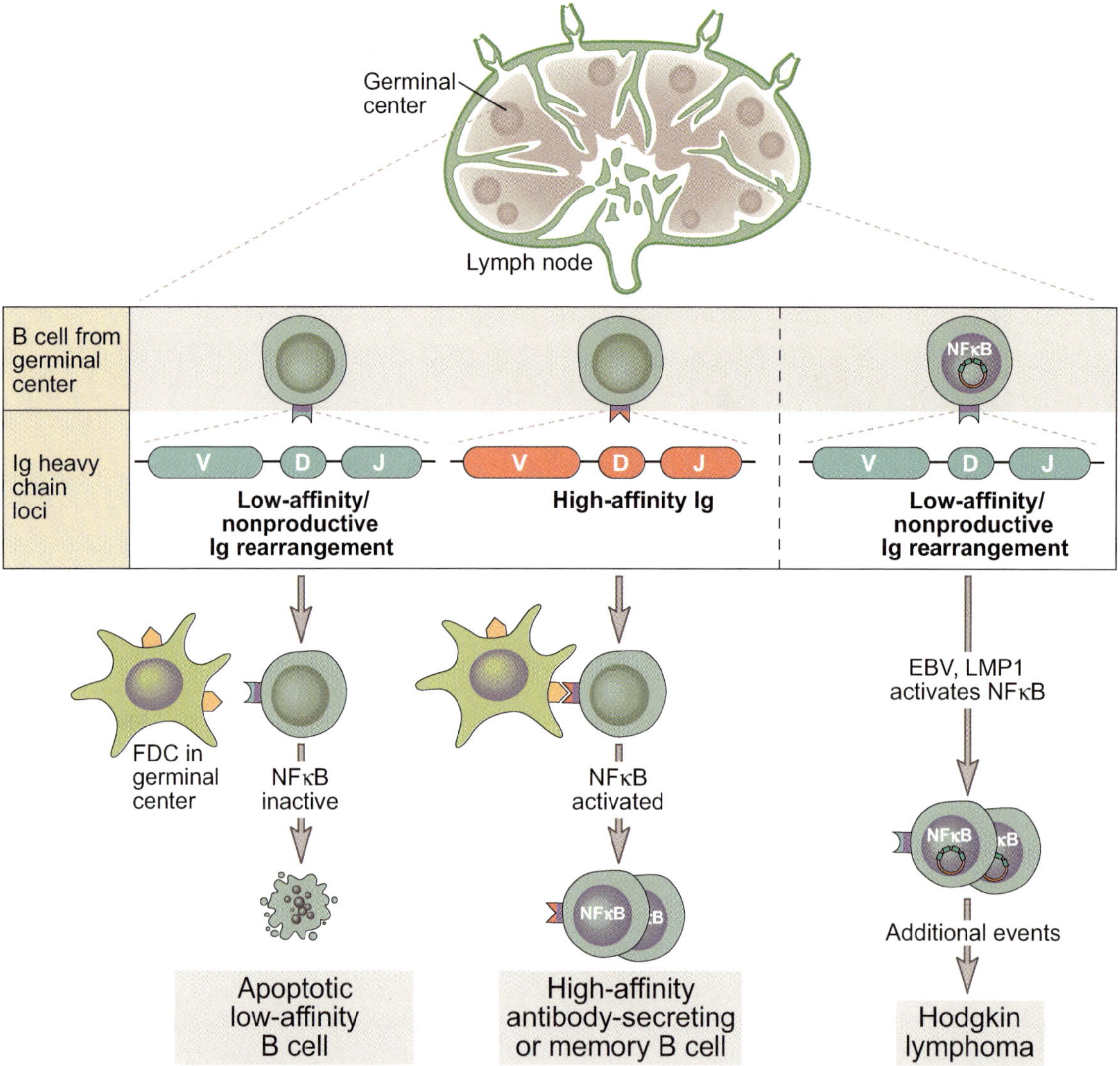

Figure 12

Hypothetical model for the role of Epstein-Barr virus (EBV) in Hodgkin lymphoma tumorigenesis. Normally, when B cells encounter antigen in the germinal center of a lymph node, they undergo the process of somatic hypermutation. This is a trial-and-error process where mutations that result in a low-affinity/nonproductive immunoglobulin (Ig) rearrangement lead to B cell apoptosis and are lost (*left*), whereas mutations that result in an Ig receptor with increased affinity for antigen and more efficient NFκB activation lead to increased B cell survival and selection for high-affinity antibodies (*middle*). Reed-Sternberg cells are derived from germinal center B cells that have acquired nonproductive Ig rearrangements, but EBV infection and latent membrane protein 1 (LMP1)-induced activation of NFκB expression rescue these cells, allowing them to accumulate additional genetic events required for the development of Hodgkin lymphoma. V, variable; D, diversity; J, joining; FDC, follicular dendritic cell.

these regions include cultural, dietary, and genetic predispositions for developing EBV-associated NPC. The keratinizing subtype is defined by the presence of keratin and a squamoid appearance. It is controversial whether EBV is present within keratinizing NPCs. Initial studies found no association of EBV with this form of NPC (77, 78); however, recent investigations have identified EBV in some cases of keratinizing NPC (81).

The potential role of the virus in NPC development depends upon an understanding of how and when EBV infects epithelial cells; however definitive information on these events has yet to be obtained. The oral cavity is clearly the primary portal of infection for EBV, and the shedding of the virus via oral secretions transmits EBV. Whether epithelial cells are persistently infected with EBV is controversial because researchers have not unequivocally identified EBV infection in oral epithelial cells from healthy hosts. NPC may arise from persistently EBV-infected epithelial cells that undergo a second genetic event, similar to the model for BL. Alternatively, EBV infection of epithelial cells in at-risk individuals may occur much later in life, with some studies suggesting that early exposure of the nasopharynx to environmental carcinogens may render the epithelium susceptible to EBV infection (82). Thus, NPC may not evolve from epithelial cells that already harbor EBV, but may instead represent a rare infection of an epithelial cell made more susceptible to EBV infection by exposure to carcinogens or other preneoplastic genetic changes (76). Although the exact stage that EBV infection occurs in the development of NPC is unknown, it is clear that all of the tumor cells in any EBV-associated NPC or high-grade dysplastic lesion carry monoclonal viral genomes (17, 83, 84). This indicates that infection must occur at least at a point before the expansion of the malignant epithelial clone.

So what role does EBV play in the malignant transformation in NPC? Latency gene expression in NPC appears intermediate between that seen in BL (latency I program) and HL (latency II program). The latent viral gene EBNA1 and the EBER genes are expressed in all EBV-positive cases. There is evidence that LMP2A may have growth-promoting effects in epithelial cells, and LMP2A and LMP2B transcripts are amplifiable in most tumors (85). However, LMP2A protein can be detected in only approximately 50% of the cases (86). LMP1 mRNA is more difficult to detect, and protein is identified readily in only 35% of cases (83, 87–89). The presence of LMP1 in all pre-invasive lesions, however, suggests that LMP1 expression is necessary in early lesions but may not be as essential in established carcinomas (84). EBV-induced proliferation of epithelial cells may increase the risk of other genetic events that may contribute to tumorigenesis.

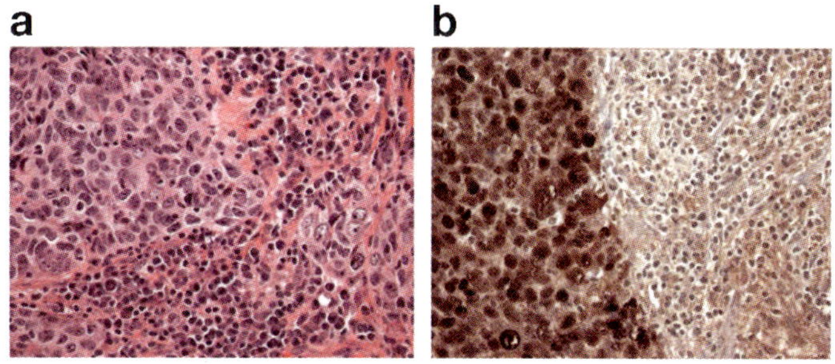

Figure 13

(*a*) Nasopharyngeal carcinoma, nonkeratinizing type with cytologically uniform round to oval vesicular nuclei, distinct medium-sized nucleoli, and admixed prominent lymphoplasmacytic infiltrate (hematoxylin and eosin stain; original magnification 200x). (*b*) Epstein-Barr virus–encoded small RNAs (EBER) in situ hybridization in an undifferentiated nasopharyngeal carcinoma showing strong nuclear reactivity within the tumor cells, but not the adjacent lymphocytes (diaminobenzidine chromogen with hematoxylin counterstain; original magnification 400x).

Occasional expression of the lytic cycle–associated protein BZLF1 has been detected in NPC samples (90); however, the absence of consistent expression of other lytic cycle–associated proteins and linear (lytic) forms of DNA within tumor cells is inidicative of a tumor not fully permissive to virus replication (17, 89). This is particularly interesting because despite the apparent absence of viral replication in the tumor, there is frequently a rise in IgA antibody titers to lytic viral proteins [e.g., viral capsid protein (VCA)

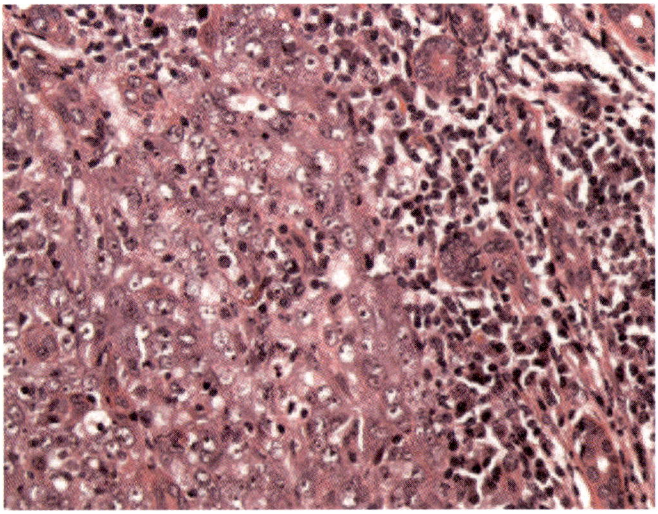

Figure 14

Lymphoepithelioma-like carcinoma of the salivary gland. Note the prominent associated lymphoplasmacytic infiltrate (hematoxylin and eosin stain; original magnification 200x).

and early antigen] and membrane antigen in patients with NPC, which can be used successfully as a clinical screening test in areas where NPC is endemic (91). In addition, cell-free DNA levels in the serum can provide diagnostic, prognostic, and therapeutic information about NPC patients (92). It is unclear whether the cell-free DNA represents naked DNA or encapsidated virions, but the resistance to DNase digestion and relatively small NPC tumor burden relative to serum DNA levels suggests that the virus may arise from active replication rather than dying tumor cells. Why these surrogate markers for viral replication are so tightly linked to NPC is unclear and suggests some unrecognized role for lytic EBV replication in the pathogenesis of NPC.

EBV-Associated Diseases in Uncommon Cellular Targets of EBV

Several additional EBV-associated neoplasms that arise in atypical cellular targets exist. These include the lymphoepithelioma-like carcinomas, a subset of gastric carcinomas, T cell lymphoproliferative disorders, follicular dendritic cell tumors, and possibly a small number of breast and hepatic carcinomas. A common theme may be that EBV infection represents a rare event in these cell types, but once infection occurs, viral gene expression drives tumorigenesis through many of the same pathways seen in B cell lymphomas.

Lymphoepithelioma-Like Carcinomas and Gastric Carcinoma

Carcinomas that share the histological features of undifferentiated NPCs (lymphoepitheliomas) have been identified in other sites, including the thymus, larynx, tonsils, salivary glands, lungs, skin, uterine cervix, bladder, and stomach. These rare tumors are often referred to as undifferentiated carcinomas of the nasopharyngeal type, or lymphoepithelioma-like carcinomas (**Figure 14**). The incidence of EBV infection in these lymphoepithelioma-like tumors from foregut-derived sites is endemic in certain populations, e.g., Southeast Asians, Greenland Eskimos, and South Americans (93–103). This is particularly true for lymphoepithelioma-like gastric carcinomas, which are always EBV-positive, irrespective of geographical origins (100, 101). The histology is reminiscent of NPC, suggesting the possibility of a similar pathogenic mechanism.

It was recognized recently that a fraction of conventional gastric carcinomas (diffuse or intestinal) without lymphoepithelioma-like morphology is also associated with EBV infection (104). When large series ($n = 970$) of gastric carcinoma cases were studied by EBER1 in situ hybridization, EBV was detected in 59 out of 961 (6.1%) poorly and moderately differentiated tumors (105). It is unknown whether the gastric epithelium is a normal target for EBV infection, and the role of EBV infection in these malignancies remains unclear.

T Cell Lymphoproliferative Diseases

Both thymocytes and mature T cells express low levels of the EBV receptor CD21/CR2 (106, 107); however, even during the acute phase of IM, EBV infection of T cells appears to be a rare event. The most constant association of EBV with T cell disorders is seen in the so-called virus-associated hemophagocytic syndrome (VAHS) T cell lymphomas and the nasal NK/T cell lymphomas, where nearly 100% of the tumors are EBV positive. VAHS T cell lymphomas are rare, monoclonal, mature T cell proliferations that occur in patients with chronic, active EBV infection or occasionally after acute primary EBV infection (10, 108–110). As the name implies, it is associated with marked hemophagocytosis that is often fulminant in nature (110). The lymphoma cells are infected with monoclonal EBV and show the latency I/II pattern of EBV gene expression, which includes EBNA1, LMP2a, and low levels of LMP1 (108). The life-threatening hemophagocytosis that accompanies the neoplastic T cell proliferations appears to be mediated by tumor necrosis factor expression from the T cells, which, in combination with interferon-γ and probably other cytokines, can activate macrophages (111).

A nearly identical pattern of latent EBV gene expression occurs in the nasal NK/T cell lymphomas (112). Like VAHS T cell lymphomas, these tumors also show clonal EBV genome in all cases (112, 113). Nasal NK/T cell lymphomas are aggressive, destructive tumors that involve the midline nasopharyngeal tissues and are most commonly seen in Southeast Asian populations (114). The lack of surface CD3 and T cell receptor in the majority of cases, together with the absence of rearranged T cell receptor genes and the presence of the NK marker CD56, indicates that these tumors are derived from NK cells (113). Little is known regarding the contribution of EBV to the pathogenesis of these diseases. EBV can, in rare instances, infect T cells in tissue culture; however, there are no in vitro models of EBV immortalization of T cells.

Inflammatory Pseudotumor-Like Follicular Dendritic Cell Tumors

Inflammatory pseudotumor-like follicular dendritic cell (FDC) tumors were recognized recently as distinctive variants of FDC tumor (115). These tumors show a marked predominance in females, selective localization in intra-abdominal sites, especially the liver and spleen, frequent presence of systemic symptoms, and indolent behavior despite an intra-abdominal location (115–118). Histologically, inflammatory pseudotumor-like FDC tumors display dispersed spindle or ovoid cells with twisted or folded, occasionally vesicular, nuclei and distinct nucleoli, present within a lymphoplasmacytic inflammatory background. The spindle cells show evidence of follicular dendritic cell derivation, expressing markers such as CD21 (CR2), CD35, CD23, R4/23, Ki-M4, and CNA.42 (115–118). These tumors are consistently associated with EBV, which likely infects the FDC via CD21 (115–118). The spindle cells show identical episomal clonal EBV upon Southern blot analysis (118) and express LMP1, EBNA1, and EBERs (115–119), but are EBNA2 negative (118).

FDC: follicular dendritic cell

Breast and Hepatic Cancer

Recently, isolated studies have reported polymerase chain reaction detection of EBV in a significant percentage of breast and hepatocellular carcinomas (120–123). However, immunohistochemical and other studies indicate that both the number of cases showing EBV involvement and the number of tumor cells that are infected are more limited (120, 123). It remains to be seen whether there could be a potential role for EBV as a cofactor in a subset of primary breast and liver cancers.

SUMMARY

Strong evidence links EBV to the development of a spectrum of human diseases, including BL, HL, post-transplant and AIDS-related lymphomas, nasopharyngeal carcinoma, and a small subset of T cell lymphomas, gastric carcinomas, leiomyosarcomas, follicular dendritic tumors, and other epithelial carcinomas. One category of EBV-related tumors involves abnormalities in the immune system's ability to control the proliferation of virally infected cells. This category includes post-transplant and AIDS-related lymphomas in immunocompromised patients. A second category of EBV-associated tumors is seen in the immunocompetent host, where EBV is one factor in a more complex multistep process. This category includes tumors such as BL, HL, and NPC. In these cases, EBV genes that affect cell proliferation and survival may contribute directly to tumorigenesis or increase the potential for genetic transformation events. In the remaining cases, such as gastric carcinomas, follicular dendritic cell carcinomas, or T cell lymphomas, it is largely unknown how EBV gains entry into these cells and how it contributes to oncogenesis. One of the most remarkable aspects of EBV infection is the broad spectrum of involved cell types and associated diseases. Our current knowledge of the EBV life cycle, EBV gene function, and the underlying molecular mechanisms of specific malignancies makes it easy to speculate how EBV can contribute to diseases such as PTLD, BL, and HL. A better understanding of the EBV life cycle, EBV gene function, and molecular mechanisms of disease is required to appreciate fully the role of EBV infection in the complete spectrum of EBV-associated diseases.

LITERATURE CITED

1. Burkitt D, O'Conor GT. 1961. Malignant lymphoma in African children. I. A clinical syndrome. *Cancer* 14:258–69
2. Burkitt D. 1962. A children's cancer dependent on climatic factors. *Nature* 194:232–34
3. Burkitt D, Wright D. 1966. Geographical and tribal distribution of the African lymphoma in Uganda. *Br. Med. J.* 5487:569–73
4. Burkitt D. 1962. Determining the climatic limitations of a children's cancer common in Africa. *Br. Med. J.* 5311:1019–23
5. Epstein MA, Achong BG, Barr YM. 1964. Virus particles in cultured lymphoblasts from Burkitt's lymphoma. *Lancet* 15:702–3
6. Epstein MA, Barr YM. 1964. Cultivation in vitro of human lymphoblasts from Burkitt's malignant lymphoma. *Lancet* 41:252–53
7. Henle G, Henle W, Diehl V. 1968. Relation of Burkitt's tumor-associated herpes-ytpe virus to infectious mononucleosis. *Proc. Natl. Acad. Sci. USA* 59:94–101
8. zur Hausen H, Schulte-Holthausen H, Klein G, Henle W, Henle G, et al. 1970. EBV DNA in biopsies of Burkitt tumours and anaplastic carcinomas of the nasopharynx. *Nature* 228:1056–58
9. Ziegler JL, Drew WL, Miner RC, Mintz L, Rosenbaum E, et al. 1982. Outbreak of Burkitt's-like lymphoma in homosexual men. *Lancet* 2:631–33
10. Jones JF, Shurin S, Abramowsky C, Tubbs RR, Sciotto CG, et al. 1988. T-cell lymphomas containing Epstein-Barr viral DNA in patients with chronic Epstein-Barr virus infections. *N. Engl. J. Med.* 318:733–41
11. Weiss LM, Movahed LA, Warnke RA, Sklar J. 1989. Detection of Epstein-Barr viral genomes in Reed-Sternberg cells of Hodgkin's disease. *N. Engl. J. Med.* 320:502–6
12. Weiss LM, Strickler JG, Warnke RA, Purtilo DT, Sklar J. 1987. Epstein-Barr viral DNA in tissues of Hodgkin's disease. *Am. J. Pathol.* 129:86–91
13. Rickinson A, Kieff E. 2001. Epstein Barr virus and its replication. In *Fields Virology*, ed. B Fields, D Knipe, P Howley, pp. 2575–628. Philadelphia: Lippincot-Raven
14. Lindahl T, Adams A, Bjursell G, Bornkamm GW, Kaschka-Dierich C, Jehn U. 1976.

Covalently closed circular duplex DNA of Epstein-Barr virus in a human lymphoid cell line. *J. Mol. Biol.* 102:511–30

15. Kaschka-Dierich C, Adams A, Lindahl T, Bornkamm GW, Bjursell G, et al. 1976. Intracellular forms of Epstein-Barr virus DNA in human tumour cells in vivo. *Nature* 260:302–6
16. Given D, Yee D, Griem K, Kieff E. 1979. DNA of Epstein-Barr virus. V. Direct repeats of the ends of Epstein-Barr virus DNA. *J. Virol.* 30:852–62
17. Raab-Traub N, Flynn K. 1986. The structure of the termini of the Epstein-Barr virus as a marker of clonal cellular proliferation. *Cell* 47:883–89
18. Fingeroth JD, Weis JJ, Tedder TF, Strominger JL, Biro PA, Fearon DT. 1984. Epstein-Barr virus receptor of human B lymphocytes is the C3d receptor CR2. *Proc. Natl. Acad. Sci. USA* 81:4510–14
19. Janz A, Oezel M, Kurzeder C, Pich D, Kost M, et al. 2000. Infectious Epstein-Barr virus lacking major glycoprotein BLLF1 (gp350/220) demonstrates the existence of additional viral ligands. *J. Virol.* 74:10142–52
20. Tugizov SM, Berline JW, Palefsky JM. 2003. Epstein-Barr virus infection of polarized tongue and nasopharyngeal epithelial cells. *Nat. Med.* 9:307–14
21. Carel JC, Myones BL, Frazier B, Holers VM. 1990. Structural requirements for C3d,g/Epstein-Barr virus receptor (CR2/CD21) ligand binding, internalization, and viral infection. *J. Biol. Chem.* 265:12293–99
22. Nemerow GR, Cooper NR. 1984. Early events in the infection of human B lymphocytes by Epstein-Barr virus: the internalization process. *Virology* 132:186–98
23. Sinclair AJ, Farrell PJ. 1995. Host cell requirements for efficient infection of quiescent primary B lymphocytes by Epstein-Barr virus. *J. Virol.* 69:5461–68
24. Jenson HB, Farrell PJ, Miller G. 1987. Sequences of the Epstein-Barr Virus (EBV) large internal repeat form the center of a 16-kilobase-pair palindrome of EBV (P3HR-1) heterogeneous DNA. *J. Virol.* 61:1495–506
25. Jenson HB, Miller G. 1988. Polymorphisms of the region of the Epstein-Barr virus genome which disrupts latency. *Virology* 165:549–64
26. Chavrier P, Gruffat H, Chevallier-Greco A, Buisson M, Sergeant A. 1989. The Epstein-Barr virus (EBV) early promoter DR contains a cis-acting element responsive to the EBV transactivator EB1 and an enhancer with constitutive and inducible activities. *J. Virol.* 63:607–14
27. Chevallier-Greco A, Gruffat H, Manet E, Calender A, Sergeant A. 1989. The Epstein-Barr virus (EBV) DR enhancer contains two functionally different domains: domain A is constitutive and cell specific, domain B is transactivated by the EBV early protein R. *J. Virol.* 63:615–23
28. Chevallier-Greco A, Manet E, Chavrier P, Mosnier C, Daillie J, Sergeant A. 1986. Both Epstein-Barr virus (EBV)-encoded trans-acting factors, EB1 and EB2, are required to activate transcription from an EBV early promoter. *EMBO J.* 5:3243–49
29. Kenney S, Holley-Guthrie E, Mar EC, Smith M. 1989. The Epstein-Barr virus BMLF1 promoter contains an enhancer element that is responsive to the BZLF1 and BRLF1 transactivators. *J. Virol.* 63:3878–83
30. Ragoczy T, Heston L, Miller G. 1998. The Epstein-Barr virus Rta protein activates lytic cycle genes and can disrupt latency in B lymphocytes. *J. Virol.* 72:7978–84
31. Holley-Guthrie EA, Quinlivan EB, Mar EC, Kenney S. 1990. The Epstein-Barr virus (EBV) BMRF1 promoter for early antigen (EA-D) is regulated by the EBV transactivators, BRLF1 and BZLF1, in a cell-specific manner. *J. Virol.* 64:3753–59

32. Quinlivan EB, Holley-Guthrie EA, Norris M, Gutsch D, Bachenheimer SL, Kenney SC. 1993. Direct BRLF1 binding is required for cooperative BZLF1/BRLF1 activation of the Epstein-Barr virus early promoter, BMRF1. *Nucleic Acids Res.* 21:1999–2007
33. Mosier DE, Gulizia RJ, Baird SM, Wilson DB. 1988. Transfer of a functional human immune system to mice with severe combined immunodeficiency. *Nature* 335:256–59
34. Rowe M, Young LS, Crocker J, Stokes H, Henderson S, Rickinson AB. 1991. Epstein-Barr virus (EBV)-associated lymphoproliferative disease in the SCID mouse model: implications for the pathogenesis of EBV-positive lymphomas in man. *J. Exp. Med.* 173:147–58
35. Gerber P, Lucas S, Nonoyama M, Perlin E, Goldstein LI. 1972. Oral excretion of Epstein-Barr virus by healthy subjects and patients with infectious mononucleosis. *Lancet* 2:988–89
36. Lemon SM, Hutt LM, Shaw JE, Li JL, Pagano JS. 1978. Replication of Epstein-Barr virus DNA in epithelial cells in vivo. *IARC Sci. Publ.* 1978:739–44
37. Sixbey JW, Vesterinen EH, Nedrud JG, Walton LA, Pagano JS. 1983. Replication of Epstein-Barr virus in human epithelial cells infected in vitro. *Nature* 306:480–83
38. Sixbey JW, Nedrud JG, Raab-Traub N, Hanes RA, Pagano JS. 1984. Epstein-Barr virus replication in oropharyngeal epithelial cells. *N. Engl. J. Med.* 310:1225–30
39. Anagnostopoulos I, Hummel M, Kreschel C, Stein H. 1995. Morphology, immunophenotype, and distribution of latently and/or productively Epstein-Barr virus-infected cells in acute infectious mononucleosis: implications for the interindividual infection route of Epstein-Barr virus. *Blood* 85:744–50
40. Niedobitek G, Agathanggelou A, Herbst H, Whitehead L, Wright DH, Young LS. 1997. Epstein-Barr virus (EBV) infection in infectious mononucleosis: virus latency, replication and phenotype of EBV-infected cells. *J. Pathol.* 182:151–59
41. Karajannis MA, Hummel M, Anagnostopoulos I, Stein H. 1997. Strict lymphotropism of Epstein-Barr virus during acute infectious mononucleosis in nonimmunocompromised individuals. *Blood* 89:2856–62
42. Klein G, Svedmyr E, Jondal M, Persson PO. 1976. EBV-determined nuclear antigen (EBNA)-positive cells in the peripheral blood of infectious mononucleosis patients. *Int. J. Cancer* 17:21–26
43. Tierney RJ, Steven N, Young LS, Rickinson AB. 1994. Epstein-Barr virus latency in blood mononuclear cells: analysis of viral gene transcription during primary infection and in the carrier state. *J. Virol.* 68:7374–85
44. Childs CC, Parham DM, Berard CW. 1987. Infectious mononucleosis. The spectrum of morphologic changes simulating lymphoma in lymph nodes and tonsils. *Am. J. Surg. Pathol.* 11:122–32
45. Tindle BH, Parker JW, Lukes RJ. 1972. "Reed-Sternberg cells" in infectious mononucleosis? *Am. J. Clin. Pathol.* 58:607–17
46. Lukes RJ, Tindle BH, Parker JW. 1969. Reed-Sternberg-like cells in infectious mononucleosis. *Lancet* 2:1003–4
47. Sayos J, Wu C, Morra M, Wang N, Zhang X, et al. 1998. The X-linked lymphoproliferative-disease gene product SAP regulates signals induced through the co-receptor SLAM. *Nature* 395:462–69
48. Coffey AJ, Brooksbank RA, Brandau O, Oohashi T, Howell GR, et al. 1998. Host response to EBV infection in X-linked lymphoproliferative disease results from mutations in an SH2-domain encoding gene. *Nat. Genet.* 20:129–35
49. Rickinson AB, Moss DJ. 1997. Human cytotoxic T lymphocyte responses to Epstein-Barr virus infection. *Annu. Rev. Immunol.* 15:405–31
50. Faulkner GC, Burrows SR, Khanna R, Moss DJ, Bird AG, Crawford DH. 1999. X-Linked

agammaglobulinemia patients are not infected with Epstein-Barr virus: implications for the biology of the virus. *J. Virol.* 73:1555–64
51. Yao QY, Rickinson AB, Epstein MA. 1985. A re-examination of the Epstein-Barr virus carrier state in healthy seropositive individuals. *Int. J. Cancer* 35:35–42
52. Thorley-Lawson DA. 2001. Epstein-Barr virus: exploiting the immune system. *Nat. Rev. Immunol.* 1:75–82
53. Kuppers R. 2003. B cells under influence: transformation of B cells by Epstein-Barr virus. *Nat. Rev. Immunol.* 3:801–12
54. Levitskaya J, Sharipo A, Leonchiks A, Ciechanover A, Masucci MG. 1997. Inhibition of ubiquitin/proteasome-dependent protein degradation by the Gly-Ala repeat domain of the Epstein-Barr virus nuclear antigen 1. *Proc. Natl. Acad. Sci. USA* 94:12616–21
55. Moghaddam A, Rosenzweig M, Lee-Parritz D, Annis B, Johnson RP, Wang F. 1997. An animal model for acute and persistent Epstein-Barr virus infection. *Science* 276:2030–33
56. Zutter MM, Martin PJ, Sale GE, Shulman HM, Fisher L, et al. 1988. Epstein-Barr virus lymphoproliferation after bone marrow transplantation. *Blood* 72:520–29
57. Knowles DM, Cesarman E, Chadburn A, Frizzera G, Chen J, et al. 1995. Correlative morphologic and molecular genetic analysis demonstrates three distinct categories of posttransplantation lymphoproliferative disorders. *Blood* 85:552–65
58. Polack A, Hortnagel K, Pajic A, Christoph B, Baier B, et al. 1996. c-MYC activation renders proliferation of Epstein-Barr virus (EBV)-transformed cells independent of EBV nuclear antigen 2 and latent membrane protein 1. *Proc. Natl. Acad. Sci. USA* 93:10411–16
59. Cesarman E, Chadburn A, Liu YF, Migliazza A, Dalla-Favera R, Knowles DM. 1998. BCL-6 gene mutations in posttransplantation lymphoproliferative disorders predict response to therapy and clinical outcome. *Blood* 92:2294–302
60. Raphael MM, Audouin J, Lamine M, Delecluse HJ, Vuillaume M, et al. 1994. Immunophenotypic and genotypic analysis of acquired immunodeficiency syndrome-related non-Hodgkin's lymphomas. Correlation with histologic features in 36 cases. French Study Group of Pathology for HIV-Associated Tumors. *Am. J. Clin. Pathol.* 101:773–82
61. Davi F, Delecluse HJ, Guiet P, Gabarre J, Fayon A, et al. 1998. Burkitt-like lymphomas in AIDS patients: characterization within a series of 103 human immunodeficiency virus-associated non-Hodgkin's lymphomas. Burkitt's Lymphoma Study Group. *J. Clin. Oncol.* 16:3788–95
62. Diebold J, Raphael M, Prevot S, Audouin J. 1997. Lymphomas associated with HIV infection. *Cancer Surv.* 30:263–93
63. van Hoeven KH, Factor SM, Kress Y, Woodruff JM. 1993. Visceral myogenic tumors. A manifestation of HIV infection in children. *Am. J. Surg. Pathol.* 17:1176–81
64. Lee ES, Locker J, Nalesnik M, Reyes J, Jaffe R, et al. 1995. The association of Epstein-Barr virus with smooth-muscle tumors occurring after organ transplantation. *N. Engl. J. Med.* 332:19–25
65. McClain KL, Leach CT, Jenson HB, Joshi VV, Pollock BH, et al. 1995. Association of Epstein-Barr virus with leiomyosarcomas in children with AIDS. *N. Engl. J. Med.* 332:12–18
66. Rogatsch H, Bonatti H, Menet A, Larcher C, Feichtinger H, Dirnhofer S. 2000. Epstein-Barr virus-associated multicentric leiomyosarcoma in an adult patient after heart transplantation: case report and review of the literature. *Am. J. Surg. Pathol.* 24:614–21
67. Rickinson A, Kieff E. 2001. Epstein Barr Virus. In *Fields Virology*, ed. B Fields, D Knipe, P Howley, pp. 2511–73. Philadelphia: Lippincot-Raven

68. Hecht JL, Aster JC. 2000. Molecular biology of Burkitt's lymphoma. *J. Clin. Oncol.* 18:3707–21
69. Gutierrez MI, Bhatia K, Barriga F, Diez B, Muriel FS, et al. 1992. Molecular epidemiology of Burkitt's lymphoma from South America: differences in breakpoint location and Epstein-Barr virus association from tumors in other world regions. *Blood* 79:3261–66
70. Kuppers R, Hansmann ML, Rajewsky K. 1998. Clonality and germinal centre B-cell derivation of Hodgkin/Reed-Sternberg cells in Hodgkin's disease. *Ann. Oncol.* 9(Suppl. 5):S17–20
71. Kuppers R, Schwering I, Brauninger A, Rajewsky K, Hansmann ML. 2002. Biology of Hodgkin's lymphoma. *Ann. Oncol.* 13(Suppl. 1):11–18
72. Kuppers R, Rajewsky K. 1998. The origin of Hodgkin and Reed/Sternberg cells in Hodgkin's disease. *Annu. Rev. Immunol.* 16:471–93
73. Jungnickel B, Staratschek-Jox A, Brauninger A, Spieker T, Wolf J, et al. 2000. Clonal deleterious mutations in the IkappaBalpha gene in the malignant cells in Hodgkin's lymphoma. *J. Exp. Med.* 191:395–402
74. Cabannes E, Khan G, Aillet F, Jarrett RF, Hay RT. 1999. Mutations in the IkBa gene in Hodgkin's disease suggest a tumour suppressor role for IkappaBalpha. *Oncogene* 18:3063–70
75. Casola S, Otipoby KL, Alimzhanov M, Humme S, Uyttersprot N, et al. 2004. B cell receptor signal strength determines B cell fate. *Nat. Immun.* 5:317–27
76. Caldwell RG, Wilson JB, Anderson SJ, Longnecker R. 1998. Epstein-Barr virus LMP2A drives B cell development and survival in the absence of normal B cell receptor signals. *Immunity* 9:405–11
77. Klein G, Giovanella BC, Lindahl T, Fialkow PJ, Singh S, Stehlin JS. 1974. Direct evidence for the presence of Epstein-Barr virus DNA and nuclear antigen in malignant epithelial cells from patients with poorly differentiated carcinoma of the nasopharynx. *Proc. Natl. Acad. Sci. USA* 71:4737–41
78. Niedobitek G, Hansmann ML, Herbst H, Young LS, Dienemann D, et al. 1991. Epstein-Barr virus and carcinomas: undifferentiated carcinomas but not squamous cell carcinomas of the nasopharynx are regularly associated with the virus. *J. Pathol.* 165:17–24
79. Niedobitek G, Agathanggelou A, Nicholls JM. 1996. Epstein-Barr virus infection and the pathogenesis of nasopharyngeal carcinoma: viral gene expression, tumour cell phenotype, and the role of the lymphoid stroma. *Semin. Cancer Biol.* 7:165–74
80. Nicholls JM, Agathanggelou A, Fung K, Zeng X, Niedobitek G. 1997. The association of squamous cell carcinomas of the nasopharynx with Epstein-Barr virus shows geographical variation reminiscent of Burkitt's lymphoma. *J. Pathol.* 183:164–68
81. Pathmanathan R, Prasad U, Chandrika G, Sadler R, Flynn K, Raab-Traub N. 1995. Undifferentiated, nonkeratinizing, and squamous cell carcinoma of the nasopharynx. Variants of Epstein-Barr virus-infected neoplasia. *Am. J. Pathol.* 146:1355–67
82. Knox PG, Li QX, Rickinson AB, Young LS. 1996. In vitro production of stable Epstein-Barr virus-positive epithelial cell clones which resemble the virus:cell interaction observed in nasopharyngeal carcinoma. *Virology* 215:40–50
83. Niedobitek G, Young LS, Sam CK, Brooks L, Prasad U, Rickinson AB. 1992. Expression of Epstein-Barr virus genes and of lymphocyte activation molecules in undifferentiated nasopharyngeal carcinomas. *Am. J. Pathol.* 140:879–87
84. Pathmanathan R, Prasad U, Sadler R, Flynn K, Raab-Traub N. 1995. Clonal proliferations of cells infected with Epstein-Barr virus in preinvasive lesions related to nasopharyngeal carcinoma. *N. Engl. J. Med.* 333:693–98

85. Morrison JA, Raab-Traub N. 2005. Roles of the ITAM and PY motifs of Epstein-Barr virus latent membrane protein 2A in the inhibition of epithelial cell differentiation and activation of {beta}-catenin signaling. *J. Virol.* 79:2375–82
86. Heussinger N, Buttner M, Ott G, Brachtel E, Pilch BZ, et al. 2004. Expression of the Epstein-Barr virus (EBV)-encoded latent membrane protein 2A (LMP2A) in EBV-associated nasopharyngeal carcinoma. *J. Pathol.* 203:696–99
87. Brooks L, Yao QY, Rickinson AB, Young LS. 1992. Epstein-Barr virus latent gene transcription in nasopharyngeal carcinoma cells: coexpression of EBNA1, LMP1, and LMP2 transcripts. *J. Virol.* 66:2689–97
88. Young LS, Dawson CW, Clark D, Rupani H, Busson P, et al. 1988. Epstein-Barr virus gene expression in nasopharyngeal carcinoma. *J. Gen. Virol.* 69(Pt. 5):1051–65
89. Gulley ML, Amin MB, Nicholls JM, Banks PM, Ayala AG, et al. 1995. Epstein-Barr virus is detected in undifferentiated nasopharyngeal carcinoma but not in lymphoepithelioma-like carcinoma of the urinary bladder. *Hum. Pathol.* 26:1207–14
90. Cochet C, Martel-Renoir D, Grunewald V, Bosq J, Cochet G, et al. 1993. Expression of the Epstein-Barr virus immediate early gene, BZLF1, in nasopharyngeal carcinoma tumor cells. *Virology* 197:358–65
91. Low WK, Leong JL, Goh YH, Fong KW. 2000. Diagnostic value of Epstein-Barr viral serology in nasopharyngeal carcinoma. *Otolaryngol. Head Neck Surg.* 123:505–7
92. Chan KC, Lo YM. 2002. Circulating EBV DNA as a tumor marker for nasopharyngeal carcinoma. *Semin. Cancer Biol.* 12:489–96
93. Saemundsen AK, Albeck H, Hansen JP, Nielsen NH, Anvret M, et al. 1982. Epstein-Barr virus in nasopharyngeal and salivary gland carcinomas of Greenland Eskimoes. *Br. J. Cancer* 46:721–28
94. Lanier AP, Clift SR, Bornkamm G, Henle W, Goepfert H, Raab-Traub N. 1991. Epstein-Barr virus and malignant lymphoepithelial lesions of the salivary gland. *Arct. Med. Res.* 50:55–61
95. Huang DP, Ng HK, Ho YH, Chan KM. 1988. Epstein-Barr virus (EBV)-associated undifferentiated carcinoma of the parotid gland. *Histopathology* 13:509–17
96. Wong MP, Chung LP, Yuen ST, Leung SY, Chan SY, et al. 1995. In situ detection of Epstein-Barr virus in non-small cell lung carcinomas. *J. Pathol.* 177:233–40
97. Higashiyama M, Doi O, Kodama K, Yokouchi H, Tateishi R, et al. 1995. Lymphoepithelioma-like carcinoma of the lung: analysis of two cases for Epstein-Barr virus infection. *Hum. Pathol.* 26:1278–82
98. Leyvraz S, Henle W, Chahinian AP, Perlmann C, Klein G, et al. 1985. Association of Epstein-Barr virus with thymic carcinoma. *N. Engl. J. Med.* 312:1296–99
99. Fujii T, Kawai T, Saito K, Fukushima K, Hasegawa T, et al. 1993. EBER-1 expression in thymic carcinoma. *Acta Pathol. Jpn.* 43:107–10
100. Burke AP, Yen TS, Shekitka KM, Sobin LH. 1990. Lymphoepithelial carcinoma of the stomach with Epstein-Barr virus demonstrated by polymerase chain reaction. *Mod. Pathol.* 3:377–80
101. Shibata D, Tokunaga M, Uemura Y, Sato E, Tanaka S, Weiss LM. 1991. Association of Epstein-Barr virus with undifferentiated gastric carcinomas with intense lymphoid infiltration. Lymphoepithelioma-like carcinoma. *Am. J. Pathol.* 139:469–74
102. Carrascal E, Koriyama C, Akiba S, Tamayo O, Itoh T, et al. 2003. Epstein-Barr virus-associated gastric carcinoma in Cali, Colombia. *Oncol. Rep.* 10:1059–62
103. Lopes LF, Bacchi MM, Elgui-de-Oliveira D, Zanati SG, Alvarenga M, Bacchi CE. 2004.

Epstein-Barr virus infection and gastric carcinoma in Sao Paulo State, Brazil. *Braz. J. Med. Biol. Res.* 37:1707–12
104. Imai S, Koizumi S, Sugiura M, Tokunaga M, Uemura Y, et al. 1994. Gastric carcinoma: monoclonal epithelial malignant cells expressing Epstein-Barr virus latent infection protein. *Proc. Natl. Acad. Sci. USA* 91:9131–35
105. Tokunaga M, Land CE, Uemura Y, Tokudome T, Tanaka S, Sato E. 1993. Epstein-Barr virus in gastric carcinoma. *Am. J. Pathol.* 143:1250–54
106. Fischer E, Delibrias C, Kazatchkine MD. 1991. Expression of CR2 (the C3dg/EBV receptor, CD21) on normal human peripheral blood T lymphocytes. *J. Immunol.* 146:865–69
107. Tsoukas CD, Lambris JD. 1988. Expression of CR2/EBV receptors on human thymocytes detected by monoclonal antibodies. *Eur. J. Immunol.* 18:1299–302
108. Kanegane H, Bhatia K, Gutierrez M, Kaneda H, Wada T, et al. 1998. A syndrome of peripheral blood T-cell infection with Epstein-Barr virus (EBV) followed by EBV-positive T-cell lymphoma. *Blood* 91:2085–91
109. Kanegane H, Miyawaki T, Yachie A, Oh-Ishi T, Bhatia K, Tosato G. 1999. Development of EBV-positive T-cell lymphoma following infection of peripheral blood T cells with EBV. *Leuk. Lymphoma* 34:603–7
110. Su IJ, Hsu YH, Lin MT, Cheng AL, Wang CH, Weiss LM. 1993. Epstein-Barr virus-containing T-cell lymphoma presents with hemophagocytic syndrome mimicking malignant histiocytosis. *Cancer* 72:2019–27
111. Lay JD, Tsao CJ, Chen JY, Kadin ME, Su IJ. 1997. Upregulation of tumor necrosis factor-alpha gene by Epstein-Barr virus and activation of macrophages in Epstein-Barr virus-infected T cells in the pathogenesis of hemophagocytic syndrome. *J. Clin. Invest.* 100:1969–79
112. Minarovits J, Hu LF, Imai S, Harabuchi Y, Kataura A, et al. 1994. Clonality, expression and methylation patterns of the Epstein-Barr virus genomes in lethal midline granulomas classified as peripheral angiocentric T cell lymphomas. *J. Gen. Virol.* 75(Pt. 1):77–84
113. Jaffe ES, Chan JK, Su IJ, Frizzera G, Mori S, et al. 1996. Report of the Workshop on Nasal and Related Extranodal Angiocentric T/Natural Killer Cell Lymphomas. Definitions, differential diagnosis, and epidemiology. *Am. J. Surg. Pathol.* 20:103–11
114. Harabuchi Y, Yamanaka N, Kataura A, Imai S, Kinoshita T, et al. 1990. Epstein-Barr virus in nasal T-cell lymphomas in patients with lethal midline granuloma. *Lancet* 335:128–30
115. Cheuk W, Chan JK, Shek TW, Chang JH, Tsou MH, et al. 2001. Inflammatory pseudotumor-like follicular dendritic cell tumor: a distinctive low-grade malignant intra-abdominal neoplasm with consistent Epstein-Barr virus association. *Am. J. Surg. Pathol.* 25:721–31
116. Selves J, Meggetto F, Brousset P, Voigt JJ, Pradere B, et al. 1996. Inflammatory pseudotumor of the liver. Evidence for follicular dendritic reticulum cell proliferation associated with clonal Epstein-Barr virus. *Am. J. Surg. Pathol.* 20:747–53
117. Horiguchi H, Matsui-Horiguchi M, Sakata H, Ichinose M, Yamamoto T, et al. 2004. Inflammatory pseudotumor-like follicular dendritic cell tumor of the spleen. *Pathol. Int.* 54:124–31
118. Shek TW, Ho FC, Ng IO, Chan AC, Ma L, et al. 1996. Follicular dendritic cell tumor of the liver. Evidence for an Epstein-Barr virus-related clonal proliferation of follicular dendritic cells. *Am. J. Surg. Pathol.* 20:313–24
119. Chen TC, Kuo TT, Ng KF. 2001. Follicular dendritic cell tumor of the liver: a clinicopathologic and Epstein-Barr virus study of two cases. *Mod. Pathol.* 14:354–60

120. Thorne LB, Ryan JL, Elmore SH, Glaser SL, Gulley ML. 2005. Real-time PCR measures Epstein-Barr virus DNA in archival breast adenocarcinomas. *Diagn. Mol. Pathol.* 14:29–33
121. Sugawara Y, Mizugaki Y, Uchida T, Torii T, Imai S, et al. 1999. Detection of Epstein-Barr virus (EBV) in hepatocellular carcinoma tissue: a novel EBV latency characterized by the absence of EBV-encoded small RNA expression. *Virology* 256:196–202
122. Bonnet M, Guinebretiere JM, Kremmer E, Grunewald V, Benhamou E, et al. 1999. Detection of Epstein-Barr virus in invasive breast cancers. *J. Natl. Cancer Inst.* 91:1376–81
123. Chu PG, Chen YY, Chen W, Weiss LM. 2001. No direct role for Epstein-Barr virus in American hepatocellular carcinoma. *Am. J. Pathol.* 159:1287–92
124. Henderson S, Huen D, Rowe M, Dawson C, Johnson G, et al. 1993. Epstein-Barr virus-coded BHRF1 protein, a viral homologue of Bcl-2, protects human B cells from programmed cell death. *Proc. Natl. Acad. Sci. USA* 90:8479–83
125. Lee MA, Yates JL. 1992. BHRF1 of Epstein-Barr virus, which is homologous to human proto-oncogene bcl2, is not essential for transformation of B cells or for virus replication in vitro. *J. Virol.* 66:1899–906
126. Rousset F, Garcia E, Defrance T, Peronne C, Vezzio N, et al. 1992. Interleukin 10 is a potent growth and differentiation factor for activated human B lymphocytes. *Proc. Natl. Acad. Sci. USA* 89:1890–93
127. Fixman ED, Hayward GS, Hayward SD. 1992. trans-acting requirements for replication of Epstein-Barr virus ori-Lyt. *J. Virol.* 66:5030–39
128. Lee MA, Diamond ME, Yates JL. 1999. Genetic evidence that EBNA-1 is needed for efficient, stable latent infection by Epstein-Barr virus. *J. Virol.* 73:2974–82
129. Kennedy G, Komano J, Sugden B. 2003. Epstein-Barr virus provides a survival factor to Burkitt's lymphomas. *Proc. Natl. Acad. Sci. USA* 100:14269–74
130. Abbot SD, Rowe M, Cadwallader K, Ricksten A, Gordon J, et al. 1990. Epstein-Barr virus nuclear antigen 2 induces expression of the virus-encoded latent membrane protein. *J. Virol.* 64:2126–34
131. Zimber-Strobl U, Kremmer E, Grasser F, Marschall G, Laux G, Bornkamm GW. 1993. The Epstein-Barr virus nuclear antigen 2 interacts with an EBNA2 responsive cis-element of the terminal protein 1 gene promoter. *EMBO J.* 12:167–75
132. Wang F, Tsang SF, Kurilla MG, Cohen JI, Kieff E. 1990. Epstein-Barr virus nuclear antigen 2 transactivates latent membrane protein LMP1. *J. Virol.* 64:3407–16
133. Wang F, Gregory CD, Rowe M, Rickinson AB, Wang D, et al. 1987. Epstein-Barr virus nuclear antigen 2 specifically induces expression of the B-cell activation antigen CD23. *Proc. Natl. Acad. Sci. USA* 84:3452–56
134. Cordier M, Calender A, Billaud M, Zimber U, Rousselet G, et al. 1990. Stable transfection of Epstein-Barr virus (EBV) nuclear antigen 2 in lymphoma cells containing the EBV P3HR1 genome induces expression of B-cell activation molecules CD21 and CD23. *J. Virol.* 64:1002–13
135. Cohen JI, Wang F, Mannick J, Kieff E. 1989. Epstein-Barr virus nuclear protein 2 is a key determinant of lymphocyte transformation. *Proc. Natl. Acad. Sci. USA* 86:9558–62
136. Yalamanchili R, Tong X, Grossman S, Johannsen E, Mosialos G, Kieff E. 1994. Genetic and biochemical evidence that EBNA 2 interaction with a 63-kDa cellular GTG-binding protein is essential for B lymphocyte growth transformation by EBV. *Virology* 204:634–41
137. Johannsen E, Miller CL, Grossman SR, Kieff E. 1996. EBNA-2 and EBNA-3C extensively and mutually exclusively associate with RBPJkappa in Epstein-Barr virus-transformed B lymphocytes. *J. Virol.* 70:4179–83

138. Robertson ES, Grossman S, Johannsen E, Miller C, Lin J, et al. 1995. Epstein-Barr virus nuclear protein 3C modulates transcription through interaction with the sequence-specific DNA-binding protein J kappa. *J. Virol.* 69:3108–16
139. Marshall D, Sample C. 1995. Epstein-Barr virus nuclear antigen 3C is a transcriptional regulator. *J. Virol.* 69:3624–30
140. Zhao B, Sample CE. 2000. Epstein-barr virus nuclear antigen 3C activates the latent membrane protein 1 promoter in the presence of Epstein-Barr virus nuclear antigen 2 through sequences encompassing an spi-1/Spi-B binding site. *J. Virol.* 74:5151–60
141. Mannick JB, Cohen JI, Birkenbach M, Marchini A, Kieff E. 1991. The Epstein-Barr virus nuclear protein encoded by the leader of the EBNA RNAs is important in B-lymphocyte transformation. *J. Virol.* 65:6826–37
142. Harada S, Kieff E. 1997. Epstein-Barr virus nuclear protein LP stimulates EBNA-2 acidic domain-mediated transcriptional activation. *J. Virol.* 71:6611–18
143. Kilger E, Kieser A, Baumann M, Hammerschmidt W. 1998. Epstein-Barr virus-mediated B-cell proliferation is dependent upon latent membrane protein 1, which simulates an activated CD40 receptor. *EMBO J.* 17:1700–9
144. Uchida J, Yasui T, Takaoka-Shichijo Y, Muraoka M, Kulwichit W, et al. 1999. Mimicry of CD40 signals by Epstein-Barr virus LMP1 in B lymphocyte responses. *Science* 286:300–3
145. Mosialos G, Birkenbach M, Yalamanchili R, VanArsdale T, Ware C, Kieff E. 1995. The Epstein-Barr virus transforming protein LMP1 engages signaling proteins for the tumor necrosis factor receptor family. *Cell* 80:389–99
146. Kulwichit W, Edwards RH, Davenport EM, Baskar JF, Godfrey V, Raab-Traub N. 1998. Expression of the Epstein-Barr virus latent membrane protein 1 induces B cell lymphoma in transgenic mice. *Proc. Natl. Acad. Sci. USA* 95:11963–68
147. Miller CL, Burkhardt AL, Lee JH, Stealey B, Longnecker R, et al. 1995. Integral membrane protein 2 of Epstein-Barr virus regulates reactivation from latency through dominant negative effects on protein-tyrosine kinases. *Immunity* 2:155–66
148. Merchant M, Swart R, Katzman RB, Ikeda M, Ikeda A, et al. 2001. The effects of the Epstein-Barr virus latent membrane protein 2A on B cell function. *Int. Rev. Immunol.* 20:805–35
149. Merchant M, Caldwell RG, Longnecker R. 2000. The LMP2A ITAM is essential for providing B cells with development and survival signals in vivo. *J. Virol.* 74:9115–24

Calcium in Cell Injury and Death*

Zheng Dong,[1] Pothana Saikumar,[2]
Joel M. Weinberg,[3]
and Manjeri A. Venkatachalam[2]

[1]Department of Cellular Biology and Anatomy, Medical College of Georgia, Augusta, Georgia 30912; Medical Research Service, Department of Veterans Affairs Medical Center, Augusta, Georgia 30904; email: zdong@mcg.edu

[2]Department of Pathology, University of Texas Health Science Center, San Antonio, Texas 78229; email: saikumar@uthscsa.edu, venkatachal@uthscsa.edu

[3]Department of Medicine, University of Michigan Medical Center and Ann Arbor VA Healthcare System, Ann Arbor, Michigan 48109; email: wnberg@umich.edu

Annu. Rev. Pathol. Mech. Dis.
2006. 1:405–34

First published online as a Review in Advance on November 4, 2005

The *Annual Review of Pathology: Mechanisms of Disease* is online at pathmechdis.annualreviews.org

doi: 10.1146/annurev.pathol.1.110304.100218

1553-4006/06/0114-0405$20.00

Key Words

mitochondrial permeability transition, ischemia-reperfusion, apoptosis, adenosine triphosphate, glycine, nonesterified fatty acids

Abstract

Loss of Ca^{2+} homeostasis, often in the form of cytoplasmic increases, leads to cell injury. Depending upon cell type and the intensity of Ca^{2+} toxicity, the ensuing pathology can be reversible or irreversible. Although multiple destructive processes are activated by Ca^{2+}, lethal outcomes are determined largely by Ca^{2+}-induced mitochondrial permeability transition. This form of damage is primarily dependent upon mitochondrial Ca^{2+} accumulation, which is regulated by the mitochondrial membrane potential. Retention of the mitochondrial membrane potential during Ca^{2+} increases favors mitochondrial Ca^{2+} uptake and overload, resulting in mitochondrial permeability transition and cell death. In contrast, dissipation of mitochondrial membrane potential reduces mitochondrial Ca^{2+} uptake, retards mitochondrial permeability transition, and delays death, even in cells with large Ca^{2+} increases. The rates of mitochondrial membrane potential dissipation and mitochondrial Ca^{2+} uptake may determine cellular sensitivity to Ca^{2+} toxicity under pathological conditions, including ischemic injury.

Ca^{2+}: ionized calcium

Mitochondrial membrane potential (Δψm): proton gradient that is maintained across the inner mitochondrial membrane

CNS: central nervous system

ATP: adenosine triphosphate

INTRODUCTION

Following the discovery that cell death during the acute phase of injury by several toxins can be dependent upon extracellular free or ionized calcium (hereafter referred to as Ca^{2+}) (1), there has been intense research on the role of Ca^{2+} in cell injury. The Calcium Hypothesis is based upon the finding of pathological increases of intracellular Ca^{2+} during diverse injury states; these increases set in motion degenerative events that can be avoided if Ca^{2+} increases are prevented (2–4). A large body of work shows that Ca^{2+}-dependent injury is context-dependent and varies between cell types and that Ca^{2+}-independent mechanisms are also important and can result in lethal outcomes. Most importantly, it is now clear that injury mechanisms and death pathways are more complex than initially thought, and experimental attempts to find universally common threads lead to oversimplification. With these considerations in mind, this review emphasizes the cellular energy context in which Ca^{2+} increases take place. Although such increases can lead to a plethora of disturbances, certain unique factors determine whether the outcome will be lethal. In particular, whether the cells are energized to maintain the mitochondrial membrane potential (Δψm) during injury and thus accumulate Ca^{2+} within mitochondria by Δψm-dependent transport appears to be a fundamental determinant of Ca^{2+} cytotoxicity. This is illustrated by differences between Ca^{2+}-induced injury in the central nervous system (CNS), heart, and kidneys.

In the CNS, where pathological Ca^{2+} fluxes occur via receptor-mediated mechanisms in neurons and glia, Δψm-dependent Ca^{2+} uptake causes mitochondrial damage and cell death. In ischemic cardiomyocytes, mitochondria are energized via glycolysis to such an extent that they permit Δψm-dependent Ca^{2+} uptake and mitochondrial damage. During reperfusion, Δψm increases owing to respiration in sublethally damaged mitochondria and drives Ca^{2+} transport further, lethally damaging the organelles. Increased Ca^{2+} is also responsible for pathological contractures in these cells. Again, adenosine triphosphate (ATP) generated by anaerobic glycolysis or oxidative mechanisms may paradoxically worsen injury by sustaining Ca^{2+}-dependent contraction, causing mechanical damage to sublethally injured membranes. In kidneys, strictly aerobic, proximal tubular cells are surprisingly resistant to high Ca^{2+} during ischemia-reperfusion. This resistance seems related to the inability of mitochondria to accumulate Ca^{2+} owing to the rapid dissipation of Δψm during ischemia and poor or slow recovery of Δψm with reperfusion. In this cell type, Ca^{2+}-independent mechanisms appear to be important determinants of lethal injury.

By necessity, this review limits its scope to general principles and the most relevant circumstances. It will first provide an overview of general mechanisms and the circumstances under which Ca^{2+} may injure cells, emphasizing Ca^{2+}-induced degenerative events that are not necessarily lethal. Thereafter, the review considers injury in three specific tissues to illustrate how Ca^{2+} cytotoxicity varies between cell types. In the interest of cogency, the authors restrict the discussion of organ-specific injury to the settings of ischemia and reperfusion.

GENERAL CONSIDERATIONS

Physiological Maintenance of Ca^{2+} Homeostasis

Normally, Ca^{2+} concentration in the cytosol ranges between 10–100 nM, whereas extracellular Ca^{2+} concentration is 1–2 mM. The result is that a nearly 10,000-fold Ca^{2+} gradient exists across the plasma membrane. This homeostasis is maintained by interplay between energy-dependent pumps and directional transporters located in plasma membranes and organelles, and Ca^{2+} binding proteins (**Figure 1**) (5, 6).

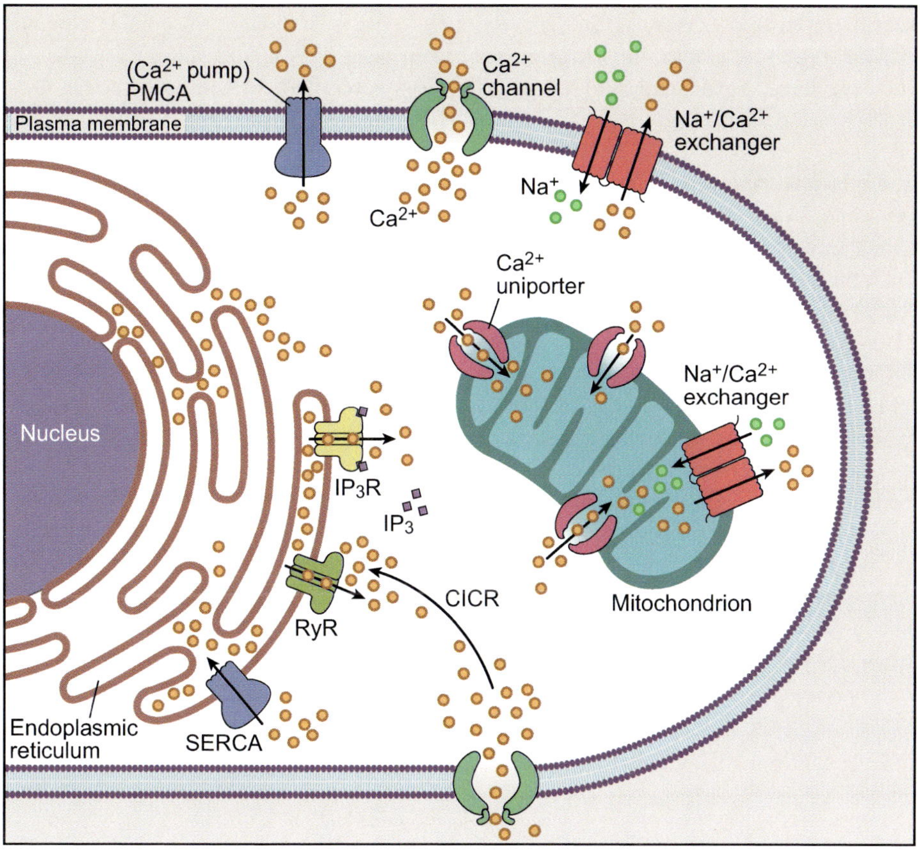

Figure 1

Calcium homeostasis in normal cells. Ionized calcium (Ca^{2+}) in the cytosol is normally maintained at 10–100 nM against steep gradients by transport of the ion to the extracellular space and cisternae of the endoplasmic reticulum (ER), and by protein binding. Physiological increases of cytosolic Ca^{2+} take place by entry through plasma membrane Ca^{2+} channels (leak channels, ligand-gated channels, and voltage-gated channels), release of Ca^{2+} from the ER or sarcoplasmic reticulum (SR) lumina upon binding of inositol trisphosphate (IP_3) to the inositol trisphosphate receptor (IP_3R), or release of Ca^{2+} from the SR (in muscle cells) upon Ca^{2+} binding to the ryanodine receptor (RyR) by a process called calcium-induced calcium release (CICR). Transport of Ca^{2+} across the plasma membrane to the extracellular space takes place via the plasma membrane calcium ATPase (PMCA) and the Na^+/Ca^{2+} exchanger. The sarco-endoplasmic reticulum calcium ATPase (SERCA) transports Ca^{2+} into the ER in nonexcitable cells, or the SR in muscle cells. Mitochondrial membranes can also buffer Ca^{2+} by transport of the ion into the mitochondrial matrix via Ca^{2+} uniporters. Abnormal increase of mitochondrial matrix Ca^{2+} concentration is prevented by transport in the reverse direction via mitochondrial Na^+/Ca^{2+} exchangers.

Plasma membrane. Transport of Ca^{2+} across the plasma membrane is tightly controlled (5, 6). Ca^{2+} influx is mediated by ligand-gated and voltage-gated channels, as well as nonselective leak channels. In resting cells, leak channels allow limited, yet continuous, Ca^{2+} influx. Two Ca^{2+}-exporting systems counter the influx. The Na^+/Ca^{2+} exchanger has low Ca^{2+} affinity but high velocity; as such, it removes Ca^{2+} when cytosolic concentrations are high. The Ca^{2+} pump, an ATPase, has high Ca^{2+} affinity and pumps

ER: endoplasmic reticulum

SR: sarcoplasmic reticulum

out Ca^{2+} even at low cytosolic Ca^{2+} concentrations. Both Ca^{2+} influx and extrusion are finely regulated to maintain large Ca^{2+} gradients across the membrane.

Endoplasmic reticulum. In normal cells, the endoplasmic reticulum, or ER, also termed sarcoplasmic reticulum or SR in muscle, is the largest reservoir of Ca^{2+}, with concentrations reaching millimolar levels. Thus, a large gradient of Ca^{2+} also exists across the ER membrane, with cytosolic Ca^{2+} concentrations $\simeq$10,000-fold lower than in the ER lumen. The gradient is maintained by the ER-specific Ca^{2+} ATPase, which drives Ca^{2+} into the ER lumen where local concentrations are buffered by Ca^{2+} binding proteins. Release of Ca^{2+} from the ER is tightly controlled by chemical or electrical signals in normal cells. The inositol trisphosphate (IP_3) receptor releases Ca^{2+} from the ER upon IP_3 binding, thus becoming a Ca^{2+} channel (7). In striated muscle, the ryanodine receptor senses electrical signals and releases Ca^{2+} from the SR (8).

Mitochondria. In resting cells, Ca^{2+} concentration in the mitochondrial matrix is low (~100 nM). However, when cytosolic Ca^{2+} rises, ion uptake by the mitochondria is rapid. This buffering action (9) allows mitochondria to regulate Ca^{2+} signals by localized interaction with the ER (10). The downward electrochemical gradient across the inner membrane directs Ca^{2+} into the mitochondria through a uniporter. Previously thought to have low Ca^{2+} affinity, becoming active only when cytosolic Ca^{2+} reaches micromolar levels (9, 11), the uniporter is now identified as a high-affinity channel (12). Mitochondria possess a Na^+/Ca^{2+} exchanger, which extrudes Ca^{2+} (9, 11). Under pathological conditions, this exchanger can operate in reverse.

Nucleus. Ca^{2+} is involved in nuclear gene transcription, DNA metabolism, and envelope turnover (13). However, control of nucleoplasmic Ca^{2+} is controversial (6). Nuclear Ca^{2+} has been thought to equilibrate rapidly with cytosolic Ca^{2+} by diffusion across nuclear pores (14). In contrast, nuclear Ca^{2+} has also been considered to be controlled independently (15), a belief supported by the identification of Ca^{2+} channels in the nuclear envelope (16).

Perturbation of Ca^{2+} Homeostasis Under Pathological Conditions

Upon stimulation, intracellular Ca^{2+} changes rapidly. The physiological increases that follow reflect the role of Ca^{2+} as a second messenger (5). For example, activation of G protein–coupled receptors leads to production of IP_3. IP_3 releases Ca^{2+} from the ER. It is conceivable that pathologically increased Ca^{2+} damages cells through the disturbance of its pivotal role in signaling. However, in most cases, injury appears to be a consequence of direct Ca^{2+}-induced damage and activation of hydrolases. Ca^{2+}-mediated injury is usually acute, rapid, and, in some circumstances, irreversible (3).

It is difficult to determine when and what types of intracellular Ca^{2+} alterations are physiological or pathogenic. A few criteria apply. First, physiological changes of Ca^{2+} are usually rapid, lasting for milliseconds, seconds, or minutes. Upon stimulation, alterations in the concentrations of cytosolic Ca^{2+} occur as spikes or oscillations. This is attributable to the cell's powerful capacity for maintaining Ca^{2+} homeostasis, without which cell injury and tissue pathology would ensue. Second, Ca^{2+} elevations during signaling usually occur in microenvironments and may spread to other areas or other cells, but are readily reversed by homeostatic mechanisms mediated by membrane transport and Ca^{2+} binding by proteins. In contrast, diffuse increases of Ca^{2+} are typical in pathological conditions. If Ca^{2+} elevations are persistent, uncontrollable, and overwhelm homeostasis, the ion becomes available in normally protected cellular environments and causes injury. Finally, functional analysis can discriminate between physiological and pathological Ca^{2+} increases: Is the cell injured, is it dying, or does it recover homeostatic function?

Although in general the Ca^{2+}-overload hypothesis is valid, Ca^{2+} depletion may also induce cell injury and death (17). In sympathetic neurons, growth-factor deprivation leads to cell death, which is prevented by membrane depolarization (18). The protective effects are attenuated by prevention of Ca^{2+} influx or by intracellular Ca^{2+} chelation, showing that Ca^{2+} can be a factor in survival (19). It is not surprising that in view of its signaling role, depletion of Ca^{2+} can be toxic.

Depletion of Ca^{2+} from the ER can also activate a stress-induced apoptotic pathway (20). The applicability of these findings to the diversity of excitable and nonexcitable cells remains to be investigated.

Differences in Ca^{2+} handling between excitable and nonexcitable cells affect their behavior during injury. In excitable cells, voltage-operated Ca^{2+} channels induce Ca^{2+} influx; in contrast, physiological Ca^{2+} increases in nonexcitable cells are mainly receptor-operated through channels in the plasma membrane and the ER. Ca^{2+} influx can activate Ca^{2+} release from internal stores such as the ER by a mechanism known as calcium-induced calcium release (CICR) (21); on the other hand, release of ER Ca^{2+} can trigger Ca^{2+} influx via capacitative Ca^{2+} entry (22). These interactions, as well as Ca^{2+} pumping mechanisms, are altered during injury. Of note, Ca^{2+} pumps in plasma membranes and the ER are ATP driven; therefore, when energy levels are low, pumping activity decreases, which results in cytosolic Ca^{2+} increases.

Perturbation of mitochondrial Ca^{2+} plays a critical role in Ca^{2+} cytotoxicity (9, 23). Normally, mitochondrial Ca^{2+} is low, but when cytosolic Ca^{2+} increases, the mitochondrial uniporter transports the ion into the mitochondrial matrix. If the mitochondrial Na^+/Ca^{2+} exchanger is overwhelmed by Ca^{2+} entry, mitochondrial matrix Ca^{2+} increases to levels high enough to trigger a process termed mitochondrial permeability transition (MPT). This involves the formation in the inner membranes of pores with permeability limits ≤1.5 kDa. Although MPT can "flicker" and be reversible (24, 25), sustained transitions lead to the collapse of $\Delta\psi m$, cessation of ATP production, and cell death by necrosis or apoptosis (24–26).

Disturbances of Ca^{2+} homeostasis in cytoplasm, the ER, or mitochondria can injure cells, but can also be reversed. However, Ca^{2+} stores are closely connected within the cells and interact with each other. As a result, dysregulation of one compartment is usually followed by responses from the others. Together, they may overwhelm the cell's capacity to maintain overall homeostasis and kill the cell.

CICR: calcium-induced calcium release

Mitochondrial permeability transition (MPT): a pore across the inner mitochondrial membrane; formed from interactions between several transmembrane proteins

Ca^{2+} Cytotoxicity and Structural Disruption

A notable feature of cellular Ca^{2+} is its versatility in binding and regulating various proteins and subcellular structures. Under pathological conditions where Ca^{2+} homeostasis is disrupted, the versatile nature of Ca^{2+} turns the ion into a powerful activator of multiple damaging processes. Most likely, not one but many injurious events are initiated, and the significance of each event is determined specifically by the nature of the insult that triggers Ca^{2+} perturbation and the cellular context. Toxicity can result from the direct effects of Ca^{2+}, indirectly through activation of degradative hydrolases, or from combinations of both processes.

Phospholipases. Phospholipases catalyze the hydrolysis of phospholipids, which are essential elements of cellular membranes. Many phospholipase isoforms require Ca^{2+} for activation and several of them can be activated directly by Ca^{2+}. For example, a role for cytosolic Ca^{2+}-dependent phospholipase A2 in ischemic injury has been demonstrated recently by gene knockout studies (27). Hydrolysis of phospholipids adversely affects the stability, fluidity, and integrity of membranes and compromises membrane-based transport. In addition, the fatty acids and lysophospholipids released during lipid hydrolysis can induce cell injury directly by disrupting cellular structures via their detergent nature and indirectly via the activation of various signaling pathways.

Calpain. Protein degradation is another prominent feature of Ca^{2+}-mediated cell injury. Calpains are cysteine proteases synthesized as inactive proenzymes, which are activated via autocatalytic proteolysis triggered by Ca^{2+}. Among calpain isoforms, the ubiquitously expressed μ- and m-calpains are activated by micro- and millimolar levels of Ca^{2+}, respectively (28). Calpains are activated during injury induced by various insults associated with Ca^{2+} increases. These enzymes degrade proteins such as spectrin to induce cytoskeleton disruption and membrane blebbing (29–31). However, their effects may also target more proximate locations in the injury cascade. For example, calpains may cleave and inactivate Bcl-2 and Bcl-XL, two important cell-death inhibitory proteins (32, 33). Bax cleavage by calpains has also been documented, producing fragments with enhanced pro-apoptotic activity (34). Even more interesting, in models of myocardial ischemia, calpains proteolytically activate the pro-apoptotic protein Bid, which then targets mitochondria, resulting in mitochondrial damage and cell death (35). Also, cross-talk between calpains and caspases, the core degradative machinery in apoptosis, has been documented in several model systems (32, 36).

Ca^{2+}-dependent endonuclease. Caspase-activated endonuclease (DNA fragment factor, or DFF) participates in apoptosis by cleaving DNA (37). Ca^{2+}-dependent endonucleases located in the nucleus become active during Ca^{2+}-mediated cell injury (38). The role of these nucleases, working alone or in combination with DFF, in the induction of DNA damage in specific cell injury models remains unclear.

Ca^{2+} and forms of cell death. The strikingly different morphologies of Ca^{2+}-related cell death suggest that disruptive processes initiated by the ion work differently depending upon pathological conditions. However, these various forms of cell death may also have some features in common. The best-recognized forms of cell death are necrosis and apoptosis. Whereas necrosis is considered an accidental and passive process, apoptosis is considered programmed and active and requires energy to progress. Morphologically, necrotic cells become swollen, with an end point indicated by loss of plasma-membrane integrity. In sharp contrast, apoptotic cells shrink, showing condensation of cytoplasm and organelles, including the mitochondria and nucleus. The plasma membrane remains intact in earlier stages of apoptosis, although it later becomes permeable by a process known as secondary necrosis. Despite these apparent differences, recent studies indicate clearly that apoptosis and necrosis are not mutually exclusive, but rather interrelated (39). First, apoptosis and necrosis can be induced by the same type of insults, e.g., Ca^{2+} overload (23). Second, these two forms of cell death seem to share signaling and regulatory mechanisms, which involve, under many circumstances, mitochondrial disruption (40). Also, cytoprotective approaches are usually effective in protecting the cells against both apoptosis and necrosis. For example, both forms of cell death are blocked by the expression of Bcl-2 (41). Finally, it is possible to switch apoptosis to necrosis in the same cells under the same stimuli. This is exemplified in experiments using caspase inhibitors (41, 42). Under such conditions, apoptosis is aborted, and yet cells are not rescued; eventually they die by necrosis. These observations suggest that, in many circumstances, the various forms of cell death may be related mechanistically. The intensity and duration of the insults may determine the morphological outcome. Another decisive factor is the condition of the cells. Without ATP, cells committed to apoptosis ultimately die by necrosis (41, 42).

Membrane blebbing. Blebbing or ballooning of the plasma membrane is a common manifestation of cell injury. Critical events for bleb formation include disruption of the cytoskeleton and its interaction with the plasma membrane (3). Ca^{2+} is a known pathophysiological regulator of actin, a major structural protein. Increased Ca^{2+} leads to fragmentation of F-actin fibers, disruption of the skeletal structure, and detachment of the cytoskeleton from the plasma membrane. Calpains, activated by Ca^{2+}, cleave cytoskeletal elements, including intermediate filaments. In addition, increased Ca^{2+} destabilizes microtubules via calmodulin. These events, collectively, lead to protrusion of the plasma membrane and formation of blebs.

Nuclear alterations. During apoptosis, the cell nucleus undergoes chromatin condensation, margination, and finally fragmentation. Although chromatin condensation and margination occur during early necrosis, the changes do not progress to nuclear fragmentation; instead, the nucleus is dissolved following the breakdown of the plasma membrane, apparently by autolysis. Do Ca^{2+} and calpain play roles in nuclear changes during apoptosis and necrosis? The answer may depend upon the experimental conditions. It would be interesting to examine whether Ca^{2+} induces nuclear reorganizaton directly or indirectly during Ca^{2+}-mediated cell injury and death, perhaps via calpain activity.

Endoplasmic reticulum stress. Relatively little is known about the structural disruptions in the ER during cell injury and death. However, the ER is the major Ca^{2+} store within the cell, and Ca^{2+} depletion from this organelle leads to stress. ER stress is now recognized as an important cause of apoptosis. Prolonged ER stress leads to the activation of caspase-12, which is localized in the ER membrane and, upon activation, can sequentially activate downstream executioner caspases to induce apoptosis (43). Under ER stress, caspase-12 can be activated by the formation of a protein complex with TRAF2 (tumor necrosis factor–associated factor 2). Importantly, caspase-12 is also activated by m-calpain (44). Release of Ca^{2+} from the ER leads to Ca^{2+} depletion in the ER and thus ER stress. The released Ca^{2+} activates calpain in cytosol, which in turn activates caspase-12, the initiator caspase of apoptosis during ER stress. In addition, the ER may regulate apoptosis via its interaction with mitochondria (see below for further discussion).

Mitochondrial disruption: two killing pores. Physiologically, mitochondria are involved in the maintenance of Ca^{2+} homeostasis mainly because of their capacity to buffer cytosolic Ca^{2+}. However, Ca^{2+} overload in mitochondria may lead to organelle damage and is an important determinant of Ca^{2+} toxicity. Morphologically, irreversible damage of mitochondria caused by Ca^{2+} overload often presents itself as severe swelling of the organelles, with calcium-containing, electron-dense deposits in the matrix and associated structural damage (**Figure 2**). Precipitation of Ca^{2+} as insoluble phosphate and hydroxyapatite has long been recognized as an important feature of mitochondrial damage and cell death. Nevertheless, only recently have pathologists been able to appreciate the significance of mitochondria in the development of tissue pathology. This is in large part attributable to insights gained from studies on the development of porous defects in the outer and inner membranes of the organelles (45).

Outer-membrane permeability. Cytochrome c, a 12–14 kDa protein normally located in the mitochondrial intermembrane space, can initiate caspase activation and apoptosis (46) when released into the

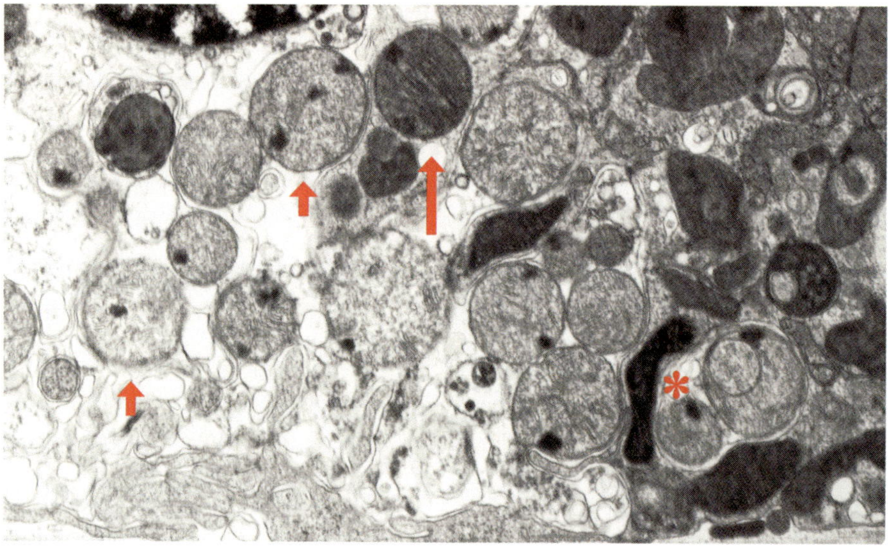

Figure 2

High-power electron micrograph of a cell injured by ischemia, showing mitochondrial swelling with electron-dense precipitates. Several mitochondria are shown. Most of the mitochondria are in various stages of swelling. A mitochondrion in condensed configuration is present just adjacent to the left of the asterisk. Two of several markedly swollen, ballooned mitochondria with amorphous electron-dense precipitates are indicated by short red arrows. When such mitochondria are examined by electron-probe microanalysis, the amorphous densities reveal the presence of calcium in pathologically high amounts. Matrix calcium also increases. Structural damage is present in some of the ballooned mitochondria. A mitochondrion with early swelling and aggregates of electron-dense material is indicated by the long red arrow.

cytosol. These findings not only identified cytochrome c as a pivotal player in signaling apoptosis, but also suggested an important role for the mitochondrial outer membrane in determining cell death and survival. We now know that loss of outer-membrane integrity results in the release of several killing molecules, including cytochrome c, apoptosis-inducing factor (AIF), Smac/Diablo, Omi/HtrA2, and others (47). How the mitochondrial outer membrane becomes permeable to intermembrane proteins during certain forms of apoptosis is being investigated. Investigators have postulated two major hypothetical models.

In the first model, outer membranes are permeabilized without decreased inner-membrane integrity. The permeabilization seems to be mediated largely by Bcl-2 family proteins, particularly Bax and Bak, two pro-apoptotic proteins with three Bcl-2 homology (BH) domains (48). These two proteins oligomerize in the outer membrane of mitochondria and, along with membrane lipids, may form pores large enough to allow leakage of intermembrane proteins (49–51). Pro-apoptotic proteins with only one BH domain (also termed BH3-only proteins, e.g., Bid, Bad, Bim, etc.) promote formation of such pores by activating Bax/Bak, whereas anti-apoptotic members, including Bcl-2 and Bcl-XL, antagonize the process (49–52).

In the second model (53), outer-membrane permeabilization is proposed to be a direct or indirect consequence of the MPT, which is primarily a pore defect of the inner membrane. In this model, MPT leads to the influx of solutes and water into mitochondria and, as a result, swelling of the matrix. Uncontrolled swelling of the matrix is thought to expand the inner membrane and break the outer membrane, thus causing leakage. Although this model is attractive because it makes a pathological connection between the inner and outer membranes, it has been challenged by several critical observations. For example, at the early stages of apoptosis, cells and cellular organelles, including mitochondria, condense and do not swell. Moreover, in well-characterized models of apoptosis, cytochrome c release occurs, whereas sufficient inner-membrane integrity is maintained to sustain $\Delta\psi m$ (54, 55). Because $\Delta\psi m$ requires transmembrane ion gradients, its presence is a reliable indicator of inner-membrane integrity and absence of MPT pores. Recent studies by separate research groups have further provided evidence to exclude a role for MPT in the development of outer-membrane permeability during apoptosis (56–58). In these studies, when cyclophilin D, a gene implicated in MPT, is knocked out, the development of MPT is suppressed. However, mitochondrial outer-membrane permeability and apoptosis induced by pro-apoptotic Bcl-2 proteins, staurosporine, and tumor necrosis factor are not affected (56–58). Nevertheless, MPT can be transient, and pharmacological inhibitors of MPT have been reported to block apoptosis in specific experimental models (59). Thus, it is likely that MPT is not necessary for apoptosis. Nevertheless, there may be conditions in which MPT can promote the development of outer-membrane permeability and apoptosis.

Mitochondrial permeability transition. As stated above, the MPT results from a development of a pore in the mitochondrial inner membrane with a size exclusion limit of $\leq$1.5 kDa, which may form transiently during physiological states but becomes permanent under injury conditions, including Ca^{2+} overload (24–26). Permanency of the MPT pore implies loss of mitochondrial homeostasis and lethal damage. MPT pores are distinct from those that leak intermembrane proteins. However, the MPT pore is not necessarily restricted to the inner membrane, and contact sites between the inner and outer mitochondrial membranes may be involved. Critical components of the MPT pore may be derived from both membranes (24–26). Thus, MPT induces permeability of the inner membrane, but its formation may involve not only events of the inner membrane, but also pathological alterations of the outer membrane.

ANT: adenine nucleotide transporter

Several proteins have been implicated in the formation of MPT pores (24, 60): adenine nucleotide translocase (ANT), located in the inner membrane; voltage-dependent anion channel (VDAC) of the outer membrane; and cyclophilin D, which interacts with ANT from the matrix side. MPT-pore formation is blocked by the ANT inhibitor bongkrekate and promoted by the ANT ligand atractyloside. In addition, cyclosporin A, the inhibitor of cyclophilin D, retards the development of MPT. The mitochondria of cyclophilin D–deficient mice exhibit a decreased, but not absent, propensity to develop the MPT and loss of sensitivity to the effects of cyclosporin A (56–58). Despite these findings, the exact structure of the MPT pore remains undefined. Recent studies have raised questions about a necessary role for ANT because mitochondria from ANT knockout animals can undergo MPT (61). Moreover, other proteins, including Bcl-2 family proteins, may interact with the MPT complex and regulate the MPT pore (62).

A role for the MPT pore in cell injury and death has long been suspected; if pore formation is not reversed, the ensuing disturbance of mitochondrial homeostasis will have destructive consequences. Dissipation of $\Delta\psi m$ will stop ATP synthesis, and the decline of cell ATP that follows will compromise overall cellular homeostasis and lead to cell death by necrosis (24–26). As discussed above, MPT is also a proposed mechanism for outer-membrane permeabilization. Importantly, MPT is promoted by intracellular pathologies such as Ca^{2+}overload, oxidative stress, phospholipid hydrolysis, diminished $\Delta\psi m$, and ATP depletion (24–26).

SERCA: sarco-endoplasmic reticulum calcium ATPase

Ca^{2+} and Mitochondrial Pathology

As discussed above, two models have been postulated for permeabilization of mitochondrial outer membranes, either with or without the participation of inner-membrane pathology. In the first model, which emphasizes outer-membrane pore formation via Bcl-2 family proteins, evidence of Ca^{2+} regulation is limited. Nevertheless, a role for Ca^{2+} has been suggested in certain forms of apoptosis through the participation of calcineurin, a Ca^{2+}/calmodulin-dependent phosphatase that can dephosphorylate and activate Bad, a BH3-only pro-apoptotic molecule (63). Dephosphorylated Bad then antagonizes Bcl-XL by heterodimerization and promotes apoptosis (63). In models of myocardial ischemia-reperfusion, Ca^{2+}-activated calpains have been reported to proteolytically process Bid into its active forms of truncated Bid or tBid (35). tBid activates Bax and Bak, which oligomerize in the outer membrane, giving rise to pore defects (64). Finally, investigators have recently suggested a direct effect of Ca^{2+} on cytochrome c release from mitochondria on the basis of the observation that the release is a two-step event involving detachment of cytochrome c from the inner membrane and permeabilization of the outer membrane (65). Ca^{2+} may play a role in causing the dissociation of cytochrome c from cardiolipin at the outside surface of the inner mitochondrial membrane. Together these studies have provided somewhat limited evidence for Ca^{2+} regulation of Bcl-2 family protein–mediated outer-membrane damage. However, there is compelling evidence that Ca^{2+} levels affect MPT: Ca^{2+} overload in the mitochondrial matrix, which is usually accompanied by energetic collapse and oxidative stress, is one of the most important inducers of MPT in vitro in isolated mitochondria and cells and in vivo during pathological conditions such as organ ischemia-reperfusion (25, 26, 60, 66).

Endoplasmic reticulum Ca^{2+} store: a determinant of mitochondrial damage and cell death? Many studies have focused on Ca^{2+} toxicity in mitochondria, whereas others have revealed an interesting cross-talk between the ER and mitochondria in Ca^{2+} regulation. More importantly, these studies now suggest an emerging role for ER-Ca^{2+} stores in determining mitochondrial damage and cell death. The initial evidence came from studies that examined Ca^{2+} regulation in cells overexpressing Bcl-2, a well-recognized anti-apoptotic protein. The ER-Ca^{2+} store, which is releasable by thapsigargin, was significantly lower in these cells (67). Subsequent studies indicated that Bcl-2 overexpression led to Ca^{2+} leak from the ER, resulting in a significant reduction of releasable Ca^{2+} (68). In the same cells, capacitative Ca^{2+} entry following ER-Ca^{2+} depletion was also suppressed. Ca^{2+} depletion in ER was proposed to be one of the cytoprotective mechanisms of Bcl-2 because the conditions that lowered Ca^{2+} in the ER also protected HeLa cells from ceramide-induced cell death, whereas treatments that increased ER Ca^{2+} showed opposite effects (69). In line with these observations, Bax/Bak-deficient cells had dramatically reduced Ca^{2+} levels in the ER, and as a result, Ca^{2+} uptake by mitochondria was inhibited and the cells became highly resistant to Ca^{2+}-dependent injury and death (70). Moreover, when the ER-Ca^{2+} defect in these cells was corrected by expressing the sarco-endoplasmic reticulum calcium ATPase (SERCA) Ca^{2+} pump, cellular sensitivity to injury was restored (70). Although the mechanism underlying ER regulation by Bcl-2 proteins remains unclear, there is evidence for direct interaction of Bcl-2 with IP_3 receptors (71), the main Ca^{2+} release channels in the ER membrane. This interaction is enhanced in the absence of Bax and Bak (71). Together these findings suggest a role for ER-Ca^{2+} level in determining mitochondrial injury and cell death. Bcl-2 family proteins, in addition to their direct regulatory effects on mitochondrial integrity, may regulate Ca^{2+} leak from the ER and Ca^{2+} level in the ER and, as a result, control Ca^{2+} uptake by mitochondria under pathological conditions.

Ca^{2+} Threshold of Cytotoxicity: A Role for Glycine in the Ca^{2+} Puzzle

An intriguing question in studies of Ca^{2+} toxicity is, how much Ca^{2+} is too much? Or, more directly, what concentrations of Ca^{2+} are lethal to the cells? Addressing this question has been difficult, mainly because of two concerns. First, as discussed above, Ca^{2+} thresholds for damage may vary between cell types and different pathological conditions. Nonexcitable and excitable cells may respond differently to Ca^{2+} toxicity. Compared with ATP-depleted cells, energized cells may accumulate much more Ca^{2+} in mitochondria owing to the presence of $\Delta\psi$m and are more likely to undergo permanent MPT, which can be lethal. Second, under various pathological conditions, Ca^{2+}-independent mechanisms of cell injury are also activated. Early plasma-membrane damage by Ca^{2+}-independent processes may lead to massive Ca^{2+} influx and set in motion secondary Ca^{2+}-mediated events postmortem, making it difficult to distinguish important premortem pathogenic mechanisms attributable to calcium from less relevant postmortem degeneration.

An important development in this area of research has been the identification of a glycine-sensitive Ca^{2+}-independent mechanism of cell injury (72). This distinctive mechanism involves the loss of glycine from energy-deprived or ATP-depleted cells, followed by plasma-membrane breakdown and cell death by necrosis. Of significance, this type of injury is abrogated by the presence of 0.25–2 mM glycine in the extracellular milieu. Glycine and related compounds have exhibited cytoprotective effects during ATP depletion in various types of cells. Importantly, glycine prevents tissue damage under pathological conditions, including ischemia-reperfusion injury of the liver, intestine, and kidneys (73). Although the molecular basis of glycine-sensitive injury remains elusive, it may be related to the deformation of a multimeric protein in the plasma membrane (74, 75).

The use of glycine to block a major form of Ca^{2+}-independent injury has permitted experimental investigation of Ca^{2+}-dependent mechanisms in a way that is not complicated by the overlay of early and lethal plasma-membrane damage, which would otherwise result in a rapid massive Ca^{2+} influx from extracellular space. Such investigations have permitted the identification of relevant Ca^{2+} increases and their consequences and the discrimination of these specific effects from confounding post-mortem phenomena. In the presence of glycine, and thus, with retention of plasma-membrane integrity, freshly isolated renal tubular cells sustain surprisingly high cytosolic Ca^{2+} (more than 100 μM) during ATP depletion by hypoxia and yet retain their structural and functional integrity (76). Moreover, ATP-depleted Madin-Darby Canine Kidney (MDCK) cells are able to survive similarly high cytosolic Ca^{2+} levels and proliferate after returning to normal culture medium. Cell death occurs only when intracellular Ca^{2+} increases beyond 100 μM, which is associated with nuclear damage and DNA breakdown (77).

Context Dependency of Lethal Injury by Calcium

A large body of research has shown that Ca^{2+}-dependent mechanisms of injury can be cell type–specific, particularly with respect to whether Ca^{2+} increases lead necessarily to lethal outcomes. Some of these studies have demonstrated unexpectedly high resistance of certain cell types to Ca^{2+} cytotoxicity. These findings are relevant to the pathological condition of ischemia-reperfusion. Does Ca^{2+} play a critical role in ischemic injury? Are there differences in Ca^{2+} cytotoxicty between various tissues and organs? What factors are responsible for such differences, if they exist?

NMDA: N-methyl D-aspartate

CALCIUM DEPENDENCY AND INJURY IN ORGAN SYSTEMS

This section describes and discusses the role played by Ca^{2+}-dependent mitochondrial damage in the causation of cell death during clinically relevant ischemia-reperfusion syndromes in three organ systems: the CNS, the heart, and the kidney. Although mechanisms differ, Ca^{2+}-mediated mitochondrial damage is of paramount importance in neuronal/glial and myocardiocyte cell death of ischemic etiology. However, kidney epithelial cells are surprisingly resistant to lethal toxicity of intracellular Ca^{2+} increase during ischemia. In ischemic kidney cells, lethality appears to be determined by persistent mitochondrial energetic dysfunction, attributable to the progressive accumulation of nonesterified fatty acids. The differences between cell types in sensitivity to Ca^{2+}-induced mitochondrial damage seem to be determined by variations in the ability of mitochondria to retain or dissipate $\Delta\psi m$.

THE CENTRAL NERVOUS SYSTEM

Increases of cytosolic Ca^{2+} in neurons can result from influx through voltage-gated Ca^{2+} channels, ligation of N-methyl D-aspartate (NMDA), kainate, and α-amino-3-hydroxy-5-methylisoxazole-4-propionic acid (AMPA) types of glutamate receptors, or from the release of ER-Ca^{2+} stores through activation of metabotropic receptors (78–81). Receptor-mediated Ca^{2+} increases play roles in neurotransmission (82), but can also cause cellular degeneration in acute and chronic CNS diseases. Prolonged and/or intense activation of NMDA receptors is a central mechanism that underlies acute neuronal injury during stroke, trauma, and epilepsy and may also be responsible for chronic neurodegeneration in Alzheimer's disease, Huntington's disease, amyotrophic lateral sclerosis, and HIV encephalopathies (**Figure 3**) (83–87). It is now known that oligodendrocytes and astrocytes in certain regions of the brain possess glutamatergic receptors for AMPA and kainate types, activation of which may also contribute to tissue damage in stroke (88). Ca^{2+} influx through glial receptors is injurious in the setting of experimental autoimmune encephalomyelitis and may participate in the pathogenesis of human demyelinating disease (88).

The best-studied pathology involving Ca^{2+}-dependent cell damage in the CNS is glutamate excitotoxicity, in which ligation of glutamate receptors leads to unphysiological and sustained increases of cellular Ca^{2+}, and cell death. The most common disease paradigm is stroke, where increased synaptic vesicular release of glutamate, failure of cellular transporters, and release of glutamate from dying cells leads to high extracellular glutamate, activation of glutamate receptors, and influx of Na^{+} and Ca^{2+} (83, 84, 87). Though release of Ca^{2+} from ER stores and influx of Ca^{2+} through voltage-dependent Ca^{2+} channels and Na^{+}/Ca^{2+} exchangers (operating in reverse) may contribute, inward transport via synaptic as well as extrasynaptic glutamate receptors is the predominant mechanism for the increase in cytosolic Ca^{2+}.

In the affected environment, cells in the center of the ischemic zone are destined to die by necrosis because they are rapidly ATP-depleted and do not reperfuse. In the peripheral zone, also known as the penumbra, respiring cells with high levels of ATP are activated by glutamate released from dead and dying cells. In these cells, mitochondria are already energized, and $\Delta\psi m$ is the primary driving force behind mitochondrial Ca^{2+} uptake (89). In the presence of energy and continued receptor-mediated Ca^{2+} influx, uncontrolled voltage-driven Ca^{2+} uptake results in irreversible mitochondrial damage and loss of function, much like in cells

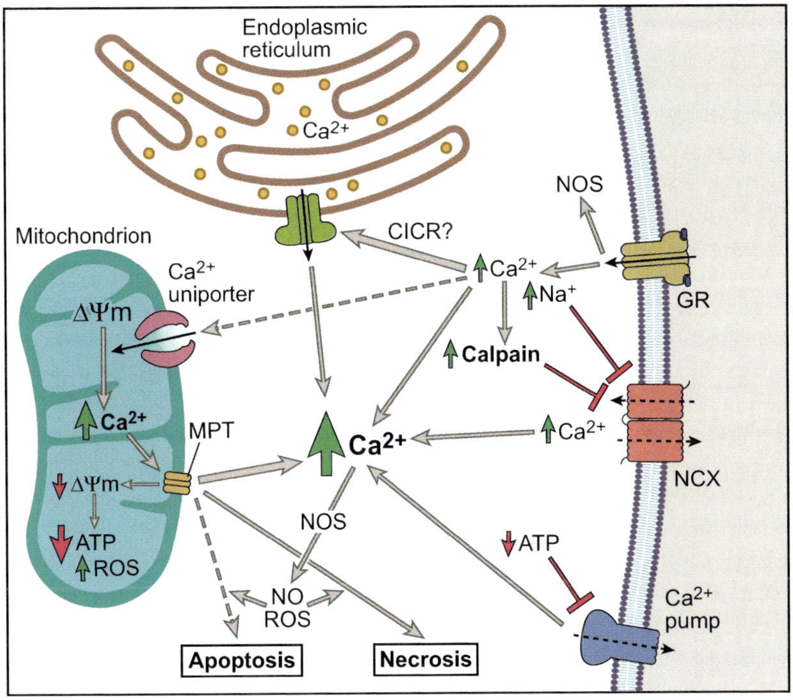

Figure 3

Excitotoxic injury in neurons. Binding of glutamate results in Na^+ and Ca^{2+} influx through plasma membrane glutamate receptors (GR). Consequently, cytosolic Na^+ and Ca^{2+} increase. Increased cytosolic Na^+ results in the consumption of adenosine triphosphate (ATP), and therefore decreases of the nucleotide. Increased Ca^{2+} leads to the activation of hydrolytic enzymes such as calpain. Ligation of glutamate to GR also stimulates production of nitric oxide (NO) by nitric oxide synthase (NOS). From the cytosol, Ca^{2+} is transported across the mitochondrial inner membranes through a Ca^{2+} uniporter into the mitochondrial matrix. This requires a proton-motive force (mitochondrial potential, $\Delta\psi m$) across the inner membrane. As long as $\Delta\psi m$ remains above threshold levels, and cytosolic Ca^{2+} is high, Ca^{2+} continues to be transported into the mitochondrial matrix. Increasing accumulation of Ca^{2+} leads to the formation of calcium precipitates within mitochondria, generation of reactive oxygen species (ROS), phospholipid hydrolysis, and, eventually, decrease of $\Delta\psi m$ and ATP, formation of mitochondrial permeability transition (MPT) pores in the inner membrane, and leakage of the accumulated Ca^{2+} back into the cytosol. Together with the failure of ATP-dependent Ca^{2+} pumps, and possibly with the participation of calcium-induced calcium release (CICR) from the endoplasmic reticulum, mitochondrial release of accumulated Ca^{2+} causes a catastrophic, delayed Ca^{2+} increase, which kills the cell. Increased cytosolic Na^+ may also be expected to inhibit Na^+ and Ca^{2+} exchange across the plasma membrane through the Na^+/Ca^{2+} exchanger (NCX) in the physiological mode, and, in addition, drive reverse exchange of Na^+ and Ca^{2+} and thus exacerbate Ca^{2+} increase in the cytosol. Proteolysis of the exchanger by calpain may also inhibit Na^+/Ca^{++} exchange. Depending on the intensity and speed of Ca^{2+}-dependent injury, determined in part by oxidant damage through ROS generation and concomitant NO production, cell death occurs by necrosis or apoptosis.

exposed to Ca^{2+} ionophores (89, 90). Receptor-mediated Ca^{2+} influx may preferentially couple with mitochondrial uptake because mitochondrial accumulation of the cation occurs at lower Ca^{2+} thresholds than for other types of Ca^{2+} channels (91). There is an initial glutamate-dependent cytosolic Ca^{2+} transient, followed after a significant delay by a sustained Ca^{2+} increase to micromolar levels in largely glutamate-independent fashion. Mitochondrial Ca^{2+} reaches millimolar levels, which results in depolarization and damage via a Ca^{2+}-dependent permeability transition, precipitation of calcium phosphate, and phospholipid hydrolysis (4, 90).

Recent work shows that the Na^+/Ca^{2+} exchanger of the plasma membrane is cleaved and inactivated by calpains during brain ischemia and neuronal excitotoxicity (92). Bano and colleagues (92) suggest that proteolytic inactivation of the Na^+/Ca^{2+} exchanger may play a large role in delayed Ca^{2+} increase and subsequent neuronal cell death (92). However, a review of all available information on the subject of neuronal excitotoxicity (89, 90, 93) still shows a predominant role for extreme mitochondrial calcium overload, development of MPT, and subsequent release of Ca^{2+} into the cytosol in the causation of delayed lethal Ca^{2+} increases. The attendant ATP depletion and homeostatic dysfunction kill the cell. Depending upon the circumstances, the pace and duration of the process, and the availability of ATP, cell death may be necrotic or apoptotic (94–96). Concurrent deregulation of the production and disposition of oxygen free radicals and NO metabolites and hydrolysis of proteins and phospholipids contribute to injury and cell demise as well. This type of damage is prevented not only by glutamate antagonism and prevention of Ca^{2+} fluxes, but also by initial depolarization of mitochondria by treatment with uncouplers (89, 97), which shows that $\Delta\psi$m-dependent Ca^{2+} uptake is indeed critical.

Several laboratories have investigated the possible relationships between Ca^{2+}-induced MPT, mitochondrial damage with cytochrome c release, and an apoptotic outcome. Cytochrome c is released from mitochondria and caspases activated during excitotoxic cell death (98, 99), but Bax and Bak, pro-apoptotic proteins that mediate mitochondrial cytochrome release during apoptosis, are not required for NMDA-mediated neuronal cell death (100). Bid, another pro-apoptotic Bcl-2 family member, has been implicated in neuronal cell death and tissue damage in experimental models of focal cerebral ischemia (101, 102). However, it is possible that severe structural damage in mitochondria that follows Ca^{2+}-induced MPT is sufficient to cause cytochrome c release secondarily. In support of this, MPT inhibitors were shown to prevent cytochrome c release not only from isolated mitochondria with Ca^{2+}-induced MPT, but also in intact cells with glutamate excitotoxicity (98). Experiments suggested that outer-membrane rupture following MPT is probably a major route for the release of mitochondrial proteins (98). The occupation of receptors by low concentrations of ligand may be followed by authentic delayed apoptosis, but the roles played by Ca^{2+}, Bcl-2 family proteins, and cytochrome c–initiated processes under these conditions remain to be investigated.

Mitochondrial pathology involving disordered Ca^{2+} homeostasis is receiving attention in research on chronic neurodegenerative diseases, but cause-and-effect relationships remain unproven. Glutamate excitotoxicity, abnormal Ca^{2+} buffering by binding proteins, free radical–mediated Ca^{2+} release from the ER, and Ca^{2+} fluxes caused by amyloid peptides are among the mechanisms that may mediate chronic toxicity in the CNS, but these issues are beyond the scope of this review.

A review of calcium in cell injury and death would be incomplete without emphasizing the seemingly paradoxical roles played by Ca^{2+} in physiological states and CNS disease. Glutamatergic neurotransmission—dependent upon cytosolic and nuclear Ca^{2+}-dependent signaling by calcium/calmodulin-dependent kinase IV, ras-extracellular signal–regulated kinase 1/2 pathway, and cyclic adenosine monophosphate response element binding protein (CREB)-dependent transcription of brain-derived neurotropic factor—is essential for neuronal survival (103). Thus, it is important to differentiate between physiological Ca^{2+} transients mediated by synaptic glutamatergic neurotransmission needed for survival, antagonism of which causes cell death by apoptosis, and the more sustained and larger Ca^{2+} increases that result from pathological ligation of extrasynaptic and synaptic glutamatergic receptors (103).

MYOCARDIUM

A major role for Ca^{2+} in the cellular pathology of myocardial infarction was suggested in the seminal work of Shen & Jennings, who found that irreversible mitochondrial damage and cell death during reperfusion injury in the heart are accompanied by the formation of calcium precipitates in the mitochondrial matrix (104). Subsequent work by Ganote and colleagues revealed that treatment with cyanide delayed cell death during reperfusion, implicating resumption of respiration as a pathogenic factor that may tip the balance between survival and death of cells injured sublethally by ischemia (105). These observations led to a line of thinking that lethality is determined by pathological Ca^{2+} transport into mitochondria, driven by $\Delta\psi m$ sustained either by reverse operation of the ATP synthase F_1F_0-ATPase during ischemia/hypoxia and/or by respiration during reperfusion or reoxygenation (**Figure 4**). A large body of work has confirmed this hypothesis (24, 106–108).

The predominant role of $\Delta\psi m$ in mitochondrial Ca^{2+} transport is key to the concept outlined in the preceding paragraph. Mitochondria participate in Ca^{2+} homeostasis by controlling $\Delta\psi m$-dependent Ca^{2+} uptake, thereby keeping intracellular free Ca^{2+} at low levels. However, mitochondrial content of the ion does not approach toxic concentrations in normal cells, as the dynamic range of Ca^{2+} in the cytosol rarely exceeds nanomolar levels. During ischemia, intracellular Na^+ rises markedly owing to failure of the plasma-membrane sodium pump, and free cytosolic Ca^{2+} increases to micromolar concentrations owing to cessation of Ca^{2+} pumping by Ca^{2+} ATPases in the plasma membrane and SR. Because intracellular Na^+ is high, normal operation of the Na^+/Ca^{2+} exchanger is also inhibited, and this transport mechanism may in fact operate in reverse, contributing to the rise of cytosolic Ca^{2+}. Under these conditions, if mitochondria can maintain a proton gradient across their inner membranes and thus $\Delta\psi m$, Ca^{2+} influx can lead to increases of mitochondrial matrix Ca^{2+} that open MPT pores (109–111). MPT pore opening is also favored by increased nonesterified fatty acids (112), which are expected to increase during ischemia owing to increased phospholipase activity (113).

ADP: adenosine diphosphate

The relationship between $\Delta\psi m$ and the MPT is complex in that decrease of $\Delta\psi m$ also lowers the Ca^{2+} threshold required for the MPT (25, 108). However, because $\Delta\psi m$ drives Ca^{2+} uptake, the most severe decreases of $\Delta\psi m$ will retard the development of the MPT by limiting increases of mitochondrial matrix Ca^{2+}. Whether sufficiently high mitochondrial Ca^{2+} concentrations to induce the MPT are reached during hypoxia/ischemia is dependent upon the extent to which $\Delta\psi m$ is retained, and this, in turn, is determined largely by the availability of ATP. If ATP declines slowly during ischemia, and particularly if ischemic cardiomyocytes generate energy by glycolysis, ATP is hydrolyzed by mitochondrial F_1F_0-ATPase to maintain $\Delta\psi m$. This notion is supported by studies of perfused hearts and isolated cardiomyocytes (110, 111). During ischemia, low pH, increased Mg^{2+}, and adenosine diphosphate (ADP) lower the probability of pore opening (106, 107).

During reperfusion, resumption of respiration in damaged cardiomyocytes increases $\Delta\psi m$. For cells that are still viable at the end of ischemia, but are damaged to a sufficient degree, there are two possible outcomes. If ATP synthesis is commensurate with recovery of Ca^{2+} homeostasis, the ions are pumped out of cells and into the SR, mitochondria avoid Ca^{2+} overload, and cells recover. If the energy status is unstable, cytosolic Ca^{2+} remains elevated, and mitochondria continue to take up Ca^{2+} because $\Delta\psi m$ is maintained to some degree by respiration. In this case, a lethal outcome is inevitable. Increased Ca^{2+}, formation

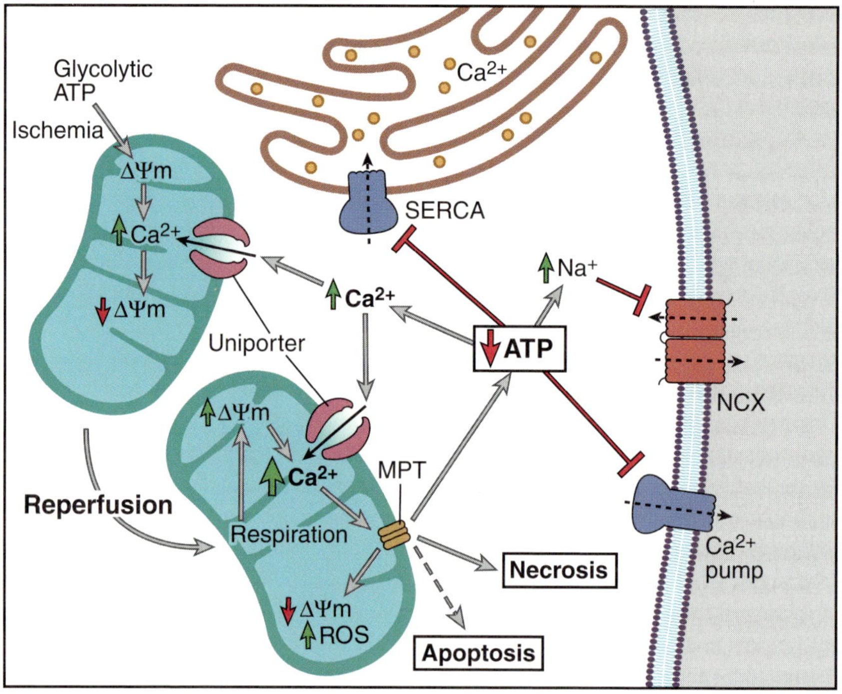

Figure 4

Ischemia-reperfusion injury of the heart. Ischemia leads to decreased adenosine triphosphate (ATP) in cells. ATP declines result in decreased activities of the Ca^{2+} pump in the plasma membrane and sarco-endoplasmic reticulum calcium ATPase (SERCA) in the sarcoplasmic reticulum and increase of intracellular sodium (Na^+) caused by failure of the sodium pump. Operation of the Na^+/Ca^{2+} exchanger (NCX) in the physiological mode is inhibited, and the exchanger may operate in reverse. Together, these events result in increase of cytosolic Ca^{2+}. Steep declines of mitochondrial potential ($\Delta\psi m$) are prevented by generation of glycolytic ATP, which is transported into mitochondria and utilized by ATP synthase operating in reverse as an ATPase to extrude protons. Preserved to some extent during ischemia, $\Delta\psi m$ drives Ca^{2+} influx into mitochondria through Ca^{2+} uniporters. Increase of Ca^{2+} in the mitochondrial matrix causes phospholipid hydrolysis with increase of nonesterified fatty acids and generation of reactive oxygen species (ROS). These events, and the direct effects of increased Ca^{2+}, may lead to the formation of mitochondrial permeability transition pores (MPT), although this destructive event is more likely to occur during reperfusion. $\Delta\psi m$ declines slowly during ischemia even in the absence of MPT. Resumption of respiration during reperfusion leads to increases of $\Delta\psi m$ in sublethally damaged mitochondria; $\Delta\psi m$-driven Ca^{2+} influx and the consequent large increases of mitochondrial Ca^{2+}, in conjunction with ROS and the damaging effects of nonesterified fatty acids resulting from phospholipid hydrolysis, deliver the coup de grace by promoting the development of MPT pores. Loss of mitochondrial function, further declines of ATP, and irreversible failure of Ca^{2+} homeostasis result in cell death by necrosis or, less commonly, by apoptosis.

of oxygen free radicals and increased Ca^{2+}-independent phospholipase A2 activity (113) together conspire to keep MPT pores open permanently (24, 106–108). A critical role for injurious $\Delta\psi m$-driven Ca^{2+} influx is demonstrated by interventions that completely depolarize mitochondria and thereby preempt Ca^{2+} fluxes and MPT. Such interventions dramatically delay or prevent cell death during reperfusion after experimental ischemia or hypoxia (108, 114), as do other maneuvers that prevent cellular and mitochondrial Ca^{2+} overload (106, 115). Cell death following MPT induction is usually necrotic, but has been associated with cytochrome c release from mitochondria and caspase activation, suggesting that apoptotic outcomes are also possible (115–117). Investigators have also found a role for calpain-mediated Bid activation following Ca^{2+} increases in mitochondrial damage and cell death during myocardial ischemia-reperfusion (35, 118).

This review considered earlier that mitochondrial ATP synthase F_1F_0-ATPase can hydrolyze glycolytic ATP to maintain $\Delta\psi m$ and drive mitochondrial Ca^{2+} influx. This mode of proton extrusion during ischemia, which can compromise the energy status further, has been referred to as cellular treason (119). These considerations are relevant to understanding the basis for protection afforded by ischemic preconditioning or stunning, interventions that significantly reduce lethal damage during subsequent ischemic episodes that may otherwise be lethal (106, 107, 110). At least in part, the protective activity of brief nonlethal periods of ischemia and agents such as diazoxide, which acts on mitochondrial ATP-sensitive K^+ channels, may be mediated by effects to limit the supply of ATP to the mitochondrial matrix for hydrolysis by the F_1F_0-ATPase during ischemia, thus decreasing $\Delta\psi m$ and Ca^{2+} accumulation and preventing Ca^{2+} overload. In this fashion, these interventions prevent MPT, and preserve the cellular nucleotide pool to promote recovery as reperfusion progresses (120, 121). Indeed, the extent of F_1F_0-ATPase activity during ischemia/hypoxia, affected by factors such as inhibitory binding proteins, may also determine the susceptibility of cardiac cells to ischemic injury in diverse species (122). Not surprisingly, current research in developing pharmacological interventions to diminish ischemic damage in myocardial cells focuses on drugs that modify ion-channel activity in the plasma membrane, SR, and mitochondrial membranes (115).

Another unique effect of Ca^{2+} overload in the reperfused heart is the occurrence of Ca^{2+}-mediated hypercontractures in cells that have been damaged sublethally during ischemia. These abnormal contractions in cells with membranes made fragile by ischemia-induced cytoskeletal defects (123, 124), loss of dystrophin (124), and Ca^{2+}-independent phospholipid hydrolysis (125) are thought to deliver a Ca^{2+}-dependent coup de grace by inducing sarcolemmal blebbing and rupture (123). As myocardial cells become ischemic, ATP is reduced but continues to be available for a short period of time. These partial reductions induce Ca^{2+}-independent rigor contractures before energy stores become totally depleted (123). Such contractures and associated cytosolic Ca^{2+} overloads predispose cardiomyocytes to develop so-called contraction band necrosis during reperfusion, which is spurred by nascent generation of ATP (126). This type of necrosis is characterized by supercontracted sarcomeres with zones of elongation in between (**Figure 5**). In any

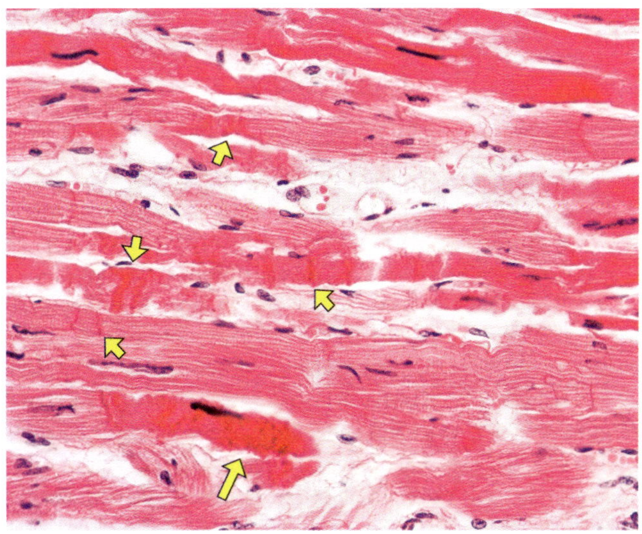

Figure 5

Section of a paraffin-embedded heart from an autopsied case of myocardial infarction showing contraction band necrosis. Several myocardial fibers exhibit dark eosinophilic bands spanning the entire width of the sarcoplasm. These bands vary in thickness and represent irregular Ca^{2+}-induced contractions during reperfusion, with the collapse of several to many sarcomeres upon themselves in the axial plane (*short yellow arrows*). Such violent contractures and the consequent pathological stretching of the sarcoplasm in between are responsible for the rupture of the sarcolemma (electron microscopy would be required to visualize the sarcolemmal pathology). A dead cardiomyocyte with condensed nucleus and severe contraction banding is indicated by the long arrow.

case, Ca^{2+} overload and regeneration of ATP are together responsible for uncontrolled, irregular contractions that mechanically tear the weakened sarcolemma. Ongoing influx of Ca^{2+} across the sarcolemma and cyclic influx into and efflux of Ca^{2+} from the SR are thought to underlie the Ca^{2+} overload contractures during reperfusion, and this mechanism is also being investigated as a target for amelioration of ischemic damage by pharmacological intervention (123).

KIDNEY

Abnormal Ca^{2+} influx and loss of cellular homeostasis have been invoked as potential pathogenic factors in kidney epithelial cell injury and cell death for more than two decades. Ca^{2+} channel antagonists have been used as putative protective agents to ameliorate ischemic/hypoxic injury (31, 127–132). However, investigation of the role played by Ca^{2+} in cell injury is fraught with pitfalls in its technical aspects and interpretation of data. Thus, the initial belief that there is a causal relationship between cytosolic Ca^{2+} increases and death of kidney cells during injury by ATP depletion/ischemia/hypoxia has been contradicted, and putative relationships between Ca^{2+} increases, mitochondrial depolarization, and cell death have been dissociated (133–135). Much of the current understanding of the relationships between Ca^{2+} and epithelial cell injury in the kidney is derived from studies on freshly isolated rabbit or rat proximal tubules, the nephron segments that bear the brunt of renal ischemic injury, and cultured kidney epithelial cells (76, 77). Failure of ion homeostasis during ischemic damage of the kidney is attributable to steep declines of ATP caused by rapid consumption of the nucleotide by transport systems in the face of failed oxidative phosphorylation, and, in the case of the well-studied proximal tubule epithelium, little or no generation of ATP by anaerobic glycolysis. Lack of energy leads to failure of ion transport, and, as outlined for the ischemic cardiomyocyte, several mechanisms contribute to the observed increases of cytosolic Ca^{2+}.

As discussed above, the use of glycine and structurally related amino acids as experimental tools that prevent the formation of glycine-sensitive pores in the plasma membrane has permitted meaningful studies of Ca^{2+} increases and their effects on cells during ATP depletion. In vivo, normal extracellular glycine concentration is borderline with respect to what would be required to prevent ATP depletion–induced membrane pore formation (136). Energy-dependent gradients of intracellular glycine (10–20 mM) are dissipated during hypoxia/ischemia (136), but total tissue concentrations do not change (137). Therefore, extracellular glycine concentrations remain above fully protective levels, preventing lethal membrane damage. The question of what happens during reperfusion remains unknown as increased ischemic levels of extracellular glycine may be "washed out" as blood flow returns and restores the borderline levels of the normal state. However, it has become clear that in vitro experiments in which cells are subjected to hypoxia/reoxygenation in the absence of glycine can yield spurious information regarding a variety of factors that impact injury and death in vivo, including the effects of Ca^{2+}. In large part, spurious interpretations of data arise from the failure to discriminate between prelethal pathogenic events and postmortem degenerations. Such methodological considerations probably underlie contradictions among published observations on the effects of agents and interventions designed to protect hypoxic cells from the deleterious effects of cytosolic Ca^{2+} increases.

Increases of free cytosolic Ca^{2+} to upper nanomolar ranges were shown to occur in metabolic inhibitor-treated rabbit proximal tubule cells and hypoxic rat proximal tubule cells using Fura-2 (129, 138); high affinity of this dye for Ca^{2+} limits accurate measurements within this range only. Measured by the low-affinity Ca^{2+} binding dyes Mag Fura-2 and Fura-2FF, free cytosolic Ca^{2+}

elevations to concentrations greater than 100 μM were shown to occur in proximal tubule cells depleted of ATP by hypoxia or respiratory blockade by Antimycin A (76); following hypoxia, the increases were fully reversible under metabolically favorable reoxygenation conditions (76). These observations indicate that hypoxic, ATP-depleted proximal tubule cells are remarkably resistant to the toxic effects of elevated cytosolic Ca^{2+} when considered in the reversibility context of these substantial calcium increases, commonly assumed ionized Ca^{2+} requirements for membrane phospholipid hydrolysis and cytoskeletal disruption, and the structural integrity maintained by hypoxic tubules with Ca^{2+} elevations (139–142). Other studies on MDCK cells confirm such observations (77).

Cultured MDCK cells depleted totally of ATP by concurrent inhibition of respiration and glycolysis resist concentrations of up to 100-μM free Ca^{2+} calcium for three hours, attested to by structural preservation and viability as measured by the ability to proliferate thereafter; cell death with Ca^{2+}-induced DNA breakdown and widespread cell damage occurs only when cytosolic free Ca^{2+} is adjusted to levels greater than 100 μM (77). These experiments argue that the biochemical and structural alterations that occur in hypoxic/ATP-depleted kidney epithelial cells with large and sustained reversible Ca^{2+} increases need not be lethal. Subsequent observations of rabbit proximal tubules that sustained major Ca^{2+} increases during hypoxia reveal the occurrence of respiratory defects and compromised ability to restore $\Delta\psi m$ in mitochondria during reoxygenation (143–146). Nevertheless, if the tubules were supplemented with specific citric acid cycle metabolites during the reoxygenation period, the affected mitochondria retained a degree of structural and functional integrity that permitted recovery of respiration, oxidative phosphorylation, and $\Delta\psi m$ (143–146).

These findings indicate that mitochondria in proximal tubules that had been energetically compromised by hypoxia do not undergo irreversible MPT, unlike reoxygenated cardiomyocytes, and that metabolic interventions can repair and reverse the hypoxic mitochondrial defects. They also show that mitochondria with persistently impaired function during reoxygenation recover without injury if appropriate measures are taken during this period (146). Protection afforded to mitochondria in this manner is associated with the recovery of entire tubule cells, as assessed by structural, biochemical, and functional criteria (143–146). Proximal tubules depleted of ATP by hypoxia or respiratory blockers exhibit marked elevations of nonesterified (free) fatty acids (NEFA) derived from phospholipid hydrolysis (133). NEFA are protonophoric, uncouple mitochondria and promote the MPT (112). The increases of NEFA in the tubule cells are predominantly Ca^{2+} independent (133). NEFA elevations persist for up to two hours of reoxygenation and correlate with persistently impaired recovery of $\Delta\psi m$; both defects are corrected if protective citric acid cycle substrates are provided during reoxygenation (150). Moreover, if NEFA are scavenged by the provision of fatty acid free albumin, $\Delta\psi m$ is fully restored (150).

NEFA: nonesterified fatty acids

The resistance of the tubule cell mitochondria to developing the MPT for long periods of time is remarkable in light of these observations on the lowering of $\Delta\psi m$ by NEFA and the large elevations of cytosolic Ca^{2+} that develop. In cardiomyocytes, hypoxic declines of $\Delta\psi m$ are slow, permitting Ca^{2+} transport, and recovery of $\Delta\psi m$ during reoxygenation can accelerate Ca^{2+} uptake catastrophically to the point where MPT is triggered, thereby killing a subpopulation of cells (24, 106–108). Unlike cardiomyocytes, proximal tubule cells can utilize glucose minimally (straight segments) or not at all (convoluted segments) for anaerobic energy metabolism (147, 148), and their ATP content falls steeply within seconds when respiration is compromised (149). Thus, it is doubtful that mitochondria in this cell type can mount $\Delta\psi m$ to a meaningful extent or substantially transport Ca^{2+} during hypoxia or ischemia (**Figure 6**). What keeps

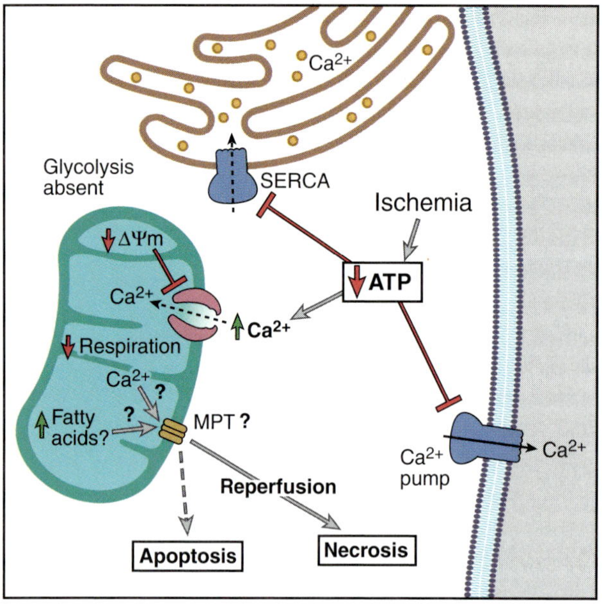

Figure 6

Ischemia-reperfusion injury of kidney proximal tubule. Unlike cardiomyocytes, proximal tubule cells have little to no capacity for anaerobic glycolysis. Acting together with rapid consumption of adenosine triphosphate (ATP) by a well-developed transport system, ischemia-associated cessation of oxidative phosphorylation and lack of glycolysis induce precipitous declines of cell ATP within seconds after the onset of ischemia. Declines of the nucleotide result in inhibition of the plasma membrane Ca^{2+} pump and sarco-endoplasmic reticulum calcium ATPase (SERCA). Together, these events result in large increases of cytosolic Ca^{2+}. Owing to the cessation of mitochondrial electron transport and lack of glycolytic ATP, mitochondrial potential ($\Delta\psi m$) falls steeply in magnitude. Although cytosolic Ca^{2+} is high, it is not actively transported through Ca^{2+} uniporters into mitochondria, owing to steep $\Delta\psi m$ declines. Intramitochondrial Ca^{2+} rises slowly by passive diffusion alone, and the concentrations do not exceed those present in the cytosol. Although cytosolic concentrations of Ca^{2+} reach levels in the range of $\sim$100 μM, cells are injured only reversibly, and lethal mitochondrial damage by formation of mitochondrial permeability transition (MPT) pores is a late event that occurs only if ischemia is not relieved. During reperfusion, mitochondria may show persistent respiratory defects, but do not undergo irreversible MPT unless the preceding duration of ischemia has been unduly prolonged or if reperfusion is also allowed to proceed in the absence of metabolic interventions that allow the mitochondria to recover normal respiration. Thus, compared with cardiomyocytes and neurons, proximal tubule cells are relatively resistant to large increases of Ca^{2+}. In large part, this resistance is likely to be due to the lack of $\Delta\psi m$-driven transport of Ca^{2+} to the much higher mitochondrial concentrations required to open MPT pores permanently. A persistent increase of nonesterified fatty acids in mitochondria and resulting respiratory defect, rather than a Ca^{2+}-induced MPT, ultimately determines lethality, unless the cells are rescued by protective metabolic interventions. With reperfusion of lethally damaged tubule cells, cell death commonly occurs by necrosis.

matrix Ca^{2+} below the threshold needed to trigger MPT during reoxygenation in the tubules is less clear because $\Delta\psi m$ recovers partially at that time to a degree that could allow some Ca^{2+} uptake despite the increased levels of NEFA. The levels reached possibly remain subthreshold because of limited net cell influx of Ca^{2+}. In this regard it is also relevant that conditions present naturally during injury, i.e., increased levels of free Mg^{2+}, high levels of ADP, and decreased pH, all serve to increase the Ca^{2+} threshold for MPT development (66, 114), and it is conceivable that there are differences from the heart with respect to the mitochondrial membrane proteins that form the MPT pore and how these proteins are regulated.

Segments other than proximal tubules of the nephron are vigorously glycolytic and are much less sensitive to necrotic damage after in vivo ischemia. The distal nephron-derived MDCK cell line develops increased levels of cytosolic free Ca^{2+} after ATP depletion produced by metabolic inhibition combined with glucose deprivation (151), and displays mitochondrial calcium uptake despite de-energization mediated by reversal of Na^+/Ca^{2+} exchange (152). However, the full role of Ca^{2+} alterations during injury to these cells is incompletely defined. The availability of glycolysis and the scarcity of necrosis in vivo indicate that apoptosis is the predominant process for lethal injury of distal nephron cells in vivo.

Despite the lack of evidence of a decisive role for Ca^{2+} in the pathogenesis of lethal tubule cell injury, Ca^{2+}-dependent, nonlethal cell damage is a factor in organ dysfunction (31). Thus, even in the presence of glycine, increases of cytosolic Ca^{2+} were shown to induce increased calpain activity (153) and cytoskeletal pathology (140), which may result in cellular dysfunction during ischemic acute renal failure. Other morphological, biochemical, and functional studies in glycine-protected cells under conditions where cytosolic Ca^{2+} is elevated agree with this assumption (77, 133, 140–142, 154). Mitochondrial calcium overload occurs prominently in the kidney as a postlethal event, and its occurrence explains increases of tissue calcium levels seen at that time, which may contribute to chronic tubulointerstitial damage (127, 155).

CONCLUDING REMARKS

Disturbances of Ca^{2+} concentrations play an important role in cell injury and death, but as with the field in general, it is more complex than originally conceived, highly nuanced in its expression in different cell types, and not predictable simply from its normal physiology. Given the potentially catastrophic effects of Ca^{2+} dysregulation, and the exquisite control over cell-death processes that have become evident in recent years, it is not surprising that the systems have evolved in this fashion.

SUMMARY POINTS

1. Mammalian cells possess a complex system that maintains Ca^{2+} homeostasis, the loss of which may lead to cell injury and tissue damage.
2. Perturbation of Ca^{2+} homeostasis activates multiple destructive processes that target subcellular structures, including the plasma membrane, cytoskeleton, mitochondria, and nucleus.
3. Mitochondrial damage involving pore defects in the inner and outer membranes is a critical determinant of cell injury and death during Ca^{2+} cytotoxicity.
4. Whether cells are energized to maintain $\Delta\psi m$ determines Ca^{2+} uptake by mitochondria and subsequent MPT and cell death.
5. The roles played by $\Delta\psi m$, mitochondrial Ca^{2+} uptake, and MPT in Ca^{2+} cytotoxicity are illustrated by cell injury and death during ischemic injury of the brain, heart, and kidneys.

FUTURE DIRECTIONS/UNRESOLVED ISSUES

1. Further studies are needed to precisely identify "the point of no return" in diverse injury systems, although MPT is known to have a prominent role in Ca^{2+} cytotoxicity.
2. Despite intensive investigations of MPT, the nature, properties, and regulation of the MPT pore remain largely unknown.
3. Whether mitochondrial outer-membrane damage develops independently or as a result of MPT during Ca^{2+} cytotoxicity remains to be determined.
4. Gene expression and deletion studies have suggested that Bcl-2 family proteins regulate ER Ca^{2+} and determine Ca^{2+} uptake by mitochondria during cell injury. It is unclear whether these findings are applicable to in vivo situations.
5. Ca^{2+} cytotoxicity is difficult to determine in vivo. Pharmacological approaches may affect cell injury and death directly via their effects on parenchymal cells or indirectly via vascular effects.

6. Ca^{2+}-independent mechanisms of cell injury are set in motion concurrently with Ca^{2+} cytotoxicity under pathological conditions. Our understanding of these mechanisms is very limited.

ACKNOWLEDGMENTS

The authors would like to acknowledge past and continued grant support for their work from the National Institutes of Health, Veterans Administration, American Heart Association, and National Kidney Foundation.

LITERATURE CITED

1. Schanne FA, Kane AB, Young EE, Farber JL. 1979. Calcium dependence of toxic cell death: a final common pathway. *Science* 206:700–2
2. Farber JL, Chien KR, Mittnacht S Jr. 1981. Myocardial ischemia: the pathogenesis of irreversible cell injury in ischemia. *Am. J. Pathol.* 102:271–81
3. Trump BF, Berezesky IK. 1995. Calcium-mediated cell injury and cell death. *FASEB J.* 9:219–28
4. Kristian T, Siesjo BK. 1998. Calcium in ischemic cell death. *Stroke* 29:705–18
5. **Berridge MJ, Bootman MD, Roderick HL. 2003. Calcium signalling: dynamics, homeostasis and remodelling. *Nat. Rev. Mol. Cell Biol.* 4:517–29**

A comprehensive review of calcium homeostasis and signaling.

6. Carafoli E, Santella L, Branca D, Brini M. 2001. Generation, control, and processing of cellular calcium signals. *Crit. Rev. Biochem. Mol. Biol.* 36:107–260
7. Patterson RL, Boehning D, Snyder SH. 2004. Inositol 1,4,5-trisphosphate receptors as signal integrators. *Annu. Rev. Biochem.* 73:437–65
8. Meissner G. 2004. Molecular regulation of cardiac ryanodine receptor ion channel. *Cell Calcium* 35:621–28
9. Duchen MR. 2000. Mitochondria and calcium: from cell signalling to cell death. *J. Physiol.* 529(Pt. 1):57–68
10. Rizzuto R, Duchen MR, Pozzan T. 2004. Flirting in little space: the ER/mitochondria Ca^{2+} liaison. *Science STKE* 2004:re1
11. Gunter TE, Yule DI, Gunter KK, Eliseev RA, Salter JD. 2004. Calcium and mitochondria. *FEBS Lett.* 567:96–102
12. Kirichok Y, Krapivinsky G, Clapham DE. 2004. The mitochondrial calcium uniporter is a highly selective ion channel. *Nature* 427:360–64
13. Hardingham GE, Cruzalegui FH, Chawla S, Bading H. 1998. Mechanisms controlling gene expression by nuclear calcium signals. *Cell Calcium* 23:131–34
14. Allbritton NL, Oancea E, Kuhn MA, Meyer T. 1994. Source of nuclear calcium signals. *Proc. Natl. Acad. Sci. USA* 91:12458–62
15. Badminton MN, Campbell AK, Rembold CM. 1996. Differential regulation of nuclear and cytosolic Ca^{2+} in HeLa cells. *J. Biol. Chem.* 271:31210–14
16. Mazzanti M, DeFelice LJ, Cohn J, Malter H. 1990. Ion channels in the nuclear envelope. *Nature* 343:764–67
17. Smith MT, Thor H, Orrenius S. 1981. Toxic injury to isolated hepatocytes is not dependent on extracellular calcium. *Science* 213:1257–59

18. Koike T, Martin DP, Johnson EM Jr. 1989. Role of Ca^{2+} channels in the ability of membrane depolarization to prevent neuronal death induced by trophic-factor deprivation: evidence that levels of internal Ca^{2+} determine nerve growth factor dependence of sympathetic ganglion cells. *Proc. Natl. Acad. Sci. USA* 86:6421–25
19. Johnson EM Jr, Koike T, Franklin J. 1992. A "calcium set-point hypothesis" of neuronal dependence on neurotrophic factor. *Exp. Neurol.* 115:163–66
20. Rao RV, Ellerby HM, Bredesen DE. 2004. Coupling endoplasmic reticulum stress to the cell death program. *Cell Death Differ.* 11:372–80
21. Kotlikoff MI. 2003. Calcium-induced calcium release in smooth muscle: the case for loose coupling. *Prog. Biophys. Mol. Biol.* 83:171–91
22. Putney JW Jr, Broad LM, Braun FJ, Lievremont JP, Bird GS. 2001. Mechanisms of capacitative calcium entry. *J. Cell. Sci.* 114:2223–29
23. **Orrenius S, Zhivotovsky B, Nicotera P. 2003. Regulation of cell death: the calcium-apoptosis link. *Nat. Rev. Mol. Cell Biol.* 4:552–65**

Summarizes a large body of information about calcium disturbances and cell death.

24. Crompton M. 1999. The mitochondrial permeability transition pore and its role in cell death. *Biochem. J.* 341(Pt. 2):233–49
25. Bernardi P. 1999. Mitochondrial transport of cations: channels, exchangers, and permeability transition. *Physiol. Rev.* 79:1127–55
26. Lemasters JJ, Nieminen AL, Qian T, Trost LC, Elmore SP, et al. 1998. The mitochondrial permeability transition in cell death: a common mechanism in necrosis, apoptosis and autophagy. *Biochim. Biophys. Acta* 1366:177–96
27. Bonventre JV, Huang Z, Taheri MR, O'Leary E, Li E, et al. 1997. Reduced fertility and postischaemic brain injury in mice deficient in cytosolic phospholipase A2. *Nature* 390:622–25
28. Goll DE, Thompson VF, Li H, Wei W, Cong J. 2003. The calpain system. *Physiol. Rev.* 83:731–801
29. Vanderklish PW, Bahr BA. 2000. The pathogenic activation of calpain: a marker and mediator of cellular toxicity and disease states. *Int. J. Exp. Pathol.* 81:323–39
30. Liu X, Van Vleet T, Schnellmann RG. 2004. The role of calpain in oncotic cell death. *Annu. Rev. Pharmacol. Toxicol.* 44:349–70
31. Edelstein CL, Ling H, Schrier RW. 1997. The nature of renal cell injury. *Kidney Int.* 51:1341–51
32. Nakagawa T, Yuan J. 2000. Cross-talk between two cysteine protease families. Activation of caspase-12 by calpain in apoptosis. *J. Cell. Biol.* 150:887–94
33. Ling YH, Liebes L, Ng B, Buckley M, Elliott PJ, et al. 2002. PS-341, a novel proteasome inhibitor, induces Bcl-2 phosphorylation and cleavage in association with G2-M phase arrest and apoptosis. *Mol. Cancer Ther.* 1:841–49
34. Cartron PF, Oliver L, Juin P, Meflah K, Vallette FM. 2004. The p18 truncated form of Bax behaves like a Bcl-2 homology domain 3-only protein. *J. Biol. Chem.* 279:11503–12
35. Chen M, He H, Zhan S, Krajewski S, Reed JC, Gottlieb RA. 2001. Bid is cleaved by calpain to an active fragment in vitro and during myocardial ischemia/reperfusion. *J. Biol. Chem.* 276:30724–28
36. Neumar RW, Xu YA, Gada H, Guttmann RP, Siman R. 2003. Cross-talk between calpain and caspase proteolytic systems during neuronal apoptosis. *J. Biol. Chem.* 278:14162–67
37. Liu X, Zou H, Slaughter C, Wang X. 1997. DFF, a heterodimeric protein that functions downstream of caspase-3 to trigger DNA fragmentation during apoptosis. *Cell* 89:175–84

38. Hughes FM Jr, Evans-Storms RB, Cidlowski JA. 1998. Evidence that non-caspase proteases are required for chromatin degradation during apoptosis. *Cell Death Differ.* 5:1017–27
39. Leist M, Jaattela M. 2001. Four deaths and a funeral: from caspases to alternative mechanisms. *Nat. Rev. Mol. Cell Biol.* 2:589–98
40. **Nieminen AL. 2003. Apoptosis and necrosis in health and disease: role of mitochondria. *Int. Rev. Cytol.* 224:29–55**

A comprehensive review of the mitochondrial role in calcium-induced cell injury.

41. Saikumar P, Dong Z, Patel Y, Hall K, Hopfer U, et al. 1998. Role of hypoxia-induced Bax translocation and cytochrome c release in reoxygenation injury. *Oncogene* 17:3401–15
42. Leist M, Single B, Castoldi AF, Kuhnle S, Nicotera P. 1997. Intracellular adenosine triphosphate (ATP) concentration: a switch in the decision between apoptosis and necrosis. *J. Exp. Med.* 185:1481–86
43. Nakagawa T, Zhu H, Morishima N, Li E, Xu J, et al. 2000. Caspase-12 mediates endoplasmic-reticulum-specific apoptosis and cytotoxicity by amyloid-beta. *Nature* 403:98–103
44. Mandic A, Hansson J, Linder S, Shoshan MC. 2003. Cisplatin induces endoplasmic reticulum stress and nucleus-independent apoptotic signaling. *J. Biol. Chem.* 278:9100–6
45. Green DR, Kroemer G. 2004. The pathophysiology of mitochondrial cell death. *Science* 305:626–29
46. Liu X, Kim CN, Yang J, Jemmerson R, Wang X. 1996. Induction of apoptotic program in cell-free extracts: requirement for dATP and cytochrome c. *Cell* 86:147–57
47. Martinou JC, Green DR. 2001. Breaking the mitochondrial barrier. *Nat. Rev. Mol. Cell Biol.* 2:63–67
48. Wei MC, Zong WX, Cheng EH, Lindsten T, Panoutsakopoulou V, et al. 2001. Proapoptotic BAX and BAK: a requisite gateway to mitochondrial dysfunction and death. *Science* 292:727–30
49. Kuwana T, Mackey MR, Perkins G, Ellisman MH, Latterich M, et al. 2002. Bid, Bax, and lipids cooperate to form supramolecular openings in the outer mitochondrial membrane. *Cell* 111:331–42
50. Mikhailov V, Mikhailova M, Degenhardt K, Venkatachalam MA, White E, Saikumar P. 2003. Association of Bax and Bak homo-oligomers in mitochondria. Bax requirement for Bak reorganization and cytochrome c release. *J. Biol. Chem.* 278:5367–76
51. Antonsson B. 2004. Mitochondria and the Bcl-2 family proteins in apoptosis signaling pathways. *Mol. Cell. Biochem.* 256/257:141–55
52. Danial NN, Korsmeyer SJ. 2004. Cell death: critical control points. *Cell* 116:205–19
53. Zamzami N, Kroemer G. 2001. The mitochondrion in apoptosis: how Pandora's box opens. *Nat. Rev. Mol. Cell Biol.* 2:67–71
54. Bossy-Wetzel E, Newmeyer DD, Green DR. 1998. Mitochondrial cytochrome c release in apoptosis occurs upstream of DEVD-specific caspase activation and independently of mitochondrial transmembrane depolarization. *EMBO J.* 17:37–49
55. Yang J, Liu X, Bhalla K, Kim CN, Ibrado AM, et al. 1997. Prevention of apoptosis by Bcl-2: release of cytochrome c from mitochondria blocked. *Science* 275:1129–32
56. Basso E, Fante L, Fowlkes J, Petronilli V, Forte MA, Bernardi P. 2005. Properties of the permeability transition pore in mitochondria devoid of cyclophilin D. *J. Biol. Chem.* 280:18558–61
57. Baines CP, Kaiser RA, Purcell NH, Blair NS, Osinska H, et al. 2005. Loss of cyclophilin D reveals a critical role for mitochondrial permeability transition in cell death. *Nature* 434:658–62

58. Nakagawa T, Shimizu S, Watanabe T, et al. 2005. Cyclophilin D-dependent mitochondrial permeability transition regulates some necrotic but not apoptotic cell death. *Nature* 434:652–58
59. Marchetti P, Castedo M, Susin SA, Zamzami N, Hirsch T, et al. 1996. Mitochondrial permeability transition is a central coordinating event of apoptosis. *J. Exp. Med.* 184:1155–60
60. Crompton M, Virji S, Ward JM. 1998. Cyclophilin-D binds strongly to complexes of the voltage-dependent anion channel and the adenine nucleotide translocase to form the permeability transition pore. *Eur. J. Biochem.* 258:729–35
61. Kokoszka JE, Waymire KG, Levy SE, Sligh JE, Cai J, et al. 2004. The ADP/ATP translocator is not essential for the mitochondrial permeability transition pore. *Nature* 427:461–65
62. Marzo I, Brenner C, Zamzami N, Jurgensmeier JM, Susin SA, et al. 1998. Bax and adenine nucleotide translocator cooperate in the mitochondrial control of apoptosis. *Science* 281:2027–31
63. Wang HG, Pathan N, Ethell IM, Krajewski S, Yamaguchi Y, et al. 1999. Ca^{2+}-induced apoptosis through calcineurin dephosphorylation of BAD. *Science* 284:339–43
64. Yi X, Yin XM, Dong Z. 2003. Inhibition of Bid-induced apoptosis by Bcl-2. tBid insertion, Bax translocation, and Bax/Bak oligomerization suppressed. *J. Biol. Chem.* 278:16992–99
65. Ott M, Robertson JD, Gogvadze V, Zhivotovsky B, Orrenius S. 2002. Cytochrome c release from mitochondria proceeds by a two-step process. *Proc. Natl. Acad. Sci. USA* 99:1259–63
66. Halestrap AP. 1999. The mitochondrial permeability transition: its molecular mechanism and role in reperfusion injury. *Biochem. Soc. Symp.* 66:181–203
67. Lam M, Dubyak G, Chen L, Nunez G, Miesfeld RL, Distelhorst CW. 1994. Evidence that BCL-2 represses apoptosis by regulating endoplasmic reticulum-associated Ca^{2+} fluxes. *Proc. Natl. Acad. Sci. USA* 91:6569–73
68. Pinton P, Ferrari D, Magalhaes P, Schulze-Osthoff K, Di Virgilio F, et al. 2000. Reduced loading of intracellular Ca^{2+} stores and downregulation of capacitative Ca^{2+} influx in Bcl-2-overexpressing cells. *J. Cell. Biol.* 148:857–62
69. Pinton P, Ferrari D, Rapizzi E, Di Virgilio F, Pozzan T, Rizzuto R. 2001. The Ca^{2+} concentration of the endoplasmic reticulum is a key determinant of ceramide-induced apoptosis: significance for the molecular mechanism of Bcl-2 action. *EMBO J.* 20:2690–701
70. Scorrano L, Oakes SA, Opferman JT, Cheng EH, Sorcinelli MD, et al. 2003. BAX and BAK regulation of endoplasmic reticulum Ca^{2+}: a control point for apoptosis. *Science* 300:135–39
71. **Oakes SA, Scorrano L, Opferman JT, Cheng EH, Sorcinelli MD, et al. 2005. Proapoptotic BAX and BAK regulate the type 1 inositol trisphosphate receptor and calcium leak from the endoplasmic reticulum. *Proc. Natl. Acad. Sci. USA* 102:105–10**

Recent developments in calcium regulation by Bcl-2 family proteins.

72. Weinberg JM, Davis JA, Abarzua M, Rajan T. 1987. Cytoprotective effects of glycine and glutathione against hypoxic injury to renal tubules. *J. Clin. Invest.* 80:1446–54
73. Zhong Z, Wheeler MD, Li X, Froh M, Schemmer P, et al. 2003. L-Glycine: a novel antiinflammatory, immunomodulatory, and cytoprotective agent. *Curr. Opin. Clin. Nutr. Metab. Care* 6:229–40

74. Dong Z, Patel Y, Saikumar P, Weinberg JM, Venkatachalam MA. 1998. Development of porous defects in plasma membranes of adenosine triphosphate-depleted Madin-Darby canine kidney cells and its inhibition by glycine. *Lab. Invest.* 78:657–68
75. Dong Z, Venkatachalam MA, Weinberg JM, Saikumar P, Patel Y. 2001. Protection of ATP-depleted cells by impermeant strychnine derivatives: implications for glycine cytoprotection. *Am. J. Pathol.* 158:1021–28
76. **Weinberg JM, Davis JA, Venkatachalam MA. 1997. Cytosolic-free calcium increases to greater than 100 micromolar in ATP-depleted proximal tubules. *J. Clin. Invest.* 100:713–22**

Remarkably high cytosolic free calcium levels are reached in hypoxic kidney cells without producing lethal injury or impairing recovery.

77. Dong Z, Saikumar P, Griess GA, Weinberg JM, Venkatachalam MA. 1998. Intracellular Ca^{2+} thresholds that determine survival or death of energy-deprived cells. *Am. J. Pathol.* 152:231–40
78. Bean BP. 1989. Classes of calcium channels in vertebrate cells. *Annu. Rev. Physiol.* 51:367–84
79. Hollmann M, Hartley M, Heinemann S. 1991. Ca^{2+} permeability of KA-AMPA–gated glutamate receptor channels depends on subunit composition. *Science* 252:851–53
80. MacDermott AB, Mayer ML, Westbrook GL, Smith SJ, Barker JL. 1986. NMDA-receptor activation increases cytoplasmic calcium concentration in cultured spinal cord neurones. *Nature* 321:519–22
81. Sucher NJ, Lei SZ, Lipton SA. 1991. Calcium channel antagonists attenuate NMDA receptor-mediated neurotoxicity of retinal ganglion cells in culture. *Brain Res.* 551:297–302
82. Gasic GP, Hollmann M. 1992. Molecular neurobiology of glutamate receptors. *Annu. Rev. Physiol.* 54:507–36
83. Choi DW. 1988. Glutamate neurotoxicity and diseases of the nervous system. *Neuron* 1:623–34
84. Lipton SA, Rosenberg PA. 1994. Excitatory amino acids as a final common pathway for neurologic disorders. *N. Engl. J. Med.* 330:613–22
85. Kaul M, Garden GA, Lipton SA. 2001. Pathways to neuronal injury and apoptosis in HIV-associated dementia. *Nature* 410:988–94
86. Lancelot E, Beal MF. 1998. Glutamate toxicity in chronic neurodegenerative disease. *Prog. Brain Res.* 116:331–47
87. **Krieger C, Duchen MR. 2002. Mitochondria, Ca^{2+} and neurodegenerative disease. *Eur. J. Pharmacol.* 447:177–88**

Excellent review of calcium neurotoxicity.

88. Matute C, Alberdi E, Ibarretxe G, Sanchez-Gomez MV. 2002. Excitotoxicity in glial cells. *Eur. J. Pharmacol.* 447:239–46
89. Nicholls DG, Budd SL. 2000. Mitochondria and neuronal survival. *Physiol. Rev.* 80:315–60
90. Nicholls DG. 2004. Mitochondrial dysfunction and glutamate excitotoxicity studied in primary neuronal cultures. *Curr. Mol. Med.* 4:149–77
91. Peng TI, Greenamyre JT. 1998. Privileged access to mitochondria of calcium influx through N-methyl-D-aspartate receptors. *Mol. Pharmacol.* 53:974–80
92. Bano D, Young KW, Guerin CJ, Lefeuvre R, Rothwell NJ, et al. 2005. Cleavage of the plasma membrane Na^+/Ca^{2+} exchanger in excitotoxicity. *Cell* 120:275–85
93. Pivovarova NB, Nguyen HV, Winters CA, Brantner CA, Smith CL, et al. 2004. Excitotoxic calcium overload in a subpopulation of mitochondria triggers delayed death in hippocampal neurons. *J. Neurosci.* 24:5611–22

94. Du Y, Bales KR, Dodel RC, Hamilton-Byrd E, Horn JW, et al. 1997. Activation of a caspase 3-related cysteine protease is required for glutamate-mediated apoptosis of cultured cerebellar granule neurons. *Proc. Natl. Acad. Sci. USA* 94:11657–62
95. Bonfoco E, Krainc D, Ankarcrona M, Nicotera P, Lipton SA. 1995. Apoptosis and necrosis: two distinct events induced, respectively, by mild and intense insults with N-methyl-D-aspartate or nitric oxide/superoxide in cortical cell cultures. *Proc. Natl. Acad. Sci. USA* 92:7162–66
96. Ankarcrona M, Dypbukt JM, Bonfoco E, Zhivotovsky B, Orrenius S, et al. 1995. Glutamate-induced neuronal death: a succession of necrosis or apoptosis depending on mitochondrial function. *Neuron* 15:961–73
97. Stout AK, Raphael HM, Kanterewicz BI, Klann E, Reynolds IJ. 1998. Glutamate-induced neuron death requires mitochondrial calcium uptake. *Nat. Neurosci.* 1:366–73
98. Brustovetsky N, Brustovetsky T, Jemmerson R, Dubinsky JM. 2002. Calcium-induced cytochrome c release from CNS mitochondria is associated with the permeability transition and rupture of the outer membrane. *J. Neurochem.* 80:207–18
99. Budd SL, Tenneti L, Lishnak T, Lipton SA. 2000. Mitochondrial and extramitochondrial apoptotic signaling pathways in cerebrocortical neurons. *Proc. Natl. Acad. Sci. USA* 97:6161–66
100. Lindsten T, Golden JA, Zong WX, Minarcik J, Harris MH, Thompson CB. 2003. The proapoptotic activities of Bax and Bak limit the size of the neural stem cell pool. *J. Neurosci.* 23:11112–19
101. Yin XM, Luo Y, Cao G, Bai L, Pei W, et al. 2002. Bid-mediated mitochondrial pathway is critical to ischemic neuronal apoptosis and focal cerebral ischemia. *J. Biol. Chem.* 277:42074–81
102. Plesnila N, Zinkel S, Le DA, Amin-Hanjani S, Wu Y, et al. 2001. BID mediates neuronal cell death after oxygen/ glucose deprivation and focal cerebral ischemia. *Proc. Natl. Acad. Sci. USA* 98:15318–23
103. Hardingham GE, Bading H. 2003. The Yin and Yang of NMDA receptor signalling. *Trends Neurosci.* 26:81–89
104. Shen AC, Jennings RB. 1972. Myocardial calcium and magnesium in acute ischemic injury. *Am. J. Pathol.* 67:417–40
105. Ganote CE, Worstell J, Kaltenbach JP. 1976. Oxygen-induced enzyme release after irreversible myocardial injury. Effects of cyanide in perfused rat hearts. *Am. J. Pathol.* 84:327–50
106. **Di Lisa F, Canton M, Menabo R, Dodoni G, Bernardi P. 2003. Mitochondria and reperfusion injury. The role of permeability transition. *Basic Res. Cardiol.* 98:235–41**
107. Halestrap AP, Clarke SJ, Javadov SA. 2004. Mitochondrial permeability transition pore opening during myocardial reperfusion–a target for cardioprotection. *Cardiovasc. Res.* 61:372–85
108. Korge P, Honda HM, Weiss JN. 2001. Regulation of the mitochondrial permeability transition by matrix Ca^{2+} and voltage during anoxia/reoxygenation. *Am. J. Physiol. Cell Physiol.* 280:C517–26
109. Griffiths EJ, Ocampo CJ, Savage JS, Rutter GA, Hansford RG, et al. 1998. Mitochondrial calcium transporting pathways during hypoxia and reoxygenation in single rat cardiomyocytes. *Cardiovasc. Res.* 39:423–33

Required reading for understanding calcium and mitochondrial damage in myocardial cell death.

110. Ylitalo KV, Ala-Rami A, Liimatta EV, Peuhkurinen KJ, Hassinen IE. 2000. Intracellular free calcium and mitochondrial membrane potential in ischemia/reperfusion and preconditioning. *J. Mol. Cell. Cardiol.* 32:1223–38
111. Di Lisa F, Blank PS, Colonna R, Gambassi G, Silverman HS, et al. 1995. Mitochondrial membrane potential in single living adult rat cardiac myocytes exposed to anoxia or metabolic inhibition. *J. Physiol.* 486(Pt. 1):1–13
112. Bernardi P, Penzo D, Wojtczak L. 2002. Mitochondrial energy dissipation by fatty acids. Mechanisms and implications for cell death. *Vitam. Horm.* 65:97–126
113. Williams SD, Gottlieb RA. 2002. Inhibition of mitochondrial calcium-independent phospholipase A2 (iPLA2) attenuates mitochondrial phospholipid loss and is cardioprotective. *Biochem. J.* 362:23–32
114. Di Lisa F, Bernardi P. 1998. Mitochondrial function as a determinant of recovery or death in cell response to injury. *Mol. Cell. Biochem.* 184:379–91
115. Eefting F, Rensing B, Wigman J, Pannekoek WJ, Liu WM, et al. 2004. Role of apoptosis in reperfusion injury. *Cardiovasc. Res.* 61:414–26
116. Borutaite V, Jekabsone A, Morkuniene R, Brown GC. 2003. Inhibition of mitochondrial permeability transition prevents mitochondrial dysfunction, cytochrome c release and apoptosis induced by heart ischemia. *J. Mol. Cell Cardiol.* 35:357–66
117. Gustafsson AB, Gottlieb RA. 2003. Mechanisms of apoptosis in the heart. *J. Clin. Immunol.* 23:447–59
118. Chen M, Won DJ, Krajewski S, Gottlieb RA. 2002. Calpain and mitochondria in ischemia/reperfusion injury. *J. Biol. Chem.* 277:29181–86
119. St-Pierre J, Brand MD, Boutilier RG. 2000. Mitochondria as ATP consumers: cellular treason in anoxia. *Proc. Natl. Acad. Sci. USA* 97:8670–74
120. Hassinen IE, Vuorinen KH, Ylitalo K, Ala-Rami A. 1998. Role of cellular energetics in ischemia-reperfusion and ischemic preconditioning of myocardium. *Mol. Cell. Biochem.* 184:393–400
121. Garlid KD, Dos Santos P, Xie ZJ, Costa AD, Paucek P. 2003. Mitochondrial potassium transport: the role of the mitochondrial ATP-sensitive K+ channel in cardiac function and cardioprotection. *Biochim. Biophys. Acta* 1606:1–21
122. Rouslin W, Broge CW, Guerrieri F, Capozza G. 1995. ATPase activity, IF1 content, and proton conductivity of ESMP from control and ischemic slow and fast heart-rate hearts. *J. Bioenerg. Biomembr.* 27:459–66
123. Piper HM, Meuter K, Schafer C. 2003. Cellular mechanisms of ischemia-reperfusion injury. *Ann. Thorac. Surg.* 75:S644–48

Discussion of calcium and myocardial injury, emphasizing their clinical aspects.

124. Armstrong SC, Latham CA, Ganote CE. 2003. An ischemic beta-dystroglycan (betaDG) degradation product: correlation with irreversible injury in adult rabbit cardiomyocytes. *Mol. Cell. Biochem.* 242:71–79
125. Hazen SL, Ford DA, Gross RW. 1991. Activation of a membrane-associated phospholipase A2 during rabbit myocardial ischemia which is highly selective for plasmalogen substrate. *J. Biol. Chem.* 266:5629–33
126. Ganote CE. 1983. Contraction band necrosis and irreversible myocardial injury. *J. Mol. Cell Cardiol.* 15:67–73
127. Weinberg JM. 1991. The cell biology of ischemic renal injury. *Kidney Int.* 39:476–500
128. Wetzels JF, Yu L, Wang X, Kribben A, Burke TJ, Schrier RW. 1993. Calcium modulation and cell injury in isolated rat proximal tubules. *J. Pharmacol. Exp. Ther.* 267:176–80

129. Kribben A, Wieder ED, Wetzels JF, Yu L, Gengaro PE, et al. 1994. Evidence for role of cytosolic free calcium in hypoxia-induced proximal tubule injury. *J. Clin. Invest.* 93:1922–29
130. Koo WS, Gengaro PE, Burke TJ, Schrier RW. 1995. Verapamil attenuates calcium-induced mitochondrial swelling and respiratory dysfunction. *J. Pharmacol. Exp. Ther.* 273:206–12
131. Chi WM, Berezesky IK, Smith MW, Trump BF. 1995. Changes in [Ca^{2+}]i in cultured rat proximal tubular epithelium: an in vitro model for renal ischemia. *Biochim. Biophys. Acta* 1243:513–20
132. Edelstein CL. 2000. Calcium-mediated proximal tubular injury-what is the role of cysteine proteases? *Nephrol. Dial. Transplant.* 15:141–44
133. Weinberg JM, Venkatachalam MA, Goldberg H, Roeser NF, Davis JA. 1995. Modulation by Gly, Ca, and acidosis of injury-associated unesterified fatty acid accumulation in proximal tubule cells. *Am. J. Physiol. Renal Physiol.* 268:F110–21
134. Peters SM, Tijsen MJ, Bindels RJ, van Os CH, Wetzels JF. 1995. Protection against hypoxic injury of rat proximal tubules by felodipine via a calcium-independent mechanism. *Pflugers Arch.* 431:20–27
135. Peters SM, Tijsen MJ, Bindels RJ, Van Os CH, Wetzels JF. 1996. Rise in cytosolic Ca^{2+} and collapse of mitochondrial potential in anoxic, but not hypoxic, rat proximal tubules. *J. Am. Soc. Nephrol.* 7:2348–56
136. Weinberg JM, Nissim I, Roeser NF, Davis JA, Schultz S, Nissim I. 1991. Relationships between intracellular amino acid levels and protection against injury to isolated proximal tubules. *Am. J. Physiol. Renal Physiol.* 260:F410–19
137. Beck FX, Ohno A, Dorge A, Thurau K. 1995. Ischemia-induced changes in cell element composition and osmolyte contents of outer medulla. *Kidney Int.* 48:449–57
138. Weinberg JM, Davis JA, Roeser NF, Venkatachalam MA. 1991. Role of increased cytosolic free calcium in the pathogenesis of rabbit proximal tubule cell injury and protection by glycine or acidosis. *J. Clin. Invest.* 87:581–90
139. Weinberg JM, Davis JA, Abarzua M, Smith RK, Kunkel R. 1990. Ouabain-induced lethal proximal tubule cell injury is prevented by glycine. *Am. J. Physiol. Renal Physiol.* 258:F346–55
140. Garza-Quintero R, Weinberg JM, Ortega-Lopez J, Davis JA, Venkatachalam MA. 1993. Conservation of structure in ATP-depleted proximal tubules: role of calcium, polyphosphoinositides, and glycine. *Am. J. Physiol. Renal Physiol.* 265:F605–23
141. Nurko S, Sogabe K, Davis JA, Roeser NF, Defrain M, et al. 1996. Contribution of actin cytoskeletal alterations to ATP depletion and calcium-induced proximal tubule cell injury. *Am. J. Physiol. Renal Physiol.* 270:F39–52
142. Sogabe K, Roeser NF, Davis JA, Nurko S, Venkatachalam MA, Weinberg JM. 1996. Calcium dependence of integrity of the actin cytoskeleton of proximal tubule cell microvilli. *Am. J. Physiol. Renal Physiol.* 271:F292–303
143. Weinberg JM, Venkatachalam MA, Roeser NF, Nissim I. 2000. Mitochondrial dysfunction during hypoxia/reoxygenation and its correction by anaerobic metabolism of citric acid cycle intermediates. *Proc. Natl. Acad. Sci. USA* 97:2826–31
144. Weinberg JM, Venkatachalam MA, Roeser NF, Saikumar P, Dong Z, et al. 2000. Anaerobic and aerobic pathways for salvage of proximal tubules from hypoxia-induced mitochondrial injury. *Am. J. Physiol. Renal Physiol.* 279:F927–43

145. Feldkamp T, Kribben A, Roeser NF, Senter RA, Kemner S, et al. 2004. Preservation of complex I function during hypoxia-reoxygenation-induced mitochondrial injury in proximal tubules. *Am. J. Physiol. Renal Physiol.* 286:F749–59
146. Feldkamp T, Kribben A, Weinberg JM. 2004. Assessment of mitochondrial membrane potential in proximal tubules after hypoxia-reoxygenation. *Am. J. Physiol. Renal Physiol.* 288:F1092–102
147. Balaban RS, Mandel LJ. 1988. Metabolic substrate utilization by rabbit proximal tubule. An NADH fluorescence study. *Am. J. Physiol. Renal Physiol.* 254:F407–16
148. Wirthensohn G, Guder WG. 1986. Renal substrate metabolism. *Physiol. Rev.* 66:469–97
149. Bastin J, Cambon N, Thompson M, Lowry OH, Burch HB. 1987. Change in energy reserves in different segments of the nephron during brief ischemia. *Kidney Int.* 31:1239–47
150. Feldkamp T, Kribben A, Roeser NF, Senter RA, and Weinberg JM. (September 13, 2005) Accumulation of nonesterified fatty acids causes the sustained energetic deficit in kidney proximal tubules after hypoxia/reoxygenation. *Am. J. Physiol. Renal Physiol.* 10.1152/ajprenal.00305.2005.

Ca^{2+}-independent mitochondrial dysfunction in hypoxic and reoxygenated proximal tubule cells is caused by accumulation of nonesterified fatty acids.

151. McCoy CE, Selvaggio AM, Alexander EA, Schwartz JH. 1988. Adenosine triphosphate depletion induces a rise in cytosolic free calcium in canine renal epithelial cells. *J. Clin. Invest.* 82:1326–32
152. Smets I, Caplanusi A, Despa S, Molnar Z, Radu M, et al. 2004. Ca^{2+} uptake in mitochondria occurs via the reverse action of the Na^+/Ca^{2+} exchanger in metabolically inhibited MDCK cells. *Am. J. Physiol. Renal Physiol.* 286:F784–94
153. Edelstein CL, Ling H, Gengaro PE, et al. 1997. Effect of glycine on prelethal and postlethal increases in calpain activity in rat renal proximal tubules. *Kidney Int.* 52:1271–78
154. Weinberg JM, Davis JA, Abarzua M, Kiani T, Kunkel R. 1990. Protection by glycine of proximal tubules from injury due to inhibitors of mitochondrial ATP production. *Am. J. Physiol. Cell Physiol.* 258:C1127–40
155. Weinberg JM, Johnson KJ, de la Iglesia FA, Allen ED. 1989. Acute alterations of tissue Ca++ and lethal tubular cell injury during HgCl2 nephrotoxicity in the rat. *Toxicol. Pathol.* 17:483–93

Genetics of Soft Tissue Tumors

Matt van de Rijn[1] and Jonathan A. Fletcher[2]

[1]Department of Pathology, Stanford University Medical Center, Stanford, California 94305; email: mrijn@stanford.edu

[2]Department of Pathology, Brigham and Women's Hospital, Boston, Massachusetts 02115; email: jfletcher@partners.org

Annu. Rev. Pathol. Mech. Dis. 2006. 1:435–66

First published online as a Review in Advance on October 28, 2005

The *Annual Review of Pathology: Mechanisms of Disease* is online at pathmechdis.annualreviews.org

doi: 10.1146/annurev.pathol.1.110304.100052

1553-4006/06/0114-0435$20.00

Key Words

sarcoma, chromosomal translocation, expression profiling, comparative genomic hybridization, tissue microarrays

Abstract

Sarcomas form a highly diverse group of rare tumors that are derived from connective tissue. More than 100 different malignant and benign soft tissue neoplasms can be recognized by histologic examination. Few diagnostic markers exist, and the cell of origin for many soft tissue tumors is unknown. The accurate diagnosis of many of these tumors therefore remains a challenge. The study of sarcomas has yielded many insights that can be applied to other neoplasms such as carcinoma. For example, the success of the treatment of gastrointestinal stromal tumor with Imatinib has led to an increased effort to find targeted therapies for other malignancies. Here we describe the known molecular changes in a number of sarcomas and focus on novel scientific approaches that can be expected to lead to improved diagnosis, prognostication, and therapy of sarcoma.

INTRODUCTION

Soft tissue tumors (STTs) are rare lesions, with approximately 15,000 new cases of malignant tumors of this type diagnosed annually in the United States (1). Slightly more than 50% of these new patients will ultimately die of this disease. This number may be an underestimate owing to underreporting; with the discovery of a new therapy for gastrointestinal stromal tumor (GIST), an extremely rapid accrual of new patients occurred, leading to a higher estimate of 5000 new cases annually for this disease alone. Previously it had been estimated that only 300–500 new cases of GIST were occurring annually in the United States (2). Regardless, the number of new sarcomas remains low and only a few clinicians (including pathologists) have extensive experience with these tumors. The situation is further complicated by the fact that within the group of STTs a large number of diagnostic entities exist. As a result of the work of many surgical pathologists, more than 100 different types of STTs now can be recognized by histologic examination (3). It should be stressed that new technologies such as genome-wide expression profiling have to a large extent confirmed the histologic separations between these different groups of STTs rather then supplanted morphologic studies. This remarkable correlation between gene expression data and histologically defined entities is indicative of the accomplishments of surgical pathologists over the past century.

Despite the success of histologic classification of STTs, conventional histology appears to have reached its limits in the subclassification or prognostication of these lesions. An example can be found in smooth muscle tumors (SMTs). Tumors derived from smooth muscle form a large subset of the STT group. SMTs are defined by the fact that in their histology they "resemble normal smooth muscle cells" (4). This definition is based entirely on morphology, and this raises problems because myofibroblasts and fibroblasts can appear similar to smooth muscle cells but give rise to different tumor types with distinct clinical behaviors. The use of actin and desmin immunostains provides only limited support for a diagnosis of SMTs, as fibroblasts and myofibroblasts can also stain for actin and even for desmin. Another difficult differential diagnostic problem involving SMTs is distinguishing between high-grade leiomyosarcoma and other high-grade sarcomas. Thus, there is a need for improved diagnostic markers for SMTs.

The clinical behavior of SMTs is dependent on the site of origin. In the deep soft tissue of the thigh, for example, even tumors with a bland histology and minimal mitotic activity can display recurrent and metastatic behavior. For tumors from a given site it can be difficult to predict clinical behavior based on histologic examination. In the uterus, some tumors with a high mitotic activity or pleomorphic nuclei can be cured by local excision. In women of childbearing age, accurate diagnosis is extremely important because diagnosis of a benign SMT will allow the patient to undergo local resection and retain her uterus. These SMTs of the uterus are quite common and frequently lead to diagnostic difficulties. Therefore, within the group of SMTs, the determination of these lesions' expected clinical behavior and the separation of these lesions from others in the differential diagnosis currently rely on the tumor cells' subtle morphologic features (5).

A novel molecular characterization of SMTs based on a genome-wide analysis of expression profiles and/or DNA copy-number changes holds promise for supplying additional information about these tumors. In addition, these studies are likely to yield additional markers to define better smooth muscle versus fibroblastic versus myofibroblastic differentiation in normal tissue. To date, several studies have appeared on gene expression profiling on relatively low numbers (13 cases or fewer) of SMTs; these are the first steps toward a molecular characterization of these lesions (6–9). Given the wide variety in sites of origin and the broad spectrum of clinical behavior that SMTs can exhibit, much larger numbers of tumors will need to be examined to specifically address these questions.

In the absence of accurate and reproducible diagnosis and prognostication of sarcomas, individualized therapy for the patients will remain impossible. Thus, there is a need for ongoing research in the field of sarcoma pathology. This review describes progress that has been made in the molecular characterization of sarcomas, both on a genome-wide basis and through more specific and detailed research of specific pathways.

MOLECULAR CHARACTERIZATION OF SARCOMAS

Various genomic mechanisms can result in activation of therapeutic targets in sarcomas (**Table 1**). Some of these aberrations are apparent using relatively low-resolution cytogenetic methods, e.g., karyotyping. One such example is the characteristic ring chromosome in dermatofibrosarcoma protuberans (DFSPs), which contains rearranged forms of chromosomes 17 and 22, resulting in an oncogenic fusion (discussed below) that activates the platelet-derived growth factor receptor β (PDGFRB) pathway (10, 11). Other sarcoma mechanisms that involve highly localized DNA perturbations can be detected by mutational analyses or indirectly, based on the mutations' effect on protein expression or function. Such mechanisms apply in the well-known KIT oncogene, found in most GISTs (12).

Although most soft tissue sarcomas contain clonal cytogenetic and molecular aberrations, only a subset of these aberrations is useful diagnostically (13–17). Indeed, many high-grade sarcomas, particularly those in the spindle-cell category, feature extremely complex genomic aberrations (**Figure 1**). The very complexity of these aberrations has confounded attempts to identify useful diagnostic or prognostic markers in many sarcomas. By contrast, small round-cell tumors and a subset of spindle-cell sarcomas (e.g., monophasic synovial sarcoma) do feature simple karyotypes. The chromosome aberrations in those tumors have entered the diagnostic lexicon (**Figures 2** and **3**) (13). Although the diagnostic significance of sarcoma genomic aberrations has been known for more than 20 years, these same aberrations have only recently become useful as therapeutic targets. However, many sarcomas have compelling molecular therapeutic targets in which the relevance to the sarcoma is clear, given that they are activated by specific genomic mutations, and the sarcoma cells retain them during clinical progression of the tumor.

In general, the mutations of greatest relevance to sarcoma-targeted therapies have been those activating an oncoprotein that can be shut down using a therapeutic inhibitor. The most compelling examples are the tyrosine kinase proteins activated by cytogenetic or molecular aberrations in various sarcomas. Although transcriptional regulators are also activated by mutations in many sarcomas, these have been less amenable to therapeutic inhibitors. Tumor suppressor mechanisms are also relatively challenging therapeutically in that it has proven more difficult to restore a lost function than to inhibit a hyperactivated (oncogenic) function. By contrast, one consequence of many tumor suppressor mutations is the activation of downstream proteins whose function normally would be inhibited by the tumor suppressor. These downstream proteins may therefore serve as therapeutic targets, thereby countering the tumor suppressor perturbation.

METHODOLOGICAL CONSIDERATIONS

The classic cytogenetic approach requires fresh, viable tumor specimens. The success of the cytogenetic analysis depends largely on the quality of the tumor specimen. The amount of tumor is less important; thus, percutaneous needle biopsies of small round-cell tumors and other cellular sarcomas can

Table 1 Typical cytogenetic aberrations in soft tissue and bone tumors

Histologic findings	Characteristic cytogenetic events	Molecular events	Frequency	Diagnostic utility?
Alveolar soft part sarcoma	t(X;17)(p11;q25)	*ASPL-TFE3* fusion	>90%	Yes
Aneurysmal bone cyst (extraosseous)	16q22 and 17p13 rearrangements	*USP6* fusion genes	>50%	Yes
Angiomatoid fibrous histiocytoma	t(12;16)(q13;p11)	*FUS-ATF1* fusion	?	Yes
Chondromyoxid fibroma	Deletion of 6q		>75%	Yes
Chondrosarcoma				
Skeletal	Complex*		>75%	?
Extraskeletal myxoid	t(9;22)(q22;q12)	*EWS-NR4A3* fusion	>75%	Yes
	t(9;17)(q22;q11)	*TAF2N-NR4A3* fusion	<10%	Yes
	t(9;15)(q22;q21)	*TCF12-NR4A3* fusion	<10%	Yes
Clear cell sarcoma	t(12;22)(q13;q12)	*EWS-ATF1* fusion	>75%	Yes
Desmoplastic small round-cell tumor	t(11;22)(p13;q12)	*EWS-WT1* fusion	>75%	Yes
Dermatofibrosarcoma protuberans	Ring form of chromosomes 17 and 22	*COL1A1-PDGFB* fusion	>75%	Yes
	t(17;22)(q21;q13)	*COL1A1-PDGFB* fusion	10%	Yes
Endometrial stromal tumor	t(7;17)(p15;q21)	*JAZF1-JJAZ1*	30%	Yes
Ewing's sarcoma	t(11;22)(q24;q12)	*EWS-FLI1* fusion	>80%	Yes
	t(21;22)(q12;q12)	*EWS-ERG* fusion	5–10%	Yes
	t(2;22)(q33;q12)	*EWS-FEV* fusion	<5%	Yes
	t(7;22)(p22;q12)	*EWS-ETV1* fusion	<5%	Yes
	t(17;22)(q12;q12)	*EWS-E1AF* fusion	<5%	Yes
	inv(22)(q12q12)	*EWS-ZSG*	<5%	Yes
Fibromatosis (Desmoid)	Trisomies 8 and 20		30%	Yes
	Deletion of 5q	*APC* inactivation	10%	Yes
Fibrosarcoma, infantile	t(12;15)(p13;q26)	*ETV6-NTRK3* fusion	>75%	Yes
	Trisomies 8, 11, 17, and 20		>75%	Yes
Gastrointestinal stromal tumor	Monosomies 14 and 22		>75%	Yes
	Deletion of 1p		>25%	No
		KIT or *PDGFRA* mutation	>90%	Yes
Giant cell tumor - bone	Telomeric associations		>50%	?
Giant cell tumor - tenosynovial	t(1;2)(p11–13;q35–36)	*CSF1* oncogene	>20%	Yes
	Trisomies 5 and 7		>25%	?
Hibernoma	11q13 rearrangement		>50%	Yes
Inflammatory myofibroblastic tumor	2p23 rearrangement	*ALK* fusion genes	50%	Yes
Leiomyoma				
Uterine	t(12;14)(q15;q24) or deletion of 7q	*HMGIC* rearrangement	40%	Yes
Extrauterine	Deletion of 1p		?	?
Leiomyosarcoma	Deletion of 1p		>50%	No
Lipoblastoma	8q12 rearrangement or polysomy 8	PLAG1 oncogenes	>80%	Yes
Lipoma				
Typical	12q15 rearrangement	*HMGIC* rearrangement	60%	Yes

(*Continued*)

Table 1 (*Continued*)

Histologic findings	Characteristic cytogenetic events	Molecular events	Frequency	Diagnostic utility?
Spindle cell or pleomorphic	Deletion of 13q or 16q		>75%	Yes
Aytpical (see well-differentiated liposarcoma)				
Chondroid	t(11;16)(q13;p12–13)		?	Yes
Liposarcoma				
Well-differentiated	Ring form of chromosome 12		>75%	Yes
Myxoid/round cell	t(12;16)(q13;p11)	*TLS-CHOP* fusion	>75%	Yes
	t(12;22)(q13;q12)	*EWS-CHOP* fusion	<5%	Yes
Pleomorphic	Complex*		90%	No
Malignant fibrous histiocytoma				
Myxoid	Ring form of chromosome 12		?	?
High-grade	Complex*		>90%	No
Myxofibrosarcoma	(see Malignant fibrous histiocytoma)			
Malignant peripheral nerve sheath tumor	(see Schwannoma)			
Mesothelioma	Deletion of 1p	*?BCL10* inactivation	>50%	Yes
	Deletion of 9p	p15, p16, and p19 inactivation	>75%	Yes
	Deletion of 22q	*NF2* inactivation	>50%	Yes
	Deletions of 3p and 6q		>50%	Yes
Neuroblastoma				
Good prognosis	Hyperdiploid, no 1p deletion		40%	Yes
Poor prognosis	1p deletion		40%	Yes
	Double-minute chromosomes	N-*myc* amplification	>25%	Yes
Osteochondroma	Deletion of 8q	*EXT1* inactivation	>25%	?
Osteosarcoma				
Low-grade	Ring chromosomes		>50%	Yes
High-grade	Complex*	Rb and p53 inactivation	>80%	?
Primitive neuroectodermal tumor	(see Ewing's sarcoma)			
Rhabdoid tumor	Deletion of 22q	*INI1* inactivation	>90%	Yes
Rhabdomyosarcoma				
Alveolar	t(2;13)(q35;q14)	*PAX3-FKHR* fusion	>75%	Yes
	t(1;13)(p36;q14), double minutes	*PAX7-FKHR* fusion	10–20%	Yes
Embryonal	Trisomies 2q, 8 and 20		>75%	Yes
		Loss of heterozygosity at 11p15	>75%	Yes
Schwannoma				
Benign	Deletion of 22q	*NF2* inactivation	>80%	Yes
Malignant, low-grade	None			
Malignant, high-grade	Complex*		>90%	No
Synovial sarcoma				
Monophasic	t(X;18)(p11;q11)	*SYT-SSX1* or *SYT-SSX2* fusion	>90%	Yes
Biphasic	t(X;18)(p11;q11)	*SYT-SSX1* fusion	>90%	Yes

*Consistent findings of extremely complex karyotypes containing multiple numerical and structural chromosomal aberrations.

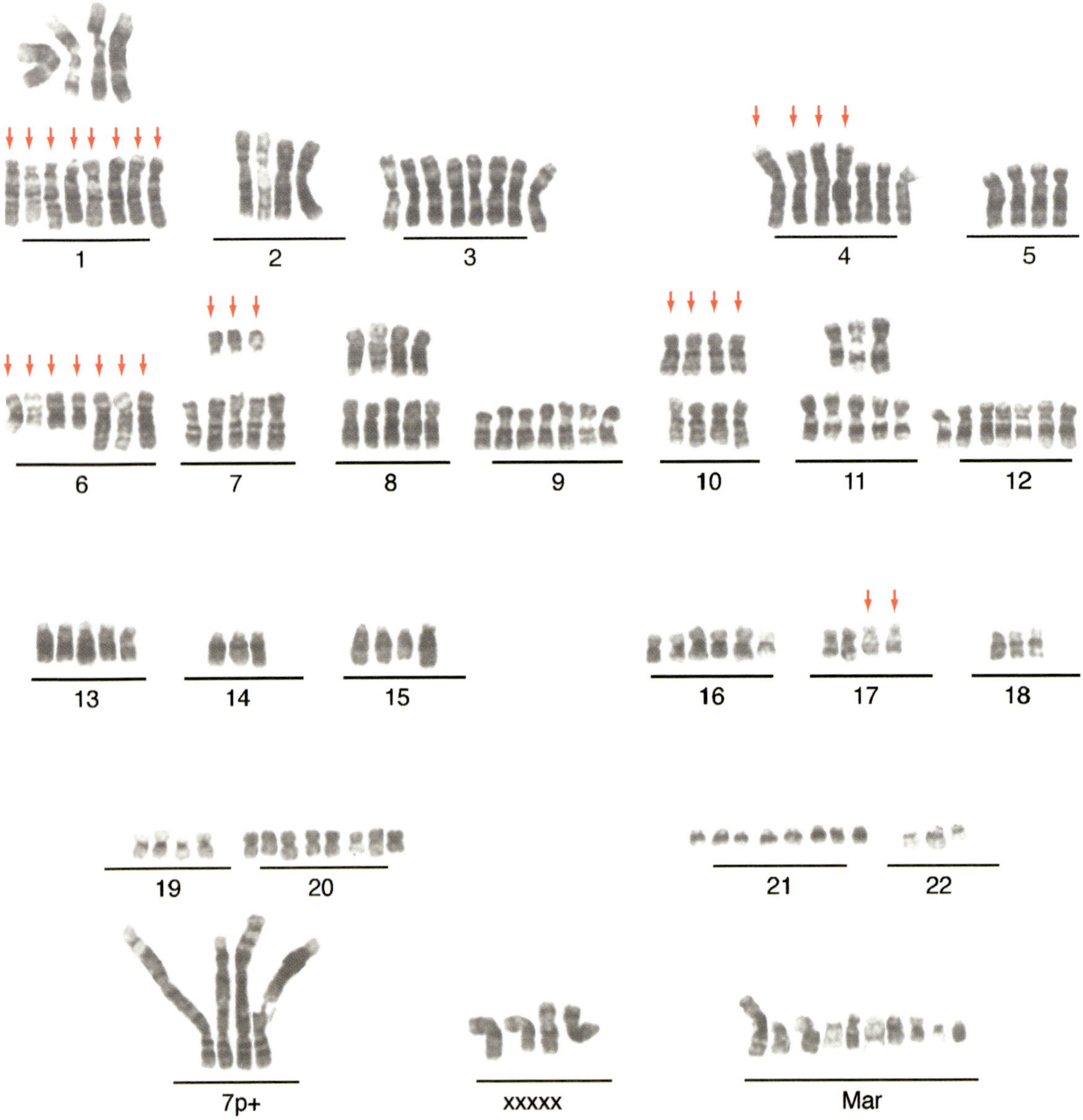

Figure 1

Karyotype of a low-grade leiomyosarcoma, showing a highly aneuploid cell with complex chromosomal aberrations. Red arrows indicate clonal chromosome rearrangements that were present in all cells analyzed from this tumor. "Mar" is an abbreviation for marker, which indicates an abnormal chromosome of uncertain origin. Chromosome rearrangements not designated by arrows (e.g., the bizarre chromosome 7 rearrangements at *lower left*) were not present in all of the tumor cells and reflect the genetic heterogeneity of this tumor.

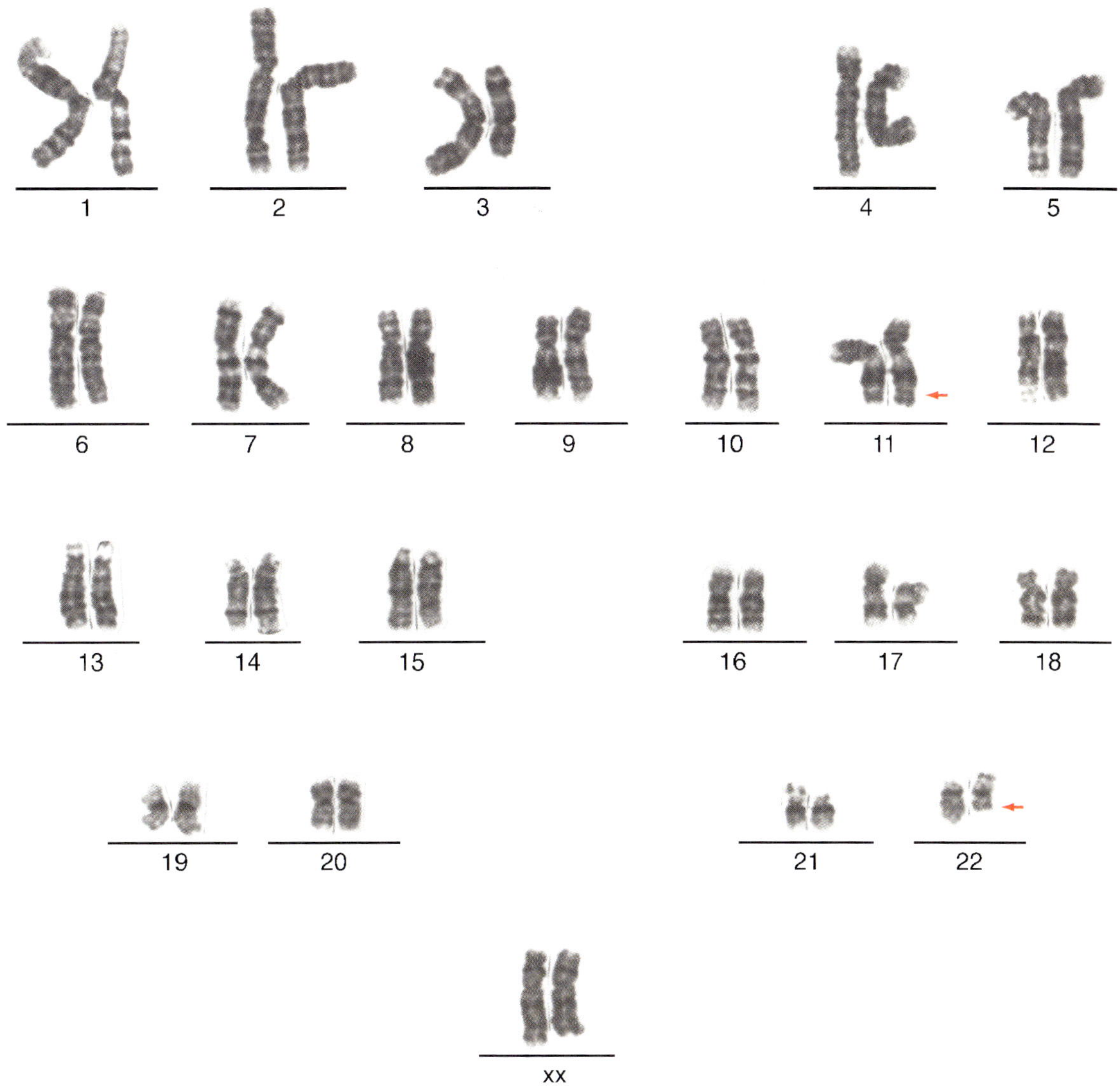

Figure 2

Karyotype of an Ewing's sarcoma, showing a diploid cell with noncomplex chromosomal aberrations. The arrows indicate the diagnostic translocation breakpoints on chromosomes 11 and 22. Deletion 3q was another clonal aberration in this tumor.

be karyotyped (13). At least 80% of all soft tissue sarcomas can be cultured successfully if the specimens are carefully selected so as to minimize necrotic and non-neoplastic components. Fluorescence in situ hybridization (FISH), PCR, and sequencing methods can be performed in archival paraffin sarcoma specimens as well as in fresh or frozen tumor specimens. FISH and molecular methods will likely play an increasing role in identifying therapeutic targets in sarcomas—as an adjunct to histological appraisal—in the near future. Several molecular cytogenetic methods have broadened the capabilities of FISH by permitting genome-wide evaluations of chromosomal aberrations. Examples include

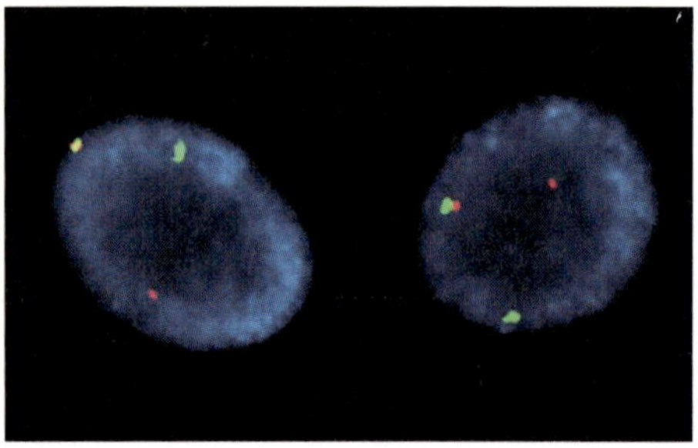

Figure 3

"Split-apart" fluorescence in situ hybridization showing SYT (SS18) rearrangement in interphase synovial sarcoma cells. Probes on the telomeric and centromeric sides of SYT are detected with FITC (*green*) and Texas Red, respectively.

comparative genomic hybridization and spectral karyotyping as well as high-throughput profiling of single-nucleotide polymorphisms. These high-throughput genomic methods are more labor-intensive than FISH and are therefore used primarily in sarcoma research rather than in clinical studies.

Cytogenetic Mechanisms

Recurring chromosome rearrangements, particularly those that serve as diagnostic and/or prognostic markers, are critical events in sarcoma tumorigenesis (**Table 1**). The nature of each chromosome rearrangement—whether involving translocation, deletion, or amplification—can identify the mechanisms by which the involved genes are altered during tumorigenesis. Certain sarcoma translocation breakpoints interrupt genes directly, resulting in novel "fusion" oncogenes. Other translocation breakpoints are adjacent to a particular gene and result in deregulated expression (typically overexpression) of the gene. Deletions of whole chromosomes or chromosomal regions generally signify loss of one or more tumor suppressor genes. Amplification events, whether extrachromosomal (double-minute chromosomes) or intrachromosomal (homogeneously staining regions) signify increased copies—and associated overexpression—of one or more oncogenes.

MOLECULAR AND CYTOGENETIC ABERRATIONS IN SARCOMAS

Adipose Tumors Have Diverse Genetic Mechanisms

Most adipose tumors contain chromosomal aberrations, with each of the various histologically different adipose tumors having its own distinctive aberrations. These aberrations include 12q rearrangement in lipoma, ring chromosomes in well-differentiated and dedifferentiated liposarcoma, t(12;16) translocations in mxyoid/round-cell liposarcoma, and cytogenetic complexity in pleomorphic liposarcomas. The most diagnostically useful aberration is the translocation of chromosomes 12 and 16, t(12;16)(q13;p11). This translocation is found in myxoid liposarcomas (18–20) and is retained in those cases that acquire round-cell features (21, 22). The t(12;16) translocation results in fusion of the CHOP gene on chromosome 12 with the TLS gene on chromosome 16 (23, 24), creating an activated transcription factor. The t(12;16) translocation is diagnostic for myxoid liposarcoma and has not been found in other types of myxoid STTs (25, 26). Either cytogenetics or reverse transcriptase PCR (RT-PCR) will detect these aberrations.

Well-differentiated liposarcomas (atypical lipomas) contain large "giant-marker" chromosomes or ring chromosomes. These abnormal chromosomes generally include chromosome 12 material, which is often admixed with components of several other chromosomes (13, 27). The ring and giant-marker chromosomes contain various amplified genes, but the essential gene amplification targets have not yet been pinpointed. These amplifications are retained when well-differentiated liposarcomas undergo dedifferentiation. Therefore, one can hope that eventual identification of the crucial gene amplification targets will reveal therapeutic targets in dedifferentiated liposarcoma. Pleomorphic liposarcomas differ cytogenetically from other liposarcomas in that they have exceedingly complex karyotypes with multiple clonal chromosome aberrations (19). The genomic complexity in pleomorphic liposarcomas has hampered attempts to define consistent chromosomal aberrations that may be of diagnostic and therapeutic utility.

PPARγ (peroxisome proliferator–activated receptor γ), a nuclear receptor and transcription factor, regulates adipose differentiation (28). PPARγ ligands have shown promise as therapeutic adjuncts in liposarcoma, particularly in myxoid/round-cell liposarcoma (29). The selectivity of PPARγ-targeted therapy is in keeping with molecular and cytogenetic evidence showing that the various types of liposarcoma are indeed distinct genetic and biologic categories. PPARγ is also highly expressed in another myxoid neoplasm, myxoid chondrosarcoma, and may function as a therapeutic target in that lesion as well (30).

Clear Cell Sarcomas (Malignant Melanomas of Soft Parts)

Clear cell sarcomas of soft tissues share many phenotypic features with cutaneous malignant melanomas. Hence, it can be difficult to distinguish histologically between clear cell sarcoma and cutaneous melanoma. Despite the histologic similarities between clear cell sarcoma and cutaneous melanoma, these two tumors are quite different clinically. Clear cell sarcomas are usually present as isolated masses located in deep soft tissues without apparent origin from skin. It is notable, therefore, that more than 75% of clear cell sarcomas contain a chromosome translocation, t(12;22)(q13;q12), that has never been reported in cutaneous melanoma. Despite the genomic differences in soft tissue and cutaneous melanomas, cDNA array studies show that clear cell sarcomas are biologically more related to melanoma than to other sarcomas (31). The t(12;22) translocation fuses the ATF1 gene on chromosome 12 with the Ewing's sarcoma gene (EWS gene) on chromosome 22 (32, 33). ATF1 encodes a transcription factor, and the biological implications of the translocation are probably similar to those discussed below in Ewing's sarcoma. The clear cell sarcoma t(12;22) translocation can be detected by karyotyping or in situ hybridization (ISH), whereas the associated ATF1-EWS fusion can be detected conveniently by RT-PCR.

Desmoplastic Small Round-Cell Tumors: Is PDGFRA a Target?

Desmoplastic small round-cell tumors are aggressive, chemotherapy-resistant neoplasms, arising predominantly, but not exclusively, from intra-abdominal soft tissues (34). These tumors are composed of undifferentiated malignant small round cells within a florid desmoplastic reaction (34). Virtually all cases express an EWS-WT1 (Wilms tumor 1) fusion oncogene (35, 36). This oncogene results from translocation between the chromosome 11 short arm and the chromosome 22 long arm, juxtaposing the WT1 and EWS genes, respectively (37, 38). Notably, the EWS-WT1 oncoprotein is a transcriptional regulator that induces expression of platelet-derived growth factor α (PDGFA) (39). PDGFA binds and activates both PDGFRβ (PDGFRB) and PDGFRα (PDGFRA), serving to activate potent mitogenic signaling pathways in fibroblasts (40). These observations suggest that the oncogenically induced PDGFA expression contributes to the prominent desmoplastic reaction in desmoplastic round-cell tumors. However, it is unclear whether PDGFA also serves an autocrine or paracrine function in directly stimulating growth of the neoplastic cells.

Ewing's Sarcomas

Most Ewing's sarcomas contain chromosome translocations involving the EWS gene. In more than 80% of cases, this translocation involves chromosomes 11 and 22, resulting in oncogenic fusion of the chromosome 11 FLI1 gene with the chromosome 22 EWS gene (41–44). FLI1 encodes a transcription factor belonging to the ETS family of transcription factors; the oncogenic EWS-FLI1 fusion gene encodes an activated version of this transcription factor. Alternatively, approximately 5%–15% of Ewing tumors have variant translocations in which the EWS gene is fused with other ETS family transcription factor genes (**Table 1**) (45–49). As they are in virtually all Ewing's sarcomas, the EWS gene translocations are considered to be essential genetic aberrations. However, targeted therapies for the EWS oncoproteins are still developmental, with no substantial clinical responses in early studies of vaccine therapies for Ewing's sarcoma (50).

Dermatofibrosarcoma Protuberans: Activated PDGFRB

Most DFSPs contain a ring chromosome composed of sequences from chromosomes 17 and 22 (51, 52). The DFSP ring chromosomes contain multiple copies of a fusion gene, COL1A1-PDGFB (platelet-derived growth factor β), in which COL1A1 (a collagen gene) is contributed by chromosome 17, and PDGFB by chromosome 22 (11, 53). The diagnostic COL1A1-PDGFB oncogene fusion can be demonstrated by FISH or RT-PCR. Occasional DFSPs have balanced t(17;22) translocations—associated with the COL1A1-PDGFB fusion gene—rather than the usual ring chromosomes. Irrespective of the cytogenetic mechanism, the COL1A1-PDGFB oncogene results in overexpression of PDGFB, which is a growth factor that activates PDGFRA and PDGFRB. Gene expression profiling studies have shown that PDGFRB is also expressed at high levels relative to other STTs, suggesting the presence of an autocrine loop in DFSP (54). These observations suggested the possibility that patients with inoperable DFSP may benefit from treatment with PDGFR inhibitors, e.g., Imatinib, and striking clinical responses in several patients have confirmed this hypothesis (55, 56).

Desmoid Tumors: Adenomatous Polyposis Coli and β-Catenin

Deep fibromatoses (desmoid tumors) can contain various cytogenetic or molecular aberrations, including adenomatous polyposis coli (APC) and β-catenin mutations (57, 58) and trisomies for chromosomes 8 or 20 (59). Cytogenetic deletions of the chromosome 5 long arm are seen in occasional desmoids, resulting in loss of the APC tumor suppressor gene, and the remaining APC allele in these cases is typically inactivated by a point mutation (60, 61). The most common mutations in sporadic desmoid tumors are activating β-catenin mutations, which Alman and colleagues (57, 58) demonstrated in 22 of 42 desmoids. These mutations stabilize the β-catenin protein, resulting in its overexpression. Therefore, it is likely that targeted therapies of the Wnt-APC-β-catenin pathway will be useful in the treatment of patients with advanced desmoid tumors. Notably, PDGFRB activation plays a highly mitogenic role in myofibroblasts. This knowledge has led to therapeutic evaluation of the Imatinib PDGFRB inhibitor in desmoids. Early data underscore the promise of this strategy (62).

Fibrosarcomas (Infantile/Congenital) and Mesoblastic Nephromas: Activated NRTK3/TRKC

Trisomies of chromosomes 8, 11, 17, and 20 are characteristic aberrations in infantile fibrosarcomas (63) and in mesoblastic nephroma, a closely related infantile renal tumor (64). In addition, most infantile fibrosarcomas and mesoblastic nephromas contain the same diagnostic chromosome translocation, t(12;15)(p13;q26) (65–67). This translocation results in fusion of the chromosome 12 ETV6 gene with the chromosome 15 NTRK3 gene. The t(12;15) translocation is difficult to detect by conventional cytogenetic banding approaches but is demonstrated readily by FISH or RT-PCR (65–67). From a clinical standpoint, infantile fibrosarcomas and most mesoblastic nephromas are undifferentiated and mitotically active, but patients with these conditions nonetheless have an excellent prognosis after excisional biopsy (68, 69). Surgical excusion cures most infantile fibrosarcomas and mesoblastic nephromas, and those that are inoperable respond well to cytotoxic therapies. A small number of cases do not respond to chemotherapy, and development of NTRK3 kinase inhibitors would doubtless be highly useful for this subgroup.

Inflammatory Myofibroblastic Tumors: Activated ALK

Inflammatory myofibroblastic tumors are composed of fascicles of bland myofibroblastic cells admixed with a prominent inflammatory infiltrate. The inflammatory component is reactive, whereas the myofibroblastic cells are neoplastic and contain clonal chromosome aberrations (70–72). A subset of inflammatory myofibroblastic tumors have cytogenetic rearrangements activating the ALK receptor tyrosine kinase gene on chromosome 2 (73). This is the same gene activated, typically by fusion with the NPM gene on chromosome 5, in many anaplastic large cell lymphomas. Inflammatory myofibroblastic tumors with ALK gene rearrangements express the ALK protein strongly and can be identified either by ALK immunohistochemical staining in paraffin sections or by FISH for ALK gene rearrangement.

Gastrointestinal Stromal Tumors: Activated KIT and PDGFRA

Most GISTs feature mutant KIT or PDGFRA oncogenes (12, 74, 75), as recent reviews have discussed (76, 77). These mutations result in constitutive activation of the KIT or PDGFRA kinases, manifested by autophosphorylation of the kinase oncoprotein (**Figure 4**) and activation of various signaling pathways for cell proliferation and survival (**Figure 5**). KIT or PDGFRA mutations can be found in the germ line, in which case the affected individuals are at risk for multiple GISTs (78). The KIT and PDGFRA oncoproteins in GISTs have been targeted with spectacular success using the small molecule kinase inhibitor, Imatinib (Gleevec) (79, 80). In addition to the KIT and PDGFRA mutations, most GISTs have distinctive karyotypes that include deletions of the long arms of chromosomes 14 and 22 (74, 81). Less often, GISTs contain deletions of the short arms of chromosomes 1, 9, and 11 (**Table 1**). KIT or PDGFRA activation results from early—and even initiating—mutational events in GISTs. These kinase activations stimulate proliferation of the neoplastic progenitor cell, resulting in hyperplasia of the GIST cell lineage (82). Subsequently, the various cytogenetic aberrations are acquired, which presumably drive the progression of the tumor toward a malignant GIST (83).

Malignant Peripheral Nerve Sheath Tumors: Ras Pathway

Benign and malignant peripheral nerve sheath tumors (MPNSTs) are seen with increased frequency in patients with the hereditary neurofibromatosis syndromes. These are the most common tumor predisposition syndromes, affecting 1 in 3500 individuals worldwide. Neurofibromas and MPNSTs are common in individuals with neurofibromatosis type 1 (NF1), whereas benign schwannomas are associated with neurofibromatosis type 2 (NF2) (central neurofibromatosis). The NF1 and NF2 genes are located on chromosomes 17 and 22, respectively, and both of these genes encode tumor suppressor proteins that normally constrain cell proliferation (84–89). MPNSTs often have deletions of the NF1 gene, which can be demonstrated by FISH assays. The NF1 gene aberrations are accompanied by a generally complex karyotype, suggesting that genetic instability plays a prominent role in the development of MPNSTs.

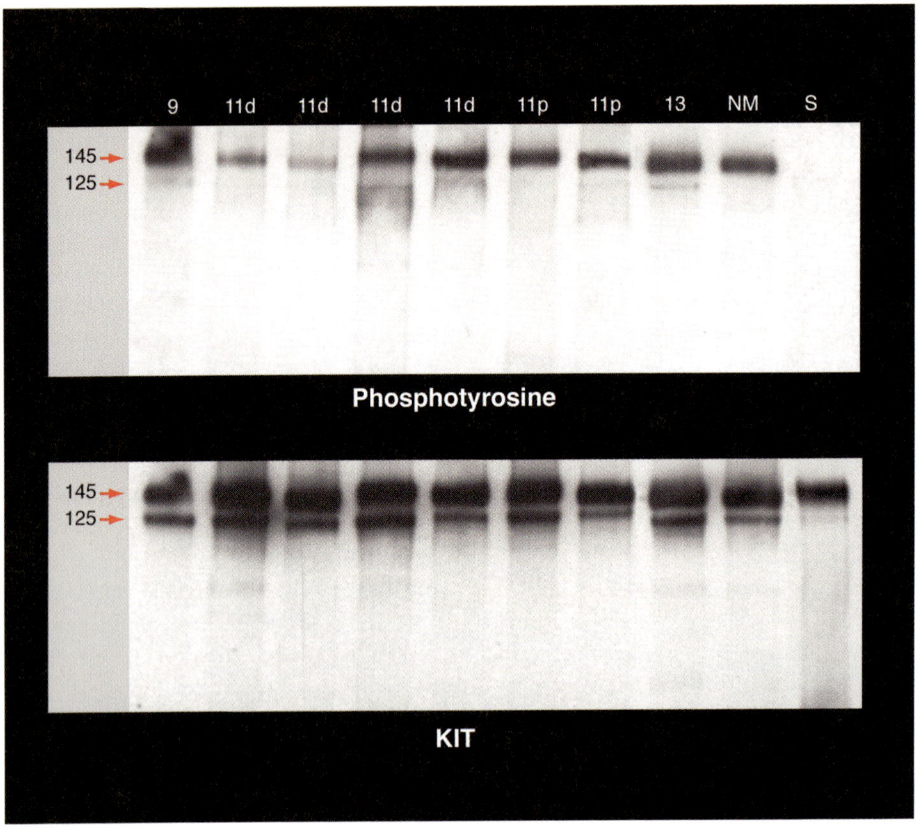

Figure 4

Immunoblot demonstration of constitutive KIT activation in gastrointestinal stromal tumors (GISTs) (lanes 1–9) and a control seminoma (S). KIT proteins were immunoprecipitated, stained for phosphotryosine (*top*), then stripped and restained for KIT (*bottom*). The lane headings—9, 11d, 11p, 13, and NM—specify the *KIT* mutation type: exon 9 mutation, exon 11 deletion, exon 11 point mutation, exon 13 mutation, and no mutation, respectively. Red arrows indicate the 125-kD newly synthesized KIT and the 145-kD membrane-associated, fully glycosylated KIT.

Notably, NF1 gene deletions can also be shown in the Schwann cell component of neurofibromas (90). This observation supports the view that neurofibromas are clonal schwannian neoplasms, whereas the other admixed cell lineages—including fibroblasts, mast cells, and perineural cells—are reactive.

The NF1 gene encodes a large protein that is related to the p120 Ras GTPase-activating protein (Ras-GAP) (91, 92). Ras-GAPs diminish signaling through the Ras pathway by stimulating the hydrolysis of GTP to GDP. This results in conversion of the active Ras-GTP complex to inactive Ras-GDP. In MPNSTs, point mutations within the NF1 Ras-binding or Ras-GAP domains can inhibit the NF1 anti-Ras function. These observations suggest that Ras inhibition may be therapeutically effective in patients with MPNSTs.

Rhabdoid Tumors

Most malignant rhabdoid tumors—whether arising in soft tissues, kidney, or the central nervous system—contain deletions of the chromosome 22 long arm. The chromosome

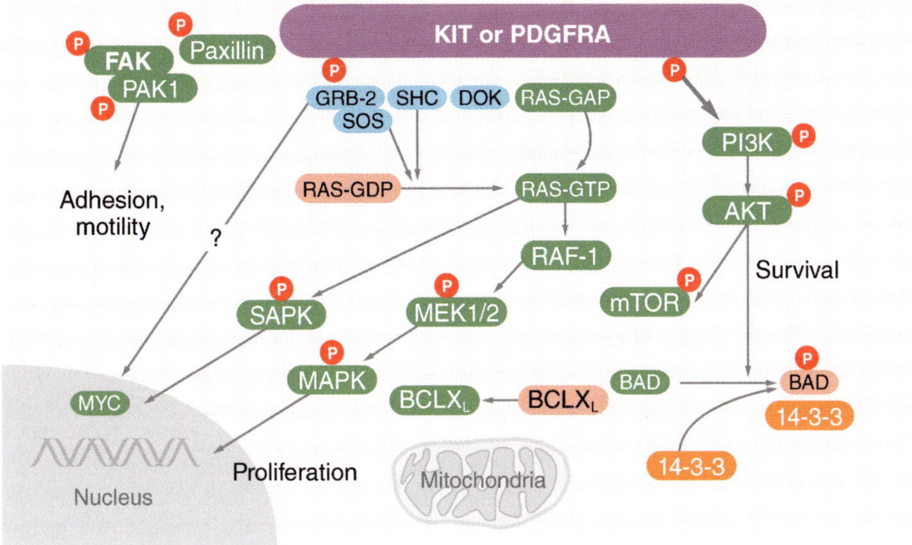

Figure 5

Cell-signaling cascades resulting from KIT or platelet-derived growth factor receptor α (PDGFRA) receptor tyrosine kinase activation in gastrointestinal stromal tumors (GISTs). This schematic is a simplified representation of the known signaling pathways activated by KIT/PDGFRA in GIST. P, phosphorylation/activation.

22 deletions target a tumor suppressor gene, INI1 (also known as SNF5 or SMARCB1), which encodes a protein involved in chromatin remodeling (93, 94). The rhabdoid tumor karyotypic profile is quite characteristic inasmuch as the chromosome 22 deletion is often the only detectable cytogenetic aberration, suggesting that INI1 inactivation is a relatively early event in rhabdoid tumorigenesis. Additional evidence of an essential tumorigenic role includes the finding of germline INI1 mutations in some individuals with rhabdoid tumors (93, 95) and the predictable development of rhabdoid tumors in mice with inactivating INI1 mutations (96). These observations suggest that novel therapies targeting the INI1 pathway may be very effective in patients with rhabdoid tumors.

Rhabdomyosarcomas

Cytogenetic analyses have been useful in reaffirming the distinct nature of embryonal and alveolar forms of rhabdomyosarcomas. Alveolar rhabdomyosarcomas contain reciprocal chromosome translocations involving the Forkhead transcription factor (FKHR) gene on chromosome 13. Generally, the FKHR gene is fused with the PAX3 gene on chromosome 2 (97–99), but some alveolar rhabdomyosarcomas contain fusions of FKHR with the PAX7 gene on chromosome 1 (100). FKHR, PAX3, and PAX7 encode transcription factors, and the PAX3-FKHR and PAX7-FKHR fusion oncogenes encode activated forms of those transcription factors (101, 102). By contrast, embryonal rhabdomyosarcomas typically lack FKHR translocations, but in experimental models they can result from activation of various receptor tyrosine kinase proteins, including MET and ERBB2 (103, 104), and can respond to inhibition of other receptor tyrosine kinase proteins, particularly IGF1R (105, 106).

Synovial Sarcomas

Most synovial sarcomas contain a translocation of chromosomes X and 18, t(X;18)(p11;q11), resulting in oncogenic fusion between one of several SSX family genes on chromosome X and the SYT (SS18) gene on chromosome 18 (107). The t(X;18) translocation is found in more than 90% of synovial sarcomas but is not found in histologic mimics such as hemangiopericytoma, mesothelioma, leiomyosarcoma, or MPNST. There are no therapies that reproducibly inhibit the t(X;18) oncogenic mechanism or the associated SYT-SSX fusion oncoproteins. However, in a preliminary report, Matsuzaki and colleagues (108) described temporary stabilization of synovial sarcoma pulmonary metastases following immunotherapy with autologous dendritic cells that had been exposed to the SYT-SSX2 junctional region. Microarray expression profiling has shown higher ERBB2 (her2/neu) expression in synovial sarcoma compared with other soft tissue sarcomas, and the ERBB2 expression is found predominantly in the glandular components of the synovial sarcomas (109). On the basis of these findings, Allander and colleagues (109) have suggested that ERBB2 might provide a therapeutic target in synovial sarcoma. A second example of a novel potential therapeutic target in synovial sarcoma stems from the observation that synovial sarcomas express high levels of EGFR compared with other tumors (110, 111). As a result an EORTC protocol (62,022) was initiated to test the efficacy of Iressa treatment in synovial sarcoma patients. This protocol began before the correlation between EGFR mutation status and Iressa response was known in lung adenocarcinoma (112). So far, no synovial sarcomas have been shown to contain a mutation in their EGFR gene (T.O. Nielsen, unpublished results). Ultimately the mutational status of the EGFR gene may be more important for response to targeted treatment than the expression level.

EXPRESSION PROFILING STUDIES

Novel Diagnostic Markers

One of the most efficient ways to detect novel tumor-specific markers is by high-throughput gene expression profiling. On high-density gene arrays the expression levels for more than 30,000 genes in a tumor sample can be determined in a single experiment. Gene filtering usually is performed to remove those genes that are either poorly measured in the array or that show no significant variation across the tumor samples tested. Unsupervised hierarchical clustering can then be used to group together those tumors that have similar expression levels across the genes in one dimension, while in the second dimension those genes that show similar reaction across the tumors are grouped. As is shown in **Figure 6**, with very few exceptions all tumors of the same diagnosis cluster together when analyzed with unsupervised hierarchical clustering. This indicates that tumors with the same diagnosis share a significant portion of their gene expression profile; this allows us to search for diagnostic markers for that particular diagnosis group. In addition to using unsupervised hierarchical clustering, one can also mine the data in a more directed way using statistical

Figure 6

Gene expression profiling using 42,000 element DNA arrays on 103 different soft tissue tumors. Data were analyzed by unsupervised hierarchical clustering. The relatedness between the different neoplasms is shown in a dendrogram, in which 9 main branches can be distinguished. In branch 1 all 8 synovial sarcomas are clustered. Branch 2 holds all 10 dermatofibrosarcoma protuberans (DFSPs), branch 3 all but 1 of 19 solitary firbrous tumors (SFTs), and branch 4 all 5 gastrointestinal stromal tumors (GISTs). Branch 5 contains mostly muscle tumors, both smooth and skeletal derived, whereas in branch 6 a mixture of leiomyosarcomas and MFH is seen. Branch 7 contains all 10 fibromatoses, and branch 8 contains all but 1 of the 12 myxoid chondrosarcomas. In branch 9, all 5 desmoplastic small round-cell tumors (DSRCT) are clustered together with 2 epithelioid sarcomas and 1 myxoid chondrosarcoma. The only tumor that shows a significant lack of clustering in this analysis is the epithelioid sarcoma. The heat map of the gene expression patterns, here shown for a selection of only 690 genes, shows a remarkable number of genes specific for the bland spindle-cell neoplasms of SFT (*white ellipse*) and fibromatosis (*yellow ellipse*).

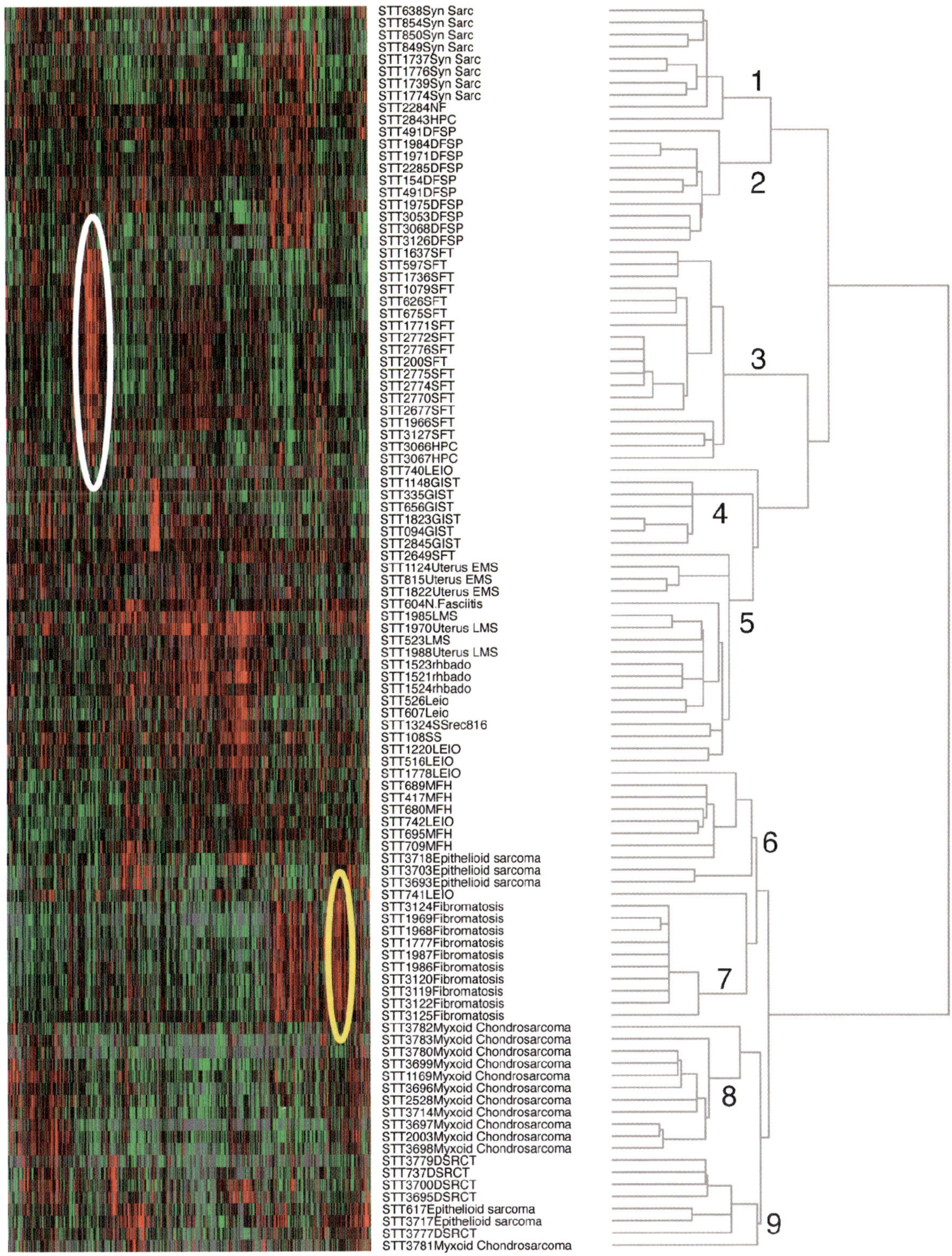
STT638Syn Sarc
STT854Syn Sarc
STT850Syn Sarc
STT849Syn Sarc
STT1737Syn Sarc
STT1776Syn Sarc
STT1739Syn Sarc
STT1774Syn Sarc
STT2284NF
STT2843HPC
STT491DFSP
STT1984DFSP
STT1971DFSP
STT2285DFSP
STT154DFSP
STT491DFSP
STT1975DFSP
STT3053DFSP
STT3068DFSP
STT3126DFSP
STT1637SFT
STT597SFT
STT1736SFT
STT1079SFT
STT626SFT
STT675SFT
STT1771SFT
STT2772SFT
STT2776SFT
STT200SFT
STT2775SFT
STT2774SFT
STT2770SFT
STT2677SFT
STT1966SFT
STT3127SFT
STT3066HPC
STT3067HPC
STT740LEIO
STT1148GIST
STT335GIST
STT656GIST
STT1823GIST
STT094GIST
STT2845GIST
STT2649SFT
STT1124Uterus EMS
STT815Uterus EMS
STT1822Uterus EMS
STT604N.Fasciitis
STT1985LMS
STT1970Uterus LMS
STT523LMS
STT1988Uterus LMS
STT1523rhbado
STT1521rhbado
STT1524rhbado
STT526Leio
STT607Leio
STT1324SSrec816
STT108SS
STT1220LEIO
STT516LEIO
STT1778LEIO
STT689MFH
STT417MFH
STT680MFH
STT742LEIO
STT695MFH
STT709MFH
STT3718Epithelioid sarcoma
STT3703Epithelioid sarcoma
STT3693Epithelioid sarcoma
STT741LEIO
STT3124Fibromatosis
STT1969Fibromatosis
STT1968Fibromatosis
STT1777Fibromatosis
STT1987Fibromatosis
STT1986Fibromatosis
STT3120Fibromatosis
STT3119Fibromatosis
STT3122Fibromatosis
STT3125Fibromatosis
STT3782Myxoid Chondrosarcoma
STT3783Myxoid Chondrosarcoma
STT3780Myxoid Chondrosarcoma
STT3699Myxoid Chondrosarcoma
STT1169Myxoid Chondrosarcoma
STT3696Myxoid Chondrosarcoma
STT2528Myxoid Chondrosarcoma
STT3714Myxoid Chondrosarcoma
STT3697Myxoid Chondrosarcoma
STT2003Myxoid Chondrosarcoma
STT3698Myxoid Chondrosarcoma
STT3779DSRCT
STT737DSRCT
STT3700DSRCT
STT3695DSRCT
STT617Epithelioid sarcoma
STT3717Epithelioid sarcoma
STT3777DSRCT
STT3781Myxoid Chondrosarcoma
1
2
3
4
5
6
7
8
9

methods such as SAM (113) and other techniques. Thus, with relatively small numbers of tumor cases from a particular diagnostic group, one can identify genes of interest as potential differential diagnostic markers. The value of these studies increases as more different tumor types can be directly compared to each other.

A number of groups have now performed these studies and have identified novel diagnostic markers (109, 111, 114–116), such as a novel marker in GIST through expression profiling. As described above, a subset of GIST has mutations in PDGFRA, a tyrosine kinase receptor related to KIT (74). These tumors do not have mutations in the KIT gene and often fail to react for KIT antibodies in immunohistochemistry (IHC). Thus, they can be mistaken for tumors other than GIST such as leiomyosarcoma. On the basis of gene microarray findings, a novel antigen, DOG1, was identified that is expressed on most GIST s, including those that harbor the PDGFRA mutation (115).

Prognostic Markers and Therapeutic Targets

The treatment of cancer patients can only improve with a move toward individualized treatment for each patient. The systematic molecular analysis of carcinomas has led to the identification of molecularly defined subgroups of patients that differ in the optimal approach to their treatment. Perhaps the best example of this is found in breast carcinoma, for which ER and HER2/Neu status have clear, direct implications for molecularly targeted treatment. More recently, DNA microarray findings highlighting novel subtypes, such as the basal subtype of breast cancer, suggest that further individualization of therapy based on accurate molecular subclassification will be possible (117–119). Tissue microarray (TMA) studies subsequently confirmed the existence of this basal group of tumors (120–122). Other studies have defined such markers in breast carcinoma through a supervised search for prognostic markers in gene microarray data (123), through the application of gene sets discovered through addressing biological questions (124, 125), by the application of RT-PCR on paraffin-embedded tissue for a limited gene set (126), and by application of cluster analyses of IHC data on TMAs (127). All of these approaches could potentially be applied to STTs.

Efforts in the field of sarcoma research have occurred on a much smaller scale. This is, at least in part, due to the low frequency of STTs such that very few research teams can accrue sufficient cases for their projects. To cope with the rarity of these lesions, networks of researchers and clinicians treating patients have been established and this has been the most productive and successful in the field of pediatric sarcomas. The novel technique of TMA analysis allows for the combination of several hundreds of paraffin-embedded tumor samples in a single paraffin block. These specimens can then be examined for the expression of proteins by IHC or by ISH for mRNA levels for specific genes. By pooling the collections of specimens from pathology archives in multiple academic centers, researchers can obtain large case numbers, even for tumors that have a very low frequency of occurrence. Sections from these TMAs can be shared by different collaborative groups. It can be expected that with time and through intense collaborations, the field of sarcoma research can ultimately overcome the challenges posed by the rarity of these lesions.

Whereas most gene array studies to date have reported on relatively small numbers of cases from a particular diagnostic group, large studies on rhabdomyosarcoma and small round blue cell tumors are under way in the laboratories of Drs. Triche and Ladanyi. In addition, GISTs were characterized as a homogeneous group of tumors, in contrast to other sarcomas (111, 128, 129). More recent studies focused on differences in expression profiles within this diagnostic entity based on either location (130) or mutation status in the KIT or PDGFRA genes (131, 132).

Comparisons Between Different Studies

Gene array analysis that is performed on a significant number of samples yields a vast and complex data set that can contain a million data points or more. The gene lists that are generated after analysis of the data are highly dependent on the type and number of samples studied, the gene filtering methods used, and the questions asked of the data set. This is one reason that it is imperative that the complete unfiltered raw data set becomes publicly available so that comparisons can be made between different groups' results. Currently not all scientific journals require that the raw data set of gene array experiments is made available upon publication. As a result for many studies only the filtered data set becomes available and often only selected genes are discussed. Marshall (133) recently commented on the lack of correlation between several expression profiling studies. When the appropriate type of questions are asked, however, a significant correlation between different studies becomes apparent. Sorlie and colleagues (119) provide an example of the tremendous benefit of comparisons between raw data sets from different publications. These researchers compared gene array data on breast carcinoma from the Stanford group with those from The Netherlands Cancer Institute and found remarkable similarities (119). More recently Chang and coworkers investigated the expression levels for the "wound-healing gene set" (125) (see also below) in the gene array data set of 295 breast carcinomas from The Netherlands Cancer Institute (123) and could confirm the prognostic significance of this gene profile (124). No similar large gene array data sets have been produced for sarcomas yet, but nevertheless, remarkable comparisons between relatively small studies can already be made. For instance, the expression of genes involved in retinoic acid response in synovial sarcoma was noted in four of five expression profiling studies. First, unsupervised hierarchical clustering of a group of diverse sarcomas showed tight grouping of synovial sarcomas that was determined by a large group of genes specifically expressed at higher levels in synovial sarcoma as compared with other tumors (111). These included two retinoic acid–binding proteins, cellular retinoic acid–binding protein 1 (CRABP1), and retinoic acid receptor-γ. SAM analysis (a supervised statistical method selecting genes most tightly associated with tumor types) (113) singled out CRABP1 as the most synovial sarcoma (SS)-specific gene in this study. These two genes resided in a cluster of 55 genes that was highly expressed in synovial sarcoma and in which eight more genes were found that are known to be induced by retinoids: the homeotic genes HOXD4, HOXD8, IRX2A, and MSX2; the chondrogenic genes BMP7 and SOX9; the neurodevelopmental gene ENC1; and the signaling factor TGFβ2. An additional 16 genes were found in this group of 55 genes that are present in retinoid-associated pathways. In a separate study Nagayama and colleagues (134) reported on expression profiling of 13 SS and 34 other sarcomas using a different expression profiling platform. They identified a list of 26 cDNAs associated with SS, of which 16 corresponded to named genes of known function (134). Of these 16 genes, 8 are retinoid-induced or involved in related pathways, and several, including CRABP1, were confirmed by semiquantitative RT-PCR (134). A third study by Allander and colleagues (109) that differed in the number and types of sarcomas examined, the platform used, and in other variables nevertheless also identified CRABP1 as being highly expressed in synovial sarcoma. Likewise, a fourth study of 51 sarcomas identified genes involved in retinoic acid–signaling among synovial sarcoma–specific gene clusters (129). Only one study performed on synovial sarcoma did not identify genes influenced by retinoids in synovial sarcomas, but this study used relatively small arrays and stringent data filtration (6). Thus, four out of five gene array studies, all using different combinations of tumors and performed on a wide variety of platforms, identified genes affected by retinoic acid as highly expressed in synovial sarcomas. Several of the studies referred to above did not publish their entire data sets, and it can be expected that a directed search would discover even more similarities than those discussed above.

Another argument for full publication of raw data is that the data sets published through gene array studies on sarcoma (or other tumors) often are so large that no single laboratory can study all aspects of the data set. An example of the validity of this statement can be found in protein kinase C-θ, which was shown to be a new marker for GIST (114), partially as a result of identifying high mRNA levels for this gene in two separate expression profiling studies of GIST (109, 111).

Other Applications of Expression Profiling Studies

Identification of translocations. As described above, the identification of translocations in STTs are not only of interest from a biological point of view; they can also be used as diagnostic tools, and in several cases the variants of translocation types found in specific sarcoma have even been shown to be associated with differences in prognosis. Furthermore, the fusion products of these tumors are likely candidates for therapeutic targeting. New translocations in STTs have most commonly been identified through conventional cytogenetic techniques. The identification of the genes involved in such new balanced translocations through chromosome walking can be a laborious process. In some sarcomas a high level of expression for one of the fusion partners is seen; this can be identified through gene expression profiling. Here we show two examples. In **Figure 7*a*** high levels of expression for SXX are seen in synovial sarcoma, but not in other tumors when genes along the breakpoint region on chromosome X are represented in the order in which they occur along the chromosome. **Figure 7*b*** shows a similar finding for desmoplastic small round-cell tumors (DSRCT), with the WT gene highly expressed in this tumor, whereas the other genes that flank it on chromosome 11 do not show an elevated expression. However, we did not observe high expression levels for known fusion partners in chromosomal translocations in several other tumors such as myxoid chondrosarcoma, rhabdomyosarcoma, and myxoid liposarcoma (S. Subbramanian, unpublished results). Thus, this approach may not be universally applicable.

Another example of how gene expression studies can lead to the identification of novel fusion partners in a sarcoma is found in the work by Wachtel and colleagues (135), in which unsupervised hierarchical clustering of gene array data revealed one case of alveolar rhabdosarcoma that did not cluster with the embryonal sarcoma. As a result, this group identified a novel variant of the translocation found in alveolar rhabdomyosarcoma.

Cell of origin and host stromal reactions to tumor. For some tumors, such as rhabdomyosarcoma, the benign precursor cell is known with reasonable certainty. The presence of cross striations in a subset of cells in rhabdomyosarcoma is clear evidence for the relationship to skeletal muscle differentiation. In SMTs, it is the shape of the cells, the expression of muscle markers, and the dense eosinophilic cytoplasm that supports derivi-ation from smooth muscle cells. In GISTs, the relationship to normal cells (in this case the pacemaker cells in the bowel, the cells of Cajal) is supported by the shared expression of a marker (the KIT tyrosine kinase receptor, CD117). In addition, families with germline KIT mutations not only suffer from frequent GIST lesions but also have hyperplastic myenteric plexus. For many soft tissue neoplasms, however, the cell of origin remains completely unknown. Examples of these tumors are synovial sarcoma, epithelioid sarcoma, and desmoplastic small round-cell tumor. For other tumors such as desmoid-type fibromatosis (DTF) and solitary fibrous tumor (SFT), there is an assumption that the

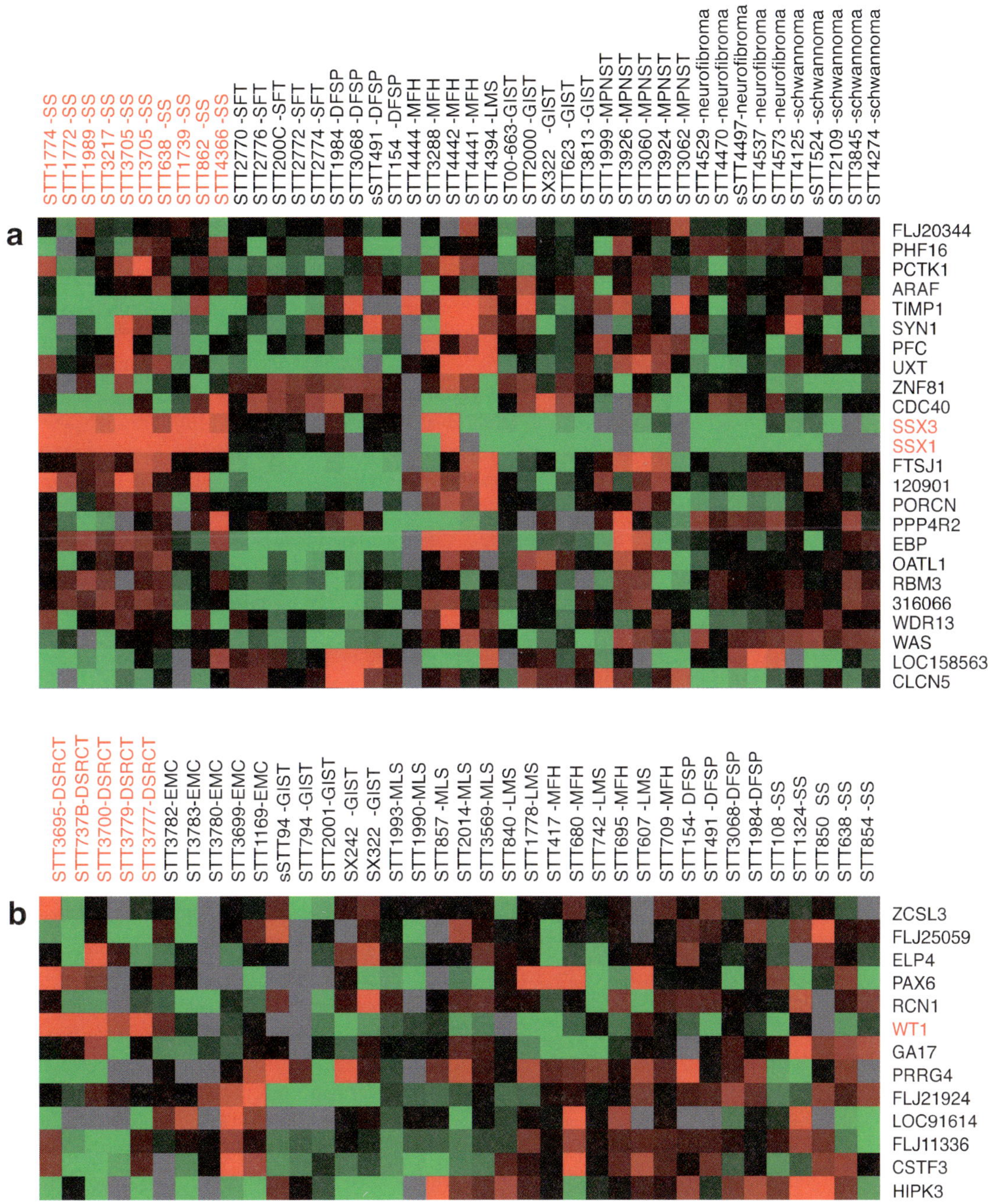

Figure 7

(*a*) Expression profiling data for a variety of 44 spindle-cell sarcomas, including 10 cases of synovial sarcoma. The genes are shown in rows and have been ordered according to their location on chromosome X. The SSX genes, involved in t(X;18), have a relatively higher level of expression in synovial sarcoma than in other tumors. Note that in this technique, mRNA levels for SSX3 and SSX1 cannot be distinguished. (*b*) A similar result is seen for the WT (Wilms tumor) gene in desmoplastic small round-cell tumors (DSRCT).

cell of origin is fibroblastic, but there is confusion about which type of fibroblast from which these two widely differing lesions derive. Currently there are no markers available to dissect normal stromal fibroblast into the subsets that may contain the precursors for these lesions. Bland spindle-shaped cells in connective tissue are currently lumped together under the terms fibroblast or myofibroblast. At the moment, very few markers exist that can be used to distinguish fibroblasts from myofibroblasts, let alone distinguish different subtypes of these cells.

A number of recent gene expression profiling studies suggest that the simple fibroblast may show a remarkable diversity of functions. For example, normal cultured fibroblasts have a distinct gene expression profile, on the basis of the site from which they were isolated (136). Likewise, endothelial and smooth muscle cells cultured from a variety of different sites in the body both show characteristic gene expression profiles that are site-specific (137). Interestingly, APOD, a marker for DFSPs (116), was found expressed at higher levels in endothelial cells from the dermis than in endothelial cells derived from other sites (137). This site-specific level of expression makes some sense when one realizes that DFSP originate in the dermis. The site-dependent variation in gene expression in these three cell types may explain, at least in part, the differences in behavior of the tumors derived from them. For example, SMTs that arise in the skin have a much better prognosis than those occurring in the deep soft tissues.

Another example of the complexity of fibroblast functions is found in the study of these cells' response to serum exposure in culture. Many of the genes induced or repressed in cultured fibroblasts upon serum exposure play a role in wound healing. This makes sense when one realizes that under physiological conditions, fibroblasts are exposed to serum only when the vascular wall has been damaged, as occurs in a wound. The genes that change expression upon exposure to serum are part of a variety of physiological responses to wounds that include, e.g., cell migration, neovascularization, hemostasis, and cytoskeletal rearrangement. Dvorak and others have proposed a long-standing hypothesis holding that carcinomas can elicit a type of wound-healing response in the surrounding stroma. This observation was based on a wide range of findings that include histologic and molecular similarities between wounds and tumor stroma, and a strong epidemiologic association between chronic wounds and cancer development (138). More recently researchers showed that tumor-associated fibroblasts enhance tumor engraftment and metastasis in nude mice (139, 140). Through analysis of global gene expression data in breast carcinoma and other epithelial malignancies, it became clear that the wound-healing program can be expressed in tumors either by the tumor cells themselves, by tumor-associated fibroblasts, or by both. More importantly, expression of these genes in a variety of epithelial malignancies, including breast carcinoma, lung carcinoma, and kidney tumors, is associated with poor clinical outcome (125). These findings indicate the complex interactions that exist between tumor cells and their surrounding stroma.

Through new marker discovery in STT s, previously unrecognized subsets of stromal cells may be identified in a manner similar to the way in which the study of lymphoma has illuminated lymphocytic differentiation pathways. We recently performed a proof-of-principle study based on the hypothesis that two similar fibroblastic tumors—SFT and DTF—can be derived by different molecular pathways from precursor cells present in normal stroma (141). If true, the markers that are differentially expressed between these two tumors would recognize different cell types in normal connective tissue. Furthermore, the differences between the gene expression patterns between SFT and DTF could provide a starting point to define distinct molecular origins of stromal proliferations in other settings, including the tumor-stroma interactions that lead to the reactive stroma in carcinomas such as breast and prostate carcinoma. DTF and SFT are composed of cells with very similar morphology, but with different histological growth patterns and dramatically different clinical behavior. SFT tends to be benign but can rarely transform into a high-grade metastatic tumor, whereas DTF shows locally aggressive recurrent behavior but never transforms into a metastatic neoplasm. In comparing the SFT and DTF gene expression profiles, we found a remarkably large number of differentially expressed genes (141). These include CTHRC1 and OSF2, highly and specifically expressed in DTF. The known SFT marker CD34 was highly expressed in SFT. In SFT we also found high levels of APOD mRNA compared to fibromatosis [although DFSP has higher levels still (116)]. In support of our hypothesis, ISH probes against CTHRC1 and OSF2 and existing antisera against CD34 and APOD showed that these markers are differentially expressed in normal connective tissue. For example, in inflammatory reactions such as those seen around fistula tracts, several DTF markers such as OSF2 are expressed in the spindle cells, but these cells fail to react for SFT markers such as CD34 (**Figures 8*a*** and ***b***). By contrast, CD34 and other SFT markers are found in spindle cells surrounding sweat glands in the dermis, and these fail to show expression for DTF markers such as CHTCR1 (**Figures 8*c*** and ***d***).

To examine the potential value of these distinct molecular signatures of stromal proliferations, we used SAM analysis to derive a model of the gene expression signatures of SFT and DTF, respectively, and searched for these signatures in large microarray gene expression data sets from 295 breast cancers (123). We found that the SFT and DTF signatures were differentially expressed among breast carcinomas and could be used to cluster breast carcinomas into different subsets (141). Among these subsets a group of breast carcinomas expressed DTF-specific genes, and a second less-well-defined group expressed predominantly SFT-specific genes. For several genes, including CTHRC1, OSF2 (DTF-specific), CD34, and APOD (SFT-specific), ISH, or IHC, confirmed the localization to the tumor stroma. For example, OSF2 was expressed in stromal, but not tumor, cells in a ductal carcinoma (**Figure 8*e***), which was negative for SFT markers (not shown). Interestingly, CTHRC1 was also recently described as expressed in tumor stroma in a SAGE analysis of breast carcinomas (142). APOD was seen in stromal cells (and in some epithelial cells) in a lobular carcinoma (**Figure 8*f***) that was negative for fibromatosis markers (not shown in **Figure 8*f***).

Thus, the two sets of genes that are expressed in SFT and DTF, respectively, appeared to show generally canonical and partly reciprocal patterns of expression in the stroma of breast carcinomas—i.e., some breast carcinomas expressed predominantly DTF-specific genes, and others expressed predominantly SFT-specific genes. Interestingly, the differential expression of these gene sets was correlated with clinical outcome. The tumors that predominantly expressed DTF genes had a much better clinical outcome compared to all other tumors, whereas those predominantly expressing SFT genes did much worse than all other tumors combined. This predictive role of tumor stroma is reminiscent of that seen with the wound-healing genes discovered on fibroblast grown in vitro in the presence or absence of serum, although the statistical significance of the DTF/SFT gene set appears less impressive than that seen with the wound-healing program. It is interesting to note that there is hardly any overlap (15 genes) between the 557 genes from the DTF/SFT gene set and the 500 genes described in the fibroblast serum response program. Although clearly further studies are needed to confirm these findings, these preliminary data indicate that the differential expression of genes in the stroma of tumors is of clinical significance. Thus, the study of sarcoma markers may indeed lead to the identification of novel stromal cell types, and these cell types may play a

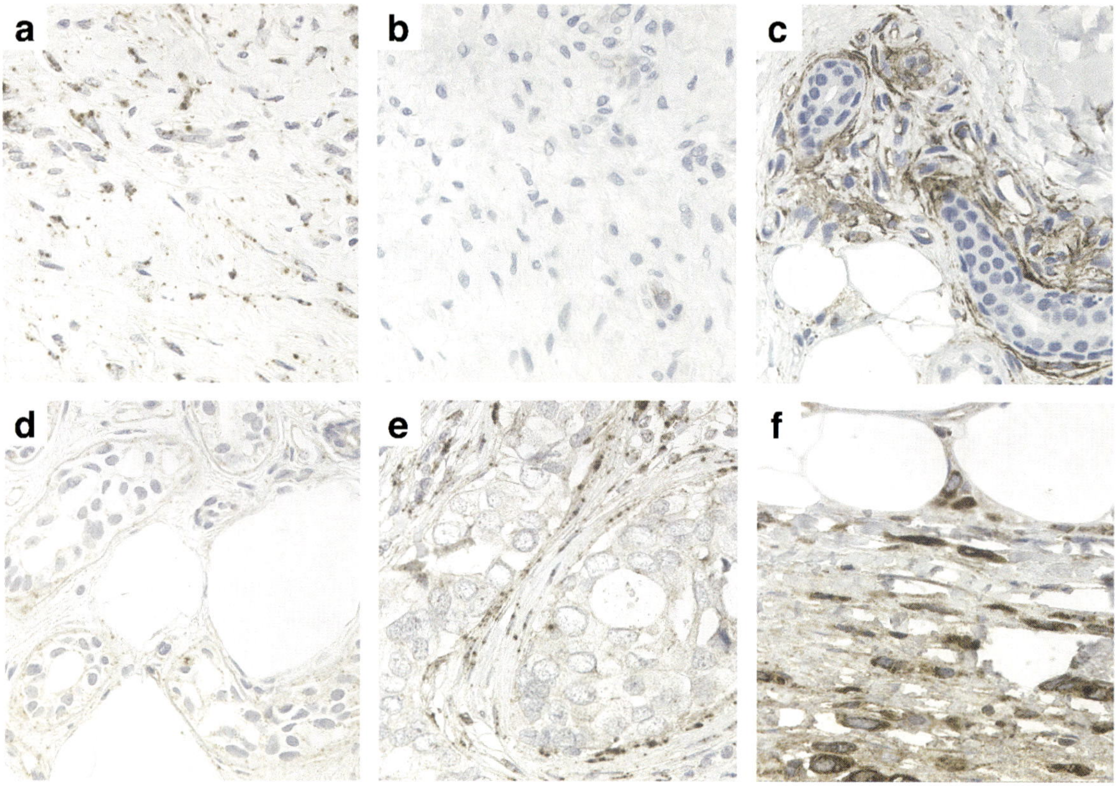

Figure 8

Differential expression of desmoid-type fribromatosis (DTF) and solitary firbrous tumor (SFT) markers in (*a*, *b*) granulation tissue, (*c*, *d*) sweat glands in skin, (*e*) ductal breast carcinoma, and (*f*) lobular breast carcinoma stained with DTF markers (OSF2-A, CTHRC1-D, and OSF2-E) and SFT markers (CD34-B, -C, and APOD-F).

role in determining the outcome of epithelial neoplasms.

Screening of Sarcoma TMAs by In Situ Hybridization

Alterations in the activation state of tyrosine kinase receptors play an important role in several STTs. As mentioned above, in DFSP, the PDGFB gene, ligand for the tyrosine kinase receptor PDGFRB, is fused through a chromosomal translocation with the COL1A1 gene. This leads to an elevated level of expression of the hybrid protein, which contains the N-terminal portion of COL1A1 and C-terminal portion of PDGFB. This hybrid protein is further processed in the cell and through proteolytic processing is transformed into a mature, biologically active PDGFB dimer that can drive the cell to tumor formation. Expression profiling has shown that in DFSP not only is the PDGFB gene highly expressed but so is its receptor, PDGFRB (54). This suggests the existence of an autocrine loop that activates the DFSP tumor cells. Within DFSP, several other genes involved in the PDGF pathway are also expressed at high levels compared to other STTs. Structurally, the PDGFRB gene is highly related to KIT and indeed, several reports have been made of the successful treatment of DFSP with Imatinib. A third example of the involvement of tyrosine kinase receptors in STTs was found in a recent study on the tyrosine kinase receptor CSF1R expression by ISH on TMAs containing 460 sarcomas. ISH allows successful interpretation of RNA levels for a large number of genes (30, 115, 132, 143, 144) on TMAs made with formalin-fixed, paraffin-embedded samples. All nine tenosynovial giant cell tumors showed high expression for CSF1R. Tenosynovial giant cell tumors are known to have a chromosomal translocation that most frequently involves chromosome 1 and 2, but the fusion partners on the chromosome have not yet been identified. Whereas CSF1R is not located on either chromosome, its ligand CSF1 is located in the area in which the translocation occurs on chromosome 1, as identified by conventional cytogenetics. Subsequent FISH studies showed that the translocation indeed involves CSF1 on chromosome 1 (R.B. West, manuscript in preparation). It therefore appears that an extensive search for the expression of other tyrosine kinase receptors in sarcoma may well lead to additional discoveries.

FUTURE

The past 10 years have witnessed a progressive interest in experimental studies of sarcomas. Certainly the success story of Imatinib in GIST, which was in turn enabled by the elucidation of the crucial KIT oncogenic roles in that tumor, has contributed to this interest. In addition, STTs continue to present diagnostic and therapeutic challenges, and the need for better biologic markers and therapeutic targets is ever pressing. Several aspects of sarcoma biology underscore just how well these rare tumors have served in providing insights into cancer biology. First, many sarcomas feature characteristic chromosomal rearrangements, and the mapping and cloning of these rearrangements have led to the identification of dozens of novel oncogenes. Second, sarcomas often feature demonstrable aberrations in kinase pathway signaling that have proved to be exceptional therapeutic targets. In this sense, sarcomas serve in general as a model for successful targeted therapy methods in solid tumor oncology. Third, sarcomas account for most of the non-CNS solid tumors in children, and therefore the continued study of sarcomas has been particularly important for progress in pediatric oncology. Fourth, the experimental characterization of those basic aspects of sarcoma biology—including identification of the transformed progenitor cell and the oncogenic mechanisms of sarcoma cell growth, survival, and differentiation—has much to contribute to a broader understanding of mesenchymal biology. For example, one can anticipate that the growth-promoting pathways in sarcomas may also be relevant in nonneoplastic disorders ranging from atherosclerotic disease to chronic inflammation. Indeed, in recent years four meetings were organized by the National Cancer Institute to support sarcoma research (State of the Science meeting, July 17–18, 2002; Sarcoma Progress Review Group planning meeting, June 30, 2003; Sarcoma Progress Review Group roundtable meeting, October 8–10, 2003; and Sarcoma-Mesenchymal Stem Cell Workshop, September 27–28, 2004). The most recent meeting, which convened researchers from the fields of sarcoma and mesenchymal stem cell research, was a tangible step in broadening the already considerable impact of sarcoma science.

ACKNOWLEDGMENTS

The authors would like to thank Drs. Blake Gilks, Torsten Nielsen, and Subbaya Subramanian for helpful comments.

LITERATURE CITED

1. Borden EC, Goldblum JR. 2002. Molecular characterization of soft tissue tumors. *Curr. Oncol. Rep.* 4:497–98
2. Fletcher CD, Berman JJ, Corless C, Gorstein F, Lasota J, et al. 2002. Diagnosis of gastrointestinal stromal tumors: A consensus approach. *Hum. Pathol.* 33:459–65
3. Weiss SW, Goldblum JR, eds. 2001. *Enzinger and Weiss's Soft Tissue Tumors*. Philadelphia: Mosby. 1632 pp. 4th ed.
4. Kempson RL, Fletcher CD, Evans HE, Hendrickson MR, Sibley RK. 2001. *Tumors of the Soft Tissues*. Bethesda, MD: Armed Forces Inst. Pathol.
5. Bell SW, Kempson RL, Hendrickson MR. 1994. Problematic uterine smooth muscle neoplasms. A clinicopathologic study of 213 cases. *Am. J. Surg. Pathol.* 18:535–58
6. Lee YF, John M, Edwards S, Clark J, Flohr P, et al. 2003. Molecular classification of synovial sarcomas, leiomyosarcomas and malignant fibrous histiocytomas by gene expression profiling. *Br. J. Cancer* 88:510–15
7. Quade BJ, Wang TY, Sornberger K, Dal Cin P, Mutter GL, Morton CC. 2004. Molecular pathogenesis of uterine smooth muscle tumors from transcriptional profiling. *Genes Chromosomes Cancer* 40:97–108
8. Ren B, Yu YP, Jing L, Liu L, Michalopoulos GK, et al. 2003. Gene expression analysis of human soft tissue leiomyosarcomas. *Hum. Pathol.* 34:549–58
9. Skubitz KM, Skubitz AP. 2003. Differential gene expression in leiomyosarcoma. *Cancer* 98:1029–38
10. Greco A, Roccato E, Miranda C, Cleris L, Formelli F, Pierotti MA. 2001. Growth-inhibitory effect of STI571 on cells transformed by the COL1A1/PDGFB rearrangement. *Int. J. Cancer* 92:354–60
11. O'Brien KP, Seroussi E, Dal Cin P, Sciot R, Mandahl N, et al. 1998. Various regions within the α-helical domain of the COL1A1 gene are fused to the second exon of the PDGFB gene in dermatofibrosarcomas and giant-cell fibroblastomas. *Genes Chromosomes Cancer* 23:187–93
12. Hirota S, Isozaki K, Moriyama Y, Hashimoto K, Nishida T, et al. 1998. Gain-of-function mutations of c-kit in human gastrointestinal stromal tumors. *Science* 279:577–80
13. Fletcher JA, Kozakewich HP, Hoffer FA, Lage JM, Weidner N, et al. 1991. Diagnostic relevance of clonal cytogenetic aberrations in malignant soft-tissue tumors. *N. Engl. J. Med.* 324:436–42
14. Heim S, Mitelman F. 1995. *Cancer Cytogenetics*. New York: Wiley-Liss. 536 pp. 2nd ed.
15. Sandberg AA, Bridge JA. 1995. *The Cytogenetics of Bone and Soft Tissue Tumors*. Austin: R.G. Landes. 469 pp.
16. Sandberg AA, Turc-Carel C, Gemmill RM. 1998. Chromosomes in solid tumors and beyond. *Cancer Res.* 48:1049–59
17. Sreekantaiah C, Ladanyi M, Rodriguez E, Chaganti RS. 1994. Chromosomal aberrations in soft tissue tumors. Relevance to diagnosis, classification, and molecular mechanisms. *Am. J. Pathol.* 144:1121–34
18. Fletcher CD, Akerman M, Dal Cin P, de Wever I, Mandahl N, et al. 1996. Correlation between clinicopathological features and karyotype in lipomatous tumors. A report of 178 cases from the Chromosomes and Morphology (CHAMP) Collaborative Study Group. *Am. J. Pathol.* 148:623–30
19. Sreekantaiah C, Karakousis CP, Leong SP, Sandberg AA. 1992. Cytogenetic findings in liposarcoma correlate with histopathologic subtypes. *Cancer* 69:2484–95

20. Turc-Carel C, Limon J, Dal Cin P, Rao U, Karakousis C, Sandberg AA. 1986. Cytogenetic studies of adipose tissue tumors. II. Recurrent reciprocal translocation t(12;16)(q13;p11) in myxoid liposarcomas. *Cancer Genet. Cytogenet.* 23:291–99
21. Hisaoka M, Tsuji S, Morimitsu Y, Hashimoto H, Shimajiri S, et al. 1998. Detection of TLS/FUS-CHOP fusion transcripts in myxoid and round cell liposarcomas by nested reverse transcription-polymerase chain reaction using archival paraffin-embedded tissues. *Diagn. Mol. Pathol.* 7:96–101
22. Kuroda M, Ishida T, Horiuchi H, Kida N, Uozaki H, et al. Chimeric TLS/FUS-CHOP gene expression and the heterogeneity of its junction in human myxoid and round cell liposarcoma. *Am. J. Pathol.* 147:1221–27
23. Aman P, Ron D, Mandahl N, Fioretos T, Heim S, et al. 1992. Rearrangement of the transcription factor gene CHOP in myxoid liposarcomas with t(12;16)(q13;p11). *Genes Chromosomes Cancer* 5:278–85
24. Crozat A, Aman P, Mandahl N, Ron D. 1993. Fusion of CHOP to a novel RNA-binding protein in human myxoid liposarcoma. *Nature* 363:640–44
25. Mandahl N, Heim S, Arheden K, Rydholm A, Willen H, Mitelman F. 1988. Rings, dicentrics, and telomeric association in histiocytomas. *Cancer Genet. Cytogenet.* 30:23–33
26. Turc-Carel C, Dal Cin P, Rao U, Karakousis C, Sandberg AA. 1998. Recurrent breakpoints at 9q31 and 22q12.2 in extraskeletal myxoid chondrosarcoma. *Cancer Genet. Cytogenet.* 30:145–50
27. Pedeutour F, Forus A, Coindre JM, Berner JM, Nicolo G, et al. 1999. Structure of the supernumerary ring and giant rod chromosomes in adipose tissue tumors. *Genes Chromosomes Cancer* 24:30–41
28. Tontonoz P, Singer S, Forman BM, Sarraf P, Fletcher JA, et al. 1997. Terminal differentiation of human liposarcoma cells induced by ligands for peroxisome proliferator-activated receptor γ and the retinoid X receptor. *Proc. Natl. Acad. Sci. USA* 94:237–41
29. Demetri GD, Fletcher CD, Mueller E, Sarraf P, Naujoks R, et al. 1999. Induction of solid tumor differentiation by the peroxisome proliferator-activated receptor-γ ligand troglitazone in patients with liposarcoma. *Proc. Natl. Acad. Sci. USA* 96:3951–56
30. Subramanian S, West RB, Marinelli RJ, Nielsen TO, Rubin BP, et al. 2005. Gene expression profile of extraskeletal myxoid chondrosarcoma. *J. Pathol.* 206:433–44
31. Segal NH, Pavlidis P, Noble WS, Antonescu CR, Viale A, et al. 2003. Classification of clear-cell sarcoma as a subtype of melanoma by genomic profiling. *J. Clin. Oncol.* 21:1775–81
32. Brown AD, Lopez-Terrada D, Denny C, Lee KA. 1995. Promoters containing ATF-binding sites are de-regulated in cells that express the EWS/ATF1 oncogene. *Oncogene* 10:1749–56
33. Zucman J, Delattre O, Desmaze C, Epstein AL, Stenman G, et al. 1993. EWS and ATF-1 gene fusion induced by t(12;22) translocation in malignant melanoma of soft parts. *Nat. Genet.* 4:341–45
34. Gerald WL, Miller HK, Battifora H, Miettinen M, Silva EG, Rosai J. 1991. Intra-abdominal desmoplastic small round-cell tumor. Report of 19 cases of a distinctive type of high-grade polyphenotypic malignancy affecting young individuals. *Am. J. Surg. Pathol.* 15:499–513
35. Gerald WL, Ladanyi M, de Alava E, Cuatrecasas M, Kushner BH, et al. 1998. Clinical, pathologic, and molecular spectrum of tumors associated with t(11;22)(p13;q12): desmoplastic small round-cell tumor and its variants. *J. Clin. Oncol.* 16:3028–36

36. Ladanyi M, Gerald W. 1994. Fusion of the EWS and WT1 genes in the desmoplastic small round cell tumor. *Cancer Res.* 54:2837–40
37. Biegel JA, Conard K, Brooks JJ. 1993. Translocation (11;22)(p13;q12): primary change in intra-abdominal desmoplastic small round cell tumor. *Genes Chromosomes Cancer* 7:119–21
38. Rodriguez E, Sreekantaiah C, Gerald W, Reuter VE, Motzer RJ, Chaganti RS. 1993. A recurring translocation, t(11;22)(p13;q11.2), characterizes intra-abdominal desmoplastic small round-cell tumors. *Cancer Genet. Cytogenet.* 69:17–21
39. Lee SB, Kolquist KA, Nichols K, Englert C, Maheswaran S, et al. 1997. The EWS-WT1 translocation product induces PDGFA in desmoplastic small round-cell tumour. *Nat. Genet.* 17:309–13
40. Kelly JD, Haldeman BA, Grant FJ, Murray MJ, Seifert RA, et al. Platelet-derived growth factor (PDGF) stimulates PDGF receptor subunit dimerization and intersubunit trans-phosphorylation. *J. Biol. Chem.* 266:8987–92
41. Delattre O, Zucman J, Plougastel B, Desmaze C, Melot T, et al. 1992. Gene fusion with an ETS DNA-binding domain caused by chromosome translocation in human tumours. *Nature* 359:162–65
42. Ewen ME, Ludlow JW, Marsilio E, DeCaprio JA, Millikan RC, et al. An N-terminal transformation-governing sequence of SV40 large T antigen contributes to the binding of both p110Rb and a second cellular protein, p120. *Cell* 58:257–67
43. Turc-Carel C, Aurias A, Mugneret F, Lizard S, Sidaner I, et al. 1988. Chromosomes in Ewing's sarcoma. I. An evaluation of 85 cases of remarkable consistency of t(11;22)(q24;q12). *Cancer Genet. Cytogenet.* 32:229–38
44. Turc-Carel C, Philip I, Berger MP, Philip T, Lenoir GM. 1984. Chromosome study of Ewing's sarcoma (ES) cell lines. Consistency of a reciprocal translocation t(11;22)(q24;q12). *Cancer Genet. Cytogenet.* 12:1–19
45. Buckler AJ, Chang DD, Graw SL, Brook JD, Haber DA, et al. 1991. Exon amplification: a strategy to isolate mammalian genes based on RNA splicing. *Proc. Natl. Acad. Sci. USA* 88:4005–9
46. Ishida S, Yoshida K, Kaneko Y, Tanaka Y, Sasaki Y, et al. 1998. The genomic breakpoint and chimeric transcripts in the EWSR1-ETV4/E1AF gene fusion in Ewing sarcoma. *Cytogenet. Cell Genet.* 82:278–83
47. Jeon IS, Davis JN, Braun BS, Sublett JE, Roussel MF, et al. 1995. A variant Ewing's sarcoma translocation (7;22) fuses the EWS gene to the ETS gene ETV1. *Oncogene* 10:1229–34
48. Kaneko Y, Yoshida K, Handa M, Toyoda Y, Nishihira H, et al. 1996. Fusion of an ETS-family gene, EIAF, to EWS by t(17;22)(q12;q12) chromosome translocation in an undifferentiated sarcoma of infancy. *Genes Chromosomes Cancer* 15:115–21
49. Peter M, Couturier J, Pacquement H, Michon J, Thomas G, et al. 1997. A new member of the ETS family fused to EWS in Ewing tumors. *Oncogene* 14:1159–64
50. Dagher R, Long LM, Read EJ, Leitman SF, Carter CS, et al. 2002. Pilot trial of tumor-specific peptide vaccination and continuous infusion interleukin-2 in patients with recurrent Ewing sarcoma and alveolar rhabdomyosarcoma: an inter-institute NIH study. *Med. Pediatr. Oncol.* 38:158–64
51. Naeem R, Lux ML, Huang SF, Naber SP, Corson JM, Fletcher JA. 1995. Ring chromosomes in dermatofibrosarcoma protuberans are composed of interspersed sequences from chromosomes 17 and 22. *Am. J. Pathol.* 147:1553–58

52. Pedeutour F, Simon MP, Minoletti F, Sozzi G, Pierotti MA, et al. 1995. Ring 22 chromosomes in dermatofibrosarcoma protuberans are low-level amplifiers of chromosome 17 and 22 sequences. *Cancer Res.* 55:2400–2403
53. Simon MP, Pedeutour F, Sirvent N, Grosgeorge J, Minoletti F, et al. 1997. Deregulation of the platelet-derived growth factor B-chain gene via fusion with collagen gene COL1A1 in dermatofibrosarcoma protuberans and giant-cell fibroblastoma. *Nat. Genet.* 15:95–98
54. Linn SC, West RB, Pollack JR, Zhu S, Hernandez-Boussard T, et al. 2003. Gene expression patterns and gene copy number changes in dermatofibrosarcoma protuberans. *Am. J. Pathol.* 163:2383–95
55. Maki RG, Awan RA, Dixon RH, Jhanwar S, Antonescu CR. 2002. Differential sensitivity to imatinib of 2 patients with metastatic sarcoma arising from dermatofibrosarcoma protuberans. *Int. J. Cancer* 100:623–26
56. Rubin BP, Schuetze SM, Eary JF, Norwood TH, Mirza S, et al. 2002. Molecular targeting of platelet-derived growth factor B by imatinib mesylate in a patient with metastatic dermatofibrosarcoma protuberans. *J. Clin. Oncol.* 20:3586–91
57. Alman BA, Li C, Pajerski ME, Diaz-Cano S, Wolfe HJ. 1997. Increased β-catenin protein and somatic APC mutations in sporadic aggressive fibromatoses (desmoid tumors). *Am. J. Pathol.* 151:329–34
58. Tejpar S, Nollet F, Li C, Wunder JS, Michils G, et al. 1999. Predominance of β-catenin mutations and β-catenin dysregulation in sporadic aggressive fibromatosis (desmoid tumor). *Oncogene* 18:6615–20
59. Fletcher JA, Naeem R, Xiao S, Corson JM. 1995. Chromosome aberrations in desmoid tumors. Trisomy 8 may be a predictor of recurrence. *Cancer Genet. Cytogenet.* 79:139–43
60. Miyaki M, Konishi M, Kikuchi-Yanoshita R, Enomoto M, Tanaka K, et al. Coexistence of somatic and germ-line mutations of APC gene in desmoid tumors from patients with familial adenomatous polyposis. *Cancer Res.* 53:5079–82
61. Sen-Gupta S, Van der Luijt RB, Bowles LV, Meera Khan P, Delhanty JD, et al. 1993. Somatic mutation of APC gene in desmoid tumour in familial adenomatous polyposis. *Lancet* 342:552–53
62. Mace J, Sybil Biermann J, Sondak V, McGinn C, Hayes C, et al. 2002. Response of extraabdominal desmoid tumors to therapy with imatinib mesylate. *Cancer* 95:2373–79
63. Schofield DE, Fletcher JA, Grier HE, Yunis EJ. 1994. Fibrosarcoma in infants and children. Application of new techniques. *Am. J. Surg. Pathol.* 18:14–24
64. Schofield DE, Yunis EJ, Fletcher JA. 1993. Chromosome aberrations in mesoblastic nephroma. *Am. J. Pathol.* 143:714–24
65. Knezevich SR, Garnett MJ, Pysher TJ, Beckwith JB, Grundy PE, Sorensen PH. 1998. ETV6-NTRK3 gene fusions and trisomy 11 establish a histogenetic link between mesoblastic nephroma and congenital fibrosarcoma, *Cancer Res.* 58:5046–48
66. Knezevich SR, McFadden DE, Tao W, Lim JF, Sorensen PH. 1998. A novel ETV6-NTRK3 gene fusion in congenital fibrosarcoma. *Nat. Genet.* 18:184–87
67. Rubin BP, Chen CJ, Morgan TW, Xiao S, Grier HE, et al. Congenital mesoblastic nephroma t(12;15) is associated with ETV6-NTRK3 gene fusion: cytogenetic and molecular relationship to congenital (infantile) fibrosarcoma. *Am. J. Pathol.* 153:1451–58
68. Bolande RP. 1973. Congenital mesoblastic nephroma of infancy. *Perspect. Pediatr. Pathol.* 1:227–50
69. Chung EB, Enzinger FM. 1976. Infantile fibrosarcoma. *Cancer* 38:729–39
70. Snyder CS, Dell'Aquila M, Haghighi P, Baergen RN, Suh YK, Yi ES. 1995. Clonal changes in inflammatory pseudotumor of the lung: a case report. *Cancer* 76:1545–49

71. Su LD, Atayde-Perez A, Sheldon S, Fletcher JA, Weiss SW. 1998. Inflammatory myofibroblastic tumor: cytogenetic evidence supporting clonal origin. *Mod. Pathol.* 11:364–68
72. Treissman SP, Gillis DA, Lee CL, Giacomantonio M, Resch L. 1994. Omental-mesenteric inflammatory pseudotumor. Cytogenetic demonstration of genetic changes and monoclonality in one tumor. *Cancer* 73:1433–37
73. Lawrence B, Perez-Atayde A, Hibbard MK, Rubin BP, Dal Cin P, et al. 2000. TPM3-ALK and TPM4-ALK oncogenes in inflammatory myofibroblastic tumors. *Am. J. Pathol.* 157:377–84
74. Heinrich MC, Corless CL, Duensing A, McGreevey L, Chen CJ, et al. 2003. PDGFRA activating mutations in gastrointestinal stromal tumors. *Science* 299:708–10
75. Rubin BP, Singer S, Tsao C, Duensing A, Lux ML, et al. 2001. KIT activation is a ubiquitous feature of gastrointestinal stromal tumors. *Cancer Res.* 61:8118–21
76. Duensing A, Heinrich MC, Fletcher CD, Fletcher JA. 2004. Biology of gastrointestinal stromal tumors: KIT mutations and beyond. *Cancer Invest.* 22:106–16
77. Heinrich MC, Blanke CD, Druker BJ, Corless CL. 2002. Inhibition of KIT tyrosine kinase activity: a novel molecular approach to the treatment of KIT-positive malignancies. *J. Clin. Oncol.* 20:1692–1703
78. Nishida T, Hirota S, Taniguchi M, Hashimoto K, Isozaki K, et al. 1998. Familial gastrointestinal stromal tumours with germline mutation of the KIT gene. *Nat. Genet.* 19:323–24
79. Demetri GD, von Mehren M, Blanke CD, Van den Abbeele AD, Eisenberg B, et al. 2002. Efficacy and safety of imatinib mesylate in advanced gastrointestinal stromal tumors. *N. Engl. J. Med.* 347:472–80
80. van Oosterom AT, Judson I, Verweij J, Stroobants S, Donato di Paola E, et al. 2001. Safety and efficacy of imatinib (STI571) in metastatic gastrointestinal stromal tumours: a phase I study. *Lancet* 358:1421–23
81. Sarlomo-Rikala M, El-Rifai W, Lahtinen T, Andersson LC, Miettinen M, Knuutila S. 1998. Different patterns of DNA copy number changes in gastrointestinal stromal tumors, leiomyomas, and schwannomas. *Hum Pathol.* 29:476–81
82. Sommer G, Agosti V, Ehlers I, Rossi F, Corbacioglu S, et al. 2003. Gastrointestinal stromal tumors in a mouse model by targeted mutation of the Kit receptor tyrosine kinase. *Proc. Nat. Acad. Sci. USA* 100:6706–11
83. Heinrich MC, Rubin BP, Longley BJ, Fletcher JA. 2002. Biology and genetic aspects of gastrointestinal stromal tumors: KIT activation and cytogenetic alterations. *Hum. Pathol.* 33:484–95
84. Basu TN, Gutmann DH, Fletcher JA, Glover TW, Collins FS, Downward J. 1992. Aberrant regulation of ras proteins in malignant tumour cells from type 1 neurofibromatosis patients. *Nature* 356:713–15
85. DeClue JE, Papageorge AG, Fletcher JA, Diehl SR, Ratner N, et al. 1992. Abnormal regulation of mammalian p21ras contributes to malignant tumor growth in von Recklinghausen (type 1) neurofibromatosis. *Cell* 69:265–73
86. Legius E, Marchuk DA, Collins FS, Glover TW. 1993. Somatic deletion of the neurofibromatosis type 1 gene in a neurofibrosarcoma supports a tumour suppressor gene hypothesis. *Nat. Genet.* 3:122–26
87. Lutchman M, Rouleau GA. 1995. The neurofibromatosis type 2 gene product, schwannomin, suppresses growth of NIH 3T3 cells. *Cancer Res.* 55:2270–74
88. Rouleau GA, Merel P, Lutchman M, Sanson M, Zucman J, et al. 1993. Alteration in a new gene encoding a putative membrane-organizing protein causes neuro-fibromatosis type 2. *Nature* 363:515–21

89. Twist EC, Ruttledge MH, Rousseau M, Sanson M, Papi L, et al. 1994. The neurofibromatosis type 2 gene is inactivated in schwannomas. *Hum. Mol. Genet.* 3:147–51
90. Kluwe L, Friedrich R, Mautner VF. 1999. Loss of NF1 allele in Schwann cells but not in fibroblasts derived from an NF1-associated neurofibroma. *Genes Chromosomes Cancer* 24:283–85
91. Xu GF, Lin B, Tanaka K, Dunn D, Wood D, et al. 1990. The catalytic domain of the neurofibromatosis type 1 gene product stimulates ras GTPase and complements ira mutants of *S. cerevisiae*. *Cell* 63:835–41
92. Xu GF, O'Connell P, Viskochil D, Cawthon R, Robertson M, et al. 1990. The neurofibromatosis type 1 gene encodes a protein related to GAP. *Cell* 62:599–608
93. Biegel JA, Zhou JY, Rorke LB, Stenstrom C, Wainwright LM, Fogelgren B. 1999. Germline and acquired mutations of INI1 in atypical teratoid and rhabdoid tumors. *Cancer Res.* 59:74–79
94. Versteege I, Sevenet N, Lange J, Rousseau-Merck MF, Ambros P, et al. 1998. Truncating mutations of hSNF5/INI1 in aggressive paediatric cancer. *Nature* 394:203–206
95. Sevenet N, Sheridan E, Amram D, Schneider P, Handgretinger R, Delattre O. 1999. Constitutional mutations of the hSNF5/INI1 gene predispose to a variety of cancers. *Am. J. Hum. Genet.* 65:1342–48
96. Roberts CW, Galusha SA, McMenamin ME, Fletcher CD, Orkin SH. 2000. Haploinsufficiency of Snf5 (integrase interactor 1) predisposes to malignant rhabdoid tumors in mice. *Proc. Natl. Acad. Sci. USA* 97:13796–800
97. Barr FG, Galili N, Holick J, Biegel JA, Rovera G, Emanuel BS. 1993. Rearrangement of the PAX3 paired box gene in the paediatric solid tumour alveolar rhabdomyosarcoma. *Nat. Genet.* 3:113–17
98. Galili N, Davis RJ, Fredericks WJ, Mukhopadhyay S, Rauscher FJ III, et al. 1993. Fusion of a fork head domain gene to PAX3 in the solid tumour alveolar rhabdomyosarcoma. *Nat. Genet.* 5:230–35
99. Shapiro DN, Sublett JE, Li B, Downing JR, Naeve CW. 1993. Fusion of PAX3 to a member of the forkhead family of transcription factors in human alveolar rhabdomyosarcoma. *Cancer Res.* 53:5108–12
100. Davis RJ, D'Cruz CM, Lovell MA, Biegel JA, Barr FG. 1994. Fusion of PAX7 to FKHR by the variant t(1;13)(p36;q14) translocation in alveolar rhabdomyosarcoma. *Cancer Res.* 54:2869–72
101. Bennicelli JL, Fredericks WJ, Wilson RB, Rauscher FJ III, Barr FG. 1995. Wild type PAX3 protein and the PAX3-FKHR fusion protein of alveolar rhabdomyosarcoma contain potent, structurally distinct transcriptional activation domains. *Oncogene* 11:119–30
102. Fredericks WJ, Galili N, Mukhopadhyay S, Rovera G, Bennicelli J, et al. 1995. The PAX3-FKHR fusion protein created by the t(2;13) translocation in alveolar rhabdomyosarcomas is a more potent transcriptional activator than PAX3. *Mol. Cell. Biol.* 15:1522–35
103. Nanni P, Nicoletti G, De Giovanni C, Croci S, Astolfi A, et al. 2003. Development of rhabdomyosarcoma in HER-2/neu transgenic p53 mutant mice. *Cancer Res.* 63:2728–32
104. Sharp R, Recio JA, Jhappan C, Otsuka T, Liu S, et al. 2002. Synergism between INK4a/ARF inactivation and aberrant HGF/SF signaling in rhabdomyosarcomagenesis. *Nat. Med.* 8:1276–80
105. Kalebic T, Blakesley V, Slade C, Plasschaert S, Leroith D, Helman LJ. 1998. Expression of a kinase-deficient IGF-I-R suppresses tumorigenicity of rhabdomyosarcoma cells constitutively expressing a wild type IGF-I-R. *Int. J. Cancer* 76:223–27

106. Kalebic T, Tsokos M, Helman LJ. 1994. In vivo treatment with antibody against IGF-1 receptor suppresses growth of human rhabdomyosarcoma and down-regulates p34cdc2. *Cancer Res.* 54:5531–34
107. Clark J, Rocques PJ, Crew AJ, Gill S, Shipley J, et al. 1994. Identification of novel genes, SYT and SSX, involved in the t(X;18)(p11.2;q11.2) translocation found in human synovial sarcoma. *Nat. Genet.* 7:502–8
108. Matsuzaki A, Suminoe A, Hattori H, Hoshina T, Hara T. 2002. Immunotherapy with autologous dendritic cells and tumor-specific synthetic peptides for synovial sarcoma. *J. Pediatr. Hematol. Oncol.* 24:220–23
109. Allander SV, Illei PB, Chen Y, Antonescu CR, Bittner M, et al. 2002. Expression profiling of synovial sarcoma by cDNA microarrays: association of ERBB2, IGFBP2, and ELF3 with epithelial differentiation. *Am. J. Pathol.* 161:1587–95
110. Nielsen TO, Hsu FD, O'Connell JX, Gilks CB, West RB, et al. 2003. Tissue microarray analysis of novel synovial sarcoma immunohistochemical markers. *Am. J. Pathol.* 163:1449–56
111. Nielsen TO, West RB, Linn SC, Alter O, Knowling MA, et al. 2002. Molecular characterisation of soft tissue tumours: a gene expression study. *Lancet* 359:1301–7
112. Lynch TJ, Bell DW, Sordella R, Gurubhagavatula S, Okimoto RA, et al. 2004. Activating mutations in the epidermal growth factor receptor underlying responsiveness of non-small-cell lung cancer to gefitinib. *New Engl. J. Med.* 350:2129–39
113. Tusher VG, Tibshirani R, Chu G. 2001. Significance analysis of microarrays applied to the ionizing radiation response. *Proc. Nat. Acad. Sci. USA* 98:5116–21. Erratum. 2001. *Proc. Natl. Acad. Sci. USA* 98:10515
114. Duensing A, Joseph NE, Medeiros F, Smith F, Hornick JL, et al. 2004. Protein kinase C θ (PKCθ) expression and constitutive activation in gastrointestinal stromal tumors (GIST s). *Cancer Res.* 64:5127–31
115. West RB, Corless CL, Chen X, Rubin BP, Subramanian S, et al. 2004. The novel marker, DOG1, is expressed ubiquitously in gastrointestinal stromal tumors irrespective of KIT or PDGFRA mutation status. *Am. J. Pathol.* 165:107–13
116. West RB, Harvell J, Linn SC, Lui CL, Prapong W, et al. 2004. Apo D in soft tissue tumors: a novel marker for dermatofibrosarcoma protuberans. *Am. J. Surg. Pathol.* 28:1063–69
117. Perou CM, Jeffrey SS, van de Rijn M, Rees CA, Eisen MB, et al. 1999. Distinctive gene expression patterns in human mammary epithelial cells and breast cancers. *Proc. Nat. Acad. Sci. USA* 96:9212–17
118. Perou CM, Sorlie T, Eisen MB, van de Rijn M, Jeffrey SS, et al. 2000. Molecular portraits of human breast tumours. *Nature* 406:747–52
119. Sorlie T, Tibshirani R, Parker J, Hastie T, Marron JS, et al. 2003. Repeated observation of breast tumor subtypes in independent gene expression data sets. *Proc. Natl. Acad. Sci. USA* 100:8418–23
120. Abd El-Rehim DM, Pinder SE, Paish CE, Bell J, Blamey RW, et al. 2004. Expression of luminal and basal cytokeratins in human breast carcinoma. *J. Pathol.* 203:661–71
121. Nielsen TO, Hsu FD, Jensen K, Cheang M, Karaca G, et al. 2004. Immunohistochemical and clinical characterization of the basal-like subtype of invasive breast carcinoma. *Clin. Cancer Res.* 10:5367–74
122. van de Rijn M, Perou CM, Tibshirani R, Haas P, Kallioniemi O, et al. 2003. Expression of cytokeratins 17 and 5 identifies a group of breast carcinomas with poor clinical outcome. *Am. J. Pathol.* 161:1991–96

123. van de Vijver MJ, He YD, van't Veer LJ, Dai H, Hart AA, et al. 2002. A gene-expression signature as a predictor of survival in breast cancer. *New Engl. J. Med.* 347:1999–2009
124. Chang HY, Nuyten DSA, Sneddon JB, Hastie T, Tibshirani R, et al. 2005. Robustness, scalability, and integration of a wound-response gene expression signature in predicting breast cancer survival. *Proc. Natl. Acad. Sci. USA* 102:3738–43
125. Chang HY, Sneddon J, Alizadeh A, Sood R, West R, et al. 2004. Gene expression signature of fibroblast serum response predicts human cancer progression: similarities between tumors and wounds. *PLoS Biol.* 2:e7
126. Paik S, Shak S, Tang G, Kim C, Baker J, et al. 2004. A multigene assay to predict recurrence of tamoxifen-treated, node-negative breast cancer. *New Engl. J. Med.* 351:2817–26
127. Makretsov N, Huntsman D, Nielsen TO, Yorida E, Peacock M, et al. 2004. Identification of prognostically significant subgroups in breast carcinoma by clustering of immunostain results. *Clin. Cancer Res.* 10:6143–51
128. Allander SV, Nupponen NN, Ringner M, Hostetter G, Maher GW, et al. 2001. Gastrointestinal stromal tumors with KIT mutations exhibit a remarkably homogeneous gene expression profile. *Cancer Res.* 61:8624–28
129. Segal NH, Pavlidis P, Antonescu CR, Maki RG, Noble WS, et al. Classification and subtype prediction of adult soft tissue sarcoma by functional genomics. *Am. J. Pathol.* 163:691–700
130. Antonescu CR, Viale A, Sarran L, Tschernyavsky SJ, Gonen M, et al. 2004. Gene expression in gastrointestinal stromal tumors is distinguished by KIT genotype and anatomic site. *Clin. Cancer Res.* 10:3282–90
131. Kang HJ, Nam SW, Kim H, Rhee H, Kim NG, et al. 2005. Correlation of KIT and platelet-derived growth factor receptor alpha mutations with gene activation and expression profiles in gastrointestinal stromal tumors. *Oncogene* 24:1066–74
132. Subramanian S, West RB, Corless CL, Ou W, Rubin BP, et al. 2004. Gastrointestinal stromal tumors (GISTs) with KIT and PDGFRA mutations have distinct gene expression profiles. *Oncogene* 23:7780–90
133. Marshall E. 2004. Getting the noise out of gene arrays. *Science* 306:630–31
134. Nagayama S, Katagiri T, Tsunoda T, Hosaka T, Nakashima Y, et al. 2002. Genome-wide analysis of gene expression in synovial sarcomas using a cDNA microarray. *Cancer Res.* 62:5859–66
135. Wachtel M, Dettling M, Koscielniak E, Stegmaier S, Treuner J, et al. 2004. Gene expression signatures identify rhabdomyosarcoma subtypes and detect a novel t(2;2)(q35;p23) translocation fusing PAX3 to NCOA1. *Cancer Res.* 64:5539–45
136. Chang HY, Chi JT, Dudoit S, Bondre C, van de Rijn M, et al. 2002. Diversity, topographic differentiation, and positional memory in human fibroblasts. *Proc. Nat. Acad. Sci. USA* 99:12877–82
137. Chi J, Chang HY, Haraldsen G, Jahnsen FL, Troyanskaya OG, et al. 2003. Endothelial cell diversity revealed by global expression profiling. *Proc. Nat. Acad. Sci. USA* 100:10623–28
138. Dvorak HF. 1986. Tumors: wounds that do not heal. Similarities between tumor stroma generation and wound healing. *New Engl. J. Med.* 315:1650–59
139. Elenbaas B, Weinberg RA. 2001. Heterotypic signaling between epithelial tumor cells and fibroblasts in carcinoma formation. *Exp. Cell Res.* 264:169–84
140. Olumi AF, Grossfeld GD, Hayward SW, Carroll PR, Tlsty TD, Cunha GR. 1999. Carcinoma-associated fibroblasts direct tumor progression of initiated human prostatic epithelium. *Cancer Res.* 59:5002–11

141. West RB, Nuyten DS, Subramanian S, Nielsen TO, Corless CL, et al. 2005. Determination of stromal signatures in breast carcinoma. *PLoS Biol.* 3:e187
142. Allinen M, Beroukhim R, Cai L, Brennan C, Lahti-Domenici J, et al. 2004. Molecular characterization of the tumor microenvironment in breast cancer. *Cancer Cell* 6:17–32
143. Iacobuzio-Donahue CA, Maitra A, Olsen M, Lowe AW, van Heek NT, et al. 2003. Exploration of global gene expression patterns in pancreatic adenocarcinoma using cDNA microarrays. *Am. J. Pathol.* 162:1151–62
144. St Croix B, Rago C, Velculescu V, Traverso G, Romans KE, et al. 2000. Genes expressed in human tumor endothelium. *Science* 289:1197–202

Severe Sepsis and Septic Shock: The Role of Gram-Negative Bacteremia

Robert S. Munford

Departments of Internal Medicine and Microbiology, University of Texas Southwestern Medical Center, Dallas, Texas 75390-9113;
email: Robert.munford@utsouthwestern.edu

Annu. Rev. Pathol. Mech. Dis. 2006. 1:467–96

The *Annual Review of Pathology: Mechanisms of Disease* is online at pathmechdis.annualreviews.org

doi: 10.1146/annurev.pathol.1.110304.100200

1553-4006/06/0114-0467$20.00

Key Words

compartmentalization, lipopolysaccharide, endotoxemia, inflammation, endotoxin, neuroendocrine

Abstract

Although Gram-negative bacteria have often been implicated in the pathogenesis of severe sepsis and septic shock, how they trigger these often lethal syndromes is uncertain. In particular, the role played by blood-borne bacteria is controversial. This review considers two alternatives. In the first, circulating Gram-negative bacteria induce toxic reactions directly within the vasculature; in the second, the major inflammatory stimulus occurs in local extravascular sites of infection and circulating bacteria contribute little to inducing toxic responses. Evidence for each alternative is found in the literature. Bacteremia and severe sepsis are not so closely linked that the most striking cases can be a model for the rest. Intravascular and extravascular triggers may warrant different approaches to prevention and therapy.

INTRODUCTION

Sepsis: the body's normal systemic responses to proven or suspected infection; these typically include fever, tachypnea, tachycardia, and leukocytosis (1, 2)

Severe sepsis: sepsis accompanied by dysfunction of one or more organs, with tissue hypoperfusion and/or hypotension; the most recent consensus definitions do not clearly distinguish between sepsis and severe sepsis (1, 2)

Septic shock: a severe response to proven or suspected infection in which hypotension requires therapy with vasopressor drugs (1, 2)

Systemic inflammation: increased vascular permeability, leukocyte infiltration, and microthrombosis in tissues distant from a site of local infection/inflammation (1–3)

Local inflammation: tissue response in which vasodilation, increased vascular permeability, and leukocyte infiltration may cause pain, swelling, redness, and warmth (1–3)

An effective circulation requires an inflammation-free bloodstream. To this end, highly conserved mechanisms prevent bloodstream invasion by microbes, clear them rapidly from the circulation, and dampen their ability to elicit toxic intravascular responses. As bacterial infection of the circulating blood is usually transient and unnoticed, these mechanisms must be extremely effective. Nonetheless, blood-borne bacteria can sometimes induce the catastrophic systemic reactions known as severe sepsis and septic shock. Similarly, injecting bacterial toxins into the bloodstream can elicit widespread tissue injury, shock, and death.

Of the various microbes that can induce these toxic reactions in humans, Gram-negative bacteria have been studied most thoroughly. How do they do it? A confident answer will be possible when the biochemical basis for infection-induced organ dysfunction and shock is understood. Short of this goal, however, there is evidence to support two different theories about how, or at least where, Gram-negative bacteria induce harmful systemic responses.

One widely accepted possibility is that Gram-negative bacteria, having withstood the host's local inflammatory defenses, make their way into the bloodstream (**Figure 1*a***). Their lipopolysaccharides (LPSs, also termed endotoxins) and other agonistic molecules then activate leukocytes, platelets, and vessel-lining cells; in turn, these responses induce systemic inflammation (e.g., increased vascular permeability, leukocyte-endothelial adhesion, and activation of complement and clotting pathways), which causes organs throughout the body to fail (4–7). The second notion is that Gram-negative bacteria and endotoxin elicit inflammation principally within infected extravascular tissues rather than in the bloodstream (**Figure 1*b***). Multi-organ dysfunction and shock are then induced by neuroendocrine dysregulation, mediators released into the blood from the infected tissue, or other mechanisms. According to this hypothesis, circulating bacteria or endotoxin need not be direct stimuli for intravascular inflammation—the harmful systemic reaction is triggered within the local tissue, not the blood.

In both theories, local inflammation is the first line of defense when bacteria cross an epithelial barrier and enter the underlying tissue. The ideas differ in how they view the systemic response. In the first theory, local and systemic defenses are a functional continuum in which inflammatory responses within the local tissue may extend into the bloodstream and propagate throughout the body (7). Bacteria that enter the bloodstream can thus trigger toxic systemic reactions. The proponents of this hypothesis assume that some degree of systemic inflammation is a frequent response to local infection and that intravascular responses to circulating bacteria and/or endotoxin often precipitate organ dysfunction and shock (6, 8). In this view, the proinflammatory mediators induce anti-inflammatory ones, both in local tissues and in the blood, and these counter-regulatory molecules help restore homeostasis. Severe sepsis and septic shock occur when there is an imbalance that allows unregulated activation of complement, coagulation, leukocyte adhesion, and other processes within the vasculature.

In contrast, the second theory assumes a functional compartmentalization in which local inflammation is normally accompanied by systemic responses that prevent inflammation in the bloodstream and uninfected organs (9) (**Figure 2**). When bacteria enter the bloodstream from an infected local site, they meet numerous factors that limit their ability to trigger inflammatory responses. Within the systemic compartment, anti-inflammation predominates and may contribute to immunosuppression, which further dampens intravascular responses to bacterial agonists (4, 9). Bacteria can directly stimulate reactions within the bloodstream, but only if they are able to bypass or overcome these normal defenses. How local inflammation triggers

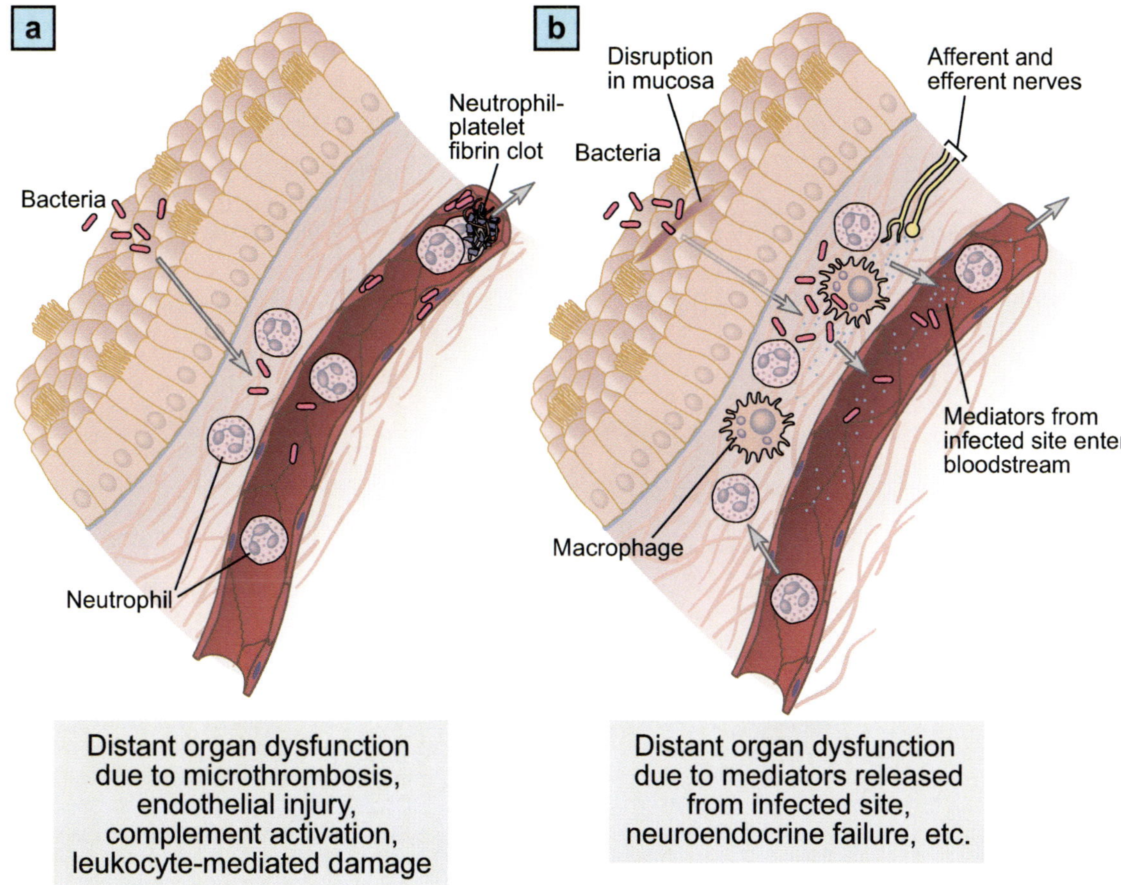

Figure 1

The contribution of Gram-negative bacteremia to severe sepsis: two hypotheses. (*a*) The intravascular stimulus hypothesis. Bacteria invade through a normal or damaged epithelium, transit the underlying tissue space, and enter a blood vessel. They then may infect and/or activate vascular endothelial cells, trigger the production of inflammatory mediators within the vasculature, and promote intravascular clotting. In many cases, there is little inflammatory reaction at the local invasion site; the pathology is found in the vasculature and distant organs. In others, there is blood-borne propagation of inflammation from the local site throughout the body. In all, circulating bacteria directly induce systemic activation of complement and coagulation and produce distant organ dysfunction. (*b*) The extravascular stimulus hypothesis. Bacteria invade through a break in an epithelial surface and enter the subepithelial tissue space where they elicit, and are normally contained by, local inflammation. Failure of the local inflammatory response to kill the bacteria allows them to enter the bloodstream, where they circulate but do little to induce intravascular damage. Dysfunction of distant organs may be produced by neuroendocrine effectors, mediators released into the blood from the local site of infection, or other mechanisms.

dysfunction in distant organs is unclear, though both humoral and neural mechanisms may be involved.

The two viewpoints thus suggest very different routes to severe sepsis and shock. This review uses data from the literature to examine these hypotheses and attempt a synthesis. Although most cases of severe sepsis seem more consistent with the second theory, there are convincing instances in which circulating Gram-negative bacteria directly trigger toxic reactions within the circulation. Both

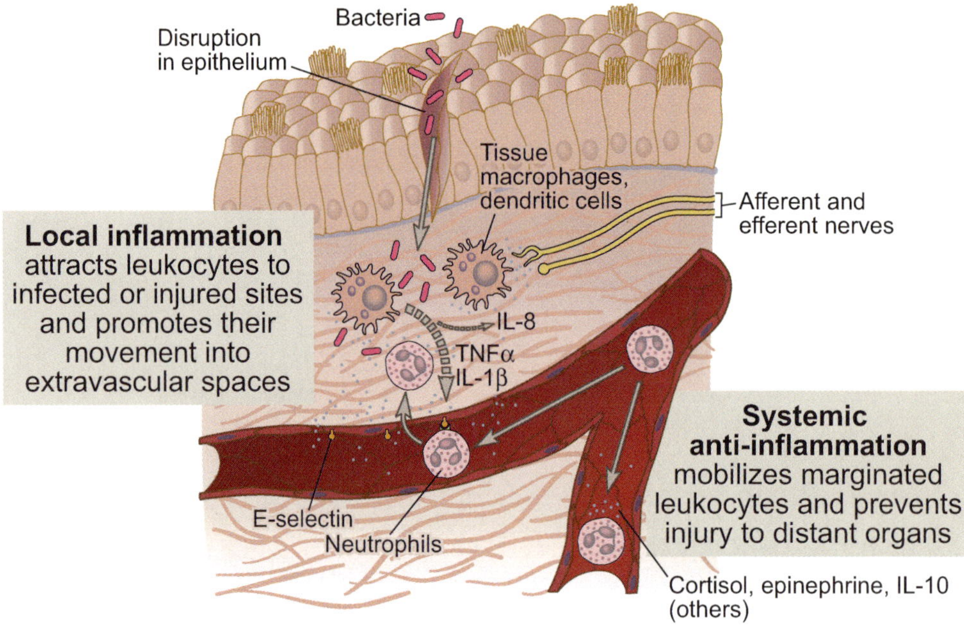

Figure 2

Local inflammation and systemic anti-inflammation hypothesis. When bacteria invade through an epithelial barrier, they are usually sensed by tissue-resident macrophages, dendritic cells, and/or mast cells. These cells release mediators that attract neutrophils to the site of infection, promote adhesion of the neutrophils to local vascular endothelium, and facilitate their diapedesis into the infected site. Local capillary permeability increases and enhances the entry of antibodies, complement, and microbe-sensing molecules into the extravascular space. Mediators released from efferent nerve endings contribute to the local inflammatory response, whereas activation of afferent nerves signals to the central nervous system that infection has occurred. Systemic responses mobilize neutrophils into the circulation and allow them to travel to the local site(s) where they are needed. Leukocyte-endothelial adhesion in these sites is promoted by the expression of E-selectin and other adhesion molecules on local endothelial cells. The same mediators that stimulate leukocyte demargination [e.g., cortisol, epinephrine, and interleukin (IL)-10] prevent neutrophils from adhering indiscriminately to vascular beds where there is no inflammation. Systemic anti-inflammatory responses may thus assist local proinflammatory defenses while minimizing injury to uninvolved organs. TNF, tumor necrosis factor.

microbial and host factors may determine where the septic response is elicited in a particular individual.

Bacteremia: isolation of bacteria in one or more blood cultures (excluding contaminants) (1–3)

GRAM-NEGATIVE BACTEREMIA AND SEVERE SEPSIS

Analysis Limitations

The clinical definition of Gram-negative bacteremia is the isolation of Gram-negative bacteria from one or more blood cultures. Whereas Gram-negative bacteria are relatively unusual blood culture contaminants (there are few false positives), the actual incidence of false negatives is not known; not only may the currently used culture media fail to grow some bacteria, but Gram-negative bacteria may enter the bloodstream intermittently or be present in very low numbers, and thus avoid detection. In a recent study of the blood of children with *Neisseria meningitidis* bacteremia, Hackett and colleagues found as many as 1.6×10^8 DNA copies ml^{-1} (10). This number greatly exceeds the bacterial concentrations previously estimated by using quantitative blood cultures and raises the possibility that most of the bacteria in the peripheral blood of patients with meningococcemia are either dead or unable to grow in artificial media. The extent to which this observation applies to other Gram-negative bacteria is not known.

Measurements of endotoxin concentrations in plasma should also provide information regarding the presence of Gram-negative bacteria in the circulation (11). The correlation between positive blood cultures and positive endotoxin tests has often been weak, however, and the specificity of the endotoxin assays has been questioned (12, 13).

Blood culture results and endotoxin measurements thus provide imperfect estimates of the true occurrence of Gram-negative bacteremia and endotoxemia. If one wants to assess the impact of Gram-negative bacteremia or endotoxemia on host physiology, an equally formidable obstacle is the absence of consistent diagnostic criteria for severe sepsis and septic shock. In addition, it is not known with certainty that severe sepsis and septic shock are a pathophysiological continuum; some investigators think that the mechanisms that produce organ dysfunction and shock are significantly different (3, 14). In much of the older clinical literature, the only surrogate clinical descriptor is hypotension or shock, and mortality is the only proxy outcome. This review assumes that severe sepsis and septic shock are equivalent endpoints. As the attributable mortality of severe sepsis approximates 25% and that of septic shock is typically near 50%, the absence of attributable mortality is taken as evidence that the cases in a given clinical series experienced few or no episodes of these syndromes.

Routes of Entry into the Blood

Gram-negative bacteremia occurs intermittently. This presumably reflects both a limited invasive potential and the efficacy of the host's mechanisms for clearing the bloodstream of bacteria (15, 16). When blood cultures remain positive for prolonged periods of time, there is usually an unresolved extravascular infection, extensive epithelial damage (e.g., burn wound), obstruction to a critical drainage route, an infected intravascular device, endocarditis, ineffective antimicrobial chemotherapy, or an infected intravenous fluid (17–19).

The ability of circulating Gram-negative bacteria to trigger severe sepsis may be related to how they enter the bloodstream. There are three major routes into the bloodstream: movement across an intact epithelial barrier, movement through damaged epithelia, and movement from extravascular sites of infection or inflammation. In each instance bacteria may enter the blood via either venous or lymphatic channels.

Movement across an epithelial barrier, with minimal local inflammation. The best-recognized example of this phenomenon is *N. meningitidis*, which colonizes the normal nasopharynx, crosses the mucosa, enters the bloodstream without eliciting clinically apparent local inflammation, infects vascular endothelial cells, and then multiplies within the vasculature. Other bacteria in this category include *Brucella* species, *Francisella tularensis*, and *Salmonella typhi*, which may cross the intestinal epithelium without eliciting symptoms, enter the bloodstream either directly or via lymphatic channels, widely infect tissue macrophages, and continuously seed the circulation (20). In general, the bacteria in this category are human pathogens; they have mechanisms that allow them to bypass normal immune defenses and establish distinctive niches within the healthy human body.

Movement across damaged epithelia with minimal local infection/inflammation. The break in the epithelial barrier may be due to mechanical or thermal trauma, a plastic catheter, or drug-induced epithelial injury. In some cases, the bacteria are potential human pathogens with a defined reservoir in the environment (e.g., *Burkholderia pseudomallei*, which is found in soil, and *Capnocytophaga* species and *Vibrio vulnificus*, which are found in animals), but more often they are derived from the patient's commensal flora or from the hospital environment (e.g., *Enterobacter*, *Klebsiella*, *Serratia*, and *Pseudomonas*). Although there may be a local tissue response to bacterial invasion, transit to the bloodstream often seems to occur with little or no local inflammation. Neutropenic patients with bacteremia are in this category, as are most patients with infected intravascular catheters.

Movement from extravascular sites of infection/inflammation. The initial tissue infection may arise following a break in the epithelium but it is initially contained by the local inflammatory response. When local tissue defenses fail, invasion of the bloodstream may occur via direct entry into a draining vein, by erosion of a vessel during ongoing inflammation, or by transit along lymphatics to regional lymph nodes, the thoracic duct, and into the blood. It is also possible that such bacteria may be carried into the circulation by phagocytes. In any of these situations, bacteremia reflects failure of local immune defenses to contain the offending microbes, often despite vigorous local inflammation. In other instances, bacteremia may complicate manipulation of the infected extravascular tissue. Although some pathogens (e.g., *Yersinia pestis*) fall into this category, the bacteria are typically commensals and the hosts are ill with an underlying disease (21). The infecting bacteria may have virulence factors that favor their survival and multiplication in humans, but it is uncertain that these factors confer a greater ability to stimulate toxic reactions within the bloodstream. Extravascular infection, usually in the abdomen, kidney, or lung, is the likely source for most patients with Gram-negative bacteremia diagnosed in developed societies today.

Appearance in Blood Cultures

In several case series of patients with Gram-negative bacteremia, *Enterobacteriaceae* and *Pseudomonadaceae* were isolated from blood cultures in more than 90% of the episodes (22–25); commensals thus dominated in the blood cultures. In general, the spectrum of Gram-negative bacteria in positive blood cultures of patients with severe sepsis has been similar to that found in less-ill patients. In a large multivariate analysis of risk factors for developing severe sepsis, the kind of Gram-negative blood culture isolate was not a significant variable (26).

Association with Severe Sepsis and Septic Shock

In their landmark prospective study of the natural history of the systemic inflammatory response syndrome, Rangel-Frausto and colleagues found positive blood cultures in 16% of patients with sepsis, 25% of those with severe sepsis, and 69% of those with septic shock (27). Similarly, Sands and colleagues found that 153 of 336 patients (45%) with severe sepsis due to Gram-negative bacterial infections had documented bloodstream infection (24). In a large retrospective survey in France, 43% of the patients with severe sepsis due to Gram-negative bacteria had positive blood cultures (26). A high percentage of patients in whom Gram-negative bacterial infection induces severe sepsis thus have circulating cultivatable bacteria at the time of diagnosis. However, one fourth to one half may not; the explanations often offered to explain this observation include the prior administration of antibiotics and the intermittent nature of bacteremia. In keeping with these ideas, Sleigh and colleagues found that amplification of 16S rDNA gene sequences can detect bacterial genomes in the blood of septic patients with negative blood cultures but a positive culture from other site(s) (28).

Gram-negative bacteremia can also be asymptomatic. Most such episodes are not detected because blood cultures are not performed. When Gram-negative bacteremia is documented, it is almost always in an individual who has developed symptoms and signs of infection. In these individuals, a positive blood culture is often associated with severe sepsis or septic shock. In retrospective studies of hospitalized patients with Gram-negative bacteremia, septic shock has been noted in 7% to 50% of the cases (22, 25, 29–31). The extent to which bacteremia directly triggers septic shock is uncertain, however. In one illustrative instance, Blot and colleagues found that patients with nosocomial *Enterobacter bacteremia* were somewhat more likely than matched intensive care unit (ICU) controls to require blood pressure support during the course of their ICU stay (78% versus 60%, $p < 0.015$) (32). Were the circulating *Enterobacter* a direct stimulus for inducing hypotension, or were they merely a marker for uncontrolled inflammation in an infected tissue bed?

WHERE DO GRAM-NEGATIVE BACTERIA INDUCE SEVERE SEPSIS/SEPTIC SHOCK?

If circulating Gram-negative bacteria directly induce severe sepsis and septic shock (the intravascular stimulus hypothesis), one would expect to find that (*a*) bacteria that enter the bloodstream without eliciting local inflammation can trigger the syndromes, (*b*) patients with severe sepsis are more likely to die if they have bacteremia, (*c*) bacteremia and local infection are independent risk factors for developing the syndromes, and (*d*) there is a direct relationship between bacterial density in the blood and the occurrence of severe sepsis and septic shock. In addition, killing circulating bacteria (thus releasing their endotoxin) might induce or worsen systemic reactions. Each of these possibilities is discussed below.

Can Circulating Bacteria and Endotoxin Cause Severe Sepsis and Septic Shock?

There are several clinical situations in which bacteria or endotoxin may enter the bloodstream without eliciting extravascular inflammation.

TNF: tumor necrosis factor

Intravenous infusion of endotoxin into volunteers. Infusion of a low bolus dose of LPS (4 nanograms kg^{-1} of patient weight) into healthy volunteers reproducibly elicits many of the usual systemic responses to infection, including fever, chills, myalgias, and headache. This model has been used frequently to define the cytokines and other mediators that contribute to the systemic inflammatory reponse in humans (33). [That administration of a larger dose can induce septic shock was dramatically illustrated by a patient who injected herself with a *Salmonella* endotoxin (34).] Despite its utility as an investigational tool, volunteer endotoxemia does not mimic several important aspects of infection-induced endotoxemia, which usually occurs in individuals who are already sick and have a primary extravascular infection, is intermittent (35) and is not the result of a bolus infusion into an arm vein. As will be discussed below, there is evidence that much of the tumor necrosis factor (TNF) that appears in the blood of endotoxin-challenged volunteers is produced by the liver and spleen and not by circulating blood cells.

Infusion-related bacteremia. When contaminated intravenous fluids are administered unintentionally to hospitalized patients, the initial responses to the bacteria presumably occur within the vasculature. In one dramatic instance, infusion of heavily contaminated dextrose solutions induced profound shock in five patients, four of whom died (36). The other published episodes of contaminated infusions do not indicate how often the infusates induced severe sepsis or septic shock. If one uses mortality as a

CRP: C-reactive protein

surrogate for septic shock, however, the impact of infusion-related bacteremia seems to be much less than that of bacteremia that is secondary (i.e., from a site of primary extravascular infection within the host). In a large outbreak of Gram-negative rod (*Enterobacter* species) bacteremia associated with contaminated intravenous infusion equipment, for example, the case-fatality rate was 13.4% overall and 7.4% in patients with nonfatal underlying diseases (37). These case-fatality rates were substantially lower than those found for Gram-negative bacteremia in contemporaneous studies of hospitalized patients (38, 39). In other incidents of infusion-associated bacteremia, the case-fatality rates were 12.5% or less [zero or one of eight cases (*Pseudomonas thomasii*) (40)], 12% [three of 26 cases (*Serratia marcescens*) (41)], and 0% [none of 12 cases (*S. marcescens*) (42)]. As noted by Maki (38), patients who become bacteremic in infusion-related epidemics tend to be younger and are less likely to have fatal underlying diseases than are patients who develop bacteremia from endogenous sites of infection; in addition, the infusion is usually terminated promptly when contamination is suspected. In the only case-control analysis of risk, mortality in the infused patients was not different from that in the control population, and none of the deaths in the cases could be attributed directly to the infusion (41).

These experiences indicate that the direct introduction of Gram-negative bacteria into the bloodstream is sufficient to trigger pyrogenic and other systemic reactions. The ability of these bacteria to induce severe sepsis or septic shock is less predictable; the important factors may include (*a*) the size of the inoculum, (*b*) the rate at which it is introduced, (*c*) the potency of the infused bacteria's endotoxin (or other agonistic molecules), (*d*) the ability of the bacteria to survive and grow in human blood, and (*e*) the fitness of the host.

Fulminant meningococcemia. *N. meningitidis* usually invades the bloodstream without eliciting clinically apparent local inflammation. Once in the circulation, the bacteria multiply within the blood and vascular lining cells and often release large amounts of endotoxin-containing cell-wall blebs (43, 44). That toxic intravascular and perivascular inflammatory reactions occur in patients with fulminant meningococcemia is undisputed; there is a virtual explosion of both pro- and anti-inflammatory mediators in the blood (45, 46). It is noteworthy that meningococcemia occurs typically in previously healthy young individuals and runs its course over a period of a few hours to a few days. Mortality in meningococcemia has been associated with low levels of C-reactive protein (CRP) at the time of presentation to a hospital (47); this finding perhaps reflects either the rapid course of the infection in susceptible individuals or the protection conferred by quickly mounting an acute-phase response.

Haemophilus influenzae type b may occasionally cause a fulminant intravascular infection (48). Other Gram-negative bacteria may also be considered intravascular human pathogens, though they typically also produce abscesses in numerous tissues, and some may cause fasciitis and other soft-tissue infections. The list includes *B. pseudomallei*, *Capnocytophaga* species, and *V. vulnificus*.

Catheter-associated bacteremia. As catheter tunnel infections and septic thrombophlebitis are relatively uncommon, patients who develop intravenous catheter-associated bacteremia offer another opportunity to assess the impact of circulating bacteria on systemic responses. Case-control studies have found no outcome difference between ICU patients who experienced catheter-associated bacteremia and those who did not (49, 50). Gram-negative bacteria were isolated from few (less than 25%) of the cases in these studies, but there is no evidence that the risk of developing severe sepsis during an episode of catheter-associated Gram-negative bacteremia is higher than the risk associated with coagulase-negative *Staphylococci*. The case-fatality rate for severely septic patients whose focus of infection is an intravenous catheter is substantially lower than that for patients who have pulmonary, abdominal, or unknown infection sites (22). Intravenous catheter infections usually arise in individuals whose anti-inflammatory systemic defenses have already been mobilized by injury, illness, or other stresses, and the bacterial density in the blood may be low (51). In most cases, catheter removal promptly removes the source.

Endocarditis. Gram-negative bacilli account for only 5%–10% of the cases in recent series. As with the better-studied Gram-positive bacterial etiologies of subacute endocarditis, however, severe sepsis and septic shock have rarely been described, despite the likely occurrence of continuous, low-level bacteremia for days.

Neutropenia. Aerobic Gram-negative bacilli are the most common blood culture isolates found in febrile neutropenic patients (52). In various series, positive blood cultures have been associated with severe sepsis or shock in 10%–20% of the cases; in one recent retrospective case series, the case-fatality rate observed for patients with neutropenia-associated bacteremia was 30% (52). The presumed route of entry into the blood is from the gastrointestinal tract, where the absence of neutrophils prevents effective containment of bacteria that transit the abnormal gut epithelium.

In summary, some of these experiences leave no doubt that circulating Gram-negative bacteria and endotoxin can induce septic shock, in keeping with the traditional (intravascular stimulus) view of sepsis pathogenesis. However, the low attributable mortality associated with most episodes of infusion-associated Gram-negative bacteremia suggests that bacteremia per se is not sufficient to trigger serious systemic reactions in many instances. The infrequent occurrence of severe sepsis or septic shock in patients with Gram-negative bacterial endocarditis supports this conclusion, as does the occurrence of Gram-negative bacteremia that resolves without treatment or adverse consequences.

Are Patients with Severe Sepsis and Gram-Negative Bacteremia More Likely to Develop Septic Shock or Die Than Patients with Culture-Negative Severe Sepsis?

As noted above, cultures have been negative in approximately one fourth to one half of the reported patients with severe sepsis or septic shock. If circulating bacteria trigger toxic reactions directly in the bloodstream, patients with positive cultures should be more likely to develop severe sepsis or die than those with negative cultures. Brun-Buisson and colleagues studied more than 11,800 admissions to adult ICUs in France to identify risk factors for adverse outcome in patients with severe sepsis. They concluded that "patients with clinically suspected sepsis but without microbiological documentation and patients with documented infection share common risk factors and are at similarly high risk of death" (53). In the prospective observational study of Rangel-Frausto and colleagues, septic patients with negative cultures and those with positive cultures had similar morbidity and mortality rates (27). The same result was found by Saez-Llorens and colleagues in a study of Latin American children with severe sepsis (54) and in the placebo group of a clinical trial of patients with severe sepsis (**Table 1**) (55).

Is the Primary Infection Site an Important Risk Factor for Severe Sepsis?

If circulating bacteria are the dominant stimuli for severe sepsis, the site of primary infection may not influence the outcome. Having invaded the bloodstream, the bacteria would multiply, release their endotoxin, and trigger harmful systemic responses in various organs. In fact, the large multivariate analysis of

Table 1 Culture-positive and culture-negative patients with severe sepsis/septic shock have similar mortality

Study	Clinical status	Culture-documented severe sepsis or septic shock: Total studied	Culture-documented severe sepsis or septic shock: CFR[a] (%)	Clinically suspected severe sepsis or septic shock, negative cultures: Total studied	Clinically suspected severe sepsis or septic shock, negative cultures: Fraction of total cases (%)	Clinically suspected severe sepsis or septic shock, negative cultures: CFR (%)	Comment
Rangel-Frausto et al. (27)	Severe sepsis	358	20	457	56.1	16	Adults, medical and surgical wards
	Septic shock	110	46	84	53.8	46	Most patients with negative cultures had been treated with antibiotics for ~3 days prior to the onset of severe sepsis
Brun-Buisson et al. (53)	Severe sepsis	742	56	310	29.4	60	Adults Multicenter survey Included patients who developed septic shock
Fisher et al. (55)	Severe sepsis	246	34	56	18.5	34	Adults Multicenter clinical trial Placebo recipients Culture-negative group included those with no culture results
Saez-Llorens et al. (54)	Sepsis	212	40	603	73.9	39	Children
	Severe sepsis						Included patients with each sepsis definition (stage)
	Septic shock MODS[b]						

[a]Case-fatality rate [deaths (total cases)$^{-1}$ $\times$ 100] 28 days after onset of severe sepsis, unadjusted for cause of death.
[b]MODS: multiple organ dysfunction syndrome.

bacteremic patients by Brun-Buisson and colleagues (26) found that the site of infection was the second most important variable for predicting risk of severe sepsis; only the patient's age was more significant. When each patient's infection site was included in the analysis, the kind of microbe isolated from the blood was not a significant determinant of risk. In several other case series, mortality was significantly higher in patients with bacteremia arising from pulmonary or abdominal infection than in those with urosepsis or catheter-associated bacteremia (22, 65, 66). Perhaps bacteria reach higher density in the blood or are more likely to reseed the circulation from foci in the lungs or abdomen; infection in these organs may also be more difficult to treat. Alternatively, inflammation that arises in these tissue beds may be more intense and/or more likely to elicit systemic reactions.

Can Bacteremia be Predicted in Patients with Severe Sepsis?

If circulating bacteria contribute directly to the pathogenesis of severe sepsis, patients with severe sepsis who are bacteremic might be distinguishable at the bedside from severely septic patients whose blood cultures are negative. In the prospective study by Bates and colleagues (67) of 1342 cases of severe sepsis in eight academic medical centers in the northeastern United States, chills and focal abdominal signs were the indices of the host response that were associated with Gram-negative bacteremia in a multivariate analysis. Peduzzi and colleagues (68) reviewed 465 cases of severe sepsis in a Veterans Administration Cooperative Study Group trial and found that a classification model that included elevated temperature, low systolic blood pressure, and thrombocytopenia could predict bacteremia, but misclassification was also high (sensitivity of 5%). These studies provide little support for the notion that Gram-negative bacteremia contributes in a distinctive way to the clinical manifestations of severe sepsis.

DOES SEVERE SEPSIS HAVE ENDOGENOUS TRIGGERS?

How does infection induce severe sepsis when no microbes can be grown from any tissue site? Perhaps the infecting microbes cannot be cultured with the techniques used, or the infected site has not been sampled for culture, or the bacteria were killed by prior antimicrobial therapy. But effective antimicrobial therapy is known to be lifesaving in patients with positive cultures; if the infecting bacteria are already dead by the time the diagnosis is suspected and cultures are drawn, why should the clinical outcome be so poor?

Perhaps many culture-negative patients considered to have severe sepsis are not infected. Indeed, students of trauma-associated multiple organ dysfunction syndrome (MODS) have realized for many years that infection is not required to produce dysfunction of organs distant from a site of injury (57, 58). As most of the known host microbial pattern-recognition proteins also have endogenous ligands (59–61), might the pathophysiological states known as severe sepsis and MODS be induced by one or more of these molecules? Might endogenous and exogenous ligands be additive, or even synergistic, stimuli (61, 62)? The best candidate for a proinflammatory endogenous ligand is currently high-mobility group box 1 (HMGB1), a secreted nuclear factor that was recently reported to induce ischemia-perfusion injury in a toll-like receptor 4 (TLR4)-dependent fashion (63).

Is there a Relationship Between Bacterial Density in the Blood and the Occurrence of Severe Sepsis/Septic Shock?

If severe sepsis is triggered principally by circulating bacteria or their products, the risk of developing severe sepsis may be related directly to the concentration of bacteria in the patient's blood. Du Pont & Spink did quantitative blood cultures in hospitalized adults and found that the concentration of bacteria in venous blood correlated with mortality but not with septic shock (39). Kreger and colleagues (69) found that case-fatality rates were higher in patients whose blood cultures grew more colony-forming units (cfu) ml^{-1}, but only when underlying disease was not factored into the analysis. There was no relationship between severity of underlying disease and the magnitude of bacteremia. In a more recent study, Kellog and colleagues found no relationship between the fraction of eight blood cultures that were positive and the occurrence of sepsis syndrome (severe sepsis) (70).

In most of the cases in these series, as in most cases of bacteremic severe sepsis diagnosed today, the blood cultures grew commensal bacteria that rarely caused disease in healthy humans. Even for some classical human pathogens, however, there has not been a strong relationship between bacterial density in the blood and the risk of developing severe sepsis. One prominent example is *S. typhi*, which seeds the bloodstream from lymphatic sites during the first week or two of infection and can reach moderate densities (10^2–10^3 cfu ml^{-1}) in the blood. Whereas typhoid patients with higher-level bacteremia may be more likely to experience high fever and delirium (20), severe sepsis occurs infrequently and has no reported relationship to bacterial density in the blood. [Most of the *S. typhi* that circulate in the blood of patients with typhoid fever are intracellular and thus may not stimulate other cells within the vascular compartment. In fact, the cells in the blood of typhoid patients have reduced ability to release TNF when they are exposed to endotoxin ex vivo (71).]

Studies on several pediatric pathogens are also germane. Higher blood concentrations of *H. influenzae* type b were found in children with meningitis than in those with epiglottitis (which typically occurs in older children) or bacteremia (72, 73), but no relationship between bacterial density and severe sepsis was noted. In their analysis of quantitative blood cultures from children with meningococcal disease, Sullivan & LaScolea found no relationship between bacterial density and clinical syndrome; children with meningococcemia and those with meningitis had overlapping concentrations of circulating (cultivatable) meningococci and two children with more than 100 cfu ml^{-1} recovered spontaneously without antibiotic treatment (74).

An obvious problem with analyses of bacterial density in the blood is the possibility that blood-borne bacteria may not be cultivatable ex vivo. As noted above, Hackett and colleagues recently found that bacterial load, as determined using the polymerase chain reaction, was higher in children with severe meningococcal disease than those with mild disease; their estimates of the numbers of circulating bacteria, based on DNA copies, were much higher than those reported previously using quantitative blood cultures (10). Similar studies are needed in patients infected with other kinds of Gram-negative bacteria.

High bacterial density may be found in the blood of patients with fatal septicemic plague (75) or melioidosis (76), in asplenic patients who experience high-level meningococcal or *H. influenzae* type b bacteremia, or in some neutropenic patients who develop bacteremia (77). When viewed as part of the overall spectrum of severe sepsis, however, these unusual experiences may have unduly influenced medical opinion in favor of the "more circulating Gram-negative bacteria, worse outcome" notion.

Does Killing Circulating Gram-Negative Bacteria Induce Harmful Systemic Reactions?

Scientific interest in endotoxin as a trigger for septic shock received an enormous boost in 1948, when Spink and colleagues (78) described the development of fever and a shock-like picture within eight to twelve hours after initiating aureomycin therapy in patients with brucellosis. A similar phenomenon, also reminiscent of the Jarisch-Herxheimer reaction, was reported following the initiation of chloramphenicol therapy for typhoid fever (79). These studies suggested that bacterial lysis, by releasing endotoxin and/or other molecules, could trigger deleterious systemic responses in the infected host. During the half century since these reports appeared in the literature, antibiotic-induced release of endotoxin has received much attention. In a careful review of the topic, Hurley concluded in 1992 that "there is no evidence to support and some evidence to refute the concern that the rapid destruction of Gram-negative bacteria can result in an adverse outcome" (80). Subsequent observations have not significantly challenged this assessment (81).

In volunteers infected with *S. typhi*, induction of pyrogenic tolerance to repeated intravenous doses of endotoxin had no discernible impact on the febrile course of typhoid fever; this result led Greisman and colleagues to conclude that circulating endotoxin plays no role in the pathogenesis of the sustained fever and toxemia of this human disease (83). It thus seems unlikely that antibiotic treatment–induced deterioration in typhoid patients (79) would be due to circulating endotoxin; it is more likely that hypersensitivity to endotoxin occurs in extravascular tissues (see the discussion in Reference 84). Even in patients with fulminant meningococcemia in whom the pathological impact of circulating bacteria and endotoxin is undisputed, the available evidence strongly suggests that antibiotic treatment does not enhance endotoxin release or worsen outcome (43). On the other hand, antibiotic-induced release of endotoxin within infected tissue beds (or within infected cells?) may account for the untoward reactions observed in some patients. Evidence for this notion comes from studies of rabbits and humans with bacterial meningitis, in whom antibiotic-induced lysis of bacteria can trigger inflammation within the cerebrospinal fluid compartment (85, 86) and possibly induce shock (87).

The Evidence From Pathology

Pathologists studying the organs of patients with severe sepsis often report few abnormalities. There is little or no tissue necrosis. Microthrombi, although occasionally present, are linked infrequently to organ dysfunction (88–91). Significant foci of infection are also uncommon (92). Impressive apoptosis occurs in the spleen and gastrointestinal epithelium, but not in other dysfunctional organs (93, 94). The microscopic examination usually does not suggest why a particular organ has failed or identify a cause of death (4). These findings are consistent with the clinical observation that organ function usually returns to baseline in patients who survive an episode of severe sepsis or septic shock. They are also in keeping with the idea that organ dysfunction is due to a reversible derangement of the microcirculation, with abnormal oxygen utilization by cells within the dysfunctional organ (3, 95). Although some authors have invoked transient thrombus-induced ischemia-reperfusion injury to account for the microcirculatory derangement (90), there is also evidence that chemical modulators of vascular tone are probably involved (96).

In dramatic contrast, the histopathology of the skin lesions of patients with fulminant meningococcemia is striking. There is endothelial cell swelling, local thrombosis, perivascular infiltration by leukocytes, and, often, surrounding hemorrhage (44, 97). Similar changes have been noted in other organs at autopsy. Another impressive skin lesion is ecthyma gangrenosum, in which vessel walls are replaced by Gram-negative bacteria, usually *Pseudomonas aeruginosa*. This lesion occurs in profoundly neutropenic patients. These disparate experiences again suggest that there is more than one route to severe sepsis. Intravascular pathogens may not be suitable models for cases caused by most commensal Gram-negative bacteria, and vice versa.

MODS: multiple organ dysfunction syndrome

That Gram-negative bacteria or endotoxin can elicit systemic intravascular reactions directly is undeniable when one considers how patients react to unintended infusions of bacteria. However, several observations suggest that the major trigger for systemic responses can also occur in extravascular sites of infection/inflammation: the similar mortality rates seen in septic patients with positive or negative cultures, the difficulty with which bacteremia can be predicted at the bedside of a patient with severe sepsis, the strong association of severe sepsis risk with the primary infection site, and the absence of a convincing relationship between bacterial density in the blood and the occurrence of severe sepsis. The intravascular stimulus hypothesis also cannot account for severe sepsis triggered by noninfectious extravascular processes such as pancreatitis, or for the multiple organ dysfunction syndrome (MODS) that may follow major trauma.

INNATE IMMUNE DEFENSE OF THE BLOODSTREAM

A synthesis may possibly be reached by considering a major difference between the two hypotheses: the notion that systemic

MBL: mannose-binding lectin

TLR4: toll-like receptor 4

responses to infection or injury normally prevent, rather than propagate, inflammation within the bloodstream.

Mechanisms that Prevent Gram-Negative Bacteremia

Microbes enter an animal's internal milieu by crossing an epithelial barrier. The most effective internal mechanisms for preventing invasion of the bloodstream are those that sense microbes in tissues and mobilize local inflammatory responses to kill the invaders before they can enter the circulation. Enormous advances in understanding these mechanisms have occurred since the discovery of the toll-like receptors that sense microbial molecules and initiate inflammatory responses. These advances have recently been reviewed (60, 98) and will not be detailed here.

In addition, the blood contains several elements that help prevent bacteremia and/or clear bacteria from the circulation. These elements also need little discussion here. They include some of the most ancient and highly conserved defense molecules: antibodies [including natural immunoglobulin (Ig) M antibodies], CRP, mannose-binding lectin (MBL), and complement. Inflammation-induced clotting at local sites of infection may also help prevent bacteremia (**Table 2**).

Mechanisms that May Prevent Systemic Responses to Endotoxin

Several innate immune mechanisms seem to prevent or dampen responses to endotoxin and Gram-negative bacteria within the bloodstream.

Preventing endotoxin-sensing. That elements of plasma can block toxic responses to endotoxin has been known for many years. The reported mechanisms now include binding endotoxin to circulating lipoproteins, endotoxin clearance from the circulation by natural or acquired antibodies, neutralization of some endotoxins by MBL, CRP, or bactericidal permeability-increasing protein, and efflux of LPS from the surfaces of monocytes. Somewhat surprisingly, there may also be interference with LPS activation of toll-like receptor 4 (TLR4)-expressing blood cells by high plasma concentrations of three molecules that promote LPS sensing in extravascular sites: soluble CD14, LPS-binding protein, and MD-2. All of these mechanisms are more active in the blood of critically ill patients (99–101). Even when large amounts of endotoxin are present in the blood of severely septic patients, their plasma inhibits the ability of reporter cells to respond to LPS ex vivo (102). See Reference 84 for a review of these phenomena.

Modulating systemic responses to endotoxin. Systemic responses to endotoxin may occur in both solid organs and circulating cells. Fong and colleagues found that 25%–50% of the TNF that appears in the blood of healthy volunteers following an intravenous endotoxin challenge is produced in the splanchnic bed (103). Using the same endotoxin challenge model, Spek and colleagues found little correspondence between the pattern of peripheral blood cytokines and the pattern of cytokine messenger RNAs produced by cells in the same blood samples (104). They concluded that blood cells seem to make a minor contribution to the cytokine response to endotoxin. The major site at which endotoxin stimulates cells within the systemic compartment is probably the liver, the organ that clears most Gram-negative bacteria and endotoxin from the bloodstream. Hepatic responses to endotoxin include the production of numerous cytokines and acute-phase proteins. Several of these molecules neutralize proinflammatory cytokines or other potentially toxic products of local inflammation (9, 105); they include cytokine antagonists [e.g., soluble interleukin (IL)-1 receptor antagonist and soluble TNF receptors], protease inhibitors, and antioxidants.

Table 2 Innate immune defense of the bloodstream

Mechanisms that help prevent Gram-negative bacteremia
Local defenses
Phagocytic cells
Oxygen-dependent and -independent intracellular bactericidal mechanisms
Secreted proteins
Bactericidal permeability-increasing protein
Lactoferrin
Defensins
Microbial pattern-recognition molecules
Toll-like receptors (TLR), particularly TLR4
Lipopolysaccharide (LPS)-binding protein, CD14, MD-2
Local clotting
Blood-borne defenses
Natural (and acquired) antibodies
Serum complement
Microbe-associated pattern-recognition molecules
C-reactive protein
Mannose-binding lectin
Bactericidal permeability-increasing protein
Others
Mechanisms that may prevent systemic responses to endotoxin
Preventing endotoxin sensing in the blood
Phagocytic cell enzymes that detoxify LPS within local tissues (acyloxyacyl hydrolase, ? phosphatases)
Mechanisms that neutralize and/or clear LPS from the tissues and blood:
Antibodies, mannose-binding lectin, C-reactive protein
Bactericidal permeability-increasing protein
Mechanisms that prevent LPS activation of cells within the vasculature:
High concentrations of soluble CD14, LPS-binding protein, and MD-2
Factors that transfer LPS to plasma lipoproteins (e.g., CD14)
Plasma factors that promote efflux of LPS from monocyte cell surfaces
Modulating systemic responses to endotoxin
Mechanisms that reprogram cells in the circulation and splanchnic bed to diminish proinflammatory responses to LPS while maintaining or augmenting anti-inflammatory ones
Acute-phase increases in the blood concentrations of numerous anti-inflammatory and anti-infective molecules

Coordinating Local and Systemic Responses to Infection: The Role of the Nervous System

Studies performed recently in rodents suggest that communication between an infected local tissue and the central nervous system may occur at three levels (**Figure 3*a***). First, microbial molecules or inflammatory mediators stimulate local sensory fibers within the infected tissue; these fibers rapidly induce central nervous system responses in the absence of circulating cytokines (106). Second, low amounts of cytokines, prostaglandin E_2 or microbial agonists may diffuse from the infected tissue into the blood; once in the blood, these factors can be sensed in the liver, where they initiate afferent traffic along the vagus nerve that activates the hypothalamic-pituitary-adrenal axis (HPA) and induces fever (107, 108). Third, larger amounts of these molecules achieve blood concentrations that can directly influence the brain stem and hypothalamus (109).

HPA: hypothalamic-pituitary-adrenal

In each instance, the central nervous system responds by mobilizing neurohormonal mechanisms that should prevent inflammation within the bloodstream and

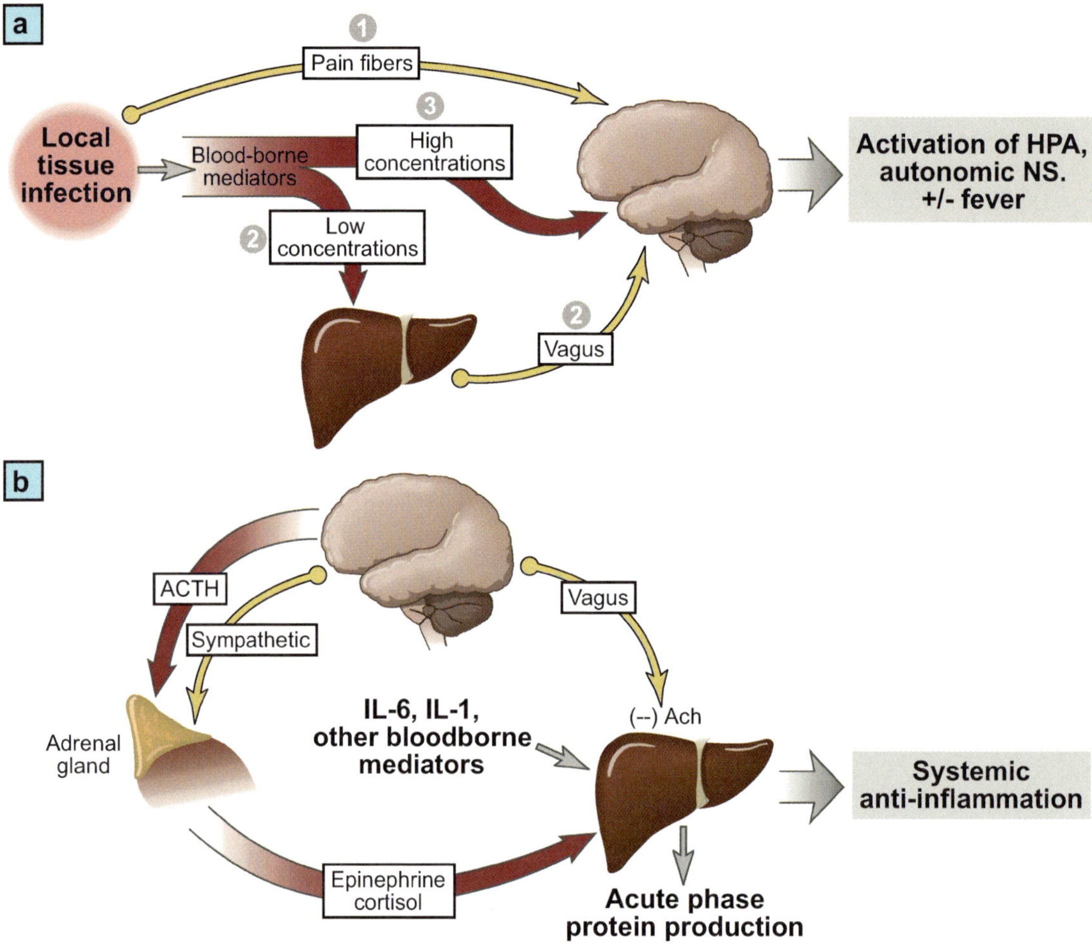

Figure 3

The systemic anti-inflammatory reflexes. (*a*) Studies in rodents have found that communication between an infected tissue and the brain may occur in at least three ways. In increasing order of activation threshold, they are (*1*) afferent nociceptive or small sensory fibers, (*2*) production of mediators that, when present in low concentrations in the blood, may activate vagal afferents in the liver, and (*3*) delivery of higher concentrations of mediators via the bloodstream to the hypothalamus/brain stem. Each of these paths may activate the hypothalamic-pituitary-adrenal axis (HPA), the autonomic nervous system, and the thermoregulatory center. (*b*) Activation of the central nervous system triggers numerous changes that seem to prevent inflammation within the bloodstream via the sympathetic (e.g., epinephrine, norepinephrine) and parasympathetic (e.g., acetylcholine) nervous systems (NS) and the HPA [e.g., α-MSH (alpha-melanocyte-stimulating hormone), ACTH (adrenocorticotrophic hormone), and cortisol]. In addition, cortisol is permissive for the production of acute-phase proteins, whereas epinephrine can increase circulating concentrations of interleukin (IL)-6, a major blood-borne stimulus to acute-phase-protein production and the HPA. When commensal bacteria enter the bloodstream from an extravascular local infection site, the second (extravascular stimulus) hypothesis holds that these and other systemic anti-inflammatory mechanisms can often prevent the bacteria from directly inducing toxic responses within the vasculature and distant organs. It is also possible that mechanisms that may have evolved to prevent excessive systemic anti-inflammation, such as mediator tachyphylaxis and the production of counteracting hormones [e.g., macrophage migration inhibitory factor (MIF) and possibly high-mobility group box 1 (HMGB1)], contribute to the pathogenesis of organ dysfunction and shock (142). Ach, acetylcholine.

in uninfected organs (**Figure 3*b***) (9). The anti-inflammatory hormones include ACTH (adrenocorticotrophic hormone), α-MSH (alpha-melanocyte-stimulating hormone), epinephrine, cortisol, vasoactive intestinal polypeptide, and others. It seems likely that endotoxin sensing in the bloodstream is normally modulated by neurohumoral mediators in ways that diminish endotoxin-induced TNF production while enhancing, or maintaining, the production of IL-10, IL-1 receptor antagonist, and other modulatory molecules. The most compelling demonstration of this phenomenon has been the ability of epinephrine or cortisol infusion to alter cytokine responses to intravenous endotoxin infusion in volunteers (110, 111). At least in rats, vagal stimulation can also diminish TNF production in response to intravenous endotoxin (112); Tracey's lab has recently reported that acetylcholine also inhibits LPS-induced production of high-mobility group box 1 (HMGB1), the most prominent late proinflammatory mediator, by macrophages (113).

In summary, many mechanisms that should prevent inflammation within the bloodstream can be activated by injury, infection, and illness (9). Whether circulating Gram-negative bacteria or endotoxin triggers severe sepsis may be determined, at least in part, by the extent to which these mechanisms have been mobilized prior to the entry of bacteria or endotoxin into the bloodstream.

Are Innate Immune Responses to Infection Compartmentalized?

In the above discussion, it is assumed that responses to infection and injury are compartmentalized within the body. Infection and/or inflammation in an extravascular tissue site (local compartment) are accompanied by responses that normally prevent inflammation in the bloodstream and other organs (systemic compartment) (**Figure 2**). Many clinical observations and experimental results are consistent with this notion. In one prominent clinical study, Dugernier and colleagues (114) measured cytokine concentrations in the ascitic fluid, lymph, and plasma of patients with severe pancreatitis who had developed multiorgan dysfunction. Although both pro- and anti-inflammatory cytokine levels were highest in ascitic fluid and lowest in plasma, cell-free ascitic fluid stimulated a reporter cell line to increase adhesion molecule expression (a marker of inflammation), whereas lymph and plasma did not. In fact, both lymph and plasma inhibited the ability of TNF and IL-1β to activate the reporter cells, presumably because these fluids contained high concentrations of inhibitors. These authors concluded that "the pancreas and the splanchnic area are sites of a proinflammatory response and that an early, dominant, and sustained anti-inflammatory activity takes place in circulating compartments."

Evidence for compartmentalization of inflammation has also been found in patients with early, localized infection. Rivera-Chavez and colleagues (115) found that individuals experiencing acute appendicitis had elevated levels of TNF in the peritoneal fluid but not in plasma; in contrast, their plasma contained high concentrations of IL-4, IL-6, and IL-10 and inhibited the release of IL-8 by reporter cells in response to LPS. These changes were more pronounced in patients with complicated appendicitis (e.g., perforation and gangrene). In patients with septic shock caused by cellulitis, Annane and colleagues found that increased activity of inducible nitric oxide synthase was confined to areas of putrescent skin; there was no evidence for propagation of the inflammatory response to adjacent tissue or the bloodstream (116).

In a study of rabbits with experimental *E. coli* peritonitis, Matue-Bello and colleagues found that bacteremia was insufficient to trigger inflammation within the lung; only when intraperitoneal infection was uncontrolled did lung injury become evident (117). They proposed the existence of local and systemic compartments. Support for the

ACTH: adrenocorticotrophic hormone

α-MSH: alpha-melanocyte stimulating hormone

HMGB1: high-mobility group box 1

Systemic compartment: the bloodstream and organs distant from a local tissue site of infection or inflammation

Local compartment: a tissue or organ in which infection has occurred, usually via inoculation or invasion across an epithelial surface (1–3)

compartmentalization model has also come from Kurahashi and colleagues, who found that sustained, high-level (10^4 cfu ml^{-1}) *P. aeruginosa* bacteremia did not induce hypotension in previously healthy rabbits (118). In contrast, when the same bacterial strain was inoculated into the lungs, hypotension began before bacteremia could be detected. They implicated TNF, produced within the lungs, as the most important mediator of shock, and they found that it induced hypotension only when it was able to diffuse into the blood. With experimental peritonitis in mice (119), intraperitoneal concentrations of proinflammatory mediators were higher within the peritoneal fluid than in plasma, whereas IL-10 concentrations were higher in plasma, in keeping with the clinical observations of Rivera-Chavez and colleagues (115) cited above.

As discussed above, the neurohumoral response to infection and other stresses seems to be anti-inflammatory and dampens responses to endotoxin within the systemic compartment. In contrast, the neural contribution to local inflammation is often proinflammatory and mediated by substance P and other neuropeptides. Indeed, some neuroendocrine mediators, such as corticotrophin-releasing hormone and catecholamines, can have context-dependent actions (120, 121); they generally promote inflammation in extravascular sites while preventing it within the circulation.

The compartmentalization model has several limitations. Clear-cut functional or anatomical compartmental boundaries are difficult to define, particularly because the blood flowing through an infected tissue could be considered both local and systemic. It seems likely that there are gradients between an inflamed tissue and the systemic circulation in which both venous and lymphatic effluents participate (114, 116, 122), but the nature of these gradients is not well established. Another weakness is the absence of definitive criteria for pro- and anti- inflammation within a given fluid or compartment (9). Indeed, the simple pro- and anti-inflammation dichotomy may mask several levels of complexity (123). There are also findings that do not fit easily into a compartmentalization model. For example, Funayama and colleagues found that intragingival injection of LPS induced histidine-decarboxylase activity in the liver, lung, and spleen of mice with a magnitude and time course similar to those seen with intravenous injection (124). They proposed that LPS is readily transported from the gingiva to extra-oral tissues. There is also evidence from a mouse model that cytokines do not diffuse from infected peritoneal fluid into the bloodstream; this evidence suggests that "at least part of the circulating (proinflammatory) cytokines are produced systemically" (125).

There is no doubt that cells within the peripheral blood of normal humans can respond to endotoxin and Gram-negative bacteria. That the normally protective mechanisms within the systemic compartment can be exceeded by intravascular pathogens or intravenously infused bacterial endotoxin should not be surprising, particularly when these challenges occur in previously healthy persons whose systemic responses have not been induced by prior stress or illness. It is less certain that intravascular reactions to endotoxin and Gram-negative bacteria can be so profoundly suppressed by the body's responses to stress that they do not occur in patients who have primary extravascular infections and eventually develop bacteremia or endotoxemia. If this is the case, as it seems to be, there must be mechanisms by which local inflammation can trigger severe sepsis and septic shock. Understanding these mechanisms is a major challenge for sepsis research.

Another Hypothesis

It is widely accepted that septic patients can progress sequentially from mild to severe over a period of hours to days (from sepsis to severe sepsis to septic shock) (27). Ulloa & Tracey (14) have recently proposed that, in contrast, severe sepsis and septic shock are distinct clinical entities: In their view, septic shock occurs abruptly, without previous severe sepsis, and leads to death within hours, whereas severe sepsis takes much longer to develop, may last days, and is not often a prodrome for septic shock. Fulminant meningococcemia is their prototype for septic shock. Whereas TNF is the dominant blood-borne cytokine in septic shock, Ulloa & Tracey note that it is typically absent in the blood of patients with severe sepsis; HMGB1, which they consider the necessary and sufficient proinflammatory cytokine in patients with severe sepsis, appears hours after the peak of TNF (14). Their emphasis is thus on the time course of the systemic response, not on where or how it is elicited within the body, and they argue that cytokine profiles based on TNF and HMGB1 can be used to categorize patients for clinical trials. This interesting hypothesis is consistent with the ability of TNF, but not HMGB1, to induce shock in experimental animals, and it has the advantage that it may readily be tested. However, it is hard to reconcile this idea with Rangel-Frausto's prospective observation that 71% of patients who developed septic shock had experienced sepsis and/or severe sepsis on previous days in the hospital, with a median interval from severe sepsis to septic shock of more than 28 days (27). In addition, some patients with severe sepsis may have persistently high TNF levels (126); this evidence suggests that the cytokine profile for severe sepsis may not be so clear-cut. An attractive feature of their hypothesis is its emphasis upon HMGB1, which is currently the most promising target for therapeutics intended to interrupt the pathophysiology of severe sepsis (127).

DEVELOPING SEVERE SEPSIS/ SEPTIC SHOCK: THE ROLE OF GRAM-NEGATIVE BACTEREMIA

When one considers the broad spectrum of patients who develop severe sepsis or septic shock, several factors seem to influence the ability of Gram-negative bacteria and endotoxin to elicit inflammation within the vasculature.

The Microbes

Gram-negative bacteria are most likely to elicit inflammatory reactions within the bloodstream when they are able to infect vascular endothelial cells and/or perivascular tissue and can release large amounts of endotoxin-containing membrane blebs. Although this description best fits *N. meningitidis*, other Gram-negative intravascular human pathogens (e.g., *Haemophilus influenzae* type b) may share these attributes. In contrast to these bacteria that can potently trigger intravascular inflammation, *B. pseudomallei* and *Y. pestis* may reach high concentrations in human blood partly because their endotoxin is so poorly sensed that protective innate defenses are not mobilized (128, 128a); these bacteria may also produce molecules that dampen inflammation. Still other human pathogens may be considered extravascular because they largely inhabit tissue macrophages. They elicit severe sepsis or septic shock infrequently, even when blood cultures are positive, possibly because the bacteria circulate within monocytes; *S. typhi* and *Brucellae* species are in this category. Finally, when commensal Gram-negative bacteria enter the bloodstream of an individual in whom systemic anti-inflammatory defenses have been induced by illness, they may not trigger significant intravascular responses unless the host is severely compromised (for example, by profound neutropenia) or the inoculum is large or abruptly delivered (as with infusion of contaminated fluid).

The Site and Duration of Infection

When the infecting bacterium is a commensal, it matters whether the primary infection site is intravascular or extravascular. Whereas catheter-associated infections infrequently induce severe sepsis, in part because the infected source can be readily removed, primary infection in the abdomen or lungs often does so whether there is bacteremia or not.

PAI-1: plasminogen activator inhibitor-1

The Status of the Host

Several features of the host are also important. First, activation of acute-phase responses by injury or illness should, as discussed above, help prevent inflammatory responses within the circulation. All of the known mechanisms for preventing endotoxin sensing are more active in the blood of ill individuals. High plasma concentrations of anti-inflammatory molecules should also decrease the ability of circulating bacteria to stimulate intravascular inflammation. Although this anti-inflammatory milieu would be predicted to benefit most patients, there is evidence that it may also be harmful. Indeed, mortality in patients with either community-acquired infections or severe sepsis has been related to a high ratio of IL-10 to TNF in the plasma (129, 130). Does this ratio reflect exuberant yet ineffective systemic anti-inflammation, or do excessive anti-inflammatory systemic responses contribute directly to outcome? Can a prompt anti-inflammatory systemic response allow more rapid bacterial growth in the bloodstream (as has been suggested in patients with meningococcemia) (131)? Are cytokine levels or ratios valuable clues to pathogenesis? Unfortunately, the available investigative tools do not allow definitive answers to these questions.

Second, it has been appreciated since the seminal observations of McCabe & Jackson (132) that, in patients with Gram-negative bacteremia, the risk of dying increases with the severity of the patient's underlying disease. Age is the second most important predictor of early mortality in such patients. Although these associations have been confirmed in many studies, how they interact to influence the systemic impact of bacteremia is not certain.

Third, genetic predispositions may be important risk factors for developing severe sepsis. To take the best-studied example, approximately 80% of individuals with *N. meningitidis* bacteremia develop meningitis rather than the fulminant syndrome discussed above. In various small clinical series, single nucleotide polymorphisms in several genes have been associated with the risk of developing fulminant meningococcemia. These associations suggest important roles for phagocytosis [e.g., FcγRIIA (Fc gamma receptor IIA) (133)], proinflammatory cytokines [e.g., IL-1β (134)], clotting [plasminogen activator inhibitor-1 (PAI-1)], and blood pressure regulation [angiotensin II–converting enzyme (135)] in the systemic reaction to *N. meningitidis* (136). Although these observations require confirmation, they suggest an important role for inherited factors in determining whether this pathogen elicits toxic reactions within the vasculature. In other studies, polymorphisms in the TLR4, PAI-1, TNF, and caspase-12 genes have been associated with risk of developing severe sepsis and/or mortality in various populations of patients, most of whom were infected with commensal bacteria (137, 138). In the case of the Factor V Leiden mutation, which confers resistance to the natural anticoagulant protein C, it is interesting that heterozygotes may be more likely to develop arterial thrombosis as a complication of fulminant meningococcemia (139), yet are protected from dying should they develop severe sepsis triggered by commensal bacteria (140). These observations suggest that an increased tendency to clot is harmful in intravascular infections yet beneficial in primary extravascular ones.

IMPLICATIONS FOR RESEARCH AND THERAPY

There are impressive challenges for sepsis research. Most importantly, the biochemical basis for both multi-organ dysfunction and septic shock must be determined. There are probably many routes to these endpoints, however, and correctly mapping these routes may also be important for improving prevention and therapy.

It is essential to find out how local inflammation contributes to the pathogenesis of severe sepsis and septic shock. Although studies in experimental animals have shown that mediators released into the blood from infected local tissues can cause shock (118), there is much more to be learned. To test the extravascular stimulus theory, it will be important to develop experimental models in which distant organ injury and shock can be induced by local infection (or other local stimuli) in the absence of bacteremia. Of the models in use today, zymosan-induced peritonitis may be the most satisfactory for this purpose (141).

Does a dysfunctional (autonomic) nervous system contribute significantly to sepsis pathogenesis? Recent experiments using orthogonal polarization spectroscopy to study the microcirculation of the tongue have suggested that this may be the case (96), as have various observations in both experimental animals and human patients (142). Having begun to understand the neural pathways by which local infection is communicated to the brain in rodents, it is important now to confirm these findings in higher animals. In addition, more must be learned about how efferent nerves influence responses to infection and inflammation within both infected tissues and distant organs.

Even in patients with fulminant meningococcemia or septic shock, anti-inflammatory molecules seem to dominate in both plasma and blood cells (102, 143). How do circulating endotoxin and Gram-negative bacteria directly elicit toxic reactions within the bloodstream despite the presence of strong anti-inflammatory forces in the blood? As noted above, there is also evidence that an exuberant anti-inflammatory cytokine response can be associated with increased risk of dying. Is this response insufficient to control the proinflammatory response, does it contribute somehow to organ dysfunction and/or shock, or is it an epiphenomenon? There are abnormal concentrations of more than 50 molecules in the blood of septic patients. Which, if any, of these molecules is the key target for intervention?

The two hypotheses discussed above have different implications for therapy. Agents that may kill Gram-negative bacteria or neutralize endotoxin in the circulation, such as IgM antibodies, should be most effective when Gram-negative bacteria or endotoxin stimulate toxic reactions within the vasculature. When the dominant inflammatory stimulus occurs within an extravascular tissue, in contrast, it may be advantageous to give drugs that can more effectively neutralize endotoxin or kill bacteria outside the bloodstream. Finding foci of infection and implementing effective drainage or excision are also urgent goals when the major stimulus is extravascular.

SUMMARY POINTS

1. Patients who develop severe sepsis and septic shock may arrive at these endpoints in different ways.
2. In some patients, pathogenic Gram-negative bacteria induce severe sepsis by invading the bloodstream, infecting vascular endothelial cells and intra/perivascular structures, releasing endotoxin, and stimulating toxic reactions within the circulation. The prototype in this category is *N. meningitidis*.

3. In other patients, uncontrolled local inflammation may trigger severe sepsis. The primary infection is often in the lungs or abdomen, and the infecting bacteria typically arise from the patient's own flora (e.g., *Enterobacteriaceae*). In these patients, bacteremia and endotoxemia may contribute little to the systemic response; the major stimulus arises within the infected local tissue. No microbial etiology can be identified in 20% to 50% of the cases of severe sepsis and septic shock, raising the possibility that endogenous mediators can also trigger or intensify the syndromes.
4. The two different pathogenetic pathways may be interpreted in terms of a functional compartmentalization of the body's responses to infection. In this model, local inflammatory responses are normally contained by systemic mechanisms that prevent inflammation within the bloodstream. Systemic responses to injury, infection and/or illness augment the anti-inflammatory state, which reduces the stimulatory impact of bacteria or endotoxin that enter the blood from extravascular primary sites of infection. The anti-inflammatory mechanisms can be overcome by intravascular pathogens such as *N. meningitidis*, or in exceptional cases in which there is abrupt or very high-grade bacteremia or endotoxemia.
5. Several factors influence the pathogenesis of severe sepsis in patients infected with Gram-negative bacteria: the nature of the microbe (i.e., pathogen versus commensal), the site of primary infection (i.e., intravascular versus extravascular), the prior status of the host (e.g., healthy versus ill and severity of illness), and polymorphisms in genes that influence innate immunity and the microcirculation.
6. The pathophysiology of severe sepsis is not a simple continuum in which the most striking cases can serve as a model for the rest. Incorporating microbe- and host-specific variables into the design and analysis of clinical trials may help identify agents that can benefit patients who become severely septic via different pathogenetic routes.

ACKNOWLEDGMENTS

The author is supported by grant AI18188 from the National Institute for Allergy and Infectious Diseases and by the Jan and Henri Bromberg Chair in Internal Medicine of the University of Texas Southwestern Medical Center, Dallas, Texas.

LITERATURE CITED

1. Cohen IL. 1993. Definitions for sepsis and organ failure: The ACCP/SCCM Consensus Conference Committee report. *Chest* 103:656
2. Levy MM, Fink MP, Marshall JC, Abraham E, Angus D, et al. 2003. 2001 SCCM/ESICM/ACCP/ATS/SIS International Sepsis Definitions Conference. *Crit. Care Med.* 31:1250–56
3. Munford RS. 2005. Sepsis, severe sepsis and septic shock. In *Principles and Practice of Infectious Diseases*, ed. GL Mandell, JE Bennett, R Dolin, pp. 906–26. Philadelphia: Elsevier Churchill-Livingstone
4. **Hotchkiss RS, Karl IE. 2003. Medical progress: The pathophysiology and treatment of sepsis. *N. Engl. J. Med.* 348:138–50**

Excellent overall review of severe sepsis, emphasizing the role of apoptosis in immunosuppression.

5. Riedemann NC, Guo RF, Ward PA. 2003. The enigma of sepsis. *J. Clin. Invest.* 112:460–67

6. Cohen J. 2002. The immunopathogenesis of sepsis. *Nature* 420:885–91
7. Bone RC, Grodzin CJ, Balk RA. 1997. Sepsis: A new hypothesis for pathogenesis of the disease process. *Chest* 112:235–43
8. Bone RC. 1996. Immunologic dissonance: a continuing evolution in our understanding of the systemic inflammatory response syndrome (SIRS) and the multiple organ dysfunction syndrome (MODS). *Ann. Intern. Med.* 125:680–87
9. Munford RS, Pugin J. 2001. Normal responses to injury prevent systemic inflammation and can be immunosuppressive. *Am. J. Respir. Crit. Care Med.* 163:316–21
10. **Hackett SJ, Guiver M, Marsh J, Sills JA, Thomson AP, et al. 2002. Meningococcal bacterial DNA load at presentation correlates with disease severity. *Arch. Dis. Child* 86:44–46**

Evidence for bacterial genomes in the blood of septic patients whose blood cultures were negative.

11. van Deventer SJH, Buller HR, ten Cate JW, Sturk A, Pauw W. 1988. Endotoxaemia: an early predictor of septicaemia in febrile patients. *Lancet* 1:605–9
12. Bates DW, Parsonnet J, Ketchum PA, Miller EB, Novitsky TJ, et al. 1998. Limulus amebocyte lysate assay for detection of endotoxin in patients with sepsis syndrome. *Clin. Infect. Dis.* 27:582–91
13. Hurley JC. 2003. Endotoxemia and Gram-negative bacteremia as predictors of outcome in sepsis: a meta-analysis using ROC curves. *J. Endotoxin Res.* 9:271–79
14. Ulloa L, Tracey KJ. 2005. The 'cytokine profile': a code for sepsis. *Trends Mol. Med.* 11:56–63
15. Rogers DE. 1960. Host mechanisms which act to remove bacteria from the blood stream. *Bacteriol. Rev.* 24:50–66
16. Felty AR, Keefer CS. 1924. Bacillus coli sepsis. *JAMA* 82:1430–33
17. Harris JA, Cobb CG. 1973. Persistent gram-negative bacteremia. Observations in twenty patients. *Am. J. Surg.* 125:705–17
18. Weinstein MP, Reller LB. 1984. Clinical importance of "breakthrough" bacteremia. *Am. J. Med.* 76:175–80
19. Chowers MY, Gottesman B, Paul M, Weinberger M, Pitlik S, Leibovici L. 2003. Persistent bacteremia in the absence of defined intravascular foci: Clinical significance and risk factors. *Eur. J. Clin. Microbiol. Infect. Dis.* 22:592–96
20. Wain J, Pham VB, Ha V, Nguyen NM, To SD, et al. 2001. Quantitation of bacteria in bone marrow from patients with typhoid fever: relationship between counts and clinical features. *J. Clin. Microbiol.* 39:1571–76
21. Murono K, Hirano Y, Koyano S, Ito K, Fujieda K. 2003. Molecular comparison of bacterial isolates from blood with strains colonizing pharynx and intestine in immunocompromised patients with sepsis. *J. Med. Microbiol.* 52:527–30
22. Weinstein MP, Murphy JR, Reller LB, Lichenstein KA. 1983. The clinical significance of positive blood cultures: A comprehensive analysis of 500 episodes of bacteremia and fungemia in adults. II. Clinical observations, with special reference to factors influencing prognosis. *Rev. Infect. Dis.* 5:54–70
23. Jones GR, Lowes JA. 1996. The systemic inflammatory response syndrome as a predictor of bacteraemia and outcome from sepsis. *Q. J. Med.* 89:515–22
24. Sands KE, Bates DW, Lanken PN, Graman PS, Hibberd PL, et al. 1997. Epidemiology of sepsis syndrome in 8 academic medical centers. *JAMA* 278:234–40
25. Bates DW, Pruess KE, Lee TH. 1995. How bad are bacteremia and sepsis? Outcomes in a cohort with suspected bacteremia. *Arch. Intern. Med.* 155:593–98
26. Brun-Buisson C, Doyon F, Carlet J, Bedock B, Annonay CH, et al. 1996. Bacteremia

and severe sepsis in adults: A multicenter prospective survey in ICUs and wards of 24 hospitals. *Am. J. Respir. Crit. Care Med.* 154:617–24
27. Rangel-Frausto MS, Pittet D, Costigan M, Hwang T, Davis CS, Wenzel RP. 1995. The natural history of the systemic inflammatory response syndrome (SIRS). *JAMA* 273:117–23
28. Sleigh J, Cursons R, La Pine M. 2001. Detection of bacteraemia in critically ill patients using 16S rDNA polymerase chain reaction and DNA sequencing. *Intensive Care Med.* 27:1269–73
29. Kreger BE, Craven DE, McCabe WR. 1980. Gram-negative bacteremia. IV. Re-evaluation of clinical features and treatment in 612 patients. *Am. J. Med.* 68:344–55
30. Leibovici L, Greenshtain S, Cohen O, Mor F, Wysenbeek AJ. 1991. Bacteremia in febrile patients. A clinical model for diagnosis. *Arch. Intern. Med.* 151:1801–6
31. Mitchell AE, Derrington P, Turner P, Hunt LP, Oakhill A, Marks DI. 2004. Gram-negative bacteraemia (GNB) after 428 unrelated donor bone marrow transplants (UD-BMT): risk factors, prophylaxis, therapy and outcome. *Bone Marrow Transplant.* 33:303–10
32. Blot SI, Vandewoude KH, Colardyn FA. 2003. Evaluation of outcome in critically ill patients with nosocomial Enterobacter bacteremia-Results of a matched cohort study. *Chest* 123:1208–13
33. Suffredini AF, Hochstein HD, McMahon FG. 1999. Dose-related inflammatory effects of intravenous endotoxin in humans: Evaluation of a new clinical lot of *Escherichia coli* O:113 endotoxin. *J. Infect. Dis.* 179:1278–82
34. Taveira da Silva AM, Kaulbach HC, Chuidian FS, Lambert DR, Suffredini AF, Danner RL. 1993. Brief report: Shock and multiple-organ dysfunction after self-administration of Salmonella endotoxin. *N. Engl. J. Med.* 328:1457–60
35. Danner RL, Elin RJ, Hosseini JM, Wesley RA, Reilly JM, Parillo JE. 1991. Endotoxemia in human septic shock. *Chest* 99:169–75
36. Meers PD, Calder MW, Mazhar MM, Lawrie GM. 1973. Intravenous infusion of contaminated dextrose solution: The Deveonport incident. *Lancet* 2:1189–92
37. Maki DG, Rhame FS, Mackel DC, Bennett JV. 1976. Nationwide epidemic of septicemia caused by contaminated intravenous products I. Epidemiologic and clinical features. *Am. J. Med.* 60:471–85
38. Maki DG. 1981. Nosocomial bacteremia. An epidemiologic overview. *Am. J. Med.* 70:719–32
39. DuPont HL, Spink WW. 1969. Infections due to Gram-negative organisms: an analysis of 860 patients with bacteremia at the University of Minnesota Medical Center, 1958–1966. *Medicine* 48:307–32
40. Phillips I, Eykyn S, Laker M. 1972. Outbreak of hospital infection caused by contaminated autoclaved fluids. *Lancet* 1:1258–60
41. Ostrowsky BE, Whitener C, Bredenberg HK, Carson LA, Holt S, et al. 2002. Serratia marcescens bacteremia traced to an infused narcotic. *N. Engl. J. Med.* 346:1529–37
42. Grohskopf LA, Roth VR, Feikin DR, Arduino MJ, Carson LA, et al. 2001. Serratia liquefaciens bloodstream infections from contamination of epoetin alfa at a hemodialysis center. *N. Engl. J. Med.* 344:1491–97
43. Brandtzaeg P, Kierulf P, Gaustad P, Skulberg A, Bruun JN, et al. 1989. Plasma endotoxin as a predictor of multiple organ failure and death in systemic meningococcal disease. *J. Infect. Dis.* 159:195–204

44. Harrison OB, Robertson BD, Faust SN, Jepson MA, Goldin RD, et al. 2002. Analysis of pathogen-host cell interactions in purpura fulminans: Expression of capsule, type IV Pili, and PorA by Neisseria meningitidis in vivo. *Infect. Immun.* 70:5193–201
45. Kirsch EA, Barton RP, Kitchen L, Giroir BP. 1996. Pathophysiology, treatment and outcome of meningococcemia: a review and recent experience. *Pediatr. Infect. Dis. J.* 15:967–79
46. Lehmann AK, Halstensen A, Sornes S, Rokke O, Waage A. 1995. High levels of interleukin 10 in serum are associated with fatality in meningococcal disease. *Infect. Immun.* 63:2109–12
47. Marzouk O, Bestwick K, Thomson APJ, Sills JA, Hart CA. 1993. Variation in serum C-reactive protein across the clinical spectrum of meningococcal disease. *Acta Paediatr.* 82:729–33
48. Jacobs RF, Hsi S, Wilson CB, Benjamin D, Smith AL, Morrow R. 1983. Apparent meningococcemia: clinical features of disease due to Haemophilus influenzae and Neisseria meningitidis. *Pediatrics* 72:469–72
49. Rello J, Ochagavia A, Sabanes E, Roque M, Mariscal D, et al. 2000. Evaluation of outcome of intravenous catheter-related infections in critically ill patients. *Am. J. Respir. Crit. Care Med.* 162:1027–30
50. DiGiovine B, Chenoweth C, Watts C, Higgins M. 1999. The attributable mortality and costs of primary nosocomial bloodstream infections in the intensive care unit. *Am. J. Respir. Crit. Care Med.* 160:976–81
51. Quilici N, Audibert G, Conroy MC, Bollaert PE, Guillemin F, et al. 1997. Differential quantitative blood cultures in the diagnosis of catheter-related sepsis in intensive care units. *Clin. Infect. Dis.* 25:1066–70
52. Velasco E, Byington R, Martins CA, Schirmer M, Dias LM, Goncalves VM. 2003. Prospective evaluation of the epidemiology, microbiology, and outcome of bloodstream infections in hematologic patients in a single cancer center. *Eur. J. Clin. Microbiol. Infect. Dis.* 22:137–43
53. Brun-Buisson C, Doyon F, Carlet J, Dellamonica P, Gouin F, et al. 1995. Incidence, risk factors, and outcome of severe sepsis and septic shock in adults—A multicenter prospective study in intensive care units. *JAMA* 274:968–74
54. Saez-Llorens X, Vargas S, Guerra F, Coronado L. 1995. Application of new sepsis definitions to evaluate outcome of pediatric patients with severe systemic infections. *Pediatr. Infect. Dis. J.* 14:557–61
55. Fisher CJ Jr, Dhainaut J-FA, Opal SM, Pribble JP, Balk RA, et al. 1994. Recombinant human interleukin 1 receptor antagonist in the treatment of patients with sepsis syndrome: Results from a randomized, double-blind, placebo-controlled trial. *JAMA* 271:1836–43
56. Deleted in proof
57. Nuytinck JK, Goris JA, Redl H, Schlag G, van Munster PJ. 1986. Posttraumatic complications and inflammatory mediators. *Arch. Surg.* 121:886–90
58. Goris RJ, te Boekhorst TP, Nuytinck JK, Gimbrere JS. 1985. Multiple-organ failure. Generalized autodestructive inflammation? *Arch. Surg.* 120:1109–15
59. Gordon S. 2002. Pattern recognition receptors: Doubling up for the innate immune response. *Cell* 111:927–30
60. Beutler B. 2004. Inferences, questions and possibilities in Toll-like receptor signalling. *Nature* 430:257–63
61. Hoebe K, Georgel P, Rutschmann S, Du X, Mudd S, Crozat K, et al. 2005. CD36 is a sensor of diacylglycerides. *Nature* 433:523–27

62. Sato S, Nomura F, Kawai T, Takeuchi O, Muhlradt PF, et al. 2000. Synergy and cross-tolerance between toll-like receptor (TLR) 2- and TLR4-mediated signaling pathways. *J. Immunol.* 165:7096–101
63. Tsung A, Sahai R, Tanaka H, Nakao A, Fink MP, et al. 2005. The nuclear factor HMGB1 mediates hepatic injury after murine liver ischemia-reperfusion. *J. Exp. Med.* 201:1135–43
64. Deleted in proof
65. Bryan CS, Reynolds KL, Brenner ER. 1983. Analysis of 1,186 episodes of gram-negative bacteremia in non-university hospitals: the effects of antimicrobial therapy. *Rev. Infect. Dis.* 4:629–38
66. McCue JD. 1985. Improved mortality in gram-negative bacillary bacteremia. *Arch. Int. Med.* 145:1212–16
67. Bates DW, Sands K, Miller E, Lanken PN, Hibberd PL, et al. 1997. Predicting bacteremia in patients with sepsis syndrome. *J. Infect. Dis.* 176:1538–51
68. Peduzzi P, Shatney C, Sheagren J, Sprung C. 1992. Predictors of bacteremia and gram-negative bacteremia in patients with sepsis. VA Syst.Sepsis Coop. Study Group. *Arch. Intern. Med.* 152:529–35
69. Kreger BE, Craven DE, Carling PC, McCabe WR. 1980. Gram-negative bacteremia. III. Reassessment of etiology, epidemiology and ecology in 612 patients. *Am. J. Med.* 68:332–43
70. Kellogg JA, Bankert DA, Manzella JP, Parsey KS, Scott SL, Cavanaugh SH. 1995. Occurrence and documentation of low-level bacteremia in a community hospital's patient population. *Am. J. Clin. Pathol.* 104:524–29
71. House D, Chinh NT, Hien TT, Parry CP, Ly NT, et al. 2002. Cytokine release by lipopolysaccharide-stimulated whole blood from patients with typhoid fever. *J. Infect. Dis.* 186:240–45
72. LaScolea LJ Jr, Rosales SV, Welliver RC, Ogra PL. 1985. Mechanisms underlying the development of meningitis or epiglottitis in children after Haemophilus influenzae type b bacteremia. *J. Infect. Dis.* 151:1162–65
73. Santosham M, Moxon ER. 1977. Persistent Gram-negative bacteremia. *J. Pediatr.* 91:719–21
74. Sullivan DT, LaScolea LJ Jr. 1987. Neisseria meningitidis bacteremia in children: quantitation of bacteremia and spontaneous clinical recovery without antibiotic therapy. *Pediatrics* 80:63–67
75. Butler T, Levin J, Linh NN, Chau DM, Adickman M, Arnold K. 1976. Yersinia pestis infection in Vietnam. II. Quantiative blood cultures and detection of endotoxin in the cerebrospinal fluid of patients with meningitis. *J. Infect. Dis.* 133:493–99
76. Walsh AL, Smith MD, Wuthiekanun V, Suputtamongkol Y, Chaowagul W, et al. 1995. Prognostic significance of quantitative bacteremia in septicemic melioidosis. *Clin. Infect. Dis.* 21:1498–500
77. Shenep JL, Flynn PM, Barrett FF, Stidham GL, Westenkirchner DF. 1988. Serial quantitation of endotoxemia and bacteremia during therapy for gram-negative bacterial sepsis. *J. Infect. Dis.* 157:565–68
78. Spink WW, Braude AI, Castaneda MR, Goytia RS. 1948. Aureomycin therapy in human brucellosis due to *Brucella melitensis*. *JAMA* 138:1145–48
79. Reilly J, Compagnon A, Tournier P, Bastin R, Du Buit H. 1950. Les accidents du traitement des fievres typhoides par la chloromycetine. *Ann. Med.* 51:597–629

80. Hurley JC. 1992. Antibiotic-induced release of endotoxin: A reappraisal. *Clin. Infect. Dis.* 15:840–54
81. Simpson AJ, Opal SM, Angus BJ, Prins JM, Palardy JE, et al. 2000. Differential antibiotic-induced endotoxin release in severe melioidosis. *J. Infect. Dis.* 181:1014–19
82. Deleted in proof
83. Greisman SE, Hornick RB, Woodward TE. 1964. The role of endotoxin during typhoid fever and tularemia in man. *J. Clin. Invest.* 43:1747–57
84. Munford RS. 2005. Detoxifying endotoxin: time, place and person. *J. Endotoxin. Res.* 11:69–84
85. Mertsola J, Ramilo O, Mustafa MM, Saez-Llorens X, Hansen EJ, McCracken GH Jr. 1989. Release of endotoxin after antibiotic treatment of Gram-negative bacterial meningitis. *Pediatr. Infect. Dis. J.* 8:904–6
86. Arditi M, Ables L, Yogev R. 1989. Cerebrospinal fluid endotoxin levels in children with *H. influenzae* meningitis before and after administration of intravenous ceftriaxone. *J. Infect. Dis.* 160:1005–11
87. Berkowitz FE, Vallabh P, Altman DI, Diamantes F, Van Wyk HJP, Stroucken JMM. 1983. Jarisch-Herxheimer reaction in meningococcal meningitis. *Am. J. Dis. Child.* 137:599
88. Mant MJ, King EG. 1979. Severe, acute disseminated intravascular coagulation. A reappraisal of its pathophysiology, clinical significance and therapy based on 47 patients. *Am. J. Med.* 67:557–63
89. Robboy SJ, Major MC, Colman RW, Minna JD. 1972. Pathology of disseminated intravascular coagulation (DIC). Analysis of 26 cases. *Hum. Pathol.* 3:327–43
90. Ten Cate H, Schoenmakers SH, Franco R, Timmerman JJ, Groot AP, et al. 2001. Microvascular coagulopathy and disseminated intravascular coagulation. *Crit. Care. Med.* 29:S95–97
91. Shimamura K, Oka K, Nakazawa M, Kojima M. 1983. Distribution patterns of microthrombi in disseminated intravascular coagulation. *Arch. Pathol. Lab. Med.* 107:543–47
92. Marshall JC, Christou NV, Horn R, Meakins JL. 1988. The microbiology of multiple organ failure. The proximal gastrointestinal tract as an occult reservoir of pathogens. *Arch. Surg.* 123:309–15
93. Hotchkiss RS, Swanson PE, Freeman BD, Tinsley KW, Cobb JP, et al. 1999. Apoptotic cell death in patients with sepsis, shock, and multiple organ dysfunction [see comments]. *Crit. Care Med.* 27:1230–51
94. Hotchkiss RS, Tinsley KW, Swanson PE, Schmieg RE Jr, Hui JJ, et al. 2001. Sepsis-induced apoptosis causes progressive profound depletion of B and $CD4^+$ T lymphocytes in humans. *J. Immunol.* 166:6952–63
95. Fink M. 1997. Cytopathic hypoxia in sepsis. *Acta Anaesthesiol. Scand.* 110:87–95
96. De Backer D, Creteur J, Preiser JC, Dubois MJ, Vincent JL. 2002. Microvascular blood flow is altered in patients with sepsis. *Am. J. Respir. Crit. Care Med.* 166:98–104
97. Sotto MN, Langer B, Hoshino-Shimizu S, de Brito T. 1976. Pathogenesis of cutaneous lesions in acute meningococcemia in humans: light, immunofluorescent, and electron microscopic studies of skin biopsy specimens. *J. Infect. Dis.* 133:506–14
98. Vogel SN, Fenton M. 2003. Toll-like receptor 4 signalling: new perspectives on a complex signal-transduction problem. *Biochem. Soc. Trans.* 31:664–68
99. Hamann L, Alexander C, Stamme C, Zahringer U, Schumann RR. 2005. Acute-phase concentrations of lipopolysaccharide (LPS)-binding protein inhibit innate immune cell

activation by different LPS chemotypes via different mechanisms. *Infect. Immun.* 73:193–200

100. Kitchens RL, Thompson PA, O'Keefe GE, Munford RS. 2000. Plasma constituents regulate LPS binding to, and release from, the monocyte cell surface. *J. Endotoxin. Res.* 6:482
101. Kitchens RL, Thompson PA, Munford RS, O'Keefe GE. 2003. Acute inflammation and infection maintain circulating phospholipid levels and enhance lipopolysaccharide binding to plasma lipoproteins. *J. Lipid Res.* 44:2339–48
102. Brandtzaeg P, Osnes L, Ovstebo R, Joo GB, Westvik A-B, Kieruf P. 1996. Net inflammatory capacity of human septic shock plasma evaluated by a monocyte-based target cell assay: identification of interleukin-10 as a major functional deactivator of human monocytes. *J. Exp. Med.* 184:51–60
103. Fong Y, Marano MA, Moldawer LL, Wei H, Calvano SE, et al. 1990. The acute splanchnic and peripheral tissue metabolic response to endotoxin in humans. *J. Clin. Invest.* 85:1896–904
104. Spek CA, Verbon A, Aberson H, Pribble JP, McElgunn CJ, et al. 2003. Treatment with an anti-CD14 monoclonal antibody delays and inhibits lipopolysaccharide-induced gene expression in humans *in vivo*. *J. Clin. Immunol.* 23:132–40
105. Tilg H, Dinarello CA, Mier JW. 1997. IL-6 and APPs: anti-inflammatory and immunosuppressive mediators. *Immunol. Today* 9:428–32
106. Campisi J, Hansen MK, O'Connor KA, Biedenkapp JC, Watkins LR, et al. 2003. Circulating cytokines and endotoxin are not necessary for the activation of the sickness or corticosterone response produced by peripheral *E. coli* challenge. *J. Appl. Physiol.* 95:1873–82
107. Székely M, Balaskó M, Kulchitsky VA, Simons CT, Ivanov AI, Romanovsky AA. 2000. Multiple neural mechanisms of fever. *Auton. Neurosci.* 85:78–82
108. Gaykema RPA, Goehler LE, Hansen MK, Maier SF, Watkins LR. 2000. Subdiaphragmatic vagotomy blocks interleukin-1β-induced fever but does not reduce IL-1β levels in the circulation. *J. Auton. Nerv. Syst.* 85:72–77
109. Netea MG, Kullberg B-J, Van der Meer JWM. 2000. Circulating cytokines as mediators of fever. *Clin. Infect. Dis.* 31:S178–84
110. Barber AE, Coyle SM, Fischer E, Smith C, van der Poll T, et al. 1995. Influence of hypercortisolemia on soluble tumor necrosis factor receptor II and interleukin-1 receptor antagonist responses to endotoxin in human beings. *Surgery* 118:406–11
111. van der Poll T, Coyle SM, Barbosa K, Braxton CC, Lowry SF. 1996. Epinephrine inhibits tumor necrosis factor-α and potentiates interleukin 10 production during human endotoxemia. *J. Clin. Invest.* 97:713–19
112. Borovikova LV, Ivanova S, Zhang M, Yang H, Botchkina GI, et al. 2000. Vagus nerve stimulation attenuates the systemic inflammatory response to endotoxin. *Nature* 405:458–62
113. Wang H, Liao H, Ochani M, Justiniani M, Lin X, et al. 2004. Cholinergic agonists inhibit HMGB1 release and improve survival in experimental sepsis. *Nat. Med.* 10:1216–21
114. **Dugernier TL, Laterre PF, Wittebole X, Roeseler J, Latinne D, et al. 2003. Compartmentalization of the inflammatory response during acute pancreatitis: correlation with local and systemic complications. *Am. J. Respir. Crit. Care Med.* 168:148–57**

The inflammatory response to pancreatitis may be compartmentalized.

115. Rivera-Chavez FA, Wheeler H, Lindberg G, Munford RS, O'Keefe GE. 2003. Regional

and systemic cytokine responses to acute inflammation of the vermiform appendix. *Ann. Surg.* 237:408–16

116. Annane D, Sanquer S, Sébille V, Faye A, Djuranovic D, et al. 2000. Compartmentalised inducible nitric-oxide synthase activity in septic shock. *Lancet* 355:1143–48
117. Matute-Bello G, Frevert CW, Kajikawa O, Skerrett SJ, Goodman RB, et al. 2001. Septic shock and acute lung injury in rabbits with peritonitis - Failure of the neutrophil response to localized infection. *Am. J. Respir. Crit. Care Med.* 163:234–43
118. **Kurahashi K, Kajikawa O, Sawa T, Ohara M, Gropper MA, et al. 1999. Pathogenesis of septic shock in *Pseudomonas aeruginosa* pneumonia. *J. Clin. Invest.* 104:743–50**

Evidence that local inflammation can induce septic shock.

119. Ebong S, Call D, Nemzek J, Bolgos G, Newcomb D, Remick D. 1999. Immunopathologic alterations in murine models of sepsis of increasing severity. *Infect. Immun.* 67:6603–10
120. Elenkov IJ, Wilder RL, Chrousos GP, Vizi ES. 2000. The sympathetic nerve–an integrative interface between two supersystems: the brain and the immune system. *Pharmacol. Rev.* 52:595–638
121. Webster EL, Barrientos RM, Contoreggi C, Isaac MG, Ligier S, et al. 2002. Corticotropin releasing hormone (CRH) antagonist attenuates adjuvant induced arthritis: Role of CRH in peripheral inflammation. *J. Rheumatol.* 29:1252–61
122. Lemaire LCJM, Van Lanschot JB, van der Poll T, Buurman WA, van Deventer SJH, Gouma DJ. 1998. Lymph of patients with a systemic inflammatory response syndrome inhibits lipopolysaccharide-induced cytokine production. *J. Infect. Dis.* 178:883–86
123. Kushner I. 1998. Semantics, inflammation, cytokines and common sense. *Cytokine Growth Factor Rev.* 9:191–96
124. Funayama H, Mayanagi H, Takada H, Endo Y. 2001. Inflammatory reactions in extraoral tissues in mice after intragingival injection of lipopolysaccharide. *J. Infect. Dis.* 184:1566–71
125. Zanetti G, Heumann D, Gerain J, Kohler J, Abbet P, et al. 1992. Cytokine production after intravenous or peritoneal gram-negative bacterial challenge in mice. *J. Immunol.* 148:1890–97
126. Calandra T, Baumgartner J-D, Grau GE, Wu M-M, Lambert P-H, et al. 1990. Prognostic values of tumor necrosis factor/cachectin, interleukin-1, interferon-α, and interferon-gamma in the serum of patients with septic shock. *J. Infect. Dis.* 161:982–87
127. Wang H, Yang H, Tracey KJ. 2004. Extracellular role of HMGB1 in inflammation and sepsis. *J. Intern. Med.* 255:320–31
128. Matsuura M, Kawahara K, Ezaki T, Nakano M. 1996. Biological activities of lipopolysaccharide of Burkholderia (Pseudomonas) pseudomallei. *FEMS Microbiol. Lett.* 137:79–83

128a. Kawahara K, Tsukano H, Watanabe H, Lindner B, Matsuura M. 2002. Modification of the structure and activity of lipid A in Yersinia pestis lipopolysaccharide by growth temperature. *Infect. Immun.* 70:4092–98

129. Van Dissel JT, van Langevelde P, Westendorp RG, Kwappenberg K, Frolich M. 1998. Anti-inflammatory cytokine profile and mortality in febrile patients. *Lancet* 351:950–53
130. Gogos CA, Drosou E, Bassaris HP, Skoutelis A. 2000. Pro- versus anti-inflammatory cytokine profile in patients with severe sepsis: A marker for prognosis and future therapeutic options. *J. Infect. Dis.* 181:176–80
131. Westendorp RGJ, Langermans JAM, Huizinga TWJ, Elouali AH, Verweij CL, et al.

1997. Genetic influence on cytokine production and fatal meningococcal disease. *Lancet* 349:170–73

132. McCabe WR, Jackson GG. 1962. Gram-negative bacteremia I. Etiology and ecology. *Arch. Intern. Med.* 110:83–91
133. Platonov AE, Shipulin GA, Vershinina IV, Dankert J, Van de Winkel JG, Kuijper EJ. 1998. Association of human FcgammaRIIa (CD32) polymorphism with susceptibility to and severity of meningococcal disease. *Clin. Infect. Dis.* 27:746–50
134. Read RC, Camp NJ, Di Giovine FS, Borrow R, Kaczmarski EB, et al. 2000. An interleukin-1 genotype is associated with fatal outcome of meningococcal disease. *J. Infect. Dis.* 182:1557–60
135. Harding D, Baines PB, Brull D, Vassiliou V, Ellis I, et al. 2002. Severity of meningococcal disease in children and the angiotensin-converting enzyme insertion/deletion polymorphism. *Am. J. Respir. Crit. Care Med.* 165:1103–6
136. Emonts M, Hazelzet JA, De Groot R, Hermans PW. 2003. Host genetic determinants of Neisseria meningitidis infections. *Lancet Infect. Dis.* 3:565–77
137. Saleh M, Vaillancourt JP, Graham RK, Huyck M, Srinivasula SM, et al. 2004. Differential modulation of endotoxin responsiveness by human caspase-12 polymorphisms. *Nature* 429:75–79
138. Texereau J, Pene F, Chiche JD, Rousseau C, Mira JP. 2004. Importance of hemostatic gene polymorphisms for susceptibility to and outcome of severe sepsis. *Crit. Care Med.* 32:S313–19
139. Kondaveeti S, Hibberd ML, Booy R, Nadel S, Levin M. 1999. Effect of the Factor V Leiden mutation on the severity of meningococcal disease. *Pediatr. Infect. Dis. J.* 18:893–96
140. Kerlin BA, Yan SB, Isermann BH, Brandt JT, Sood R, et al. 2003. Survival advantage associated with heterozygous factor V Leiden mutation in patients with severe sepsis and in mouse endotoxemia. *Blood* 102:3085–92
141. Von Asmuth EJU, Maessen JG, Van der Linden CJ, Buurman WA. 1990. Tumour necrosis factor alpha (TNF-α) and interleukin 6 in a zymosan-induced shock model. *Scand. J. Immunol.* 32:313–19
142. Munford RS, Tracey KJ. 2002. Is severe sepsis a neuroendocrine disease? *Mol. Med.* 8:437–42
143. Ertel W, Kremer J-P, Kenney J, Steckholzer U, Jarrar D, et al. 1995. Downregulation of proinflammatory cytokine release in whole blood from septic patients. *Blood* 85:1341–47

Proteases in Parasitic Diseases

James H. McKerrow, Conor Caffrey, Ben Kelly, P'ng Loke, and Mohammed Sajid

Department of Pathology and the Sandler Center, University of California, San Francisco, San Francisco, California 94143; email: jmck@cgl.ucsf.edu, caffrey@cgl.ucsf.edu, bkelly@itsa.ucsf.edu, ploke@itsa.ucsf.edu, sajid@cgl.ucsf.edu

Annu. Rev. Pathol. Mech. Dis. 2006. 1:497–536

First published online as a Review in Advance on October 31, 2005

The *Annual Review of Pathology: Mechanisms of Disease* is online at pathmechdis.annualreviews.org

doi: 10.1146/annurev.pathol.1.110304.100151

1553-4006/06/0114-0497$20.00

Key Words

parasite, protease inhibitor, invasion, host, immune response

Abstract

Parasitic diseases represent major global health problems of immense proportion. Schistosomiasis, malaria, leishmaniasis, Chagas disease, and African sleeping sickness affect hundreds of millions of people worldwide, cause millions of deaths annually, and present an immense social and economic burden. Recent advances in genomic analysis of several of the major global parasites have revealed key factors involved in the pathogenesis of parasite diseases. Among the major virulence factors identified are parasite-derived proteases. This review focuses on the direct role of proteases in disease pathogenesis. Well-characterized examples of the roles proteases play in pathogenesis include their involvement in invasion of the host by parasite migration through tissue barriers, degradation of hemoglobin and other blood proteins, immune evasion, and activation of inflammation.

INTRODUCTION

Parasitic diseases, caused by a diverse spectrum of eukaryotic organisms, represent a major global health problem. Age-adjusted disability years, a measure of the effect of disease morbidity, are greater for seemingly exotic parasitic diseases than for well-known entities like diabetes (1). Currently, malaria infects more than 500 million people worldwide, schistosomiasis more than 200 million, and hookworm or *Ascaris* close to a billion. Elimination of these diseases is probably not feasible in our lifetime. Even control is hampered by the relative lack of interest shown by the pharmaceutical industry in vaccine or drug development for human parasitic diseases. This lack of interest is largely owing to the fact that these diseases primarily affect poor people in poor countries.

If we are to make any headway in developing new drugs or vaccines for human parasitic diseases, it is clear that our understanding of the pathogenesis of these diseases must be significantly more sophisticated than it is today. Part of the problem in making headway in this regard is a relative lack of research funding, and, as a consequence, less active research in this area compared with research on diseases of the wealthier nations of the world. Our lack of understanding of parasitic disease pathogenesis is compounded by the problem that the biology of host-parasite relationships is extremely complex. In contrast to most other infectious diseases, parasitic infections may be long-lived (individual schistosome parasites can live longer than a decade in their host), and as parasites are eukaryotic organisms, their cellular and biochemical machinery is complex.

Some headway has been made in identifying factors that are key to parasite virulence and the pathogenesis of the diseases they produce. Among the most widely studied of these factors are parasite-derived proteases. As in other infections, proteases can play a variety of roles in establishing, maintaining, and exacerbating an infection. This review focuses on our current state of knowledge concerning the role of parasite proteases in the pathogenesis of parasitic diseases. Inasmuch as recent reviews have covered in depth the biochemical properties and molecular evolution of parasite proteases (2), these topics will not be addressed. Rather, the role of proteases in virulence and pathogenesis is emphasized. Attention is given to identifying the gaps in our knowledge and predicting what future research must be done to fill these gaps.

PROTEASES IN PARASITE TISSUE INVASION

Parasitic worms, or helminthes, are large, multicellular organisms that can reside in and migrate through a variety of tissues and organs. In most cases, the migratory stage of the parasite is larval (**Figure 1**). In nematodes, there are two stages that have the capacity to traverse tissue barriers during invasion or dissemination. L3, the infective third larval stage, is the larval stage that penetrates the intact host skin in the case of hookworms and *Strongyloides*, or the intestinal wall by *Anisakis*. Human pathology associated with nematode larval migration is often seen in cases where nonhuman parasites inadvertently invade a human host. For example, invasion and migration of *Anisakis* L3 larvae following ingestion of raw or poorly cooked seafood can elicit an intense inflammatory response characterized by eosinophil infiltration, edema, and pain (3, 4). There are many case reports of individuals misdiagnosed with peptic ulcer disease or appendicitis following an *Anisakis* larval invasion. Often, the most intense immune response is to dead or dying parasites, which release antigens not normally recognized by the vertebrate host. Alternatively, accidental invasion of the human host by a nonhuman parasite can elicit an inflammatory response in the human host owing to the fact that the parasite has evolved effective mechanisms for immune invasion only in the definitive (not human) host.

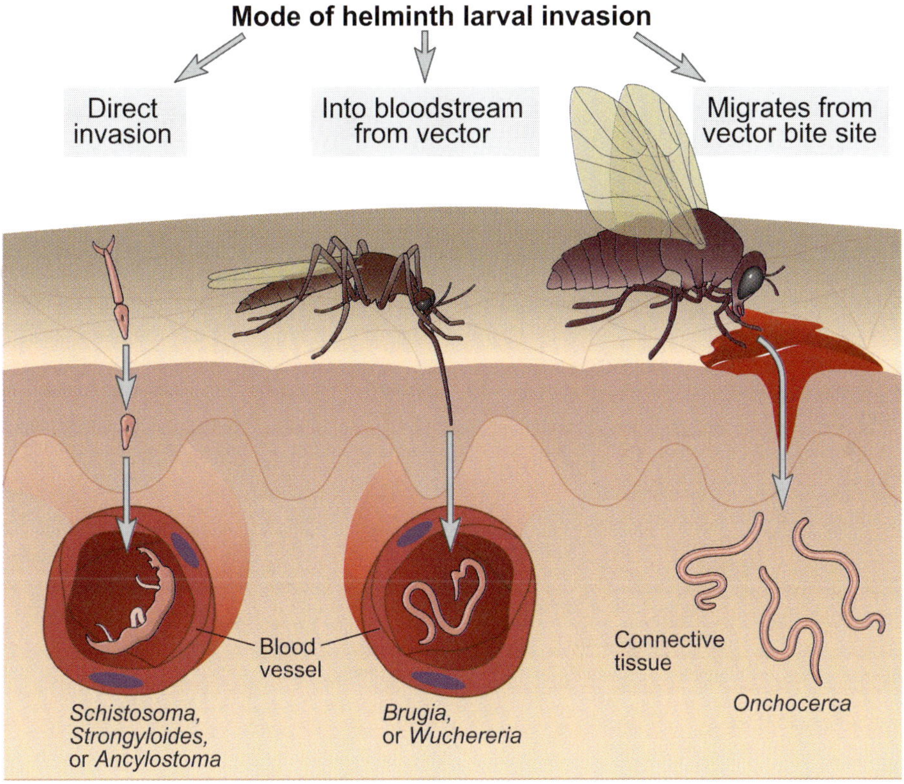

Figure 1

Different modes of invasion of host by helminth larvae. Invasion may be direct from the environment (schistosomes, hookworm), along vector bite path (*Brugia*), or dispersed from vector bite (*Onchocerca*).

Cases of larval migration into the intestinal wall [in the case of *Anisakis* (2, 3)] or through skin or subcutaneous tissue [in the case of hookworms (5), *Strongyloides* (6), and *Toxocara* (7)] are frequently reported. In some cases, migration through the host tissue is rapid enough that the term *larva currens* (from the Latin participle for running) is used to describe this phenomenon. It is assumed that such migration is mediated by the release of proteolytic enzymes that can degrade tissue barriers. Potent proteolytic enzymes of the serine and metalloprotease classes have been identified in secretory products of virtually all of these nematode larvae (8). Unfortunately, to date, there is no method to alter these parasites genetically to examine whether protease-deficient larvae can still invade. Nevertheless, in some cases, class-specific protease inhibitors have been shown, at least in vitro, to arrest larval invasion of the skin (e.g., by *Strongyloides* parasites) (9).

Another nematode parasite stage that often has widespread tissue migration is the microfilaria of *Onchocerca* and related filarial parasites (10). This stage of the parasite disseminates in order to optimize the probability of being taken up by an insect vector as the insect takes a blood meal. Again, although no direct evidence has emerged to implicate proteases in this migration, protease expression has been reported at this parasite stage (10).

Cysteine proteases: enzymatic proteins utilizing a cysteine thiol group to hydrolyze peptide bonds

Among trematode parasites or flukes, there are several examples of secretion of potent proteolytic enzymes during the tissue-invasive stage of the life cycle (**Figure 2**). In the liver fluke *Fasciola*, for example, juvenile worms release a potent cathepsin B–like cysteine protease (11), which is thought to play a role in the invasion of liver capsule and hepatic parenchyma akin to the role of cathepsin B in tumor cell invasion (2). Similar enzymes have been reported in tissue invasive stages of *Paragonimus*, the lung fluke

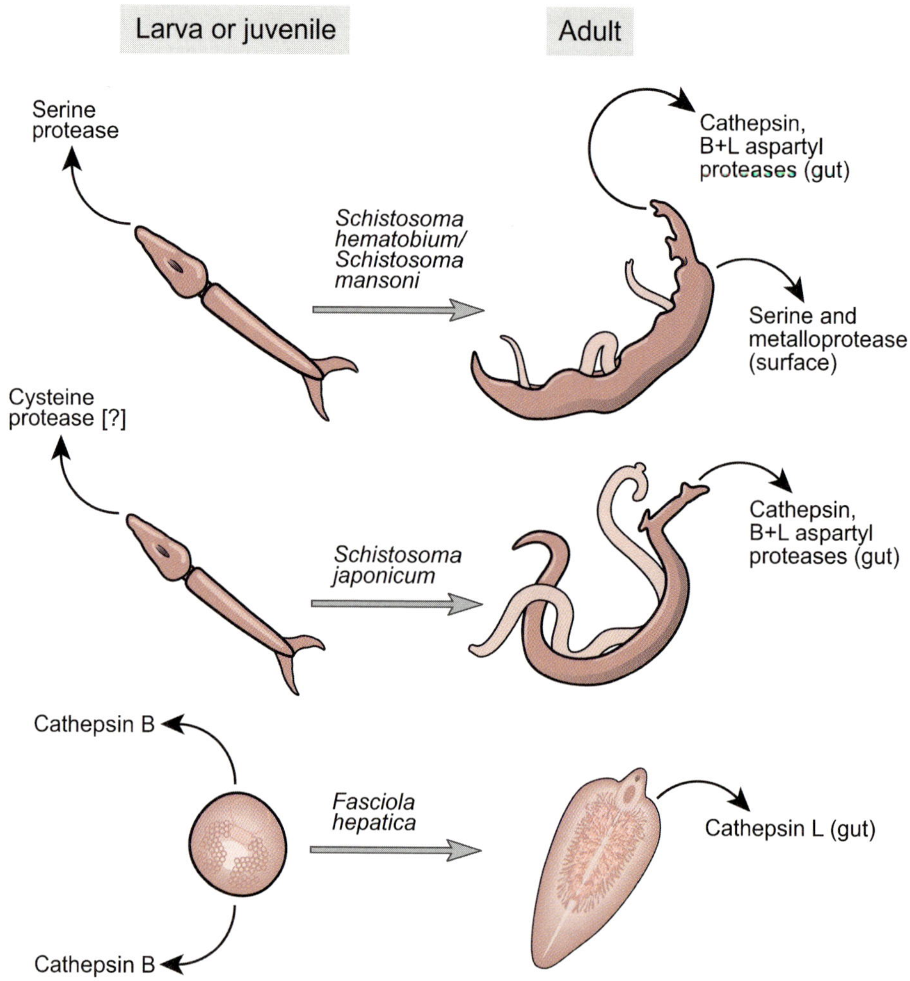

Figure 2

Comparison of protease release by larval versus adult helminth parasites. In larvae, proteases function primarily in tissue invasion or immune evasion. In adults, they function in gut degradation of host proteins, anticoagulation, and immune evasion (see text for details).

IL: interleukin

(12, 13), and *Clonorchis*, the Chinese liver fluke (14). In the lung fluke, larval proteases have also been proposed to play a role in immune evasion by degrading immunoglobulin (Ig) G and altering interleukin (IL)-8 production (15, 16).

The schistosome blood fluke is the best characterized of the trematode parasites. Proteases have been implicated directly or indirectly in pathology caused by several stages of this parasite. Eggs produced by female parasites elicit an intense granulomatous response, which is the basis of disease pathogenesis in chronic schistosomiasis. Among the products of the embryonic larva (miracidium) in the egg is a cysteine protease known to be released into the extracellular milieu (17). Although there is no direct evidence at this time for participation of this protease in eliciting the T helper 2 (Th2)-like response that characterizes granuloma, cysteine proteases are often immunogenic or allergenic (2).

A broad spectrum of proteases is produced in the gut of developing adult schistosomes. These proteases are used, presumably, to degrade hemoglobin and other host proteins during intravascular residence (1, 18). Interestingly, two of these proteases, both from the Clan CA cysteine protease family (2), were originally discovered because of their immunogenicity (19). These proteases characteristically elicit an antibody response in virtually every host and have even been explored as serodiagnostic agents for schistosomiasis (20). What role this immune response may play in host protection or pathogenesis is currently unknown. Similar gut-associated proteases are found in other trematodes including *Paragonimus* (21) and *Fasciola* (17, 22, 23). Of note is that the *Fasciola* gut proteases are promising vaccine candidates. Less well characterized, but also intriguing, are proteases thought to be present at or near the surface of developing or adult schistosomes. These proteases are proposed to play a role in anticoagulation or elimination of bound IgG and complement (24).

Perhaps the most extensively studied helminth protease is the serine protease secreted by the larvae of *Schistosoma mansoni* (termed cercariae). Recent reviews have discussed the potential role of this enzyme in tissue invasion (25–27). However, a second proposed function is in immune evasion (28). Initial invasion of the keratinized layer of the surface of skin probably requires little proteolytic digestion. This most superficial layer of skin is well hydrated in the aqueous environment in which infection is initiated. However, microscopic analysis has demonstrated clear destruction of the epidermal layer by degradation of desmosome structures and lysis or apoptosis of epidermal cells. Both light and electron microscopic studies have demonstrated degradation of the dermal/epidermal basement membrane (**Figure 3**). It is thought that the larvae, termed schistosomula at this stage of development, break through the basement membrane and continue migrating through the superficial dermis to enter small venules or lymphatics.

Aside from the potential histolytic role of secreted proteases in cercarial invasion, it has been proposed that, by degrading protein anchors for the glycocalyx the cercarial serine protease may also function to remodel the invading larva to a form that can evade immune detection. The glycocalyx is a complex carbohydrate surface coat that protects the organism from osmotic shock in hypotonic fresh water, into which the larvae emerge from snails and swim to the exposed mammalian host (29). The glycocalx is known to be a potent activator of complement and so must be jettisoned before cercariae are well into the skin.

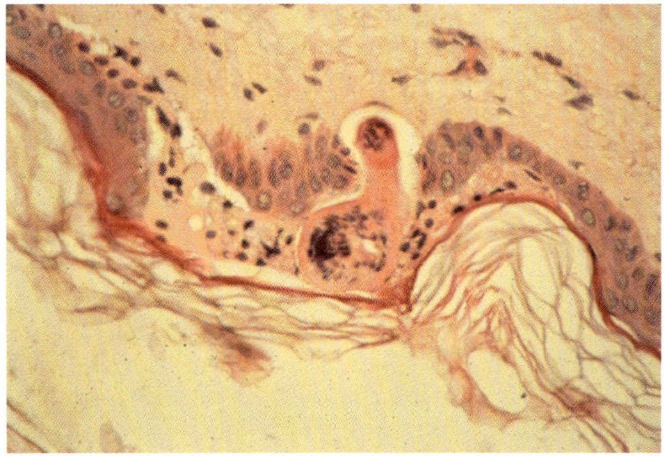

Figure 3

Schistosome cercaria invading human skin. Note the destruction of epidermis in the wake of migrating larva, which has now breached the dermal/epidermal basement membrane.

Schistosomula: stage of schistosome parasite following entry into mammalian host

Proteins released by invading schistosome larvae, or present on their surface, are the first to be seen by the host's immune system. Recent mass spectrometric analysis of the proteins released during cercarial invasion of skin has shown that the serine protease released by the cercaria is one of the most, if not the most, abundant proteins seen by the host (29). Interestingly, whereas bird or small mammal parasites cause an intense inflammatory response when they invade human skin, the larvae of human-specific schistosomes invade and reach the blood stream with relatively little immune response (26). However, recent studies have documented that even in this relatively unrecognized invasion process, dendritic cells appear to migrate to regional lymph nodes, and some agents of the innate immune response, possibly including mast cell products and prostaglandins, are released (26). Does the serine protease released during cercarial invasion play a role in immune evasion for human schistosomes, and are there significant differences between human and nonhuman schistosomes in activity

Kinetoplastid: protozoan organism that possesses a kinetoplast

or immunogenicity of this enzyme? Although these questions are active subjects in current research, the answers are at present unknown.

PROTOZOAN PARASITE PROTEASES

Leishmania

Leishmania are kinetoplastid protozoan parasites of vertebrate macrophages that cause the chronic sandfly-borne disease leishmaniasis, which impacts approximately 12 million people in 88 countries. Upon taking a blood meal, *Leishmania*-infected sandflies transmit the flagellated insect vector stage (promastigote) through the skin of the vertebrate host. Following uptake of promastigotes by host macrophages, the parasites differentiate into ovoid, aflagellate forms (amastigotes) that replicate in the macrophage phagolysosome. Rupture of the infected macrophage leads to dissemination of amastigotes to neighboring macrophages and eventual lesion development. The life cycle is completed when a sandfly feeds on an infected vertebrate host. The following section of this review highlights recent findings demonstrating the contributions of the GP63 proteases and members of the cysteine protease family to *Leishmania* pathogenesis (**Table 1**).

Table 1 Examples of proposed roles for proteases in pathogenesis

Protease/ activity	Parasite	Experimental strategy	Pathogenic function	Proposed mechanism	References
GP63	*Leishmania major*	Gene knockout	Complement resistance	Degradation of complement	(33)
GP63	*Leishmania amazonensis*	Antisense RNA	Macrophage infection	Facilitating macrophage binding/intramacrophage viability	(32)
GP63	*L. amazonensis*	Overexpression	Migration through extracellular matrix	Degradation of extracellular matrix	(36)
CPA	*Leishmania mexicana*	Gene knockout	None confirmed	—	(46)
CPB	*L. mexicana*	Gene knockout	Macrophage infection	Facilitating promastigote entry	(49, 50)
CPB	*L. mexicana*	Gene knockout	Th1 suppression	Degradation of innate immune signaling components	(53)
CPC	*L. mexicana*	Gene knockout	Macrophage infection	Facilitating promastigote entry	(47)
EhCP1	*Entamoeba histolytica*	No data	—	—	—
EhCP2	*E. histolytica*	Overexpression	Enteric cytopathology	Intestinal layer disruption	(64)
EhCP1	*E. histolytica*	Biochemical assay	Dysregulated inflammation	Inducing pathologic inflammation	(65)
EhCP5	*E. histolytica*	Antisense RNA suppression	Enteric cytopathology	Intestinal layer disruption	(68)
EhCP5	*E. histolytica*	Antisense RNA suppression	Dyregulated inflammation/hepatic pathology	Promoting pathologic inflammation	(67, 68)
Serine protease activity	*Schistosoma mansoni*	Biochemical assay	Depletion of immunoglobulins	Immunoglobulin degradation	(71)

Leishmania Leishmanolysin

Since the finding that the glycosyl phosphatidyl inositol (GPI)-anchored zinc metalloprotease leishmanolysin (GP63, 63 kDa glycoprotein) is a highly abundant protein on the surface of *Leishmania* (30, 31), a number of pathogenic roles have been proposed for this protein, including uptake and invasion of host macrophages and resistance against host complement–mediated lysis. In support of GP63's role in macrophage parasitization, it was shown that expression of a *gp63* antisense RNA construct in *Leishmania amazonensis* led to impaired parasitization of macrophages (32). In contrast to these findings, however, *gp63−/− Leishmania major*, which lacks all seven of the *gp63* genes found in this species, showed no defects in macrophage infection (33). Analyses of *gp63−/− L. major* promastigotes confirmed a role for GP63 in resistance to host complement, as these mutant parasites were dramatically more susceptible to lysis by human serum and showed delayed pathogenesis in susceptible mice (33). Although these studies definitively demonstrate a role for GP63 in protection against complement, they do not discriminate between an enzymatic versus a structural role for GP63. Earlier studies, however, with the purified C3 component of complement showed that GP63 is certainly able to cleave complement directly (34). Because mouse complement is considerably less lytic than human complement (35), and given the absence of a role for *L. major* GP63 in macrophage parasitization, the delayed lesion development in mice infected with *gp63−/− L. major* implies that GP63 could be involved in additional pathogenic pathways such as migration through the extracellular matrix (36). Deletion of the gene encoding GPI8 (component 8 of GPI protein transamidase), a component of the GPI protein transamidase complex in *Leishmania mexicana* (a species closely related to *L. amazonensis*), resulted in parasites that lack the capacity to anchor GPI-linked molecules such as GP63 (37). Unexpectedly, *gpi8−/−* mutants showed no lesion development or impairment of macrophage infection in mice (37). Such findings leave open the possibility that GP63 may have a role in pathogenesis that is independent of GPI anchoring in the cell membrane, which has previously been considered important for allowing GP63 to protect against microbicidal host responses at the parasite cell surface.

Taken together, these data suggest there may be species-specific differences in GP63 function. In agreement with these interpretations, the complexity of GP63 genes has been found to vary widely among *Leishmania* species, with *L. major* showing the simplest arrangement (38, 39). For example, *Leishmania chagasi* shows a higher *gp63* gene complexity than *L. major*, which leads to a more heterogeneous population of protein products (40). Subtle biochemical differences between these GP63 isoforms may underlie *Leishmania* species–specific pathologies. Indeed, diverse species of *Leishmania* show distinct sensitivities to human complement (35), although it is important to bear in mind that this could be attributed to parasite molecules other than GP63 that vary with species that have also been implicated in complement resistance, such as lipophosphoglycan (41–43). In summary, it appears that the role of GP63 in *Leishmania* pathogenesis is a complex and varied one that remains to be fully understood. To discriminate between species-specific functions and how they may relate to species-specific pathologies, some future experimental approaches are outlined below.

To test whether GP63 may provide a structural versus an enzymatic function in resistance to complement, catalytically active versus inactive GP63 could be introduced into *L. major* GP63-null mutants. Establishing whether functional differences exist amongst *Leishmania* GP63 proteins that correlate with the studies undertaken thus far could be addressed using gene targeting to generate additional *gp63−/−* species, including *L. mexicana* and *Leishmania donovani*, together with cross-transfection of GP63 genes between species and into *gp63−/− L. major*. Because other GPI-anchored *Leishmania* molecules, such as lipophosphoglycan and the leucine-rich repeat protein GP46 (a 46 kDa surface glycoprotein) (44), have been shown to have roles in complement resistance, deletion of GP63 and GP46 genes in GPI8 mutants should aid determination of the relative contribution of GP63 to complement resistance and pathogenesis and clarify whether these molecules have GPI-linkage-independent roles. The number of selectable genetic markers available for *Leishmania* (45) should allow the generation of such mutants with relative ease. These approaches, however, may be technically difficult in certain species, such as *Leishmania brasiliensis*, that possess a particularly high number of *gp63* genes, which are typically located on more than one chromosome (39).

Leishmania Cysteine Proteases

Leishmania species, especially those that belong to the *L. mexicana* complex, express high levels of cysteine proteases. The best characterized of these enzymes are the cathepsin L–like A (CPA) and B (CPB) families of cysteine proteases and the cathepsin B–like C (CPC) family of cysteine proteases, which are found in large lysosomal organelles, termed megasomes, in amastigote stages (46–48).

The CPA proteases appear to be redundant in *L. mexicana* infection, as deletion of the *L. mexicana cpa* genes (46) showed no effect on either macrophage infection or lesion development in mice. Deletion of the *L. mexicana cpc* genes led to modest defects in lesion development in vivo despite greatly impaired macrophage infection by promastigote forms of this mutant in vitro (47). This result suggests that the primary role of the CPC proteases is to facilitate promastigote invasion.

Like GP63, the CPB proteases are encoded by a tandem gene array whose complexity is species dependent; the number of gene copies in the array ranges from 8 to 19 for *L. major* and *L. mexicana*, respectively (48). Studies of *L. mexicana cpb−/−* mutants that lack all *cpb* genes suggest that the role of this type of protease in pathogenesis is more profound than that of either the CPA or CPC proteases. Because the *cpb* genes are predominantly expressed in the amastigote stage, the impaired macrophage infection phenotype of *L. mexicana cpb−/−* promastigotes but not amastigotes seems surprising (49). Detailed analyses of *cpb* gene expression (50), however, revealed that CPB-1 and CPB-2 are homologous proteases expressed predominantly in infectious metacyclic promastigote stages of *L. mexicana*. Although this result suggests that these CPBs should be critical during promastigote invasion, transfection of *cpb−/−* promastigotes with *cpb-1* failed to restore macrophage infection by *cpb−/− L. mexicana* promastigotes (50). Instead, members of the *cpb-3* to *-18* gene class partially rescued the promastigote infection defect. This result suggests that these genes, although expressed predominantly in amastigotes, also have a role in promastigote invasion of macrophages (50).

One of the most interesting but poorly understood features of *Leishmania* infections are the species-specific pathologies that occur in both human patients and experimentally infected mice. For instance, infection with *L. mexicana* leads to lesion development in most strains of mice, including C57/BL6 and C3H, that robustly heal *L. major* infections via protective CD4+ Th1 immunity. Conversely, lesion development in *L. major* infection is generally restricted to mouse strains, such as BALB/c, that are genetically predisposed to mounting a Th2 CD4+ T cell response to *Leishmania*. Previous investigations with *cpb−/− L. mexicana* have suggested a role for CPBs in the species specificity of these *Leishmania* pathologies. These studies showed highly attenuated lesion development in BALB/c mice infected with *cpb−/− L. mexicana* that correlated with a shift from a susceptible Th2 response toward a protective Th1 response (51, 52). Furthermore, recent data (53, 54) suggest that *L. mexicana* causes lesion development in *L. major*–resistant mouse strains because, unlike *L. major*, *L. mexicana* amastigotes are able to suppress protective Th1 responses by cleaving components of the nuclear factor for κB transcription factor (NFκB) and mitogen-activated protein kinase signaling pathways that drive transcription of Th1-inducing cytokines (such as IL-12) in infected phagocytes. Although these studies showed that wild-type but not *cpb−/−* *L. mexicana* amastigotes were able to suppress bacterial lipopolysaccharide-induced IL-12 production from cultured macrophages and attenuate protective IL-12-dependent Th1 responses in vivo, infection of macrophages with either wild-type or *cpb−/−* *L. mexicana* elicited similar levels of IL-12. These data suggest that, rather than inhibiting IL-12 expression in macrophages, CPB proteases may suppress IL-12 in other antigen-presenting cells (APCs) (such as dendritic cells) or even modulate other Th1-inducing cytokines (such as IL-18) that can augment the effects of IL-12 on Th1 responses (55). As *Leishmania* amastigotes reside within infected host cells in phagolysosomal compartments, the ability of *Leishmania* proteases to degrade cytokine-signaling components located in the host cell cytoplasm (such as NFκB) would seem unlikely. However, recent findings that infected phagocytes can export parasite proteins from the phagolysosome into the host cell cytoplasm (56) suggest a route through which interactions between *L. mexicana* CPB and host cytoplasmic proteins can occur (48).

The ability of *L. mexicana* CPB to attenuate Th1 responses through the suppression of Th1-inducing cytokines implies that such modulation is independent of Th2 responses (48, 54). However, analyses of *STAT* (signal transducer and activator of transcription)-*6−/−* mice (57) show that Th2 responses are required for susceptibility to *L. mexicana*. It remains possible that differences in the route of parasite inoculation and the use of different parasite life cycle stages could account for these conflicting conclusions. Although recent data discussed here show that *L. mexicana* CPBs can interfere with lipopolysaccharide-induced inflammatory cytokine production in infected macrophages, further research is needed to clarify the extent to which these findings have relevance to *L. mexicana* infections in vivo.

Cytokine: a low-molecular-weight protein that modulates (stimulates or inhibits) the differentiation, proliferation, or function of immune cells

Entamoeba histolytica

Ingestion of water or food contaminated with cysts (dormant, spore-like stages) of *Entamoeba histolytica* causes amebiasis, a parasitic disease characterized by colitis and diarrhea. Invasive forms of this disease may lead to peritonitis and liver abscesses and result in approximately 100,000 fatalities per year. This section of our review focuses on recent studies that demonstrate the role of *E. histolytica* proteases in the pathogenesis of amebiasis (**Table 1**).

Entamoeba histolytica Proteases

E. histolytica trophozoites (the replicative form) can cleave human and mouse IgG and completely degrade human IgA (58, 59). This result suggests that *E. histolytica* possesses a highly specific IgG proteolytic activity and a distinct, broad-specificity IgA proteolytic activity. A number of studies have established a critical role for cysteine proteases in *E. histolytica* virulence, including recent work (60) that shows that co-inoculation of *E. histolytica* with the broad-specificity cysteine protease inhibitor E64 [N-(trans-epoxysuccinyl)-L-leucyl 4 guanidobutylaminide] into hamsters resulted in rapid parasite clearance that correlated with decreased parasite erythrophagocytosis in vitro.

A recent survey predicted a total of 20 cysteine proteases in the *E. histolytica* genome (61). However analyses of protease activity in cultured *E. histolytica* trophozoites attribute most of the total cysteine protease activity to only three cysteine proteases: *E. histolytica* cysteine protease 1 (EhCP1), *E. histolytica* cysteine protease 2 (EhCP2), and *E. histolytica* cysteine protease 5 (EhCP5) (62). The apparent absence of fully functional orthologues

SCID: severe combined immunodeficient

of EhCP1 and EhCP5 in *Entamoeba dispar*, a closely related nonpathogenic species (62, 63), suggests that these two cysteine proteases may be especially important in *E. histolytica* pathogenesis.

Studies of infected Chinese hamster ovary cell monolayers with non-cell-permeable and cell-permeable forms of E64 suggest that *E. histolytica* cysteine proteases account for approximately 50% of intestinal cytopathic activity (64). Furthermore, overexpression of EhCP2 in *E. histolytica* transfectants (64) showed that, although liver abscesses remained unaffected compared with wild-type infections, moderate destruction of Chinese hamster ovary cell monolayers was observed. This observation suggests that *E. histolytica* cysteine proteases can contribute to host cell layer disruption. EhCP2 may also facilitate pathologic host inflammatory responses as cleavage by purified EhCP2 can enhance the activity of host chemokines such as CXCL8 (65) and cause increased chemotaxis of granulocytes.

Although functional studies of EhCP1 and EhCP5 have been impeded by technical difficulties in overexpressing these cysteine proteases in *E. histolytica* (64), RNA antisense suppression of EhCP5 led to reduced parasite phagocytic activity that correlated with attenuated liver abscesses in infected hamsters despite showing no impairment of cytopathic activity (66, 67). Recently, however, infections of human intestinal xenografts in severe combined immunodeficient (SCID) mice with EhCP5-deficient parasites showed reduced IL-1β and IL-8 induction, decreased neutrophil recruitment, and reduced cytopathic damage (68). These data suggest that EhCP5 may act, at least in humans, to disrupt intestinal integrity by invoking host inflammatory responses. In this instance, EhCP5 may be proteolytically activating pro-interleukin-1β in analogous fashion to mammalian IL-1β converting enzyme (68).

In summary, significant advances have been made toward understanding the importance of cysteine proteases in amebiasis. Both EhCP2 and EhCP5 may have cytopathologic roles in colitis and impact host inflammatory responses. EhCP5 also appears to have a role in the development of liver abscesses; this role may involve activation of caspase cascades that cause apoptosis of hepatocytes (68). The role of EhCP5-dependent phagocytosis in pathogenesis, however, remains unclear.

Although distinct roles for *E. histolytica* cysteine proteases in intestinal barrier disruption, inflammation, and liver pathogenesis are emerging, controversies and a number of gaps in our understanding of amebiasis remain. For instance, there are data supporting both activating and suppressive effects of *E. histolytica* cysteine proteases on inflammatory events (65). Furthermore, recent studies show that EhCP5 can inactivate the host proinflammatory cytokine IL-18 (69). One interpretation that reconciles these data is that *E. histolytica* may tailor components of the host inflammatory response to favor invasion and dissemination, as opposed to mediating generalized elevation or suppression of inflammation. Further characterization of host inflammatory cytokine profiles and host inflammatory cell activities in response to *E. histolytica* infection will help clarify whether this scenario holds true.

Additional deficiencies in our understanding of amebiasis that need to be addressed include the pathogenic contributions of EhCP1 and characterizing the serine proteases of this protozoan pathogen. Such issues will no doubt be addressed in the near future through further use of *E. histolytica* transgenic approaches, including RNA interference (70) and human xenograft mouse models (**Table 1**).

IMMUNOGLOBULIN DEGRADATION: PROTEASES OF PARASITIC WORMS

Studies by Pleass and colleagues (71) (**Table 1**) have demonstrated that schistosomula stages of *S. mansoni* release an elastase-like serine protease activity that degrades IgE from both humans and rodents, but not human IgG. Although worm infections are typically associated with increased levels of IgE, the role of this class of immunoglobulin in host infections is still controversial. Depletion of IgE in *S. mansoni*–infected mice suggests that IgE may actually contribute to host pathogenesis, rather than protection (72). Conversely, recent studies of IgE-deficient mice showed delayed clearance of both *S. mansoni* (73) and *Brugia malayi* infections (74). Secondary infections of these mice, however, resulted in accelerated worm clearance similar to secondary infections of wild-type mice, indicating that worm antigen–specific responses were generally unimpaired. Because these mice also showed defects in IgG expression during primary infections, it is possible that, during a primary response, nonspecific IgG has a more critical role in worm expulsion than nonspecific IgE (74). Validation of the role of serine protease activity of parasitic nematodes in immunoglobulin degradation (71, 75) will be greatly facilitated by transgenic approaches that are being developed for these complex metazoan parasites (18).

ROLE OF THE *TRYPANOSOMA CRUZI* PROTEASE, CRUZAIN, IN IMMUNE EVASION AND DISEASE PATHOGENESIS

The American trypanosome *Trypanosoma cruzi* causes Chagas disease, which is a common cause of fatal dilated cardiomyopathy in many Latin American countries. *T. cruzi* is an intracellular parasite that lives free in the cytoplasm. Proteases produced by the amastigote (intracellular) stage of this parasite are on the surface of amastigotes and are directly in contact with the host cell cytoplasm (76).

T. cruzi is transmitted by insects from the *Reduviidae* family through insect feces, which are released reflexively while the bug takes a blood meal from humans. Entry of even a few parasites can cause a systemic and acute infection. During this acute phase all types of nucleated cells in the body can potentially be infected by the parasite (77). In the majority of cases, this systemic infection is almost completely controlled by the immune response (78). However, the parasite is rarely completely eliminated, and low-level parasitemia and infection of specific tissues, such as cardiac muscle or enteric ganglia, can persist for decades.

Parasite persistence eventually leads to a debilitating heart disease that kills more than 50,000 people every year. Although tissue damage that occurs in cardiac muscle with Chagas disease is clearly related to persistent parasite infection, there is no consensus as to whether tissue damage is caused entirely by the parasite or is exacerbated by an autoimmune response (79, 80). In both these models of disease progression, the major protease of *T. cruzi* has been suggested to play an important role.

Cruzain (also known as Cruzipain and GP57/51) is a cysteine protease that accounts for the major proteolytic activity of *T. cruzi* (**Figure 4**). It is expressed at every stage of the parasitic life cycle, but is differentially localized to carry out stage-specific functions. In the epimastigote (insect vector) stage, Cruzain is localized to lysosome-like organelles, where it serves to degrade endocytosed nutrients. Cruzain is localized to the flagellar pocket of the free-swimming extracellular trypomastigotes within infected human hosts. Upon entry into new host cells, trypomastigotes transform into the replicative amastigotes. At this stage, Cruzain is relocated to the cell surface and presumably functions in the cytoplasm of the host cell. Recently, Cruzain has also been shown to mediate invasion of host cells by trypomastigotes through two different pathways (81, 82). One pathway involves the triggering of the B2 kinin receptor (B2R), whereas the other pathway is independent of the kinin receptors.

In chronic Chagas disease patients, as well as in experimental animal models, Cruzain is a highly immunogenic antigen. Although there is considerable controversy about whether the clinical effects of Chagas disease are exacerbated by auto-immunity, there is no

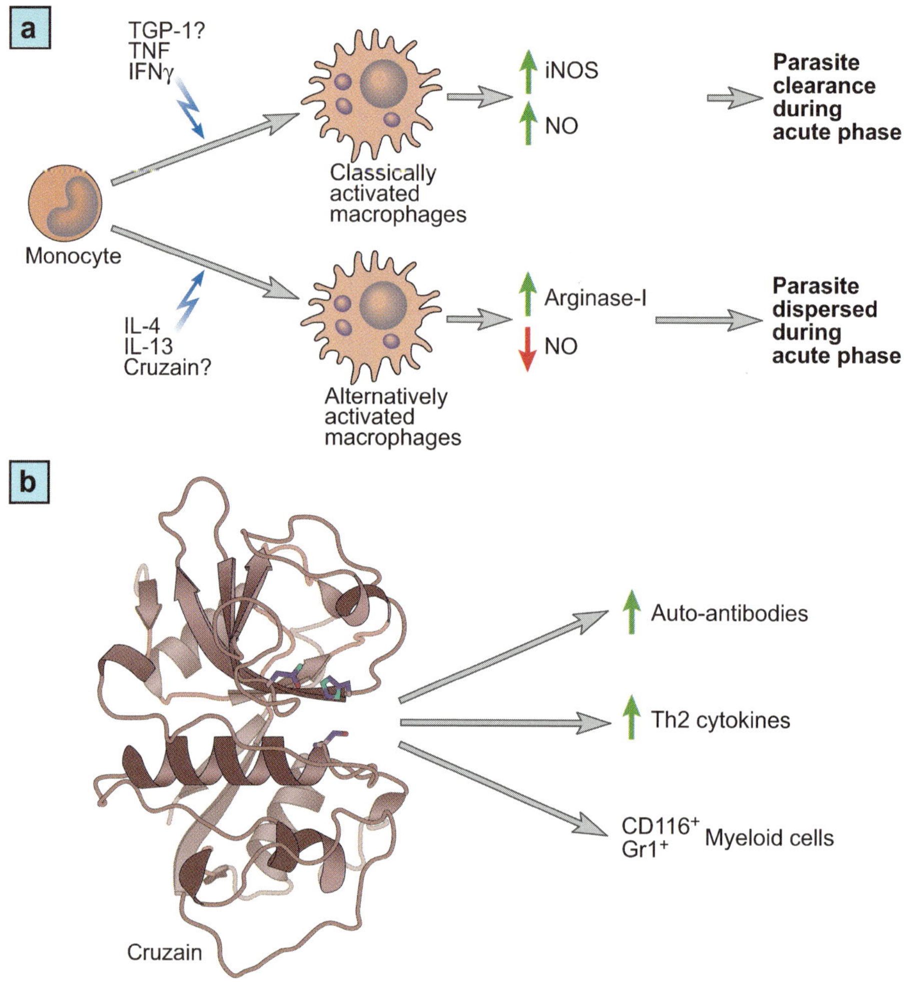

Figure 4

(*a*) Inflammatory monocytes can be either classically activated by T helper 1 (Th1) or inflammatory cytokines or alternatively activated by Th2 cytokines such as interleukin (IL)-4 and IL-13. Purified glycolipid anchors (TGP-1) from *Trypanosoma cruzi* can classically activate macrophages, whereas Cruzain/Cruzipain can alternatively activate macrophages. The induction of inducible nitric oxide synthase (iNOS) results in increased production of nitric oxide (NO) and may contribute to rapid clearance of parasites during the acute phase of the infection. Conversely, increased arginase-1 activity may lead to reduced NO production and contribute to parasite dispersal during the acute phase of infection. (*b*) Immunization of mice with the purified enzyme Cruzain increases auto-antibodies against heart and skeletal muscle through some unknown mechanism. Immunization of mice with Cruzain also leads to increased hematopoiesis of $CD11b^{+}$ and $Gr1^{+}$ myeloid cells associated with increased Th2 cytokines in BALB/c mice. The mechanism for this correlation is also unknown.

doubt that anti-self responses are present during chronic *T. cruzi* infection. Sera (serine repeat antigen 7) from Chagas disease patients as well as *T. cruzi*–infected mice react to heart and skeletal muscle, as well as to some other antigens (83–86). More recently, there has been a series of studies showing that immunization with Cruzain and complete Frend's adjuvent led to cellular and antibody responses against skeletal muscle myosin and cardiac myosin; these responses were associated with tissue abnormalities (87, 88). Interestingly, this result was not observed on the C57/6 mice background (89). C57BL/6 mice generated a more Th1 bias towards Cruzain with more interferon-γ (IFNγ) and less IL-4 production. These results implicated a Th2 response directed at Cruzain associated with purified Cruzain-induced autoimmunity. Further studies are needed to confirm these observations. BALB/c mice immunized with purified Cruzain exhibited other interesting characteristics such as splenomegaly, owing to increased hematopoiesis and expansion of Cd11b+ Gr1+ myeloid cells. These cells were also associated with increased Th2 cytokine (IL-4 and IL-13) production (90).

The term alternatively activated macrophages was originally used to describe macrophages that have an activated surface-marker phenotype but do not upregulate inducible nitric oxide synthase (iNOS) (91). It was later found that the Th2 cytokines (IL-4 and IL-13) direct alternatively activated macrophages to skew L-arginine metabolism towards the production of polyamines (92, 93). In contrast, macrophages activated by Th1 cytokines [e.g., IFNγ and tumor necrosis factor (TNF)] direct L-arginine metabolism towards production of NO. Th2 cytokines upregulate arginase-1, whereas Th1 cytokines upregulate iNOS. Arginase-1 and iNOS compete for their common substrate, L-arginine. The production of radical oxygen species by iNOS is of key importance in the antimicrobicidal properties of classically activated macrophages. There are many parasitic diseases where the balance between classical and alternative macrophage activation could play an important role in pathogenesis (94).

An interesting hypothesis that has emerged from recent studies is that *T. cruzi* alternatively activates infected macrophages through the effects of Cruzain. When macrophages are cultured with purified parasite-derived Cruzain in vitro, they exhibit signs of alternative activation (95). These signs include increased arginase-1 activity and secretion of IL-10 and transforming growth factor β (TGFβ). This phenotype was associated with an increased intracellular growth of the parasite as well as increased survival. Tyrosine kinases, protein kinase A, and p38 mitogen-activated protein kinase are implicated as signaling components of this macrophage activation pathway (96). However, the hypothesis that Cruzain can alternatively activate macrophages has yet to be tested with live parasite infections in vitro and in vivo. One of the limitations of the studies done to date is the lack of a Cruzain-deficient parasite. Efforts by several laboratories to make a Cruzain-deficient parasite by homologous recombination have been unsuccessful, probably because Cruzain is an essential protein.

TNF: tissue necrosis factor

There are two implications of alternative macrophage activation in the pathogenesis of Chagas disease. Although not experimentally demonstrated, it is implied that alternatively activated macrophages do not have the trypanocidal activity of classically activated macrophages because the L-arginine pathway is skewed away from production of NO. During the acute phase of infection, this mechanism could promote survival and replication of the parasite (97) followed by increased systemic dispersal. It is especially interesting that the stronger Th1 response in C57BL/6 mice immunized with Cruzain is associated with the lack of an auto-immune response against heart myosin; in addition, the immunized C57BL/6 mice have normal numbers of myeloid cells expressing the receptors Mac-1 and Gr1 (89) that could potentially be precursors to alternatively activated macrophages.

Because Cruzain is responsible for the major proteolytic activity of the parasite and could be playing important roles in pathology, it is an attractive drug target (98). A cysteine protease inhibitor (K777) targets this enzyme and blocks the parasite life cycle both in vitro (99) and in experimental animals (76). This drug is currently in late preclinical development. Drug-resistant parasites have

Filarial nematodes: worms of the *Filarioidea* family, which includes invasive worms found in the lymphatic vessels

MEROPS: the Peptidase Database

been isolated that secrete large amounts of unprocessed inactive Cruzain (100). In analysis of different strains of immunodeficient mice, results suggest that the Cruzain inhibitor could be protecting *T. cruzi*–infected mice by reversing the immune evasion mechanisms of the parasite, in addition to directly inhibiting the replication of the parasite. *T. cruzi* is adept at silently infecting host cells without inducing changes in gene expression (101). One of our hypotheses is that the innate and adaptive immune components, especially macrophages, are awakened to the presence of the parasite when Cruzain is inhibited by K777.

THE OTHER SIDE OF THE MIRROR: PARASITE-DERIVED PROTEASE INHIBITORS AND DISEASE

Given the chronicity of infection associated in general with helminths (schistosomes may remain for the life of the human host), it is not surprising that these parasites have evolved elegant strategies to modulate the host immune response via molecular mechanisms that are recently beginning to be understood (102, 103). Much of this research has focused on filarial nematodes, which reside in close proximity to host immune effector cells in the lymphatic system and skin. Immunomodulatory molecules actively released from filarial nematodes can manipulate the cytokine network, intracellular signal transduction pathways, and host enzyme function in immune cell targets such as T cells, macrophages, and APCs. These molecules include phosphorylcholine, which is found on many parasite proteins that interfere with activation and proliferation of T and B cells (104) and is known to polarize the T helper response to the Th2 type by upregulating IL-10 release from B cells (105). Filarial worms also produce orthologues of cytokines [e.g., a macrophage-migratory inhibitory factor (106) that can directly bind to and modulate immune effector cells]. Finally, inhibitors of cysteine (cystatins) and serine (serpins) proteases have been described for nematodes and are believed to downregulate the host immune response at key junctures (see References 107 and 108 for reviews).

Cystatins

Cystatins are tight-binding and reversible protein inhibitors of cysteine proteases belonging to the MEROPS (the Peptidase Database) inhibitor family I25, clan IH (109). In vertebrates, cystatins are ubiquitously expressed both extra- and intracellularly in tissues and body fluids. A succinct review of the three main types of vertebrate cystatins is available (110). Two aspects of modulation of the host immune response by filarial cystatins are noteworthy: (*a*) the putative inhibition of host protease activity in APCs and (*b*) the subsequent hyporeactivity of the T cell proliferative response that may be caused by that inhibition (see Reference 107 for a comprehensive review of these and other immunomodulatory effects associated with nematode cystatins).

The first described parasite cystatin was Onchocystatin, isolated from *Onchocerca volvulus*, the filarial nematode that causes river blindness. Onchocystatin was initially thought to contribute to cuticle molting via inhibition of endogenous cathepsin-L enzyme activity (111); however, an orthologous inhibitor of cathepsin L was subsequently found to be secreted from males and microfilaria of the jird filarid *Acanthocheilonema viteae*, which do not molt (107a). This observation suggested an extracellular function for cystatins at the host-parasite interface. Secreted cystatins were then found for other filarids, including *B. malayi* (elephantiasis) (112) and the rat parasite *Litmosoides sigmodontis* (113) (**Table 2**). Cystatins have also been characterized in a number of geohelminths (a parasitic helminth that spends part of its life cycle in the soil), including the sheep gastric nematode *Haemonchus contortus* (114) and the rat intestinal parasite *Nippostrongylus brasiliensis* (115). In addition, cystatin sequences are

Table 2 Parasite protease inhibitors and their putative functions

Inhibitor type	Name	Parasite	Life-stage expressed	Function	References
Cystatin (Ov 17)	Onchocystatin	*Onchocerca volvulus*	L3[a]–L4	Molting of cuticle	(111)
Cystatin	Onchocystatin	*O. volvulus*	Adult, MF[b]	Suppresses T cell proliferation	(117)
Cystatin	Av17	*Acanthocheilonema viteae*	Adult, MF	Suppresses T cell proliferation	(107a)
Cystatin	Bm-CPI-1	*Brugia malayi*	L3	Unknown	(102)
Cystatin	Bm-CPI-2	*B. malayi*	L3, adult, MF	Suppressed T cell proliferation via major histocompatibility complex antigen presentation	(112)
Cystatin	Ls-Cystatin	*Litmosoides sigmodontis*	L3, adult, MF	Suppresses T cell proliferation	(113)
Serpin	Bm-SPI-1	*B. malayi*	All	Regulation of proteolysis	(135)
Serpin	Bm-SPI-2	*B. malayi*	MF	Unknown, but is noninhibitory	(136, 137)
Serpin	Smpi56	*Schistosoma mansoni*	Adults	Inhibits coagulation?	(140)
Serpin	SHSPI	*Schistosoma haematobium*	Adults	Inhibits coagulation?	(142, 143)
Ascaris-type protease inhibitor	Multiple forms	*Ascaris suum* v. *lumbriocoides*	L3, adult, eggs	Inhibit host intestinal trypsin and chymotrypsin	(145, 149, 151)
Ascaris-type protease inhibitor	AcAP5 and AcAp6	*Ancylostoma caninum*	Adult	Inhibit factor Xa at active site	(158, 159)
Ascaris-type protease inhibitor	AcAPc2	*A. caninum*	Adult	Inhibits factor VIIa/tissue factor via exosite binding to Xa	(160)
Ascaris-type protease inhibitor	AcAPc3 and AcAPc4	*A. caninum*	Adult	As for Ac APc2	(162)
Ascaris-type protease inhibitor	AceAP1	*Ancylostoma ceylanicum*	Adult	Inhibits both Xa active site and complex-formation with VIIa/TF	(163, 164)

[a]L3: infective third larval stage
[b]MF: microfilariae

found for a number of other animal and plant parasitic nematodes using the BLAST (basic local alignment search tool) algorithm available at **www.nematode.net** (116). Like their vertebrate counterparts, nematode cystatins inhibit the mammalian lysosomal cysteine proteases cathepsins L and S and, to a lesser extent, cathepsin B (114, 115, 117). The filarial cystatins from *B. malayi*, *L. sigmodontis*, and *O. volvulus* contain the SND (serine-asparagine-aspartate) motif required to inhibit the activity of an asparaginyl endopeptidase (AE, also known as legumain), and such inhibitory activity has been shown in vitro for the *B. malayi* cystatin Bm-CPI-2 (*B. malayi* cysteine protease inhibitor-2) (112, 118). Cystatin-mediated inhibition of host cathepsins L and S and AE would be a critical advantage to the parasite in evading host immunity, as these proteases are required

Major histocompatibility complex (MHC): a chromosomal region encoding molecules involved in antigen presentation to T cells

to (*a*) process antigen for presentation by the major histocompatability complex (MHC) class II APCs and (*b*) digest the MHC II–associated invariant chain (Ii) chaperone prior to peptide antigen loading (reviewed in References 119 and 120) (**Figure 5**). Indeed, in immature dendritic APCs, higher levels of endogenous cystatins are expressed to prevent Ii-chain processing and direct trafficking of MHC II molecules to the lysosomes (121). Interference with either or both of these functions by parasite cystatins would effectively downregulate antigen presentation and subsequent proliferation of immune effector cells. Interestingly, the *B. malayi* cystatin Bm-CPI-2 has been shown to inhibit the presentation of T cell epitopes from the tetanus toxin C fragment by APCs in vitro (the first time that a product of a eukaryotic pathogen has been demonstrated to directly interfere with antigen presentation) (112). So far, one study has attempted to investigate the immunomodulatory effect of nematode cystatins in vivo (113) by implanting osmotic pumps that released the cystatin of *L. sigmodontis* into mice. After one week of induction and then subsequent challenge with microfilariae, mice showed a decreased *L. sigmodontis* antigen–specific proliferative response in spleen cells. This effect was long lasting, as T cell reactivity was still decreased six weeks after the last of three cystatin applications. As *L. sigmodontis* cystatin contains the SND motif, it would be of interest to determine whether the decreased proliferative response is owing to a specific inhibition of host AE and whether mutation of this motif alters spleen cell reactivity.

Particular attention has focused on the contribution of host AE to antigen processing in APCs (120, 122) and its inhibition by filarial cystatins. Murray and colleagues (118) demonstrated by site-directed mutagenesis the requirement of the SND motif in Bm-CPI-2 for inhibition of human AE. On the basis of this result and their demonstration that two *Caenorhabditis elegans* cystatin orthologues lacking the SND motif do not inhibit AE, the authors hypothesized that convergent evolution at the SND site in both vertebrate and filarial type 2 cystatins has maintained the motif's integrity and functionality. However, querying the database (116) with Onchocystatin using BLAST reveals that the SND motif is not restricted to just filarial cystatins, but is also found in those from geohelminths such as *H. contortus* (Genbank accession number CB019553) and *Ostertagia ostertagi* (Genbank accession number BQ098839) and plant nematode parasites such as *Heterodera glycines* Genbank accession number BF013652) and *Globodera rostochiensis* (BM344603). Furthermore, the SND motif is changed to SNV (serine-asparagine-valine) in the cystatin from the filarial parasite *A. viteae* (L43053), which is immunomodulatory (107a), and it would be of interest to test whether this cystatin displays a similar ability to inhibit MHC II processing and antigen presentation as described above.

Onchocystatin has been shown to elicit anti-inflammatory cytokines in vitro (117). Human peripheral blood mononuclear cells stimulated with purified protein derivative produced significantly less of the Th1-inducing cytokine IL-12, whereas levels of the Th2 cytokine IL-10 were increased. The elevated IL-10 levels were associated with hyporeactivity in the proliferative response of peripheral blood mononuclear cells (decreased on average by 52%), and this outcome may or may not be due directly to host protease inhibition in APCs. Corresponding in vivo studies have documented high levels of IL-10 in filariasis patients that coincide with T cell hyporeactivity (123). In addition, Th1 cells reactive to parasite antigen are suppressed in mice infected with *Brugia pahangi* by a mechanism involving IL-10 and APCs (124). In contrast to filarial cystatins, peripheral blood mononuclear cells exposed to *C. elegans* cystatins do not increase IL-10 production and downregulate T cell proliferation (125). Rather they induce increased production of the proinflammatory cytokine TNFα, IL-12, and IFNγ. As mentioned above, it would be interesting to determine whether

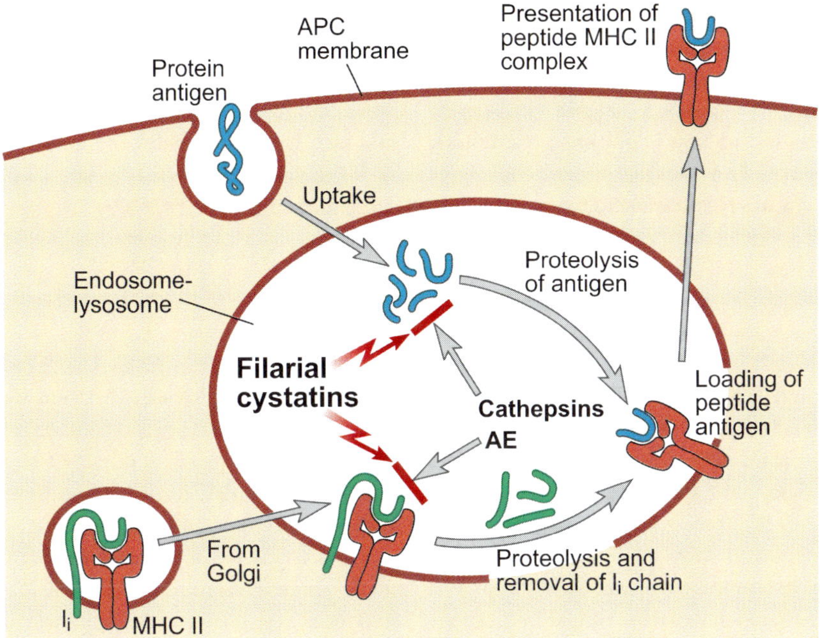

Figure 5

Secreted filarial cystatins are hypothesized to enter antigen-presenting cells (APCs) and inhibit endosomal-lysosomal APC cysteine proteases such as cathepsins L and S and asparaginyl endopeptidase (AE). Consequently, two important processes required for antigen presentation are affected adversely: (*a*) proteolysis and removal of the major histocompatibility complex (MHC) class II–associated invariant chain (I_i) prior to loading of peptide antigen and (*b*) proteolysis of exogenous protein antigens for peptide loading of MHC class II molecules (see Reference 107 for a review).

this effect is due to the specific lack of a SND motif and, therefore, inhibition of AE or to some other structural difference(s) (**Figure 5**).

Serpins

Demonstration of a direct link between the production of helminth serpins and modulation of the host immune response is more tentative than the data in hand for cystatins. However, the current information is tantalizing enough to warrant further investigation (108). Serpins comprise a large family of diverse proteins (126) that, in humans, regulate proteolysis in blood coagulation, inflammation, and complement activation (127). Serpins use an extraordinary inhibition mechanism by presenting a bait peptide, which, when cleaved, induces a massive conformational shift that deforms and irreversibly inactivates the tightly bound protease. The serpin is thus converted from its native stressed (S) conformation to a more stable, relaxed (R) form structure (128).

A hallmark of chronic inflammation is a continuous migration and degranulation of neutrophils, which release proteases such as host neutrophil elastase (HNE) and cathepsin G (catG). These proteases, when operating unchecked and because of their broad substrate specificity, can cause tissue degeneration by degrading structural proteins such as collagen and elastin. Also, catG activity is important in the inflammatory response, as the enzyme is chemotactic for monocytes and neutrophils (129) and can process chemokines (130). However, serpins, such as 1-antichymotrypsin, inhibit these proteases and, therefore, are anti-inflammatory (131, 132). Indeed, many viruses successfully interfere with inflammatory responses by producing their own serpin molecules (133, 134). Also, many tumor cell lines resist the cytolytic activities of T cells in vitro by expressing serpins that inhibit the proapoptotic granzymes. Thus, it is not difficult to imagine that parasites produce orthologous serpins to inhibit inflammatory and/or cytolytic T cell responses.

Two serpin genes, whose gene products share just 28% sequence homology (136), have been identified in *B. malayi* [*Bm-spn-1* (135) and *Bm-spn-2*] (**Table 2**). *Bm-spn-1* is expressed during most parasite life stages, but *Bm-spn-2* is expressed only in microfilariae and accounts for greater than 2% of the mRNA (136). Its restriction to the microfilariae implies a function in evasion or modulation of the host immune response, and it has been demonstrated in vitro that Bm-SPN-2 can inhibit both HNE and catG, but not a range of other serine proteases (136). Subsequently, however, an inhibitory function for Bm-SPN-2 could not be demonstrated (137). Rather, Bm-SPN-2 most likely acted as substrate for both HNE and catG and was neither capable of the S to R conformational shift required for inhibition, nor of forming stable complexes in the presence of the strong anionic detergent, sodium dodecyl sulfate. Nonetheless, the fact that Bm-SPN-2 is only secreted by microfilariae does suggest a function of possible immunomodulatory consequence. It is known that some mammalian serpins, although not inhibitory, have evolved alternative functions (138, 139).

Serpins have also been identified in schistosome flatworms (140, 141) and are postulated to inhibit host effector functions such as inflammation and complement. The best characterized serpin is a 54–58 kDa molecule, termed SHSPI (*Schistosoma haematobium* serine protease inhibitor), located on the surface of the blood fluke *S. haematobium* (142, 143). Its surface location makes it well placed to operate at the host-parasite interface. SHSPI may function to prevent clot formation around the parasite by thrombin-like enzymes in plasma. *S. mansoni* also possesses a surface-associated serpin termed Smpi56 (*S. mansoni* protease inhibitor of 56 kDa), which has been shown to inhibit HNE (140) and may function to block the in vivo action of HNE [in vitro, HNE is toxic to cultured immature schistosomes (144)].

Ascaris-Type Serine Protease Inhibitors

First described in the intestinal nematode *Ascaris* by Fraefel & Acher (145), and then in more detail by Peanasky and colleagues (146, 147), this distinct group of small (<100 amino acids) proteins (MEROPS inhibitor family I25) are characterized by possessing 10 invariant cysteinyl groups that form five disulphide bonds. The term smapin (small protease inhibitor) has also appeared in the literature describing these proteins (108). Like the serpins, target proteases become irreversibly bound to the smapins through cleavage of an exposed loop. Tertiary structures have been determined for inhibitors from *Ascaris* (148, 149) and the dog hookworm *Ancylostoma caninum* (150). In *Ascaris*, these inhibitors coat the surface of the worm gut, eggs, and larvae and so facilitate survival in the intestinal tract by inactivating host protease activities (151). These molecules are part of a larger group of orthologous proteins (either inhibitory or noninhibitory) that have been identified in other nematodes (152, 153) and phyla, including arthropods (154), amphibians (155), and humans (e.g., von Willebrand factor) (156).

However, it is the orthologous anticoagulatory molecules from blood-feeding hookworms that are the subject of intense interest due to the potential of these molecules in the therapy of various thrombotic conditions (156). For a century it had been known that hookworms produce potent anticoagulants (157), but it is in just the past decade that the molecules responsible have been identified and characterized. In *A. caninum*, the inhibitors AcAP5 (*A. caninum* anticoagulant peptide 5), AcAP6 (158, 159), and AcAPc2

(160) have evolved to specifically inhibit different serine proteases involved in the blood-coagulation cascade and thereby allow for unobstructed blood feeding. AcAP5 and AcAP6 inhibit factor Xa (fXa) by interacting directly with its catalytic site (158, 159). In contrast, AcAPc2 binds to fXa (or its precursor fX) at an exosite removed from the catalytic site prior to binding of fXa to the tissue factor/fVIIa complex. The resulting quaternary complex prevents the subsequent processing of prothrombin to thrombin (160). In this way AcAPc2 interferes specifically with the critical junction point for the both intrinsic and extrinsic coagulation pathways. The use of an exosite on fXa for binding by AcAPc2 differs from the binding observed with the endogenous inhibitor, tissue-factor pathway inhibitor, which binds directly to the active site of fXa (161). Other anticoagulants in *A. caninum* (e.g., AcAPc3 and 4) have since been identified and are believed to act like AcAPc2 (162). Some of these anticoagulants are localized in different organs of the worm, including the buccal capsule (the site of attachment to the host intestinal epithelium) and the esophagus (162). This observation suggests, therefore, that the individual inhibitors have different functions within the worm, rather than merely act to increase functional redundancy. For the related *Ancylostoma ceylanicum*, which, unlike *A. caninum*, can complete development in humans, just one orthologue (AceAP1) has been characterized (163). This molecule seems to combine the properties of both AcAP5 and AcAPc2 by binding to and inhibiting the active site of fXa and forming a quaternary complex with fVIIa/tissue factor via exosite binding (163, 164). Interestingly, the binding affinity of AceAP1 to the fXa active site (73 nM) is much lower than that of AcAP5 (0.56 nM), and it has been proposed that this difference may be responsible for the differing abilities of the worms to feed on blood, with *A. caninum* being the more voracious (165).

The remarkable specificity and potency of AcAPc2 makes it an ideal candidate for drug development to treat partial or occlusive thrombi associated with deep-vein thrombosis and ischemic stroke (166). For the past 50 years, the primary parenteral anticoagulant has been heparin or derivatives thereof, known as low-molecular-weight heparins. However, side effects associated with heparin, such as prolonged bleeding and thrombocytopenia, have maintained momentum in the search for improved therapeutics, especially those targeting coagulation proteases upstream of thrombin. AcAPc2 (also termed NAPc2 for nematode anticoagulant protein) may fulfill this need with its unique mechanism of inhibiting fVIIa/tissue factor. The pharmacokinetic profile of AcAP2 is governed by its binding to fX with a long elimination half-life of >50 hours (166). Subsequent Phase I and II clinical trials have demonstrated the efficacy of AcAPc2 to reduce postoperative thrombosis without an increased incidence of bleeding complications (167, 168). Clinical studies are ongoing.

GETTING IN AND OUT: THE ROLE OF *APICOMPLEXA* PROTEASES

In *Apicomplexa* parasites, proteases function in a diverse assortment of processes such as nutrient catabolism, housekeeping, and protein activation—enzyme activities that are key to a successful parasitic lifestyle. This review focuses on the protease classes utilized by *Apicomplexa* during initiation and propagation of infection in vertebrate hosts, specifically highlighting the role of resident proteases during host cell invasion (ingress) and exit (egress) pathways. Protease orthologues, which are conventionally considered to be highly catabolic and enzymatically promiscuous in vertebrate and bacterial systems, can surprisingly be functionally selective and have an apparent restricted substrate preference in *Apicomplexa*. Unique uses of proteases, including trafficking lysosomal cathepsin-like proteases into extralysosomal compartments using serine proteases that resemble bacterial

***Apicomplexa*:** intracellular parasitic protozoa that possess an apical complex of organelles

Parasitophorous vacuole (PV): organelle-like structure formed as a parasite actively invades a target cell; the membrane is generally comprised of both parasite and host material

orthologues, curious hybrid cysteinyl-serinyl proteases, and aspartyl proteases that function at or around a neutral pH, have been brought into play by this highly successful group of parasites. Understanding the detailed molecular aspects of this host-parasite interface may serve to expose vulnerabilities that can be beset by selective immuno- and/or pharmacological lines of attack.

THE *APICOMPLEXA*

Several thousand species of *Apicomplexa* comprise a remarkably diverse group of protozoa that reside and proliferate within one or more type of vertebrate cell (169). This intracellular parasitic predisposition was the evolutionary driving force to developing an efficient entry (as well as egress) system in target metazoan cells. Although the specific host cell type may vary tremendously between parasites, the elaborate apical multi-organellar complex (hence, *Apicomplexa*) associated with the invasion process is remarkably conserved morphologically (see The Zoite below). Regulated sequential discharge of the apical complex organelles is conditional for successful vacuolar invasion during which numerous parasite-derived structural proteins and proteases are released and play critical roles in this dynamic progression. Proteolytic hydrolysis of proteins within and/or from micronemes, rhoptries, and dense granules has been demonstrated, and it is now recognized that selective chemotherapeutic targeting of these enzymes can thwart the invasion process, as well as exit strategies, and so blockade the parasite's passage and dissemination through the vertebrate host. To this end, much work has gone into identifying and characterizing key *Apicomplexa*-derived, invasion-associated and exit-resident proteases.

There are numerous excellent current reviews dealing with motility, organellar biogenesis, parasite-derived actin-myosin motors, and formation of the parasitophorous vacuole (PV) in the context of invasion in *Plasmodium* and *Toxoplasma*, the two most studied and clinically significant human pathogens in this group (170–174). *Plasmodium* kills approximately two to three million children a year and *Toxoplasma* infects approximately 50% of the world's population. This review, in addition to the aforementioned *Apicomplexa*, draws attention to other members of the group that pose considerable veterinary health problems and economic burden, including *Theileria*, *Neospora*, *Cryptosporidium*, *Eimeria*, *Sarcocystis*, and *Babesia*. The comparative role of proteases in cellular invasion and exit of these organisms are discussed. Although the cell-penetration strategies undertaken by most *Apicomplexa* appear to be conserved, it is evident that disparate classes of proteases, located in distinct compartments, are utilized to accomplish the same biological function.

THE ZOITE

In *Apicomplexa*, the zoite is highly adapted to penetrate and parasitize vertebrate cells. In general, it is avocado-shaped and can vary in length between 8 μm for *Toxoplasma* tachyzoites to approximately 1.5 μm for *Theileria* sporozoites and *Plasmodium* merozoites. The polarized organelles required for attachment and invasion consist of an apical conoid and associated microtubules, numerous micronemes (up to 40 in *Plasmodium*), two to eight rhoptries, and a subpopulation of apical dense granules (**Figure 6**). Slight variations occur in *Babesia* parasites that possess dense granule-like organelles termed spherical bodies and *Theileria* sporozoites that have additional microspheres, also associated with the establishment of intracellular parasites. Micronemes are the invasion organelles and contain numerous adhesion proteins or complexes (see below). Rhoptries are acidic organelles (immature at approximately pH 4 and mature at approximately pH 6) that add material to the growing invasion cavity (also referred to as PV) that is formed around the parasite during the invasion process. Dense granules (termed such because of their

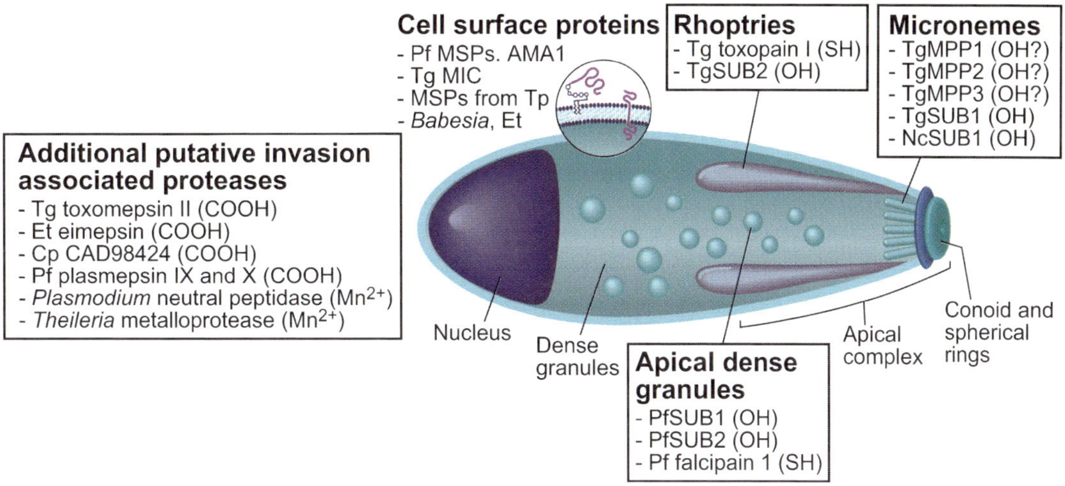

Figure 6

Schematic drawing showing a generic *Apicomplexa* invasion stage (zoite), highlighting the peptidase (*boxed*) and their subcellular locations and peptidase catalytic type when known. Pf, *Plasmodium falciparum*; Tg, *Toxoplama gondii*; Nc, *Neospora caninum*; Et, *Eimeria tenella*; Cp, *Cryptosporidium parvum*; Tp, *Theileria parvum*; MSP, merozoite surface protein; AMA, apical membrane antigen; MPP, microneme processing peptidase; SUB, subtilase; MIC, microneme protein; OH, serine peptidase; SH, cysteine peptidase; COOH, aspartyl peptidase; Mn^{2+}, metalopeptidase.

appearance under electron microscopy) are released post invasion and play a role in adapting the PV for effective parasite survival (**Figure 6**).

Initial Protein Processing

A range of proteins, or protein complexes, in *Apicomplexa* is peptidolytically processed en route to, or within, the apical organelles prior to invasion or exit. Single or multiple processing of membrane-bound or soluble proteins are thought to be necessary for correct organellar biosynthesis, intracellular targeting, and functional assembly of protein complexes or generation of adhesive domains (175, 176). In *Toxoplama gondii* a number of microneme proteins, including members of the microneme protein (MIC) family and TgAMA1 (*T. gondii* apical membrane antigen), are transprocessed at their N termini prior to invasion. The serine protease TgSUB1 is also processed; however, this is likely to be autocatalytic (177). The sissile bond (the specific peptide bond that is hydrolyzed) and flanking subsite residues have been mapped for a number of microneme protein substrates and reveal a single cleavage with no observable consensus (173), which suggests that the activity is regulated by the accessibility of a spatially restricted membrane resident protease (spacio-specificity), the identity of which is unknown. Proteins produced from the micronemes of the zoite prior to invasion include MIC proteins (in *Neospora*), TRAP (thrombospondin-related adhesive protein) and SCRP (super cysteine-rich protein) proteins (in *Plasmodium* and *Cryptosporidium*), and circumsporozoite proteins and EBA175 (erythrocyte binding antigen 175) family (in *Plasmodium*). Microneme proteins from other *Apicomplexa* such as *Sarcocystis*, SML (sarcocystis muris lection), and MIC family proteins from *Theileria*, *Eimeria*, and *Neopsora* may also serve as potential substrates for proteolytic activities. This activity has been linked to a serine or cysteine protease activity, as evidenced by sensitivity to either a subtilisin inhibitor or a selective cathepsin B inhibitor, respectively.

MIC: microneme protein

Rhoptry: large, paired, acidic tear drop–shaped secretory organelles that are part of the apical complex

Intracellular inhibition of the only resident cysteine protease characterized to date, the cathepsin B–like enzyme toxopain 1, interferes with rhoptry biogenesis, rhoptry protein processing, and targeting (specifically, ROP2, 3, and 4), concomitant with a reduction in parasite proliferation (69). The rhoptry subtilisin-like serine protease, TgSUB2, has also been implicated in the cleavage of a number of ROPs (rhoptry family of protein) (178). The inability to generate *tgsub2* null parasites in *Toxoplasma* may suggest that this gene product is essential (178, 179).

In *Plasmodium*, another protein that undergoes proteolytic processing is merozoite surface protein 1 (MSP1), a highly abundant, GPI-anchored protein of approximately 190 kDa located on late schizonts and merozoites within infected erythrocytes. Lysis of the infected erythrocyte releases 16 to 32 merozoites, each of which invades new red blood cells and so propagates the asexual part of the malaria life cycle. At or prior to the lysis of the erythrocyte, MSP1 is proteolytically processed at three discrete cleavage sites. Intriguingly the polypeptides generated do not dissociate from each other (as is the case with the majority of proteolytic events) but instead form a noncovalently associated complex (180). This so-called primary processing is sensitive to inhibitors of cysteine and serine proteases and is thought to be essential for progression of the asexual cycle. The identity of the protease remains unknown and may well be the same as the activity involved in parasite egress (see below).

Cell Invasion

Invasion of *Apicomplexa* zoites into target cells is an active process quite distinct from induced uptake or phagocytosis as seen with other parasitic protozoa such as *T. cruzi* and *Leishmania*. The penetration process is directly linked to the cytoskeleton and motility of the invading parasite and is facilitated by surface contact gliding at speeds of 1–10 μm s^{-1}. Cilia and flagella do not play a part in motility (181). Locating suitable cells is thought to be by chance. However, the series of events leading to invasion itself is a superbly regulated and efficient process. The infectious zoites can make primary reversible contact by means of any surface. In *Plasmodium*, inhibitors of serine and cysteine proteases can block this step. Following contact, the parasite rapidly reorients itself so that the apical end is in close contact with the host cell. In doing so, the zoite develops a protrusion of the conoid that results in the formation of a surface dimple. These features have been observed in *Eimeria* sporozoites, *Neospora* tachyzoites, *Plasmodium* merozoites, *Toxoplasma* tachyzoites, *Babesia* merozoites, and *Sarcocystis* zoites. In contrast, *Theileria* sporozoites are not motile, lack a conoid, and do not re-orientate post binding (**Figure 7**).

In *Apicomplexa*, host cell selectivity is a function of specific ligands on the target cell and the abundant surface proteins prevalent on all zoites. *Theileria* sporozoites only target cells that express T cell markers. *Plasmodium falciparum* sporozoites selectively seek out hepatocytes, whereas in *Toxoplasma* virtually any host cell can be invaded. The efficiency of infection is exemplified by *Plasmodium* sporozoites where as few as 10 parasites are thought to be injected in the wild-type state; although, only a few parasites are needed to initiate an infection under experimental conditions. Location and entry into target hepatocytes is a rapid process taking merely minutes post injection into the host. Motility, targeting, and the associated molecules in sporozoites have been well studied (182, 183). The *P. falciparum* merozoite is even more formidable and able to proceed from rupture to new invasion in a matter of seconds. However, *Theileria* sporozoites remain infectious for up to six hours in vitro.

Penetration of the host cell is carried out by an ordered discharge of the apical organelles and is triggered by an increase in intracellular Ca^{2+} and action of kinases. The microneme contents are released first and add proteins and protein complexes as well as proteases to the parasite surface (184). Host-parasite contact is made and appears as a band, formed by tight contact between the parasite surface and the host cell membrane. This band moves from anterior to posterior as the parasite invades the host cell. There is concomitant protease activity and shedding of parasite surface proteins as the invasion process progresses. In *Toxoplasma* and *Neospora*, the subtilsin-related serine proteases TgSUB1 and NcSUB1, respectively, are released (185). In addition, in *Toxoplasma*, a number of microneme-processing protease activities are also evident. The MPPs are sensitive to only a subset of serine protease inhibitors, as are rhomboids, members of another class of serine proteases that are multitransmembrane enzymes whose active sites are buried within the lipid bilayer of the membrane. A number of rhomboid family proteases have been identified in *Toxoplasma* and *Plasmodium*, and are very appealing candidates for microneme-processing protease activity (176).

Host cell entry of *Eimeria* merozoites and sporozoites has been shown to be sensitive to the serine protease inhibitors leupeptin, TPCK (N-tosyl-phenylalanine chloromethyl ketone), TLCK (N-tosyl-L-lysine chloromethyl ketone), and PMSF (phenylmethylsufonyl fluoride), whereas sporozoites are also inhibited by the inhibitor antipain (186), which inhibits serine or cysteine protease activity. A recent functional chemical knockout approach demonstrated that dense granules of *P. falciparum* merozoites contain the cysteine protease falcipain 1, which is a key component of the erythrocyte invasion pathway (187). However, falcipain 1 genetic null parasites were found to be indistinguishable from wild-type malaria parasites (188). This result suggests a possible lack of in vivo chemical specificity with the chemical-targeting approach.

Intriguingly, members of the aspartyl-protease group of enzymes in *Apicomplexa* have also been implicated in the invasion process. These enzymes are typically lysosomal and therefore function at a very low pH rather than the near neutral pH assumed necessary for invasion. Nonetheless, candidate invasion–associated aspartyl proteases include eimepsin from *Eimeria*, toxamepsin II for *Toxoplasma* and CAD98424 from *Cryptosporidium*. In *Plasmodium*, the tightly regulated increase in the number of transcripts for aspartyl proteases plasmepsin IX and X in the late schizonts stage is evidence for the involvement of these proteases in the exit or invasion process. By and large, metalloprotease activity is weakly linked with the invasion process, and to date only a single *Plasmodium* neutral metalloprotease involved in the invasion of merozoites has been described (189).

The processing and shedding of some parasite proteins is thought to be an indispensable requirement for functional entry into cells, and interfering with the sheddase activity is thought to incapacitate the infectious zoite. Noteworthy examples of such proteins include the *P. falciparum* MSP1 and the transmembrane-spanning apical membrane antigen 1, both of which are processed by a common membrane-bound, spacially restricted, Ca^{2+}-dependent serine protease activity (albeit with distinct substrate specificities) (190). PfSUB1 and PfSUB2, orthologues of bacterial subtilisins, are candidate enzymes for this activity, as both proteases are localized to subpopulations of apical dense granules (191). However, dense-granule contents are thought to be released only when invasion is at or near completion, and the direct involvement of PfSUB1 and PfSUB2 in invasion is still a matter of debate. Recent developments by Withers-Martinez and colleagues (191) used substrates and selective small chemical inhibitors of PfSUB1 to exclude PfSUB1 as the processing enzyme. Therefore, PfSUB2 may be the best candidate enzyme for MSP1 and apical membrane antigen 1 processing. Evidence for this hypothesis is indirect and includes the facts that (*a*) PfSUB2 has a transmembrane-spanning domain and (*b*) it is not possible to generate *pfsub2*-null parasites in the rodent malaria, *Plasmodium*

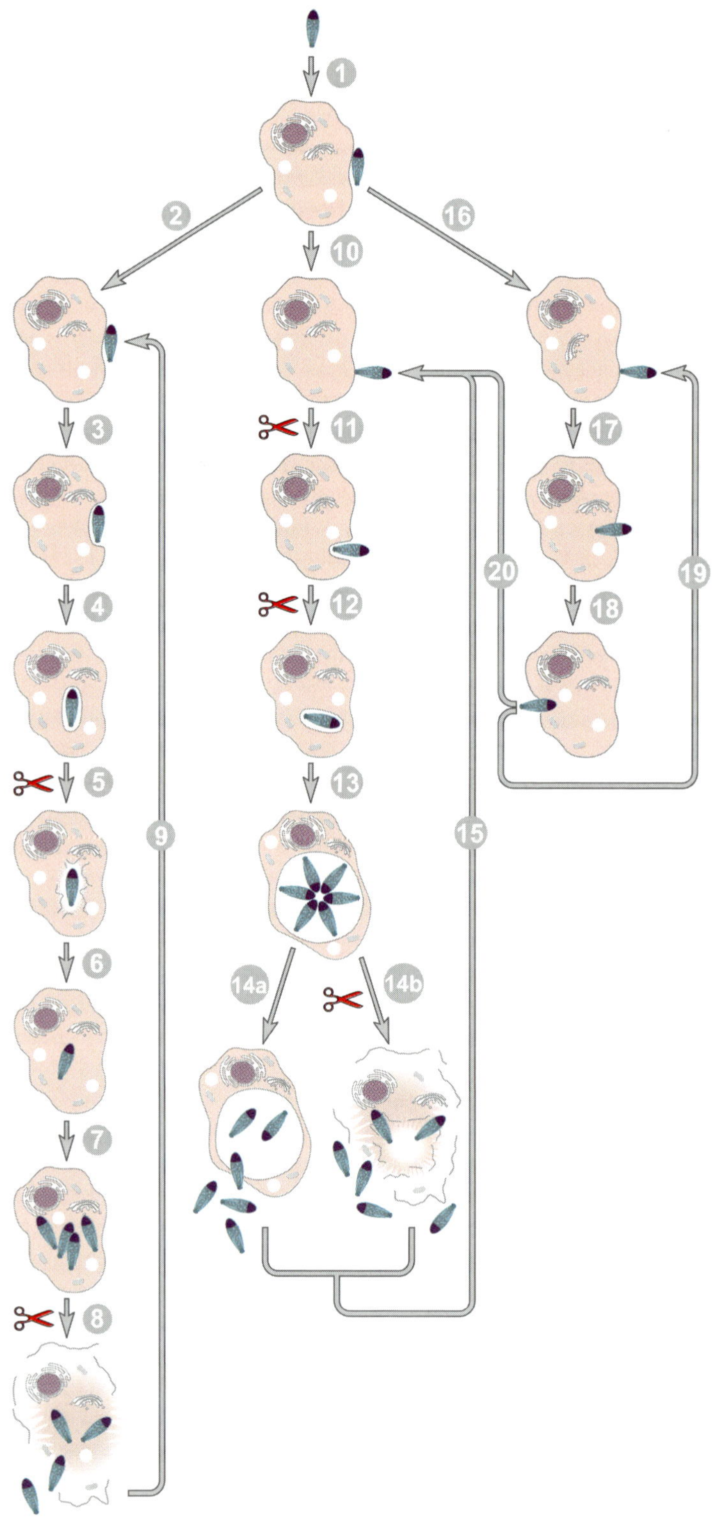
1
2
10
16
3
11
17
4
12
18
20
19
5
13
9
15
6
14a
14b
7
8

berghei (178, 179). It is worth mentioning that complete removal of surface protein by protease is not desired; indeed, GPI- or transmembrane-tethered portions remain after cleavage and are thought to play a direct role in the invasion process.

Rhoptry secretion is coincident with the formation of the newly formed PV, the cavity that surrounds the invading parasite. The released rhoptry contents are thought to subtly alter the PV, resulting in no acidification and promoting mitochondrial and endoplasmic reticulum association. The chemical cue for sequential rhoptry and dense-granule release is not known and may be due to an invasion clock triggered by the initial apical attachment and Ca^{2+} burst. Distinct from the aforementioned PfSUB1 and PfSUB2, other serine protease activities, such as p67 (in *P. falciparum*) and p68 (in *Plasmodium chaubaudi*), have been characterized in *Plasmodium* rhoptries. Unusually, these GPI-anchored proteases are activated upon release from the membrane and are linked to the formation of the PV.

Unlike the parasites we describe above, *Theileria* sporozoites invade T cells in any orientation and with no apparent discharge of the apical organelles. Nevertheless, components of the surface coat are lost during the zippering and internalization of the parasite into the PV. *Theileria* invasion is only sensitive to inhibitors of serine proteases (192). Moreover, whereas generally in *Apicomplexa* the parasitophorous vacuolar membrane (PVM) is derived from both parasite and host material, with *Theileria* the PVM is entirely host derived. In addition, pretreatment of the host cell with protease inhibitors such as 1–10 phenanthroline and EDTA (inhibitors of metalloproteases) also impairs *Theileria* sporozoite entry. This result suggests that proteases are required from both the parasite and the host for successful ingress. The observation that pretreating the parasites with trypsin results in noninvasive tight clumps of parasites suggests that a proteolytic step generates an adhesive surface necessary for the zippering process. Two sporozoite surface proteins, p67 and polymorphic immunodominant molecule (PIM) and host-derived MHC class I are implicated in the initial binding of parasite with the host (193). At approximately 10–15 minutes post invasion, internalized parasites release the contents of their micronemes and rhoptries and concomitantly escape the

Figure 7

Simplified schematic drawing of cell penetration and exit strategies undertaken by the invasive stage (zoite) of apicomplexan parasites, highlighting the steps where proteases perform an essential role (*indicated by scissors*). Once a zoite has located a target host cell, the initial binding (which is reversible) is via any surface of the parasite (*1*). Invasion follows one of three distinct penetration pathways. In one pathway the zoite does not reorientate (*2*). As is the case with *Theileria*, the parasite invades (*3*) and resides briefly in the newly formed parasitophorous vacuole (PV) (*4*). Parasite-derived proteases aid in lysis of the PV (*5*) and the parasite is then free-living in host cell cytoplasm (*6*). Following replication (*7*) the parasite ruptures the host cell (*8*) and is ready to start the invasion cycle once more (*9*). In the case of *Toxoplasma* and *Plasmodium*, the zoites are able to orientate themselves so as to make a tight junction of their apical ends with the host plasma membrane (*10*). Discharge of the apical complex components is coincident with the invasion process. Parasite-derived proteases are indispensable for the invasion step (*11*), and the parasite inhabits the PV (*12*). Following replication (*13*) within the PV, the parasites escape the confines of both the plasma membrane and the parasitophorous vacuolar membrane by one of two pathways: either actively crossing both the parasitophorous vacuole and plasma membrane and ultimately lysing the host cell (*14a*) as seen in *Toxoplasma*, or by lysing both the parasitophorous vacuole and plasma membrane (*14b*) as in the case of Plasmodium. The newly emerged parasite locates new target cells and repeats the invasion and replication cycle (*15*). Uniquely, *Plasmodium* sporozoites once bound to the host hepatocyte (*16*) can move directly into the cytoplasm without forming a vacuole (*17*). The parasite moves straight through and out of the cell (*18*) to either repeat nonvacuolar penetration (*19*) or, alternatively, to invade and replicate in the more conventional vacuolar fashion (*20*).

SERA: serine repeat antigen

nonacidified vacuole into the cytoplasm. The role of proteases in this process is currently being studied (B. Shiels & M. Sajid, work in progress).

In contrast to the above mentioned vacuolar invasion, elegant work by Mota and coworkers (195) revealed an alternative cell entry strategy, seemingly unique to *Plasmodium* sporozoites. Prior to attaching and initiating vacuolar entry into hepatocytes, the *Plasmodium* sporozoites make contact at the apical end and glide directly from the outer plasma membrane surface into the cell cytoplasm without forming a vacuole. The penetration aperture is sealed upon entry and is evident as a membrane lesion. The sporozoite passes straight through the cell cytoplasm and repeats the plasma membrane traversal on exit. This process occurs a number of times prior to settling for vacuolar invasion and is thought to have biological relevance in furnishing the parasite with the ability to traverse cells surrounding the liver (such as Kupffer cells) en route to initiating a new malaria infection. The involvement of proteases in nonvacuolar invasion is unknown; however, vacuolar invasion is sensitive to inhibitors of serine and cysteine proteases (196).

CELL EXIT

Release of *Apicomplexa* from the host cell is often considered to be a passive process that involves physical rupture of the PVM and host cell membrane. The involvement of proteases in this process has been known for a while; however, teasing out the effect of inhibitors on parasite development or directly on parasite exit has been challenging. In *Plasmodium knowlesi*, a simian malaria, chymostatin and leupeptin were effective at inhibiting exit (197), whereas in the closely related *P. falciparum*, leupeptin, antipain, and pepstatin had similar effects (198). The general cysteine protease inhibitor E64 has been shown to inhibit parasite development as well as exit (199). It is entirely feasible that the invasion and exit pathways may well have a protease in common. In *Plasmodium*, exit from within the PVM and the erythrocyte membrane has been shown to be an ordered, two-step process (199, 200). The order of events remains to be contended; nonetheless, protease inhibitors have been shown to selectively block each step, demonstrating that the initial PVM lysis within the intact erythrocyte is sensitive to E64, whereas the second step, erythrocyte plasma membrane lysis, is sensitive to leupeptin and antipain (200). In a number of late schizonts, *Plasmodium* proteases have been shown to cleave structural proteins in the erythrocyte membrane and are likely to be involved directly in the egress process. Resident proteases include the serine repeat antigens (SERAs) (particularly SERA4, 5, and 6) (201, 202), falcipain 2 (203, 204), and possibly the acid basic repeat antigens, which are cryptic serine proteases. SERA5 is an unusual hybrid protease as it has a cysteine protease scaffold and a serine residue as the catalytic amino acid. Biochemically, SERA5 is predicted to be inert; indeed, similar hybrids using human proteases generated in vitro resulted in catalytically dead enzymes (205). In spite of this, SERA5 has been shown to be catalytically active, and, even more astonishingly, the activity is sensitive to inhibitors of both serine and cysteine proteases, including E64 and leupeptin (206). An aspartyl protease from *P. falciparum*, plasmepsin II, which, unusually, is active at neutral pH, has also been suggested to be involved in the exit pathway (207). Little is known regarding the release of *Plasmodium* merozoite from hepatocytes, but it is highly likely to involve similar enzymes as above.

To summarize, *Apicomplexa* have opted to use at least one serine peptidase in the invasion and probably in exit process as well. *Toxoplasma* and *Neospora* have serine peptidases in the micronemes; *Toxoplasma* also use rhoptries whilst *Plasmodium* utilizes the apical dense granules. It is possible that the dynamic timings of discharge from micronemes, rhoptries, and dense granules vary between parasites, allowing each respective enzyme to be functional in the invasion process. In addition,

Toxoplasma has opted to also use a cathepsin B–like peptidase located in the rhoptries, a class of peptidase absent in *Plasmodium*. Even with the completion of the *Plasmodium* and *Toxoplasma* genome sequences, and the prediction of all potential proteases, functionally assigning peptidases to a discrete roll in invasion and/or exit has been problematic. This is due, in part, to identifying activities that may be present at a very low level, specificity (location and enzyme) of inhibitors used in vivo, and also difficulties in teasing out closely related activities. Advances in selective chemistries and increased sensitivities with mass spectrometry have gone a long away to addressing this shortfall. In addition, the potential involvement of catalytically inert peptidase scaffolds or macromolecular protein inhibitors in regulating the invasion and/or exit process remains unknown.

CONCLUSION

Work over the past two decades has validated the general concept that proteolytic enzymes are key factors in the interplay between parasite and host (**Table 3**). The ability of proteolytic enzymes to catalyze degradation of macromolecules, serve as regulators of protein activation, and catalyze turnover of peptides and growth factors leaves little doubt as to why they so fervently appear as key elements in both biology and pathology. In the host-parasite relationship, proteases clearly play key roles as virulence factors in many infections. Paradoxically, although proteases can function to help parasites evade the immune response, they also can induce inflammation and immune responses.

Much remains to be done to validate many of the intriguing but more specific hypotheses about the role of proteases in parasitic infections. This validation will require advancing the molecular technology that can be applied to complex parasitic systems to a new level. Although this work is clearly a challenge, there is good reason to be optimistic. *C. elegans* has proved to be a useful surrogate for the study of the roles of proteases in many helminth parasite functions, including molting and nutrition. RNA interference and transfection are being successfully applied, although the technologies are in their infancy, to many protozoan and helminth parasites. When these technologies becomes more standardized, many of the models of parasite evasion of the immune response can be directly tested by interfering with the functions of the specific enzymes and factors implicated above.

Finally, the interplay between host and parasite can also be explored from the host side through the use of many new models of immune or endocrine disruption in the mouse. Virtually all major parasitic infections

Table 3 Summary of the role of proteases in parasitic disease pathogenesis

Protease class	Role in pathogenesis	Comment
Cysteine	Tissue invasion (*Entamoeba* and *Fasciola*) Nutrient degradation (trypanosomes, helminthes, malaria) Immune evasion (*Trypanosoma cruzi*) Processing other key proteins (malaria, *Leishmania*)	Cysteine proteases most common in protozoa and primitive metazoa and may reflect a common reducing environment and anaerobic metabolism
Serine	Anticoagulation (helminthes) Tissue invasion (schistosomes) Processing other key proteins (malaria)	Trypsin family serine proteases implicated in anticoagulation and invasion Subtilisn family serine proteases in protein processing
Aspartyl	Nutrient degradation (helminthes, malaria)	Interesting parallel use by helminthes and malaria parasites for hemoglobin degradation
Metalloproteases	Anticoagulation (helminthes) Tissue invasion (helminth larvae) Nutrient degradation (malaria)	Most evidence from studies of hookworm anticoagulation and tissue invasion

can be followed through reasonable mouse models of disease. A combination of transfection technology and mouse models of infection should therefore lead to validation or dismissal of models of the host-parasite biology discussed in this review.

SUMMARY POINTS

1. Proteases play key roles in tissue invasion, immune evasion, and anticoagulation for parasitic helminths.
2. Parasite-derived protease inhibitors may protect against host-derived proteases or regulate endogenous enzymes.
3. Proteases of *Leishmania* and *Entamoeba* have critical roles in invasion and manipulation of host immune responses.
4. Cruzain is the major cysteine protease of *T. cruzi*, which may play an important role in pathology because it is involved in (*a*) host cell invasion, (*b*) auto-immunity, (*c*) immune deviation, and (*d*) immune evasion.
5. Anti-Cruzain inhibitors, under development as chemotherapy, may be reversing immune evasion mechanisms of the parasite.
6. Many helminth parasites release inhibitors of cysteine (cystatins) and serine proteases (serpins) that are believed to downregulate host immune and inflammatory responses.
7. Hookworms release serine protease inhibitors that are potent anticoagulants, and some of these are in clinical trials as antithrombotics for treatment of deep-vein thrombosis and ischemic stroke.
8. *Apicomplexa* parasites have evolved specialized organelles and hydrolytic enzymes (proteases) that are crucial for invasion and exit from target host cells.

ACKNOWLEDGMENTS

Special thanks go to the colleagues in the Tropical Disease Research Unit, funded in part by the National Institutes of Health grants AI35707 and A1053247, and the Sandler Center for Basic Research in Parasitic Diseases, funded by The Sandler Family Supporting Foundation.

LITERATURE CITED

1. Special Programme for Research and Training in Tropical Diseases. 2004. **http://www.who.int/tdr/tropics**
2. Barrett AJ. 2004. Bioinformatics of proteases in the MEROPS database. *Curr. Opin. Drug Discov. Dev.* 7:334–41
3. Sakanari JA. 1990. Anisakis—from the platter to the microfuge. *Parasitol. Today* 6:323–27
4. Daschner A, Cuellar C, Sanchez-Pastor S, Pascual CY, Martin-Esteban M. 2002. Gastro-allergic anisakiasis as a consequence of simultaneous primary and secondary immune response. *Parasite Immunol.* 24:243–51
5. Nakamura-Uchiyama F, Yamasaki E, Nawa Y. 2002. One confirmed and six suspected cases of cutaneous larva migrans caused by overseas infection with dog hookworm larvae. *J. Dermatol.* 29:104–11

6. Ly MN, Bethel SL, Usmani AS, Lambert DR. 2003. Cutaneous Strongyloides stercoralis infection: an unusual presentation. *J. Am. Acad. Dermatol.* 49:S157–60
7. Kagialis-Girard S, Mialou V, Ffrench M, Dupuis-Girod S, Pages MP, Bertrand Y. 2005. Thrombocytosis and toxocariasis: report of two pediatric cases. *Pediatr. Blood Cancer* 44:190–92
8. Tort J, Brindley PJ, Knox D, Wolfe KH, Dalton JP. 1999. Proteinases and associated genes of parasitic helminths. *Adv. Parasitol.* 43:161–266
9. McKerrow JH, Brindley P, Brown M, Gam AA, Staunton C, Neva FA. 1990. Strongyloides stercoralis: identification of a protease that facilitates penetration of skin by the infective larvae. *Exp. Parasitol.* 70:134–43
10. Lackey A, James ER, Sakanari JA, Resnick SD, Brown M, et al. 1989. Extracellular proteases of Onchocerca. *Exp. Parasitol.* 68:176–85
11. Law RH, Smooker PM, Irving JA, Piedrafita D, Ponting R, et al. 2003. Cloning and expression of the major secreted cathepsin B-like protein from juvenile Fasciola hepatica and analysis of immunogenicity following liver fluke infection. *Infect. Immun.* 71:6921–32
12. Shin MH, Lee SY. 2000. Proteolytic activity of cysteine protease in excretory-secretory product of Paragonimus westermani newly excysted metacercariae pivotally regulates IL-8 production of human eosinophils. *Parasite Immunol.* 22:529–33
13. Park H, Kim SI, Hong KM, Kim MJ, Shin CH, et al. 2002. Characterization and classification of five cysteine proteinases expressed by Paragonimus westermani adult worm. *Exp. Parasitol.* 102:143–49
14. Na BK, Lee HJ, Cho SH, Lee HW, Cho JH, et al. 2002. Expression of cysteine proteinase of Clonorchis sinensis and its use in serodiagnosis of clonorchiasis. *J. Parasitol.* 88:1000–6
15. Yamakami K, Hamajima F, Akao S, Tadakuma T. 1995. Purification and characterization of acid cysteine protease from metacercariae of the mammalian trematode parasite Paragonimus westermani. *Eur. J. Biochem.* 233:490–97
16. Shin MH, Lee SY. 2000. Proteolytic activity of cysteine protease in excretory-secretory product of Paragonimus westermani newly excysted metacercariae pivotally regulate IL-8 production of human eosinophils. *Parasite Immunol.* 22:529–33
17. Sung CK, Dresden MH. 1986. Cysteinyl proteinases of Schistosoma mansoni eggs: purification and partial characterization. *J. Parasitol.* 72:891–900
18. Caffrey CR, McKerrow JH, Salter JP, Sajid M. 2004. Blood 'n' guts: an update on schistosome digestive peptidases. *Trends Parasitol.* 20:241–48
19. Ruppel A, Shi YE, Wei DX, Diesfeld HJ. 1987. Sera of Schistosoma japonicum-infected patients cross-react with diagnostic 31/32 kD proteins of S. mansoni. *Clin. Exp. Immunol.* 69:291–98
20. Li YL, Idris MA, Corachan M, Han JJ, Kirschfink M, Ruppel A. 1996. Circulating antigens in schistosomiasis: detection of 31/32-kDa proteins in sera from patients infected with Schistosoma japonicum, S. mansoni, S. haematobium, or S. intercalatum. *Parasitol. Res.* 82:14–18
21. Yun DH, Chung JY, Chung YB, Bahk YY, Kang SY, et al. 2000. Structural and immunological characteristics of a 28-kilodalton cruzipain-like cysteine protease of Paragonimus westermani expressed in the definitive host stage. *Clin. Diagn. Lab. Immunol.* 7:932–39
22. Yamasaki K, Ishiyama H, Imaizumi T, Kanbe T, Yabuuchi Y. 1989. Effect of OPC-12759, a novel antiulcer agent, on chronic and acute experimental gastric ulcer, and gastric secretion in rats. *Jpn. J. Pharmacol.* 49:441–48

23. Smith AM, Dowd AJ, McGonigle S, Keegan PS, Brennan G, et al. 1993. Purification of a cathepsin L-like proteinase secreted by adult Fasciola hepatica. *Mol. Biochem. Parasitol.* 62:1–8
24. Skelly PJ. 2005. Intravascular schistosomes and complement. *Trends Parasitol.* In press
25. Salter JP, Choe Y, Albrecht H, Franklin C, Lim KC, et al. 2002. Cercarial elastase is encoded by a functionally conserved gene family across multiple species of schistosomes. *J. Biol. Chem.* 277:24618–24
26. Mountford AP, Trottein F. 2004. Schistosomes in the skin: a balance between immune priming and regulation. *Trends Parasitol.* 20:221–26
27. Curwen RS, Wilson RA. 2003. Invasion of skin by schistosome cercariae: some neglected facts. *Trends Parasitol.* 19:63–66
28. Fishelson Z. 1995. Novel mechanisms of immune evasion by Schistosoma mansoni. *Mem. Inst. Oswaldo Cruz* 90:289–92
29. Knudsen GM, Medzihradszky KF, Lim KC, Hansell E, McKerrow JH. 2005. Proteomic analysis of *Schistosoma mansoni* cercarial secretions. *Mol. Cell. Proteomics.* In press
30. Chang CS, Chang KP. 1986. Monoclonal antibody affinity purification of a Leishmania membrane glycoprotein and its inhibition of leishmania-macrophage binding. *Proc. Natl. Acad. Sci. USA* 83:100–4
31. Frommel TO, Button LL, Fujikura Y, McMaster WR. 1990. The major surface glycoprotein (GP63) is present in both life stages of Leishmania. *Mol. Biochem. Parasitol.* 38:25–32
32. Chen DQ, Kolli BK, Yadava N, Lu HG, Gilman-Sachs A, et al. 2000. Episomal expression of specific sense and antisense mRNAs in Leishmania amazonensis: modulation of gp63 level in promastigotes and their infection of macrophages in vitro. *Infect. Immun.* 68:80–86
33. Joshi PB, Kelly BL, Kamhawi S, Sacks DL, McMaster WR. 2002. Targeted gene deletion in Leishmania major identifies leishmanolysin (GP63) as a virulence factor. *Mol. Biochem. Parasitol.* 120:33–40
34. Brittingham A, Mosser DM. 1996. Exploitation of the complement system by Leishmania promastigotes. *Parasitol. Today* 12:444–47
35. Dominguez M, Moreno I, Lopez-Trascasa M, Torano A. 2002. Complement interaction with trypanosomatid promastigotes in normal human serum. *J. Exp. Med.* 195:451–59
36. McGwire BS, Chang KP, Engman DM. 2003. Migration through the extracellular matrix by the parasitic protozoan Leishmania is enhanced by surface metalloprotease gp63. *Infect. Immun.* 71:1008–10
37. Hilley JD, Zawadzki JL, McConville MJ, Coombs GH, Mottram JC. 2000. Leishmania mexicana mutants lacking glycosylphosphatidylinositol (GPI):protein transamidase provide insights into the biosynthesis and functions of GPI-anchored proteins. *Mol. Biol. Cell* 11:1183–95
38. Voth BR, Kelly BL, Joshi PB, Ivens AC, McMaster WR. 1998. Differentially expressed Leishmania major gp63 genes encode cell surface leishmanolysin with distinct signals for glycosylphosphatidylinositol attachment. *Mol. Biochem. Parasitol.* 93:31–41
39. Victoir K, Dujardin JC, de Doncker S, Barker DC, Arevalo J, et al. 1995. Plasticity of gp63 gene organization in Leishmania (Viannia) braziliensis and Leishmania (Viannia) peruviana. *Parasitology* 111(Pt. 3):265–73
40. Yao C, Luo J, Storlie P, Donelson JE, Wilson ME. 2004. Multiple products of the Leishmania chagasi major surface protease (MSP or GP63) gene family. *Mol. Biochem. Parasitol.* 135:171–83

41. McConville MJ, Schnur LF, Jaffe C, Schneider P. 1995. Structure of Leishmania lipophosphoglycan: inter- and intra-specific polymorphism in Old World species. *Biochem. J.* 310(Pt. 3):807–18
42. McConville MJ, Turco SJ, Ferguson MA, Sacks DL. 1992. Developmental modification of lipophosphoglycan during the differentiation of Leishmania major promastigotes to an infectious stage. *EMBO J.* 11:3593–600
43. Sacks DL. 1992. The structure and function of the surface lipophosphoglycan on different developmental stages of Leishmania promastigotes. *Infect Agents Dis.* 1:200–6
44. Lincoln LM, Ozaki M, Donelson JE, Beetham JK. 2004. Genetic complementation of Leishmania deficient in PSA (GP46) restores their resistance to lysis by complement. *Mol. Biochem. Parasitol.* 137:185–89
45. Beverley SM. 2003. Protozomics: trypanosomatid parasite genetics comes of age. *Nat. Rev. Genet.* 4:11–19
46. Souza AE, Bates PA, Coombs GH, Mottram JC. 1994. Null mutants for the lmcpa cysteine proteinase gene in Leishmania mexicana. *Mol. Biochem. Parasitol.* 63:213–20
47. Bart G, Frame MJ, Carter R, Coombs GH, Mottram JC. 1997. Cathepsin B-like cysteine proteinase-deficient mutants of Leishmania mexicana. *Mol. Biochem. Parasitol.* 88:53–61
48. Mottram JC, Coombs GH, Alexander J. 2004. Cysteine peptidases as virulence factors of Leishmania. *Curr. Opin. Microbiol.* 7:375–81
49. Mottram JC, Souza AE, Hutchison JE, Carter R, Frame MJ, Coombs GH. 1996. Evidence from disruption of the lmcpb gene array of Leishmania mexicana that cysteine proteinases are virulence factors. *Proc. Natl. Acad. Sci. USA* 93:6008–13
50. Mottram JC, Frame MJ, Brooks DR, Tetley L, Hutchison JE, et al. 1997. The multiple cpb cysteine proteinase genes of Leishmania mexicana encode isoenzymes that differ in their stage regulation and substrate preferences. *J. Biol. Chem.* 272:14285–93
51. Frame MJ, Mottram JC, Coombs GH. 2000. Analysis of the roles of cysteine proteinases of Leishmania mexicana in the host-parasite interaction. *Parasitology* 121(Pt. 4):367–77
52. Alexander J, Coombs GH, Mottram JC. 1998. Leishmania mexicana cysteine proteinase-deficient mutants have attenuated virulence for mice and potentiate a Th1 response. *J. Immunol.* 161:6794–801
53. Cameron P, McGachy A, Anderson M, Paul A, Coombs GH, et al. 2004. Inhibition of lipopolysaccharide-induced macrophage IL-12 production by Leishmania mexicana amastigotes: the role of cysteine peptidases and the NF-kappaB signaling pathway. *J. Immunol.* 173:3297–304
54. Buxbaum LU, Denise H, Coombs GH, Alexander J, Mottram JC, Scott P. 2003. Cysteine protease B of Leishmania mexicana inhibits host Th1 responses and protective immunity. *J. Immunol.* 171:3711–17
55. Fukao T, Matsuda S, Koyasu S. 2000. Synergistic effects of IL-4 and IL-18 on IL-12-dependent IFN-gamma production by dendritic cells. *J. Immunol.* 164:64–71
56. Houde M, Bertholet S, Gagnon E, Brunet S, Goyette G, et al. 2003. Phagosomes are competent organelles for antigen cross-presentation. *Nature* 425:402–6
57. Stamm LM, Raisanen-Sokolowski A, Okano M, Russell ME, David JR, Satoskar AR. 1998. Mice with STAT6-targeted gene disruption develop a Th1 response and control cutaneous leishmaniasis. *J. Immunol.* 161:6180–88
58. Tran VQ, Herdman DS, Torian BE, Reed SL. 1998. The neutral cysteine proteinase of Entamoeba histolytica degrades IgG and prevents its binding. *J. Infect. Dis.* 177:508–11
59. Kelsall BL, Ravdin JI. 1993. Degradation of human IgA by Entamoeba histolytica. *J. Infect. Dis.* 168:1319–22

60. Olivos-Garcia A, Tello E, Nequiz-Avendano M, Gonzalez-Canto A, Lopez-Vancell R, et al. 2004. Cysteine proteinase activity is required for survival of the parasite in experimental acute amoebic liver abscesses in hamsters. *Parasitology* 129:19–25
61. Bruchhaus I, Loftus BJ, Hall N, Tannich E. 2003. The intestinal protozoan parasite Entamoeba histolytica contains 20 cysteine protease genes, of which only a small subset is expressed during in vitro cultivation. *Eukaryot. Cell* 2:501–9
62. Bruchhaus I, Jacobs T, Leippe M, Tannich E. 1996. Entamoeba histolytica and Entamoeba dispar: differences in numbers and expression of cysteine proteinase genes. *Mol. Microbiol.* 22:255–63
63. Willhoeft U, Hamann L, Tannich E. 1999. A DNA sequence corresponding to the gene encoding cysteine proteinase 5 in Entamoeba histolytica is present and positionally conserved but highly degenerated in Entamoeba dispar. *Infect. Immun.* 67:5925–29
64. Hellberg A, Nickel R, Lotter H, Tannich E, Bruchhaus I. 2001. Overexpression of cysteine proteinase 2 in Entamoeba histolytica or Entamoeba dispar increases amoeba-induced monolayer destruction in vitro but does not augment amoebic liver abscess formation in gerbils. *Cell. Microbiol.* 3:13–20
65. Pertuz Belloso S, Ostoa Saloma P, Benitez I, Soldevila G, Olivos A, Garcia-Zepeda E. 2004. Entamoeba histolytica cysteine protease 2 (EhCP2) modulates leucocyte migration by proteolytic cleavage of chemokines. *Parasite Immunol.* 26:237–41
66. Ankri S, Stolarsky T, Mirelman D. 1998. Antisense inhibition of expression of cysteine proteinases does not affect Entamoeba histolytica cytopathic or haemolytic activity but inhibits phagocytosis. *Mol. Microbiol.* 28:777–85
67. Ankri S, Stolarsky T, Bracha R, Padilla-Vaca F, Mirelman D. 1999. Antisense inhibition of expression of cysteine proteinases affects Entamoeba histolytica-induced formation of liver abscess in hamsters. *Infect. Immun.* 67:421–22
68. Zhang Z, Wang L, Seydel KB, Li E, Ankri S, et al. 2000. Entamoeba histolytica cysteine proteinases with interleukin-1 beta converting enzyme (ICE) activity cause intestinal inflammation and tissue damage in amoebiasis. *Mol. Microbiol.* 37:542–48
69. Que X, Kim SH, Sajid M, Eckmann L, Dinarello CA, et al. 2003. A surface amebic cysteine proteinase inactivates interleukin-18. *Infect. Immun.* 71:1274–80
70. Kaur G, Lohia A. 2004. Inhibition of gene expression with double strand RNA interference in Entamoeba histolytica. *Biochem. Biophys. Res. Commun.* 320:1118–22
71. Pleass RJ, Kusel JR, Woof JM. 2000. Cleavage of human IgE mediated by Schistosoma mansoni. *Int. Arch. Allergy Immunol.* 121:194–204
72. Amiri P, Haak-Frendscho M, Robbins K, McKerrow JH, Stewart T, Jardieu P. 1994. Anti-immunoglobulin E treatment decreases worm burden and egg production in Schistosoma mansoni-infected normal and interferon gamma knockout mice. *J. Exp. Med.* 180:43–51
73. King CL, Xianli J, Malhotra I, Liu S, Mahmoud AA, Oettgen HC. 1997. Mice with a targeted deletion of the IgE gene have increased worm burdens and reduced granulomatous inflammation following primary infection with Schistosoma mansoni. *J. Immunol.* 158:294–300
74. Spencer LA, Porte P, Zetoff C, Rajan TV. 2003. Mice genetically deficient in immunoglobulin E are more permissive hosts than wild-type mice to a primary, but not secondary, infection with the filarial nematode Brugia malayi. *Infect. Immun.* 71:2462–67
75. Ghendler Y, Parizade M, Arnon R, McKerrow JH, Fishelson Z. 1996. Schistosoma mansoni: evidence for a 28-kDa membrane-anchored protease on schistosomula. *Exp. Parasitol.* 83:73–82

76. Engel JC, Doyle PS, Palmer J, Hsieh I, Bainton DF, McKerrow JH. 1998. Cysteine protease inhibitors alter Golgi complex ultrastructure and function in Trypanosoma cruzi. *J. Cell Sci.* 111(Pt. 5):597–606
77. Burleigh BA, Andrews NW. 1995. The mechanisms of Trypanosoma cruzi invasion of mammalian cells. *Annu. Rev. Microbiol.* 49:175–200
78. Martin D, Tarleton R. 2004. Generation, specificity, and function of CD8+ T cells in Trypanosoma cruzi infection. *Immunol. Rev.* 201:304–17
79. Engman DM, Leon JS. 2002. Pathogenesis of Chagas heart disease: role of autoimmunity. *Acta Trop.* 81:123–32
80. Tarleton RL. 2003. Chagas disease: a role for autoimmunity? *Trends Parasitol.* 19:447–51
81. Scharfstein J, Schmitz V, Morandi V, Capella MM, Lima AP, et al. 2000. Host cell invasion by Trypanosoma cruzi is potentiated by activation of bradykinin B(2) receptors. *J. Exp. Med.* 192:1289–300
82. Aparicio IM, Scharfstein J, Lima AP. 2004. A new cruzipain-mediated pathway of human cell invasion by Trypanosoma cruzi requires trypomastigote membranes. *Infect. Immun.* 72:5892–902
83. Arnholdt AC, Piuvezam MR, Russo DM, Lima AP, Pedrosa RC, et al. 1993. Analysis and partial epitope mapping of human T cell responses to Trypanosoma cruzi cysteinyl proteinase. *J. Immunol.* 151:3171–79
84. Kierszenbaum F. 1999. Chagas' disease and the autoimmunity hypothesis. *Clin. Microbiol. Rev.* 12:210–23
85. Lozykowski MG, McCormick TS, Rowland EC. 1991. Coincidence of tissue antibody and cardiac pathology in mice infected with Trypanosoma cruzi. *Trans. R. Soc. Trop. Med. Hyg.* 85:225–26
86. Laguens RP, Meckert PC, Chambo JG. 1988. Antiheart antibody-dependent cytotoxicity in the sera of mice chronically infected with Trypanosoma cruzi. *Infect. Immun.* 56:993–97
87. Giordanengo L, Maldonado C, Rivarola HW, Iosa D, Girones N, et al. 2000. Induction of antibodies reactive to cardiac myosin and development of heart alterations in cruzipain-immunized mice and their offspring. *Eur. J. Immunol.* 30:3181–89
88. Giordanengo L, Fretes R, Diaz H, Cano R, Bacile A, et al. 2000. Cruzipain induces autoimmune response against skeletal muscle and tissue damage in mice. *Muscle Nerve* 23:1407–13
89. Guinazu N, Pellegrini A, Giordanengo L, Aoki MP, Rivarola HW, et al. 2004. Immune response to a major Trypanosoma cruzi antigen, cruzipain, is differentially modulated in C57BL/6 and BALB/c mice. *Microbes Infect.* 6:1250–58
90. Giordanengo L, Guinazu N, Stempin C, Fretes R, Cerban F, Gea S. 2002. Cruzipain, a major Trypanosoma cruzi antigen, conditions the host immune response in favor of parasite. *Eur. J. Immunol.* 32:1003–11
91. Gordon S. 2003. Alternative activation of macrophages. *Nat. Rev. Immunol.* 3:23–35
92. Munder M, Eichmann K, Moran JM, Centeno F, Soler G, Modolell M. 1999. Th1/Th2-regulated expression of arginase isoforms in murine macrophages and dendritic cells. *J. Immunol.* 163:3771–77
93. Munder M, Eichmann K, Modolell M. 1998. Alternative metabolic states in murine macrophages reflected by the nitric oxide synthase/arginase balance: competitive regulation by CD4+ T cells correlates with Th1/Th2 phenotype. *J. Immunol.* 160:5347–54

94. Noel W, Raes G, Hassanzadeh Ghassabeh G, De Baetselier P, Beschin A. 2004. Alternatively activated macrophages during parasite infections. *Trends Parasitol.* 20:126–33
95. Stempin C, Giordanengo L, Gea S, Cerban F. 2002. Alternative activation and increase of Trypanosoma cruzi survival in murine macrophages stimulated by cruzipain, a parasite antigen. *J. Leukoc. Biol.* 72:727–34
96. Stempin CC, Tanos TB, Coso OA, Cerban FM. 2004. Arginase induction promotes Trypanosoma cruzi intracellular replication in Cruzipain-treated J774 cells through the activation of multiple signaling pathways. *Eur. J. Immunol.* 34:200–9
97. Piacenza L, Peluffo G, Radi R. 2001. L-arginine-dependent suppression of apoptosis in Trypanosoma cruzi: contribution of the nitric oxide and polyamine pathways. *Proc. Natl. Acad. Sci. USA* 98:7301–6
98. McKerrow JH, McGrath ME, Engel JC. 1995. The cysteine protease of Trypanosoma cruzi as a model for antiparasite drug design. *Parasitol. Today* 11:279–82
99. Engel JC, Doyle PS, Hsieh I, McKerrow JH. 1998. Cysteine protease inhibitors cure an experimental Trypanosoma cruzi infection. *J. Exp. Med.* 188:725–34
100. Engel JC, Torres C, Hsieh I, Doyle PS, McKerrow JH, Garcia CT. 2000. Upregulation of the secretory pathway in cysteine protease inhibitor-resistant Trypanosoma cruzi. *J. Cell Sci.* 113(Pt. 8):1345–54
101. Vaena de Avalos S, Blader IJ, Fisher M, Boothroyd JC, Burleigh BA. 2002. Immediate/early response to Trypanosoma cruzi infection involves minimal modulation of host cell transcription. *J. Biol. Chem.* 277:639–44
102. Maizels RM, Gomez-Escobar N, Gregory WF, Murray J, Zang X. 2001. Immune evasion genes from filarial nematodes. *Int. J. Parasitol.* 31:889–98
103. Pearce EJ, Kane CM, Sun J, Taylor JJ, McKee AS, Cervi L. 2004. Th2 response polarization during infection with the helminth parasite Schistosoma mansoni. *Immunol. Rev.* 201:117–26
104. Harnett W, Harnett MM. 2001. Modulation of the host immune system by phosphorylcholine-containing glycoproteins secreted by parasitic filarial nematodes. *Biochim. Biophys. Acta* 1539:7–15
105. Al-Qaoud KM, Fleischer B, Hoerauf A. 1998. The Xid defect imparts susceptibility to experimental murine filariosis–association with a lack of antibody and IL-10 production by B cells in response to phosphorylcholine. *Int. Immunol.* 10:17–25
106. Pastrana DV, Raghavan N, FitzGerald P, Eisinger SW, Metz C, et al. 1998. Filarial nematode parasites secrete a homologue of the human cytokine macrophage migration inhibitory factor. *Infect. Immun.* 66:5955–63
107. Hartmann S, Lucias R. 2003. Modulation of host immune response by nematode cystatins. *Int. J. Parasitol.* 33:1291–302
107a. Hartmann S, Kyewski B, Sonnenburg B, Lucius R. 1997. A filarial cysteine protease inhibitor down regulates T cell proliferation and enhances interleukin 10 production. *Eur. J. Immunol.* 27:2253–60
108. Zang X, Maizels RM. 2001. Serine proteinase inhibitors from nematodes and the arms race between host and pathogen. *Trends Biochem. Sci.* 26:191–97
109. MEROPS the Peptidase Database. Release 7.10. **http://merops.sanger.ac.uk**
110. Abrahamson M, Alvarez-Fernandez M, Nathanson CM. 2003. Cystatins. *Biochem. Soc. Symp.* 70:179–99
111. Lustigman S, Brotman B, Huima T, Prince AM, McKerrow JH. 1992. Molecular cloning and characterization of onchocystatin, a cysteine proteinase inhibitor of Onchocerca volvulus. *J. Biol. Chem.* 267:17339–46

112. Manoury B, Gregory WF, Maizels RM, Watts C. 2001. Bm-CPI-2, a cystatin homolog secreted by the filarial parasite Brugia malayi, inhibits class II MHC-restricted antigen processing. *Curr. Biol.* 11:447–51
113. Pfaff AW, Schulz-Key H, Soboslay PT, Taylor DW, MacLennan K, Hoffmann WH. 2002. Litomosoides sigmodontis cystatin acts as an immunomodulator during experimental filariasis. *Int. J. Parasitol.* 32:171–78
114. Newlands GF, Skuce PJ, Knox DP, Smith WD. 2001. Cloning and expression of cystatin, a potent cysteine protease inhibitor from the gut of Haemonchus contortus. *Parasitology* 122:371–78
115. Dainichi T, Maekawa Y, Ishii K, Himeno K. 2001. Molecular cloning of a cystatin from parasitic intestinal nematode, Nippostrongylus brasiliensis. *J. Med. Invest.* 48:81–87
116. Genome Sequencing Center. 2003. **http://www.nematode.net**
117. Schonemeyer A, Lucius R, Sonnenburg B, Brattig N, Sabat R, et al. 2001. Modulation of human T cell responses and macrophage functions by onchocystatin, a secreted protein of the filarial nematode Onchocerca volvulus. *J. Immunol.* 167:3207–15
118. Murray J, Manoury B, Balic A, Watts C, Maizels RM. 2005. Bm-CPI-2, a cystatin from Brugia malayi nematode parasites, differs from Caenorhabditis elegans cystatins in a specific site mediating inhibition of the antigen-processing enzyme AEP. *Mol. Biochem. Parasitol.* 139:197–203
119. Nakagawa TY, Rudensky AY. 1999. The role of lysosomal proteinases in MHC class II-mediated antigen processing and presentation. *Immunol. Rev.* 172:121–29
120. Antoniou AN, Blackwood SL, Mazzeo D, Watts C. 2000. Control of antigen presentation by a single protease cleavage site. *Immunity* 12:391–98
121. Pierre P, Mellman I. 1998. Developmental regulation of invariant chain proteolysis controls MHC class II trafficking in mouse dendritic cells. *Cell* 93:1135–45
122. Watts C, Moss CX, Mazzeo D, West MA, Matthews SP, Li DN. 2003. Creation versus destruction of T cell eptitopes in the class II MHC pathway. *Ann. NY Acad. Sci.* 987:9–14
123. Mahanty S, Mollis SN, Ravichandran M, Abrams JS, Kumaraswami V, et al. 1996. High levels of spontaneous and parasite antigen-driven interleukin-10 production are associated with antigen-specific hyporesponsiveness in human lymphatic filariasis. *J. Infect. Dis.* 173:769–73
124. Osborne J, Devaney E. 1999. Interleukin-10 and antigen-presenting cells actively suppress Th1 cells in BALB/c mice infected with the filarial parasite Brugia pahangi. *Infect. Immun.* 67:1599–605
125. Schierack P, Lucius R, Sonnenburg B, Schilling K, Hartmann S. 2003. Parasite-specific immunomodulatory functions of filarial cystatin. *Infect. Immun.* 71:2422–29
126. Roberts TH, Hejgaard J, Saunders NF, Cavicchioli R, Curmi PM. 2004. Serpins in unicellular Eukarya, Archaea, and Bacteria: sequence analysis and evolution. *J. Mol. Evol.* 59:437–47
127. Silverman GA, Bird PI, Carrell RW, Church FC, Coughlin PB, et al. 2001. The serpins are an expanding superfamily of structurally similar but functionally diverse proteins. Evolution, mechanism of inhibition, novel functions, and a revised nomenclature. *J. Biol. Chem.* 276:33293–96
128. Huntington JA, Read RJ, Carrell RW. 2000. Structure of a serpin-protease complex shows inhibition by deformation. *Nature* 407:923–26
129. Chertov O, Ueda H, Xu LL, Tani K, Murphy WJ, et al. 1997. Identification of human neutrophil-derived cathepsin G and azurocidin/CAP37 as chemoattractants for mononuclear cells and neutrophils. *J. Exp. Med.* 186:739–47

130. Padrines M, Wolf M, Walz A, Baggiolini M. 1994. Interleukin-8 processing by neutrophil elastase, cathepsin G and proteinase-3. *FEBS Lett.* 352:231–35
131. Murohara T, Guo JP, Lefer AM. 1995. Cardioprotection by a novel recombinant serine protease inhibitor in myocardial ischemia and reperfusion injury. *J. Pharmacol. Exp. Ther.* 274:1246–53
132. Tremblay GM, Janelle MF, Bourbonnais Y. 2003. Anti-inflammatory activity of neutrophil elastase inhibitors. *Curr. Opin. Investig. Drugs* 4:556–65
133. Ray CA, Black RA, Kronheim SR, Greenstreet TA, Sleath PR, et al. 1992. Viral inhibition of inflammation: cowpox virus encodes an inhibitor of the interleukin-1 beta converting enzyme. *Cell* 69:597–604
134. Lucas A, Dai E, Liu L, Guan H, Nash P, et al. 2000. Transplant vasculopathy: viral anti-inflammatory serpin regulation of atherogenesis. *J. Heart Lung Transpl.* 19:1029–38
135. Yenbutr P, Scott AL. 1995. Molecular cloning of a serine proteinase inhibitor from Brugia malayi. *Infect. Immun.* 63:1745–53
136. Zang X, Yazdanbakhsh M, Jiang H, Kanost MR, Maizels RM. 1999. A novel serpin expressed by blood-borne microfilariae of the parasitic nematode Brugia malayi inhibits human neutrophil serine proteinases. *Blood* 94:1418–28
137. Stanley P, Stein PE. 2003. BmSPN2, a serpin secreted by the filarial nematode Brugia malayi, does not inhibit human neutrophil proteinases but plays a noninhibitory role. *Biochemistry* 42:6241–48
138. Stein PE, Tewkesbury DA, Carrell RW. 1989. Ovalbumin and angiotensinogen lack serpin S-R conformational change. *Biochem. J.* 262:103–7
139. Dafforn TR, Della M, Miller AD. 2001. The molecular interactions of heat shock protein 47 (Hsp47) and their implications for collagen biosynthesis. *J. Biol. Chem.* 276:49310–19
140. Ghendler Y, Arnon R, Fishelson Z. 1994. Schistosoma mansoni: isolation and characterization of Smpi56, a novel serine protease inhibitor. *Exp. Parasitol.* 78:121–31
141. Modha J, Roberts MC, Kusel JR. 1996. Schistosomes and serpins: A complex business. *Parasitol. Today* 12:119–21
142. Blanton RE, Licate LS, Aman RA. 1994. Characterization of a native and recombinant Schistosoma haematobium serine protease inhibitor gene product. *Mol. Biochem. Parasitol.* 63:1–11
143. Huang W, Haas TA, Biesterfeldt J, Mankawsky L, Blanton RE, Lee X. 1999. Purification and crystallization of a novel membrane-anchored protein: the Schistosoma haematobium serpin. *Acta Crystallogr.* D 55(Pt. 1):350–52
144. Freudenstein-Dan A, Gold D, Fishelson Z. 2003. Killing of schistosomes by elastase and hydrogen peroxide: implications for leukocyte-mediated schistosome killing. *J. Parasitol.* 89:1129–35
145. Fraefel W, Acher R. 1968. The amino acid sequence of a trypsin inhibitor isolated from ascaris (Ascaris lumbricoides var. suum). *Biochim. Biophys. Acta* 154:615–17
146. Babin DR, Peanasky RJ, Goos SM. 1984. The isoinhibitors of chymotrypsin/elastase from Ascaris lumbricoides: the primary structure. *Arch. Biochem. Biophys.* 232:143–61
147. Peanasky RJ, Bentz Y, Paulson B, Graham DL, Babin DR. 1984. The isoinhibitors of chymotrypsin/elastase from Ascaris lumbricoides: isolation by affinity chromatography and association with the enzymes. *Arch. Biochem. Biophys.* 232:127–34
148. Grasberger BL, Clore GM, Gronenborn AM. 1994. High-resolution structure of Ascaris trypsin inhibitor in solution: direct evidence for a pH-induced conformational transition in the reactive site. *Structure* 2:669–78

149. Huang K, Streynadka NC, Bernard VD, Peanasky RJ, James MN. 1994. The molecular structure of the complex Ascaris chymotrypsin/elastase inhibitor with porcine elastase. *Structure* 2:679–89
150. Duggan BM, Dyson HJ, Wright PE. 1999. Inherent flexibility in a potent inhibitor of blood coagulation, recombinant nematode anticoagulant protein c2. *Eur. J. Biochem.* 265:539–48
151. Martzen MR, Geise GL, Hogan BJ, Peanasky RJ. 1985. Ascaris suum: localization by immunochemical and fluorescent probes of host proteases and parasite proteinase inhibitors in cross-sections. *Exp. Parasitol.* 60:139–49
152. Lu CC, Nguyen T, Morris S, Hill D, Sakanari JA. 1998. Anisakis simplex: mutational bursts in the reactive site centers of serine protease inhibitors from an ascarid nematode. *Exp. Parasitol.* 89:257–61
153. Rhoads ML, Fetterer RH, Hill DE, Urban JF Jr. 2000. Trichuris suis: a secretory chymotrypsin/elastase inhibitor with potential as an immunomodulator. *Exp. Parasitol.* 95:36–44
154. Bania J, Stachowiak D, Polanowski A. 1999. Primary structure and properties of the cathepsin G/chymotrypsin inhibitor from the larval hemolymph of Apis mellifera. *Eur. J. Biochem.* 262:680–87
155. Mignogna G, Pascarella S, Wechselberger C, Hinterleitner C, Mollay C, et al. 1996. BSTI, a trypsin inhibitor from skin secretions of Bombina bombina related to protease inhibitors of nematodes. *Protein Sci.* 5:357–62
156. Vlasuk GP, Rote WE. 2002. Inhibition of factor VIIa/tissue factor with nematode anticoagulant protein c2: from unique mechanism to a promising new clinical anticoagulant. *Trends Cardiovasc. Med.* 12:325–31
157. Loeb L, Smith AJ. 1904. The presence of a substance inhibiting the coagulation of blood in anchylostoma. *Proc. Natl. Acad. Sci. USA* 7:173–78
158. Cappello M, Clyne LP, McPhedran P, Hotez PJ. 1993. Ancylostoma factor Xa inhibitor: partial purification and its identification as a major hookworm-derived anticoagulant in vitro. *J. Infect. Dis.* 167:1474–77
159. Cappello M, Vlasuk GP, Bergum PW, Huang S, Hotez PJ. 1995. Ancylostoma caninum anticoagulant peptide: a hookworm-derived inhibitor of human coagulation factor Xa. *Proc. Natl. Acad. Sci. USA* 92:6152–56
160. Stassens P, Bergum PW, Gansemans Y, Jespers L, Laroche Y, et al. 1996. Anticoagulant repertoire of the hookworm Ancylostoma caninum. *Proc. Natl. Acad. Sci. USA* 93:2149–54
161. Baugh RJ, Broze GJ Jr, Krishnaswamy S. 1998. Regulation of extrinsic pathway factor Xa formation by tissue factor pathway inhibitor. *J. Biol. Chem.* 273:4378–86
162. Mieszczanek J, Harrison LM, Vlasuk GP, Cappello M. 2004. Anticoagulant peptides from Ancylostoma caninum are immunologically distinct and localize to separate structures within the adult hookworm. *Mol. Biochem. Parasitol.* 133:319–23
163. Mieszczanek J, Harrison LM, Cappello M. 2004. Ancylostoma ceylanicum anticoagulant peptide-1: role of the predicted reactive site amino acid in mediating inhibition of coagulation factors Xa and VIIa. *Mol. Biochem. Parasitol.* 137:151–59
164. Harrison LM, Nerlinger A, Bungiro RD, Cordova JL, Kuzmic P, Cappello M. 2002. Molecular characterization of Ancylostoma inhibitors of coagulation factor Xa. Hookworm anticoagulant activity in vitro predicts parasite bloodfeeding in vivo. *J. Biol. Chem.* 277:6223–39

165. Rep BH. 1980. Pathogenicity of hookworms. The significance of population regression for the pathogenicity of hookworms. *Trop. Geogr. Med.* 32:251–55
166. Vlasuk GP, Bradbury A, Lopez-Kinninger L, Colon S, Bergum PW, et al. 2003. Pharmacokinetics and anticoagulant properties of the factor VIIa-tissue factor inhibitor recombinant Nematode Anticoagulant Protein c2 following subcutaneous administration in man. Dependence on the stoichiometric binding to circulating factor X. *Thromb. Haemost.* 90:803–12
167. Lee A, Agnelli G, Buller H, Ginsberg J, Heit J, et al. 2001. Dose-response study of recombinant factor VIIa/tissue factor inhibitor recombinant nematode anticoagulant protein c2 in prevention of postoperative venous thromboembolism in patients undergoing total knee replacement. *Circulation* 104:74–78
168. Geerts WH, Heit JA, Clagett GP, Pineo GF, Colwell CW, et al. 2001. Prevention of venous thromboembolism. *Chest* 119:S132–75
169. Leander BS, Clopton RE, Keeling PJ. 2003. Phylogeny of gregarines (Apicomplexa) as inferred from small-subunit rDNA and beta-tubulin. *Int. J. Syst. Evol. Microbiol.* 53:345–54
170. Sibley LD. 2004. Intracellular parasite invasion strategies. *Science* 304:248–53
171. Soldati D, Meissner M. 2004. Toxoplasma as a novel system for motility. *Curr. Opin. Cell Biol.* 16:32–40
172. Binder EM, Kim K. 2004. Location, location, location: trafficking and function of secreted proteases of toxoplasma and Plasmodium. *Traffic* 5:914–24
173. Kim K, Weiss LM. 2004. Toxoplasma gondii: the model apicomplexan. *Int. J. Parasitol.* 34:423–32
174. Blackman MJ. 2004. Proteases in host cell invasion by the malaria parasite. *Cell. Microbiol.* 6:893–903
175. Opitz C, Di Cristina M, Reiss M, Ruppert T, Crisanti A, Soldati D. 2002. Intramembrane cleavage of microneme proteins at the surface of the apicomplexan parasite Toxoplasma gondii. *EMBO J.* 21:1577–85
176. Carruthers VB, Sherman GD, Sibley LD. 2000. The Toxoplasma adhesive protein MIC2 is proteolytically processed at multiple sites by two parasite-derived proteases. *J. Biol. Chem.* 275:14346–53
177. Miller SA, Binder EM, Blackman MJ, Carruthers VB, Kim K. 2001. A conserved subtilisin-like protein TgSUB1 in microneme organelles of Toxoplasma gondii. *J. Biol. Chem.* 276:45341–48
178. Miller SA, Thathy V, Ajioka JW, Blackman MJ, Kim K. 2003. TgSUB2 is a Toxoplasma gondii rhoptry organelle processing proteinase. *Mol. Microbiol.* 49:883–94
179. Uzureau P, Barale JC, Janse CJ, Waters AP, Breton CB. 2004. Gene targeting demonstrates that the Plasmodium berghei subtilisin PbSUB2 is essential for red cell invasion and reveals spontaneous genetic recombination events. *Cell. Microbiol.* 6:65–78
180. Holder AA, Blackman MJ. 1994. What is the function of MSP-1 on the malaria merzoite? *Parasitol. Today* 10:182–84
181. Kappe SHI, Buscaglia CA, Bergman LW, Crabb BS, Coppens I, Nussenzweig V. 2004. Apicomplexan gliding motility and host cell invasion: overhauling the motor model. *Trends Parasitol.* 20:13–16
182. Sultan AA. 1999. Molecular mechanisms of malaria sporozoite motility and invasion of host cells. *Int. Microbiol.* 2:155–60
183. Silvie O, Franetich JF, Renia L, Mazier D. 2004. Malaria sporozoite: migrating for a living. *Trends Mol. Med.* 10:97–100

184. Dowse T, Soldati D. 2004. Host cell invasion by the apicomplexans: the significance of microneme protein proteolysis. *Curr. Opin. Microbiol.* 7:388–96
185. Louie K, Nordhausen R, Robinson TW, Barr BC, Conrad PA. 2002. Characterization of Neospora caninum protease, NcSUB1 (NC-p65), with rabbit anti-N54. *J. Parasitol.* 88:1113–19
186. Fuller AL, McDougald LR. 1990. Reduction in cell entry of Eimeria tenella (Coccidia) sporozoites by protease inhibitors, and partial characterization of proteolytic activity associated with intact sporozoites and merozoites. *J. Parasitol.* 76:464–67
187. Greenbaum DC, Baruch A, Grainger M, Bozdech Z, Medzihradszky KF, et al. 2002. A role for the protease falcipain 1 in host cell invasion by the human malaria parasite. *Science* 298:2002–6
188. Eksi S, Czesny B, Greenbaum DC, Boygo M, Williamson KC. 2004. argeted disruption of Plasmodium falciparum cysteine protease, falcipain 1, reduces oocyst production, not erythrocytic stage growth. *Mol. Microbiol.* 53:243–50
189. Grellier P, Picard I, Bernard F, Mayer R, Heidrich HG, et al. 1989. Purification and identification of a neutral endopeptidase in Plasmodium falciparum schizonts and merozoites. *Parasitol. Res.* 75:455–60
190. Howell SA, Well I, Fleck SL, Kettleborough C, Collins CR, Blackman MJ. 2003. A single malaria merozoite serine protease mediates shedding of multiple surface proteins by juxtamembrane cleavage. *J. Biol. Chem.* 278:23890–98
191. Withers-Martinez C, Jean L, Blackman MJ. 2004. Subtilisin-like proteases of the malaria parasite. *Mol. Microbiol.* 53:55–63
192. Shaw MK, Tilney LG, Musoke AJ. 1991. The entry of Theileria parva sporozoites into bovine lymphocytes: evidence for MHC class I involvement. *J. Cell Biol.* 113:87–101
193. Andrews NW, Portnoy DA. 1994. Cytolysins from intracellular pathogens. *Trends Microbiol.* 2:261–63
194. Deleted in proof
195. Mota MM, Hafalla JC, Rodriguez A. 2002. Migration through host cells activates Plasmodium sporozoites for infection. *Nat. Med.* 8:1318–22
196. Coppi A, Pinzon-Ortiz C, Hutter C, Sinnis P. 2005. The Plasmodium circumsporozoite protein is proteolytically processed during cell invasion. *J. Exp. Med.* 201:27–33
197. Hadley T, Aikawa M, Miller LH. 1983. Plasmodium knowlesi: studies on invasion of rhesus erythrocytes by merozoites in the presence of protease inhibitors. *Exp. Parasitol.* 55:306–11
198. Lyon JA, Haynes JD, Diggs CL, Chulay JD, Pratt-Rossiter JM. 1986. Plasmodium falciparum antigens synthesized by schizonts and stabilized at the merozoite surface by antibodies when schizonts mature in the presence of growth inhibitory immune serum. *J. Immunol.* 136:2252–58
199. Salmon BL, Oksman A, Goldberg DE. 2001. Malaria parasite exit from the host erythrocyte: a two-step process requiring extraerythrocytic proteolysis. *Proc. Natl. Acad. Sci. USA* 98:271–76
200. Wickham ME, Culvenor JG, Cowman AF. 2003. Selective inhibition of a two-step egress of malaria parasites from the host erythrocyte. *J. Biol. Chem.* 278:37658–63
201. Bourgon R, Delorenzi M, Sargeant T, Hodder AN, Crabb BS, Speed TP. 2004. The serine repeat antigen (SERA) gene family phylogeny in Plasmodium: the impact of GC content and reconciliation of gene and species trees. *Mol. Biol. Evol.* 21:2161–71

202. Miller SK, Good RT, Drew DR, Delorenzi M, Sanders PR, et al. 2002. A subset of Plasmodium falciparum SERA genes are expressed and appear to play an important role in the erythrocytic cycle. *J. Biol. Chem.* 277:47524–32
203. Hanspal M, Dua M, Takakuwa Y, Chishti AH, Mizuno A. 2002. Plasmodium falciparum cysteine protease falcipain-2 cleaves erythrocyte membrane skeletal proteins at late stages of parasite development. *Blood* 100:1048–54
204. Dhawan S, Dua M, Chishti AH, Hanspal M. 2003. Ankyrin peptide blocks falcipain-2-mediated malaria parasite release from red blood cells. *J. Biol. Chem.* 278:30180–86
205. Vernet T, Khouri HE, Laflamme P, Tessier DC, Musil R, et al. 1991. Processing of the papain precursor. *J. Biol. Chem.* 266:21451–57
206. Hodder AN, Drew DR, Epa VC, Delorenzi M, Bourgon R, et al. 2003. Enzymic, phylogenetic, and structural characterization of the unusual papain-like protease domain of Plasmodium falciparum SERA5. *J. Biol. Chem.* 278:48169–77
207. Le Bonniec S, Deregnaucourt C, Redeker V, Banerjee R, Grellier P, et al. 1999. Plasmepsin II, an acidic hemoglobinase from the Plasmodium falciparum food vacuole, is active at neutral pH on the host erythrocyte membrane skeleton. *J. Biol. Chem.* 274:14218–23

Subject Index

B

F

G

H

M

N

O

P

R

S

T